Eggs as Functional Foods and Nutraceuticals for Human Health

Food Chemistry, Function and Analysis

Series editors:
Gary Williamson, *University of Leeds, UK*
Alejandro G. Marangoni, *University of Guelph, Canada*
Juliet A. Gerrard, *University of Auckland, New Zealand*

Titles in the series:

1: Food Biosensors
2: Sensing Techniques for Food Safety and Quality Control
3: Edible Oil Structuring: Concepts, Methods and Applications
4: Food Irradiation Technologies: Concepts, Applications and Outcomes
5: Non-extractable Polyphenols and Carotenoids: Importance in Human Nutrition and Health
6: Cereal Grain-based Functional Foods: Carbohydrate and Phytochemical Components
7: Steviol Glycosides: Cultivation, Processing, Analysis and Applications in Food
8: Legumes: Nutritional Quality, Processing and Potential Health Benefits
9: Tomato Chemistry, Industrial Processing and Product Development
10: Food Contact Materials Analysis: Mass Spectrometry Techniques
11: Vitamin E: Chemistry and Nutritional Benefits
12: Anthocyanins from Natural Sources: Exploiting Targeted Delivery for Improved Health
13: Carotenoid Esters in Foods: Physical, Chemical and Biological Properties
14: Eggs as Functional Foods and Nutraceuticals for Human Health

How to obtain future titles on publication:
A standing order plan is available for this series. A standing order will bring delivery of each new volume immediately on publication.

For further information please contact:
Book Sales Department, Royal Society of Chemistry, Thomas Graham House, Science Park, Milton Road, Cambridge, CB4 0WF, UK
Telephone: +44 (0)1223 420066, Fax: +44 (0)1223 420247,
Email: booksales@rsc.org
Visit our website at www.rsc.org/books

Eggs as Functional Foods and Nutraceuticals for Human Health

Edited by

Jianping Wu
University of Alberta, Canada
Email: jwu3@ualberta.ca

ROYAL SOCIETY OF CHEMISTRY

Food Chemistry, Function and Analysis No. 14

Print ISBN: 978-1-78801-213-3
PDF ISBN: 978-1-78801-383-3
EPUB ISBN: 978-1-78801-779-4
Print ISSN: 2398-0656
Electronic ISSN: 2398-0664

A catalogue record for this book is available from the British Library

The Royal Society of Chemistry is a charity, registered in England and Wales, Number 207890, and a company incorporated in England by Royal Charter (Registered No. RC000524), registered office: Burlington House, Piccadilly, London W1J 0BA, UK, Telephone: +44 (0) 20 7437 8656.

Visit our website at www.rsc.org/books

Printed in the United Kingdom by CPI Group (UK) Ltd, Croydon, CR0 4YY, UK

Preface

The egg has been an important food throughout human civilization and is often described as "nature's perfect food" as it contains all the necessary nutrients for a new life. For example, eggs are a rich source of choline, an essential nutrient for normal development of the brain, and carotenoids such as lutein and zeaxanthin, which can provide protection against age-related macular degeneration. Egg proteins are considered as the most nutritious and economically affordable high-quality protein and are used as the "gold standard" for assessment of the quality of other proteins. More recently, the 2015–2020 Dietary Guidelines for Americans no longer include a limit for dietary cholesterol intake and recommend eggs as part of a healthy eating pattern.

Consumers are becoming more health-conscious and are looking beyond the basic nutrition to potential disease prevention and health-enhancing components. There is promising evidence to support a beneficial role of egg consumption in weight management, cardiovascular diseases including metabolic syndrome, and prevention of muscle loss, among others. Indeed, eggs contain a diverse array of bioactive compounds with properties that are applicable to nutrition, health, and value addition for functional food development.

This book is a reflection of the trends and innovations in the area of egg nutrition, functional foods, and value addition that have been presented at the past three successful Banff Egg Symposia (2012, 2014, and 2016), and several invited papers from the authors who could not attend the symposia. The objectives of this book are to provide current evidence on the relationship between egg consumption and cardiovascular diseases, metabolic syndrome, weight management, mental development, and eye, muscle, and ageing health, to showcase the new developments of egg bioactives relevant

Food Chemistry, Function and Analysis No.14
Eggs as Functional Foods and Nutraceuticals for Human Health
Edited by Jianping Wu

Published by the Royal Society of Chemistry, www.rsc.org

to antioxidants, anti-inflammation, cardiovascular and bone health, and anti-microbial and anti-viral activities, as well as to present recent developments of processing eggs for value-added food, nutritional, biomedical, functional food, and nutraceutical applications. This book will serve a broad readership in the disciplines of egg science and technology, food science, nutrition, functional foods/nutraceuticals, biochemistry, and biotechnology. This book can also be used as a key reference for the egg industry and the egg marketing sector, or as a textbook/reference for undergraduate and graduate students.

I am grateful to all authors for their outstanding contributions, which have made the publication of this monograph possible. I would like to thank Nicki Dennis, Commissioning Editor of the Royal Society of Chemistry, for providing guidance in developing the outline of the monograph, and Katie Morrey, Editorial Assistant, for all her administrative support in preparing the book.

Jianping Wu
Edmonton, Alberta, Canada

Contents

Food Chemistry, Function and Analysis No.14
Eggs as Functional Foods and Nutraceuticals for Human Health
Edited by Jianping Wu

Published by the Royal Society of Chemistry, www.rsc.org

CHAPTER 1

Eggs as Part of a Healthy Eating Pattern

RYLEE T. AHNEN AND JOANNE L. SLAVIN*

Department of Food Science and Nutrition, University of Minnesota, 166 FSCN, 1334 Eckles Ave, St. Paul, MN 55408, USA
*E-mail: jslavin@umn.edu

1.1 Introduction

Eggs have long been regarded for their nutrient density, providing consumers with a high-quality protein source in addition to a wide variety of critical minerals, vitamins, and trace elements.[1] Compared to other significant sources of dietary proteins, eggs provide relatively high levels of folate, biotin, choline, and vitamin A for a relatively small number of calories, and also deliver an impressive combination of amino acids.[2,3] Additionally, eggs serve as an affordable protein and nutrient source. As reported in the Nutrient Rich Foods Index, and again in a review by Iannotti *et al.* in 2014, eggs are the most affordable protein source in the United States when included as part of a comprehensive food list.[4,5]

However, despite the wide acceptance that eggs are an affordable and nutrient-rich food, the American public has been reticent to accept eggs as part of a healthy eating pattern owing to concerns about cholesterol intake. In fact, recent studies examining consumer data from the National Health and Nutrition Examination Survey (NHANES) found that from 2001 to 2012

Food Chemistry, Function and Analysis No.14
Eggs as Functional Foods and Nutraceuticals for Human Health
Edited by Jianping Wu

Published by the Royal Society of Chemistry, www.rsc.org

the overall proportion of the U.S. population who consumed eggs regularly (21–22%; $p = 0.311$) remained unchanged.[6] Research examining consumer perceptions about eggs and the barriers to their consumption found that egg consumption has declined owing to the perceived association most consumers make between the consumption of eggs and dietary cholesterol.[7–9]

While the perception that egg consumption is associated with dietary cholesterol and, therefore, is associated with increased levels of plasma cholesterol has been supported by recommendations put forth by the U.S. government and reputable public health organizations in the past, recent examinations of the body of literature concerning egg consumption suggest that eggs should be considered a healthy part of the diet. In the following sections, we will discuss the history of dietary recommendations that resulted in the long-held belief that egg consumption should be undertaken in moderation, the changes in the American dietary pattern that occurred as a result of those recommendations, several of the potential health benefits associated with eggs that make them a key part of the modern healthy dietary pattern, as well as the potential for eggs to be enriched in order to even better serve as a component of healthy diets.

1.2 Dietary Recommendations Concerning Eggs

1.2.1 Introduction

Dietary recommendations concerning the consumption of eggs have been part of the public's understanding of nutrition for nearly half a century, dating back to the 1968 recommendation from the American Heart Association (AHA) that individuals limit their intake of dietary cholesterol to no more than 300 mg per day in order to reduce their risk of cardiovascular disease (CVD), and that individuals consume no more than three whole eggs per week in order to meet that recommendation.[10] That recommendation created a paradigm shift in the way the American public viewed the consumption of eggs, providing the average consumer with an easy to understand dietary intervention they could undertake in order to improve their lifestyle, and resulted in an overall decline in the *per capita* consumption of eggs in the years that followed.[11] This recommendation against the consumption of dietary cholesterol, and eggs in particular, persisted for decades.

1.2.2 Dietary Recommendations from 1950 to 2010

Dietary recommendations in the United States took their first form in a report published by the American Heart Association in 1957 that posited, in somewhat uncertain terms, that the changing diet of the average American may have contributed to the increased pathogenesis of atherosclerosis in the United States.[12] As noted by Kritchevsky in *The Journal of Nutrition*, the American Heart Association released another report four years later in 1961 which focused on dietary fats and their relationship to heart attacks and strokes, putting forth recommendations for dietary modifications that began modeling the current construction of our modern dietary recommendations.[13,14] Seven years later, in 1968, the American Heart Association put forth a report that set the standard for dietary cholesterol and egg consumption that would persist for decades – that Americans should limit dietary cholesterol to no more than 300 mg per day and should not consume more than three egg yolks per week.[10]

Less than a decade after the American Heart Association recommended that consumers limit their dietary intake of eggs in order to achieve a dietary pattern that protected them against CVD, the United States government began the process of establishing federally sanctioned dietary guidelines for every United States citizen. The first iteration of these guidelines was created and published in 1977 by the U.S. Senate Select Committee on Nutrition and Human Needs, which mirrored the American Heart Association recommendation of limiting dietary cholesterol to 300 mg per day and suggested that Americans limit their intake of eggs as a means of achieving that goal.[15] Following the publication of the report from the U.S. Select Committee on Nutrition and Human Needs, the federal government took steps to formalize the process of creating and disseminating dietary recommendations to the American public and established the Dietary Guidelines for Americans, which have been issued twice a decade since 1980 and provide citizens of the United States with recommendations for developing a healthful diet.

In 1980, the U.S. Department of Agriculture and the U.S. Department of Health and Human Services published the first edition of the Dietary Guidelines for Americans (DGA). These 1980 guidelines, published as a 19-page pamphlet, provided Americans with seven focus areas for improving their overall health through nutrition.[16] One of these focus areas, "Avoid Too Much Fat, Saturated Fat, and Cholesterol," encouraged Americans to limit their intake of dietary cholesterol in order to reduce their risk of CVD, and provided eggs as an example of a common food that consumers could moderate in their diet to achieve that goal. Recommendations that encouraged Americans to reduce their dietary cholesterol intake, specifically through a reduction in their consumption of eggs, appeared almost universally in the bidecennial DGA reports published by the federal government up to, and including, the report published in 2010.[17–22] A summary of the dietary recommendations for egg consumption and cholesterol included in each of the *Dietary Guidelines* reports can be found in Table 1.1.

1.2.3 Dietary Recommendations 2010–2015

In 2013, the American Heart Association published a report providing lifestyle management guidance for individuals aiming to reduce their risk of developing cardiovascular disease. This report included evidence-based

Table 1.1 Recommendations for egg consumption as a means of regulating dietary cholesterol from the Dietary Guidelines for Americans and its predecessor, the Dietary Goals for the United States.

Year	Source	Recommendation
1977	Dietary Goals for the United States	"Decrease consumption of butterfat, eggs and other high cholesterol sources."
1980	Dietary Guidelines for Americans	"Moderate your use of eggs and organ meats (such as liver)."
1985	Dietary Guidelines for Americans	"Moderate your use of egg yolks and organ meats."
1990	Dietary Guidelines for Americans	"Moderate the use of egg yolks and organ meats."
1995	Dietary Guidelines for Americans	"Dietary cholesterol comes from animal sources such as egg yolks, meat (especially organ meats such as liver), poultry, fish, and higher fat milk products. [···] Choosing foods with less cholesterol and saturated fat will help lower your blood cholesterol levels."
2000	Dietary Guidelines for Americans	"Use egg yolks and whole eggs in moderation. Use egg whites and egg substitutes freely when cooking since they contain no cholesterol and little or no fat."
2005	Dietary Guidelines for Americans	No specific recommendation for eggs.
2010	Dietary Guidelines for Americans	"The major sources of cholesterol in the American diet include eggs and egg mixed dishes (25% of total cholesterol intake) [···] Cholesterol intake can be reduced by limiting the consumption of the specific foods that are high in cholesterol."
2015	Dietary Guidelines for Americans	"More research is needed regarding the dose–response relationship between dietary cholesterol and blood cholesterol levels. Adequate evidence is not available for a quantitative limit for dietary cholesterol specific to the *Dietary Guidelines*. Dietary cholesterol is found only in animal foods such as egg yolk, dairy products, shellfish, meats, and poultry."

recommendations for dietary patterns that were intended to reduce risk factors for CVD, including the reduction of low-density lipoprotein cholesterol (LDL-C). In the report, the AHA stated there was "insufficient evidence to determine whether lowering dietary cholesterol reduced LDL-C."[23] This recommendation was the inverse of the dietary recommendation that the AHA and other reputable public health organizations had been making for decades, and represented a turning point in the way public health advocates, the United States federal government, and health researchers would talk about dietary cholesterol to the general public.

In 2015, amidst a growing consensus that claims concerning dietary cholesterol levels and their relationship to CVD and blood lipid levels had been overstated, the *Dietary Guidelines* revised their recommendation for dietary cholesterol and stated that there was not enough evidence to develop a quantitative limit for dietary cholesterol.[24] The 2015 *Dietary Guidelines* went on to say that more research was needed to determine what, if any, dose–response relationship existed between dietary cholesterol and blood lipid levels.[24] While this departure from decades' worth of dietary recommendations that instructed consumers to limit their intake of eggs was certainly notable to researchers and public health officials, it is unclear whether the change in recommendation has been effectively communicated to consumers and the general public.

1.3 Egg Consumption in the United States

1.3.1 Introduction

Over the past five decades, the United States federal government, along with a large number of non-profits focused on consumer health, have advocated that individuals make a concerted effort to reduce their dietary intake of cholesterol by decreasing the number of eggs they consume over the course of an average day or week. However, with the release of the 2015 DGA, those recommendations have shifted away from discouraging individuals from incorporating eggs into their dietary pattern and have instead suggested that eggs can be a key part of a healthful diet. As this shift in dietary recommendations takes place, it is important to understand that the dietary recommendations concerning egg consumption that had persisted for half a century may have dramatically altered the American dietary pattern. Furthermore, the persistence of the dietary recommendation that consumers avoid consuming or over-consuming eggs may have created difficult-to-overcome information barriers that will make it less likely that consumers will incorporate eggs into what they perceive as a healthy diet.

1.3.2 Dietary Trends of Eggs

A great deal of research has been done to study the consumption trends of eggs in the United States, helping researchers and policy makers to better understand how many Americans are regularly consuming eggs and to what degree. As reported by Wang *et al.* in 1996, early United States Department of Agriculture (USDA) data demonstrated that the average *per capita* consumption of eggs in the United States steadily declined over the course of the final four decades of the 1900s, dropping from 321 eggs in 1960 to 229 eggs in 1993.[25] More recent research examining the prevalence of egg consumption throughout the United States found that roughly 20% of the population consumed eggs on any given day.[26] This estimate, that one in five Americans consume eggs on any given day, represents a largely unchanged prevalence in egg consumption compared to similar research that examined the prevalence of egg consumption from 1988 to 1994.[27] The trend for annual egg consumption from 1960 to 2017, adjusted on a *per capita* basis, can be seen in Figure 1.1.

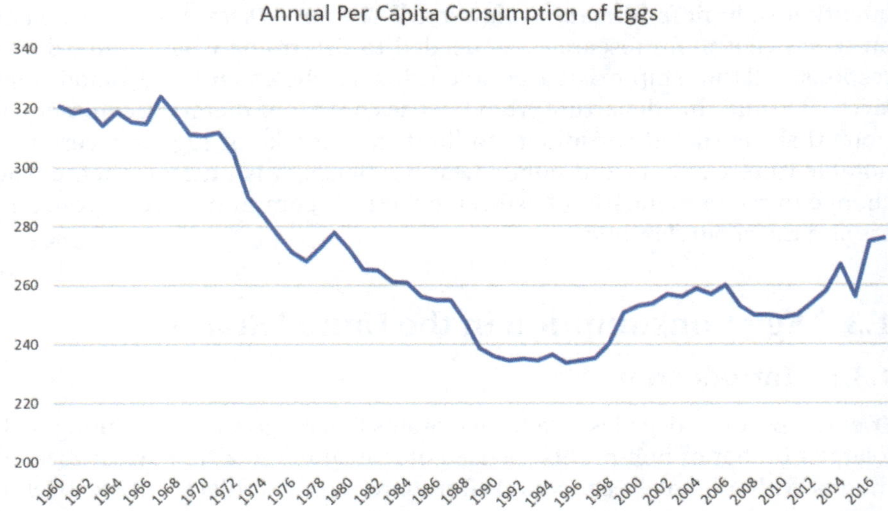

Figure 1.1 United States *per capita* consumption of shell eggs from 1960 to 2017. Data sources: USDA Economic Research Service Livestock and Meat Data, USDA Economic Research Service Poultry Yearbook.

Dietary patterns in the United States are often varied when sociodemographic indicators are examined, including an individual's level of education, their age or income level, or their socioeconomic status.[6,28,29] Owing to the relative affordability of eggs compared to other high-quality proteins available to consumers, one might expect that the presence of markers for lower socioeconomic status might be associated with a *per capita* egg consumption that was higher than average.[30] Surprisingly, the odds of egg consumption in the United States population were not impacted by multiple measures of socioeconomic status, such as level of food security, participation in the Supplemental Nutrition Assistance Program (SNAP), or individual income.[6] However, data analysis from 2003 to 2006 has indicated that the incorporation of eggs into the diet was critical for key nutrient contributions to women who were overweight and obese, and to individuals belonging to minority race or ethnic groups.[6,31,32] Taken together, this data suggests that public health workers, medical practitioners, and public health agencies must find new and effective ways to communicate the potential health benefits, and relative affordability, of eggs to populations who may be the most reliant upon them to meet their nutrient needs.

1.3.3 The Cholesterol Association

Following the decline of egg consumption in the United States in the latter half of the 20th century, some investigators questioned what had motivated Americans to reduce the number of eggs they were incorporating in their diet. Several researchers posited that the dietary recommendations that had been put forth by the American Heart Association, the DGA during the 1970s, 1980s, and 1990s, and by other public health organizations, had created a sense amongst the American public that eggs were an unhealthy food and should be avoided. In 1990, Brown and Schrader investigated how information concerning the link between cholesterol and eggs impacted *per capita* consumption of eggs in the United States and found that information linking eggs and cholesterol had resulted in 16% to 25% decreased *per capita* egg consumption by the first quarter of 1987.[33]

The theory that the public's perception of eggs as an unhealthy food, specifically owing to their association with cholesterol, had impacted U.S. egg consumption was again tested in 1996 by Wang *et al.* By examining consumer survey data from the USDA and applying a double-hurdle model of analysis, researchers determined that health concerns about cholesterol were a significant factor that affected a consumers decision about whether to purchase and consume eggs.[25] The perception that eggs should not be considered part of a healthy dietary pattern but should instead be viewed as a risky food that individuals should avoid if possible has continued well into the 21st century. As noted by Kummerow in 2015, the cholesterol hypothesis has persisted as part of America's understanding about food and has resulted in Americans consuming fewer eggs *per capita* in 2011 than in 1945 as members of the medical establishment avoid recommending eggs as a healthy protein source for their patients.[34] With the recent changes to the dietary recommendations noted above, and the understanding that beliefs about eggs and cholesterol that we now consider to be outdated are a significant barrier to their consumption, it will be critical that public health officials and medical practitioners are able to adequately and clearly explain this shift in dietary principles to the public and to their patients.

1.4 Egg Consumption and Cardiovascular Disease

1.4.1 Introduction

As dietary recommendations continued to discourage Americans from viewing eggs as part of a healthy dietary pattern and to reduce the number of eggs they were consuming, a growing number of researchers began to question the strength of the scientific data that had led to such recommendations in the first place. As noted by Fernandez and Calle in 2010, the initial recommendation of limiting dietary cholesterol to 300 mg day^{-1} for healthy individuals had little basis in scientific evidence and put the United States in the position of being one of the only nations proscribing an upper limit for dietary cholesterol to its citizens.[35] As researchers tested the strength of the association between dietary cholesterol consumption and human health, the body of scientific literature undermining the claim that Americans should actively limit their intake of dietary cholesterol grew, and eventually resulted in both the American Heart Association and the DGA reversing their stance on dietary cholesterol and removing recommendations for egg restriction from their guidelines.[23,24]

1.4.2 Epidemiological Data

Despite early recommendations that egg consumption should be restricted because increased dietary cholesterol was related to an elevated risk of CVD, the preponderance of epidemiological data that has been published subsequently does not support the claim that such an association exists.[36,37] While many epidemiological studies have been conducted in order to test the proposed relationship between egg consumption and the risk of cardiovascular disease, one of the classical epidemiological studies to do so utilized the National Nurses' Health Study dataset. This study used data collected from 37 851 men between the ages of 40 and 75 at onset and 80 082 women aged 34 to 59 at onset. Researchers identified and documented 866 cases of coronary heart disease (CHD) and 258 incident cases of stroke in men, and 939 cases of CHD and 563 incident cases of stroke in women during the 8 year follow-up period of the study. After researchers made adjustments for age, smoking, and other known CHD risk factors, they found no evidence of a significant association between consuming eggs and risk of CHD or stroke in either men or women.[38]

Additional classical epidemiological studies that sought to test the relationship between egg consumption and the risk of cardiovascular disease include the Framingham Heart Study and the NHANES data set, both of which concluded that dietary cholesterol provided by eggs in the diet had no relationship to the development of CHD.[27,39] Additionally, while some large-scale research studies have found that consumption of dietary cholesterol is associated with elevated LDL-C concentrations, Fernandez and Calle noted in 2010 that it is important to understand that for those individuals who do present a hypercholesterolemic response to dietary cholesterol, the increases are often observed in both the plasma LDL-C and the plasma high-density lipoprotein cholesterol (HDL-C) concentrations, which does not result in an altered LDL-C : HDL-C ratio.[35]

Taken together, the findings from these epidemiological research studies would suggest that a public health recommendation that associates dietary cholesterol with blood cholesterol levels, or with an elevated risk of CVD, would be ill-advised. Moreover, these findings indicate that an incredibly common dietary belief that is well known to the general public, that consuming egg raises your cholesterol levels and is bad for your heart, is likely a claim without merit. These conclusions are further supported by clinical research investigating the relationship between dietary cholesterol and risk for CHD and chronic disease in the subsequent section.

1.4.3 Clinical Research

In addition to multiple large-scale epidemiological studies that have demonstrated no connection between the intake of dietary cholesterol and the prevalence of CHD events, scores of clinical trials have been conducted to test the same hypothesis. One recent study conducted by DiMarco *et al.* examined the effect of increased egg consumption on plasma cholesterol levels in a healthy population.[40] The study observed 38 subjects, 19 men and 19 women, who participated in a 14-week crossover intervention where subjects consumed either 0, 1, 2, or 3 eggs per day for a controlled period of time. At the completion of the intervention, the researchers found that increased consumption of eggs was associated with an increase in HDL-C ($p < 0.01$) and decreased LDL-c ($p < 0.05$), and dose-dependent increases in plasma choline were also observed ($p < 0.0001$).[40] Not only do such findings suggest that the consumption of eggs is not associated with an increased risk of CHD, but findings of elevated HDL-C and increased plasma choline levels would also be considered positive health outcomes that may be beneficial to consumers.

One intervention study conducted in 2004 focused on the effects of dietary cholesterol on biomarkers for chronic disease in adolescents. The study included 54 children between the ages of 8 and 12, 29 girls and 25 boys, who participated in a crossover intervention that included one egg intervention period of two whole eggs per day, and one period that included the equivalent amount of egg whites. At the completion of the trial, biomarkers were analyzed and it was found that of the 54 children who participated in the study only 18 experienced a significant elevation in their plasma cholesterol levels.[41] Notably, those 18 children who saw an increase in plasma cholesterol saw increases in both their HDL-C and LDL-C, with no significant changes in their LDL : HDL ratio. Of the 54 children who participated in the study, 36 had no significant change in plasma cholesterol at all.[41] These findings further suggest that, for most individuals, dietary cholesterol plays little to no role in the regulation of plasma cholesterol and that for individuals who are affected by dietary cholesterol the observed changes are not likely to increase their risk factor for CVD because their LDL : HDL ratio remains unchanged.

Intervention studies have also been conducted in the elderly population to determine if individuals over 60 years of age would be more susceptible to changes in their plasma cholesterol levels based on their consumption of dietary cholesterol. One such study evaluated 42 elderly subjects, 29 postmenopausal women and 13 men, who were all free of diabetes and heart disease, and did not use reductase inhibitors. A crossover intervention was implemented that included a 1-month egg period where three large eggs were consumed per day and an intervention period where the equivalent amount of fat-free, cholesterol-free egg substitute was consumed.[42] At the completion of the trial the subjects' LDL-C and HDL-C concentrations were measured, and researchers determined that, while individual responses to the egg intervention varied amongst the participants, no alterations were observed in LDL : HDL ratios or in total cholesterol : HDL ratios. These findings suggest that dietary cholesterol, specifically the dietary cholesterol delivered through the consumption of eggs, does not result in an increased risk for heart disease in otherwise healthy elderly individuals.[42]

Intervention studies have repeatedly found that the consumption of dietary cholesterol is not associated with an increased risk for CVD and is not associated with detrimental changes in an individual's plasma cholesterol levels. The studies noted above demonstrate that this is true across age groups and genders. In fact, some intervention studies have even found that egg consumption is positively associated with increases in HDL-C, an outcome that would be considered healthful for many consumers. Much like the epidemiological data discussed earlier, human intervention studies would also suggest that public health claims advising against the consumption of eggs due to concerns about CVD risks and cholesterol levels were misguided.

1.4.4 Recommendations Lack Support

Following decades of research that questioned the credibility of a dietary recommendation that instructed consumers to limit their daily intake of dietary cholesterol in order to maintain health, the growing scientific consensus supported a shifting away from such recommendations and instead beginning to inform consumers about the potential health benefits associated with the consumption of eggs.[43] As noted earlier in this chapter, amidst this growing consensus the U.S. federal government along with consumer health advocacy groups throughout the United States began to relax their recommendations concerning dietary restrictions for eggs and removed specific calls for consumers to limit eggs in their diet.[23,24,44]

While rolling back recommendations for consumers to avoid the consumption of eggs owing to a lack of scientific evidence to support such a claim is certainly a step in the right direction, it is incumbent upon public health officials to now rectify the decades of misinformation that they have perpetuated through their dietary recommendations. The need for aggressive correction in the public perception of eggs as an unhealthy food is especially important because, as discussed in the following section, eggs provide a myriad of health benefits, including high-quality protein, choline, and help with satiety.

1.5 Positive Health Benefits

1.5.1 Introduction

Eggs have long been recognized for their nutrient density but were not thought of as part of a healthful dietary pattern owing to the common perception that consuming eggs was linked to increased cholesterol levels and, therefore, increased risk of cardiovascular disease.[2] However, as dietary

Table 1.2 Key nutrients of eggs and egg whites. Data source: USDA Nutrient Database for Standard Reference.

Key egg and egg white nutrients				
Nutrient	Per 100 g raw egg	Per large egg (50 g, raw)	Per 100 g raw egg white	Per large egg white (33 g, raw)
Protein (g)	12.56	6.28	10.9	3.6
Total Lipid (g)	9.51	4.75	0.17	0.06
Selenium (μg)	30.7	15.3	20	6.6
Riboflavin (mg)	0.457	0.229	0.439	0.145
Choline (mg)	293.8	146.9	1.1	0.4
Vitamin B12 (μg)	0.89	0.45	0.09	0.03
PUFA (g)	1.911	0.956	0	0
MUFA (g)	3.658	1.829	0	0
Vitamin A (IU)	540	270	0	0

recommendations change and the public perception of eggs alters, it is important for health experts to understand the scope of nutritional health benefits offered by eggs when they are incorporated into the diet. Eggs provide a wide variety of nutrients, acting as an excellent source of protein and delivering a rich diversity of vitamins, minerals, and fats. A brief summary of some of the key nutrients provided by whole eggs, or egg whites, can be seen in Table 1.2, which is drawn from the USDA Nutrient Database for Standard ref. 45.

1.5.2 Eggs as a Protein Source

Adequate protein consumption for individuals is an area of high concern for health professionals and is essential for an individual's overall health and wellness. The international recommendation for dietary protein intake established by the World Health Organization is 0.83 g kg^{-1} day^{-1} for the average individual, with higher intakes recommended for high activity athletes, children, and the elderly.[46–48] One of the most important factors to take into account when considering eggs as a source of protein is their relative affordability compared to other protein sources of similar quality, making them a critical dietary component for low-income individuals who are trying to establish a healthy dietary pattern.[49] This is especially important as the quality of egg protein is considered to be perfect when using the protein digestibility-corrected amino acid score (PDCAAS) for protein quality evaluation. Using the PDCAAS method to evaluate the quality of proteins, a score of less than 1 indicates the presence of a limiting amino acid, or rather, that at least one of the nine essential amino acid is not present in large enough quantities to meet consumer needs.[50,51] When compared to other proteins that are considered to be of high quality, eggs have robust scores on the PDCAAS scale, performing nearly as well as meat and fish, and outperforming soy and wheat.[5,50] The high quality of egg protein and its relative affordability suggest that it is a logical food for public health officials to recommend to consumers who are seeking to build a healthful diet on a reasonable budget.

One of the key biochemical uses of ingested protein is the synthesis of muscle, with the increased consumption of high-quality protein being associated with improved synthesis of skeletal muscle tissue as well as with muscle repair and maintenance.[52] Specific to eggs, the high quantity of the essential amino acid leucine has been associated with increased gains in muscle tissue mass and, therefore, in strength and power.[53] Research done by Moore *et al.* looked specifically at egg protein consumption in healthy young male subjects found a dose–dependent relationship between the quantity of egg protein consumed and muscle protein synthesis.[54] The association between increased protein consumption and improved muscle maintenance has also been observed in elderly populations for whom sarcopenia, or the loss of muscle tissue, is an area of concern.[47,55] This research suggests that eggs should not only be viewed as a protein source to be utilized by individuals with financial concerns, but that their high-quality and highly digestible protein should be recommended for athletes concerned with muscle development and for ageing individuals who are seeking to develop healthful diets that will help them maintain adequate muscle function in their later years. In these cases, while it may not be critical that eggs are more affordable than other sources of high-quality protein, it would certainly remain a benefit for consumers.

1.5.3 Eggs and Satiety

In addition to its association with improved muscle synthesis and muscle maintenance, protein consumption has also been positively associated with increased levels of satiety.[56,57] Dietary strategies aimed at improving post-prandial satiety response have been recognized as a critical tool for public health workers as increased levels of satiety following the consumption of a meal have been associated with an overall daily decrease in caloric intake.[58] Satiety levels have been positively associated with the levels of protein, water, and fiber found within foods, suggesting that eggs may serve as a beneficial component of meals that are designed with the aim of increasing the satiety response in consumers.[59] In fact, using a common index comparing satiety responses to specific foods, it was observed that the satiety response following egg consumption was 50% greater than the satiety response associated with a common ready-to-eat breakfast cereal or that of white bread.[60] This would suggest that as public health workers, medical practitioners, and dietitians work with individuals on putting together meal plans aimed at assisting in weight loss, breakfast plans that include eggs may be more effective and healthful options than breakfasts where cereal grains act as the staple.

One study, conducted by Vander Wal *et al.*, tested the ability of an egg-based breakfast to provide satiety to consumers when compared to a bagel breakfast. Both meals were matched for total energy and energy density. 125 men and women between the ages of 25 and 60 were assigned to one of four treatments: an egg breakfast, an egg breakfast plus a restricted calorie diet, a bagel breakfast, and a bagel breakfast plus a restricted calorie diet. After a 5 week intervention period, researchers found that the egg breakfast plus diet group had a 61% greater reduction in BMI ($p < 0.05$), a 34% greater reduction in waist circumference ($p < 0.06$), and a 65% greater reduction in weight loss ($p < 0.05$) when compared to the bagel plus diet group.[61] While no significant difference was observed between the standard egg breakfast group and the standard bagel breakfast group, the findings of this study suggest that incorporating eggs into the dietary pattern of individuals who are seeking to manage their weight may be an effective dietary intervention.[61]

Another study, also completed by Vander Wal *et al.*, examined the effect that eggs had on satiety in overweight and obese individuals.[62] Thirty women between the ages of 25 to 60 years with BMIs greater than or equal to 25 kg m^{-2} participated in a randomized crossover study to test the effect an egg breakfast had on satiety when compared to a bagel breakfast. Subjects were fed one of the two treatments for breakfast and were provided a lunch 3.5 hours later. Satiety was also measured through self-reported questionnaires. Researchers in this study found that when participants consumed the egg breakfast they experienced greater feelings of satiety compared to the bagel breakfast, and also consumed significantly less energy ($p < 0.0001$) during their lunch.[62] This data also supports the belief that incorporating eggs in a consumer's dietary pattern is not only healthful but can also help individuals better manage their energy intake through increased satiation.[62]

It is clear from the research discussed above that the incorporation of eggs into meals can serve as an effective way for consumers to improve their satiety response, which may, in turn, help them limit their overall consumption of calories throughout the day. Certainly, a common question that medical practitioners and dietitians are repeatedly faced with is how to help patients in their quest to lose or manage their weight. The ability to recommend simple dietary changes, like choosing an egg breakfast rather than a bagel breakfast, could be an effective tool to help patients reach their health goals for weight management.

1.5.4 Eggs and Choline

An essential micronutrient that has long been associated with eggs is choline.[63] Eggs are quite rich in choline, with higher choline levels than most other common foods. A comparison of choline levels between eggs and other common foods can be seen in Figure 1.2.[64] Choline must be obtained

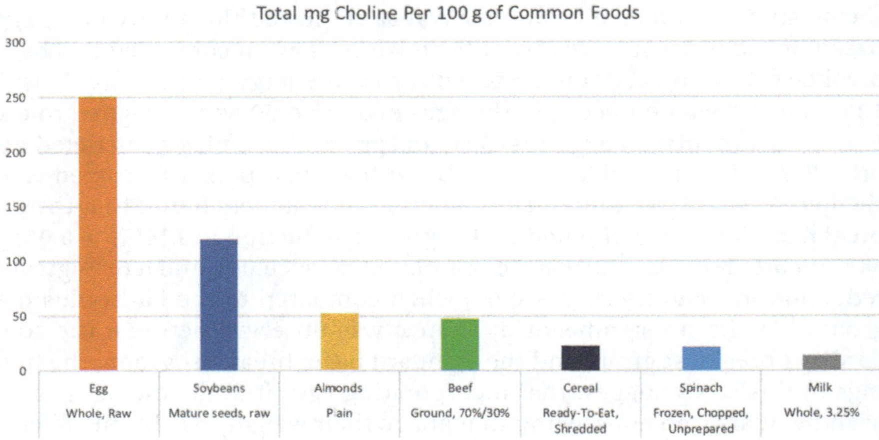

Figure 1.2 Choline levels in common foods. Data source: USDA Database for the Choline Content of Common Foods, Release Two.

in the human diet and is critical in cellular methylation reactions that are important for gene expression and the development of the neurotransmitter acetylcholine.[65,66] Not only has choline deficiency been associated with the development of non-alcoholic fatty liver disease and with neural tube defects during pregnancy, but recent epidemiological and intervention studies have suggested that maternal choline intake during pregnancy is associated with a child's cognition later in life.[66–68] In addition to its role in neurological development, choline plays a critical role in the metabolism of lipids within the body. Choline has been found to promote very low-density lipoprotein hepatic secretion and has been shown to play a role in the prevention of hepatic steatosis.[9,69]

In addition to the well-documented physiological need for choline for proper fetal development, recent research has begun to investigate if improved choline intake during pregnancy is actually associated with improved cognitive outcomes in children. One recent study tested the relationship between the level of maternal choline intake during various stages of pregnancy and the cognitive abilities of offspring as they matured. Researchers examined choline intake during pregnancy in 895 mothers participating in Project Viva and then tested the children of those mothers when the children reached the age of 7 years to determine visual memory and intelligence scores. Researchers found that an association existed between increased choline intake by the mother in the second trimester and improved cognitive scores in the child.[68] The association between choline intake during the first trimester and improved cognitive scores amongst children was also observed, but to a lesser degree.[68] While additional research is clearly required to test this potential association before it is communicated to consumers in an authoritative manner, it would certainly be of benefit for health care professionals to know that encouraging the consumption of foods high in choline during pregnancy may actually provide added benefits for the children of patients.

Despite the relative affordability and accessibility of eggs, and their ability to deliver high amounts of choline into the diet, many individuals in the United States are still susceptible to inadequate choline intake. In fact, one 2017 study that examined the NHANES datasets from 2009 to 2014, and the additional NHANES datasets for pregnant women from 2005 to 2014, found that across genders, life stages, and even in pregnancy, individuals in the United States were susceptible to suboptimal intakes of choline.[66] However, the same study found that individuals who regularly consumed eggs had nearly double the usual intake of choline compared to individuals who did not consume eggs. Researchers for the study posited that it would be incredibly difficult for individuals who do not consume eggs or did not take a choline-containing dietary supplement to achieve the suggested adequate intake levels for their life stage.[66]

1.6 Modified Eggs and the Diet

1.6.1 Introduction

As the recognition that eggs are part of a healthful dietary pattern continues to increase, it is ever more likely that researchers will continue to explore new ways through which the nutrient content of eggs can be improved. Whether these improvements are made through biotechnology, modified raising conditions for laying hens, or changes in the diet of laying hens, egg producers will seek to implement new best practices that will enhance both the nutrient density and desirability of their product.

1.6.2 Eggs and Vitamin D Fortification

Vitamin D is a critical nutrient for human vertebrates and is utilized by the body for the proper maintenance of serum calcium homeostasis.[70] The failure to achieve adequate levels of vitamin D, either through sunlight-dependent synthesis or consumption in the diet, has been connected to the development of rickets in young children and with the development of osteoporosis in grown adults.[71] Both conditions are connected to the inability for bones to properly mineralize without adequate amounts of vitamin D. Rickets is associated with growth retardation in children, deformities of the skeletal system, weakness of muscles, and, in some cases, seizures.[72] Osteoporosis, diagnosed in adults, is characterized by exceptionally low bone mass and a related increase risk of bone fractures.[73] It is widely accepted by health officials that the general public is failing to attain serum vitamin D levels that are required for healthy function, and they have therefore deemed vitamin D to be a nutrient of concern for public health.[74] As public health officials seek to address the prevalence of vitamin D insufficiency, dietary interventions involving eggs, which contain reasonable amounts of vitamin D, have been of interest.

Eggs, specifically egg yolks, contain both the D_3 and 25(OH)D_3 forms of vitamin D and are a strong candidate for increased vitamin D fortification because vitamin D provided to laying hens in their feed is easily transferred to the egg yolk, which may allow farmers to increase vitamin D concentrations in eggs through simple modifications to feed.[75,76] In recent studies, researchers have experimented with chicken feed containing various amounts of vitamin D_3 and 25(OH)D_3 to test whether supplementing feed will actually result in eggs that have consistently higher concentrations of available vitamin D for the humans that consume them. One study, conducted by Browning and Cowieson, compared nine separate treatments of an *ad libitum* mash diet, with vitamin D_3 levels ranging from 2500 IU kg^{-1} to 10 000 IU kg^{-1}, and 25(OH)D_3 levels ranging from 0 IU kg^{-1} to 2760 IU kg^{-1}.[76] After nine weeks of consuming the experimental diets, hens' eggs were analyzed for D_3 and 25(OH)D_3 and it was determined that a strong dose–dependent relationship existed between D_3 and 25(OH)D_3 levels in the diets of laying hens and the D_3 and 25(OH)D_3 levels in the yolks of the eggs that were actually laid.[76]

In addition to increasing the vitamin D levels of hen eggs through dietary supplementation, researchers have found that is it possible to increase the vitamin D levels of eggs by allowing laying hens to have greater access to the outdoors, thus stimulating sunlight-dependent synthesis of vitamin D. In 2014, Kühn *et al.* found that hens that had access to both indoor and outdoor habitats had a three- to four-fold increase in vitamin D_3 levels in their eggs compared to hens that were kept exclusively indoors.[77] Levels of vitamin D_3 in eggs reached even greater levels when laying hens were housed in exclusively outdoor environments.[77]

As public health officials and governmental agencies work to educate consumers about the potential health benefits of eggs, producers will seek to find new ways to differentiate their products or make them more attractive to consumers. As vitamin D is a nutrient of concern, and evidence suggests there are multiple ways in which egg producers can improve vitamin D content in their eggs, eggs could be well positioned to assume the role of a staple source of vitamin D in the human dietary pattern.

1.7 Conclusion and Discussion

Over 50 years ago, the United States federal government and consumer health advocacy groups initiated an information campaign that was intended to help the average consumer make healthier dietary choices by restricting their consumption of dietary cholesterol. This initiative, focused largely on providing the average consumer with easy to understand dietary guidance through the DGA, gave consumers the simple instruction to limit the number of eggs they consumed in an average week in order to maintain heart health and reduce their risk of CVD. These recommendations were made largely without scientific basis but were readily adopted by the general public throughout the United States and resulted in a precipitous decline in the overall purchase and consumption of eggs in the general population.

In the decades following these dietary recommendations, public health researchers throughout the county conducted countless epidemiological studies and clinical trials to test the relationship between the consumption of dietary cholesterol and increases in lipid and cholesterol markers associated with CVD. These studies overwhelmingly rejected the notion that dietary cholesterol was associated with plasma cholesterol levels and also found that when dietary cholesterol did impact plasma cholesterol levels, the ratio between LDL and HDL was largely unchanged. These findings resulted in a shift away from recommending restrictions in the consumption of eggs for the general population. However, the long timeframe for which dietary recommendations discouraging the use eggs existed and the relative simplicity of the dietary recommendation have already made the belief that eggs are not a healthful food nearly ubiquitous in the United States population.

Unfortunately, as noted in several studies aimed at gauging consumer attitudes towards eggs and individual willingness to purchase and consume them, the idea that eggs are linked to cholesterol levels has served as a significant deterrent for large portions of the population. This is troubling not only because the scientific community now agrees that such information is flawed, but also because eggs are able to play a critical role in the development of a healthful diet for much of the population. Not only are eggs affordable, but they provide an excellent source of protein to consumers, are rich in vitamin B12 and folate, and are high in choline.

While the public health efforts that encouraged Americans to avoid the consumption of eggs in the first place were certainly well-intentioned, the results of those recommendations over the course of the past 60 years should serve as an important lesson for individuals tasked with providing health information to the public. By telling consumers to avoid eggs for over half a century, public health officials have created large barriers to the consumption of a food we now agree is healthful, affordable, and important in a healthy dietary pattern. Not only does additional research need to be conducted that continues to demonstrate the health benefits of egg consumption, but new tactics need to be adopted for informing the public that egg consumption does not need to be restricted to ensure consumers are well informed of this dramatic change in dietary recommendations.

References

1. W. Stadelman, *Poult. Sci.*, 1999, **78**, 807–811.
2. C. H. S. Ruxton, E. Derbyshire and S. Gibson, *Nutr. Food Sci.*, 2010, **40**, 263–279.
3. D. K. Layman and N. R. Rodriguez, *Nutr. Today*, 2009, **44**, 43–48.
4. A. Drewnowski, *Am. J. Clin. Nutr.*, 2010, **91**, 1095S–1101S.
5. L. L. Iannotti, C. K. Lutter, D. A. Bunn and C. P. Stewart, *Nutr. Rev.*, 2014, **72**, 355–368.
6. Z. Conrad, L. K. Johnson, J. N. Roemmich, W. Juan and L. Jahns, *Nutrients*, 2017, **9**(4), 333.
7. M. M. Kanter, P. M. Kris-Etherton, M. L. Fernandez, K. C. Vickers and D. L. Katz, *Adv. Nutr.*, 2012, **3**, 711–717.
8. M. L. Fernandez, *Curr. Opin. Clin. Nutr. Metab. Care*, 2012, **15**, 117–121.
9. M. L. Fernandez and C. J. Andersen, in *Handbook of Eggs in Human Function*, 2015, vol. 9, pp. 15–34.
10. Committee on Nutrition American Heart Association, *Diet and Heart Disease*, Dallas, TX, USA, 1968.
11. D. J. McNamara, *Nutrients*, 2015, **7**, 8716–8722.
12. I. H. Page, F. J. Stare, A. C. Corcoran, H. Pollack and C. Wilkinson, *Circulation*, 1957, **16**, 163–178.
13. D. Kritchevsky, *J. Nutr.*, 1998, **128**, 449S–452S.
14. Central Committee for Medical and Community Program of the American Heart Association, *JAMA*, 1961, **175**, 389–391.
15. US Senate Select Committee on Nutrition and Human Needs, *Dietary Goals for the United States*, Washington, D.C., 1977.
16. US Department of Health and Human Services and US Department of Agriculture, *Nutrition and Your Health: Dietary Guidelines for Americans*, Washington, D.C., 1980.
17. US Department of Health and Human Services and US Department of Agriculture, *Nutrition and Your Health: Dietary Guidelines for Americans*, Washington, D.C., 1985.
18. US Department of Health and Human Services and US Department of Agriculture, *Nutrition and Your Health: Dietary Guidelines for Americans*, Washington, D.C., 3rd edn, 1990.
19. US Department of Health and Human Services and US Department of Agriculture, *Nutrition and Your Health: Dietary Guidelines for Americans*, Washington, D.C., 4th edn, 1995.
20. US Department of Health and Human Services and US Department of Agriculture, *Nutrition and Your Health: Dietary Guidelines for Americans*, Washington, D.C., 5th edn, 2000.
21. US Department of Health and Human Services and US Department of Agriculture, *Dietary Guidelines for Americans, 2005*, Washington, D.C., 2005.
22. US Department of Health and Human Services and US Department of Agriculture, *Dietary Guidelines for Americans, 2010*, Washington, D.C., 2010.

23. R. H. Eckel, J. M. Jakicic, J. D. Ard, J. M. de Jesus, N. Houston Miller, V. S. Hubbard, I.-M. Lee, A. H. Lichtenstein, C. M. Loria, B. E. Millen, C. A. Nonas, F. M. Sacks, S. C. Smith, L. P. Svetkey, T. A. Wadden, S. Z. Yanovski, K. A. Kendall, L. C. Morgan, M. G. Trisolini, G. Velasco, J. Wnek, J. L. Anderson, J. L. Halperin, N. M. Albert, B. Bozkurt, R. G. Brindis, L. H. Curtis, D. DeMets, J. S. Hochman, R. J. Kovacs, E. M. Ohman, S. J. Pressler, F. W. Sellke, W.-K. Shen, S. C. Smith, G. F. Tomaselli and American College of Cardiology/American Heart Association Task Force on Practice Guidelines, *Circulation*, 2014, **129**, S76–S99.
24. US Department of Health and Human Services and US Department of Agriculture, *2015–2020 Dietary Guidelines for Americans*, Washington, D.C., 2015.
25. Q. Wang, H. H. Jensen and S. T. Yen, *Appl. Econ. Lett.*, 1996, **3**, 189–191.
26. T. A. Nicklas, C. E. O'Neil and V. L. Fulgoni, *J. Nutr.*, 2015, **145**, 170S–176S.
27. W. O. Song and J. M. Kerver, *J. Am. Coll. Nutr.*, 2000, **19**, 556S–562S.
28. S. I. Kirkpatrick, K. W. Dodd, J. Reedy and S. M. Krebs-Smith, *J. Acad. Nutr. Diet.*, 2012, **112**, 624–635.e6.
29. A. K. Kant and B. I. Graubard, *Am. J. Clin. Nutr.*, 2012, **96**, 601–612.
30. C. W. Leung, E. L. Ding, P. J. Catalano, E. Villamor, E. B. Rimm and W. C. Willett, *Am. J. Clin. Nutr.*, 2012, **96**, 977–988.
31. C. E. O'Neil, T. A. Nicklas, D. R. Keast and V. L. Fulgoni, *Food Nutr. Res.*, 2014, **58**, 15784.
32. S. Vega-López, G. Pignotti, M. Todd and C. Keller, *Nutrients*, 2015, **7**, 8402–8412.
33. D. J. Brown and L. F. Schrader, *Am. J. Agric. Econ.*, 1990, **72**, 548.
34. F. A. Kummerow, in *Handbook of Eggs in Human Function*, 9th edn, 2015, pp. 53–62.
35. M. L. Fernandez and M. Calle, *Curr. Atheroscler. Rep.*, 2010, **12**, 377–383.
36. K. L. Esrey, L. Joseph and S. A. Grover, *J. Clin. Epidemiol.*, 1996, **49**, 211–216.
37. W. H. Howell, D. J. McNamara, M. A. Tosca, B. T. Smith and J. A. Gaines, *Am. J. Clin. Nutr.*, 1997, **65**, 1747–1764.
38. F. B. Hu, M. J. Stampfer, E. B. Rimm, J. E. Manson, A. Ascherio, G. A. Colditz, B. A. Rosner, D. Spiegelman, F. E. Speizer, F. M. Sacks, C. H. Hennekens and W. C. Willett, *JAMA*, 1999, **281**, 1387–1394.
39. D. J. McNamara, *J. Am. Coll. Nutr.*, 1997, **16**, 530–534.
40. D. M. DiMarco, A. Missimer, A. G. Murillo, B. S. Lemos, O. V. Malysheva, M. A. Caudill, C. N. Blesso and M. L. Fernandez, *Lipids*, 2017, **52**, 255–263.
41. M. N. Ballesteros, R. M. Cabrera, M. del Socorro Saucedo and M. L. Fernandez, *Am. J. Clin. Nutr.*, 2004, **80**, 855–861.
42. C. M. Greene, T. L. Zern, R. J. Wood, S. Shrestha, D. Aggarwal, M. J. Sharman, J. S. Volek and M. L. Fernandez, *J. Nutr.*, 2005, **135**, 2793–2798.
43. Z. Harcombe, J. S. Baker, S. M. Cooper, B. Davies, N. Sculthorpe, J. J. DiNicolantonio and F. Grace, *Open Heart*, 2015, **2**, e000196.
44. J. Gray and B. Griffin, *Nutr. Bull.*, 2009, **34**, 66–70.
45. USDA, *National Nutrient Database for Standard Reference*, https://ndb.nal.usda.gov, (accessed May 2018).

46. WHO, *Report: Protein and Amino Acid Requirements in Human Nutrition*, http://www.who.int/nutrition/publications/nutrientrequirements/WHO_TRS_935/en/, (accessed July 2017).
47. J. M. Beasley, J. M. Shikany and C. A. Thomson, *Nutr. Clin. Pract.*, 2013, **28**, 684–690.
48. D. R. Moore, D. M. Camera, J. L. Areta and J. A. Hawley, *Appl. Physiol., Nutr., Metab.*, 2014, **39**, 987–997.
49. A. Drewnowski, *Am. J. Clin. Nutr.*, 2010, **92**, 1181–1188.
50. D. Tome, *Br. J. Nutr.*, 2012, **108**, S222–S229.
51. S. Dubin, K. McKee and S. Battish, *J. Am. Diet. Assoc.*, 1994, **94**, 884–887.
52. R. R. Wolfe, *Am. J. Clin. Nutr.*, 2006, **84**, 475–482.
53. C. P. Lambert, L. L. Frank and W. J. Evans, *Sports Med.*, 2004, **34**, 317–327.
54. D. R. Moore, M. J. Robinson, J. L. Fry, J. E. Tang, E. I. Glover, S. B. Wilkinson, T. Prior, M. A. Tarnopolsky and S. M. Phillips, *Am. J. Clin. Nutr.*, 2009, **89**, 161–168.
55. L. Breen and S. M. Phillips, *Nutr. Metab.*, 2011, **8**, 68.
56. S. M. Pasiakos, *J. Food Sci.*, 2015, **80**, A2–A7.
57. J. Halkjær, A. Olsen, K. Overvad, M. U. Jakobsen, H. Boeing, B. Buijsse, D. Palli, G. Tognon, H. Du, D. L. van der A, N. G. Forouhi, N. J. Wareham, E. J. M. Feskens, T. I. A. Sørensen and A. Tjønneland, *Int. J. Obes.*, 2011, **35**, 1104–1113.
58. A. Drewnowski, *Nutr. Rev.*, 1998, **56**, 347–353.
59. S. H. Holt, J. C. Brand-Miller and P. A. Stitt, *J. Am. Diet. Assoc.*, 2001, **101**, 767–773.
60. S. H. Holt, J. C. Miller, P. Petocz and E. Farmakalidis, *Eur. J. Clin. Nutr.*, 1995, **49**, 675–690.
61. J. Vander Wal, A. Gupta, P. Khosla and N. V. Dhurandhar, *Int. J. Obes.*, 2008, **32**, 1545–1551.
62. J. S. Vander Wal, J. M. Marth, P. Khosla, K.-L. C. Jen and N. V. Dhurandhar, *J. Am. Coll. Nutr.*, 2005, **24**, 510–515.
63. S. H. Zeisel and K.-A. da Costa, *Nutr. Rev.*, 2009, **67**, 615–623.
64. K. Y. Patterson, S. A. Bhagwat, J. R. Williams, J. C. Howe and J. M. Holden, USDA Database for the Choline Content of Common Foods, Release Two, USDA, Beltsville, MD, USA, 2008.
65. Institute of Medicine US Standing Committee on the Scientific Evaluation of Dietary Reference Intakes and its Panel on Folate Other B Vitamins and Choline, *Dietary Reference Intakes for Thiamin, Riboflavin, Niacin, Vitamin B6, Folate, Vitamin B12, Pantothenic Acid, Biotin, and Choline*, National Academies Press, Washington, D.C., 1998.
66. T. C. Wallace and V. L. Fulgoni, *Nutrients*, 2017, **9**(8), 839.
67. R. M. Pitkin, *Am. J. Clin. Nutr.*, 2007, **85**, 285S–288S.
68. C. E. Boeke, M. W. Gillman, M. D. Hughes, S. L. Rifas-Shiman, E. Villamor and E. Oken, *Am. J. Epidemiol.*, 2013, **177**, 1338–1347.
69. M. E. Rinella, M. S. Elias, R. R. Smolak, T. Fu, J. Borensztajn and R. M. Green, *J. Lipid Res.*, 2008, **49**, 1068–1076.
70. S. Christakos, C. Gabrielides and W. B. Rhoten, *Endocr. Rev.*, 1989, **10**, 3–26.

71. M. F. Holick, *N. Engl. J. Med.*, 2007, **357**, 266–281.
72. M. F. Holick, *J. Clin. Invest.*, 2006, **116**, 2062–2072.
73. S. R. Cummings, J. L. Kelsey, M. C. Nevitt and K. J. O'Dowd, *Epidemiol. Rev.*, 1985, **7**, 178–208.
74. D. A. Hanley and K. S. Davison, *J. Nutr.*, 2005, **135**, 332–337.
75. D. B. Parrish and E. F. Richter, *CRC Crit. Rev. Food Sci. Nutr.*, 1979, **12**, 29–57.
76. L. C. Browning and A. J. Cowieson, *J. Sci. Food Agric.*, 2014, **94**, 1389–1396.
77. J. Kühn, A. Schutkowski, H. Kluge, F. Hirche and G. I. Stangl, *Nutrition*, 2014, **30**, 481–484.

CHAPTER 2

Eggs are a Natural Functional Food

MARIA LUZ FERNANDEZ* AND BRUNO LEMOS

Department of Nutritional Sciences, University of Connecticut Storrs, CT 06269, USA
*E-mail: maria-luz.fernandez@uconn.edu

2.1 Introduction

In spite of the United States (US) dietary guidelines released in January of 2016 where the upper limits for dietary cholesterol were removed,[1] there is still a perceived association between cholesterol content in eggs and risk for coronary heart disease (CHD). It is interesting to note that several countries in Asia and Europe removed the upper limit for dietary cholesterol several years before the US.[2] It is critical that dietary cholesterol is not recognized as the only component of eggs but that the focus shifts to the high nutritional value of eggs. Eggs are excellent sources of vitamins D and E and selenium,[3] plus eggs also contain components whose function in the human body goes beyond nutrition, including lutein and zeaxanthin,[4] and choline.[5] Eggs are also characterized by having high-quality protein contributing to satiety, which could be beneficial for those who want to lose weight.[6,7]

The risk for heart disease is not increased by egg intake, as has been shown in numerous epidemiological studies[8,9] as well as in clinical interventions with healthy[10,11] and at-risk populations.[12,13] On the contrary, eggs

Food Chemistry, Function and Analysis No.14
Eggs as Functional Foods and Nutraceuticals for Human Health
Edited by Jianping Wu

Published by the Royal Society of Chemistry, www.rsc.org

appear to have beneficial effects against heart disease risk, as exemplified by their effects of decreasing insulin resistance in individuals with metabolic syndrome[12] and inflammation in diabetic patients,[14] and consistent increases in high-density lipoprotein cholesterol (HDL-C) in various populations.[15]

The perception of the public regarding eggs needs to move from eggs being an icon for dietary cholesterol to eggs having a number of nutritious components. In the following paragraphs, we will discuss the forgotten nutritional benefits of eggs as well as the protective effects of eggs against chronic disease.

2.2 Eggs and Carotenoids (Lutein and Zeaxanthin)

2.2.1 Plasma Concentrations of Lutein and Zeaxanthin

The carotenoids lutein and zeaxanthin are surrounded by the lipid matrix in eggs, facilitating their solubilization into micelles, absorption in the small intestine and incorporation into chylomicrons for delivery to extra-hepatic tissues and the liver.[16] Compared to other foods including spinach, broccoli and kale, eggs are not a remarkable source of these carotenoids, which are in the range of 200 to 300 μg per egg. However, these carotenoids in eggs are highly bioavailable[17] and in many studies we have seen substantial increases in plasma lutein and zeaxanthin following egg intake.[18–20] Furthermore, egg intake also results in the formation of larger high-density lipoprotein (LDL) and HDL particles, which facilitate the circulation of lutein and zeaxanthin,[21] and the larger HDL has been demonstrated to increase reverse cholesterol transport.[22] Lutein and zeaxanthin, by being more fat-soluble carotenoids, are mainly transported in HDL[23] and a possible mechanism by which they are delivered into eyes and other tissues may be through scavenger receptor class B-1 (SR-B1).[24] The role of HDL in transporting lutein into the retina has been elucidated by studying WHAM chicks.[25]

2.2.2 Antioxidant Properties of Lutein and Zeaxanthin

Very few studies on the antioxidant properties of lutein and zeaxanthin have been conducted directly with egg yolk. Fernandez-Robredo *et al.*,[26] however, reported a decrease in lipid peroxidation with egg yolk in apo E (−/−) knockout mice. Other studies reported the antioxidant properties of lutein in guinea pig liver[27] and the reductions of oxidized LDL in both the plasma and aortas of guinea pigs,[28] and protection against atherosclerosis in Japanese quails.[29] Serpeloni *et al.*[30] reported that lutein induces the expression of antioxidant genes and reactive oxygen species (ROS) in mice. Clearly, the most salient antioxidant properties of lutein and zeaxanthin are related to their protective effects against age-related macular degeneration (AMD).

The retina of the eye is constantly exposed to UV light, which leads to the generation of ROS[31] and ultimately to oxidation of the retina, known as AMD.[32] AMD is irreversible and affects people over 65 years of age. It is closely associated with heredity, although exposure to the sun, iris color and nutritional status are other factors that might accelerate AMD.[33,34] The protective role of lutein and zeaxanthin was demonstrated in an early study, which showed that high intake, as well as high plasma concentrations of these carotenoids, were related to lower rates of AMD.[35]

Lutein and zeaxanthin are selectively taken up by the eye, where they reduce the generation of oxidant species,[36] indicating their important role in protecting against AMD.[37,38] The concentrations of lutein and zeaxanthin can be measured by calculating macular pigment optical density (MPOD) in the eyes. Some studies have demonstrated a higher concentration of MPOD following egg consumption.[39,40] Further, lutein- or zeaxanthin-enriched eggs have been reported to have the same effect on MPOD as supplements of these carotenoids with a concentration as high as 5 mg.[41] In addition, there are important clinical trials[42,43] that clearly support the role of lutein and zeaxanthin in protecting against AMD. Wu *et al.* recently reported from the Nurses' Health study that comparing the highest to the lowest quintile for lutein and zeaxanthin intake resulted in a 40% risk reduction for AMD in both men and women.[44] Thus, there is a consensus in the literature from clinical studies and epidemiological observations that lutein and zeaxanthin play a key role in protecting against the formation of ROS in the eyes, the subsequent oxidation and the generation of AMD.

2.2.3 Anti-inflammatory Properties of Lutein and Zeaxanthin

Lutein and zeaxanthin in eggs may also be associated with decreased inflammation. There are several studies performed in cells, animal models and diverse populations that document the anti-inflammatory properties of these carotenoids. Studies in ARPE-2 cells demonstrated that lutein and zeaxanthin accumulate in the retinal epithelial cells from 2–14-fold, indicating that these cells effectively internalize these carotenoids.[45] Further, compared to untreated cells, there was a significant decrease in the expression of inflammatory cytokines monocyte chemoattractant protein-1 (MCP-I) and complement factor H (CFH). From this study, it was concluded that protection of the proteasome from oxidative inactivation is the main mechanism by which lutein and zeaxanthin modulate the inflammatory response, explaining why these carotenoids are so effective in reducing AMD.[45] Other studies have shown that *meso*-zeaxanthin, a derivative of zeaxanthin, decreases the expression of tumor necrosis factor α (TNF-α), interleukin (IL)-6 and IL-1β in mice macrophages, confirming its potent anti-inflammatory effects.[46]

In guinea pigs, lutein supplementation has been shown to decrease inflammation in the liver and to decrease hepatic steatosis.[47] Reduction in inflammatory cytokines in aortas, as well as lipid accumulation and reduction of early atherosclerosis development, has been observed in guinea pigs by adding only 3 mg d^{-1} of lutein to the diet.[28] Other studies have shown that lutein inhibits inflammatory gene expression mediated by nuclear factor (NF)-kB in mice.[48]

Some human studies have demonstrated the anti-inflammatory effects of eggs. For example, in obese individuals, lowering of C reactive protein (CRP),[49] serum amyloid A and TNF-α[13] was observed in patients with metabolic syndrome following the consumption of three eggs per day for 12 weeks. In addition, compared to an oatmeal breakfast, intake of one egg per day resulted in lower concentrations of TNF-α and of the liver enzyme aspartate amino transferase.[14] All of these reductions in the biomarkers of inflammation were observed in individuals with well-characterized chronic inflammation. The fact that those decreases in inflammation were observed in individuals with metabolic syndrome and type-2 diabetes, with well-established low-grade chronic inflammation,[50,51] supports the role of the components of eggs in protecting against factors associated with chronic disease.

The beneficial effects of lutein on oxidative stress, inflammation and AMD derived from human and animal studies are depicted in Figure 2.1.

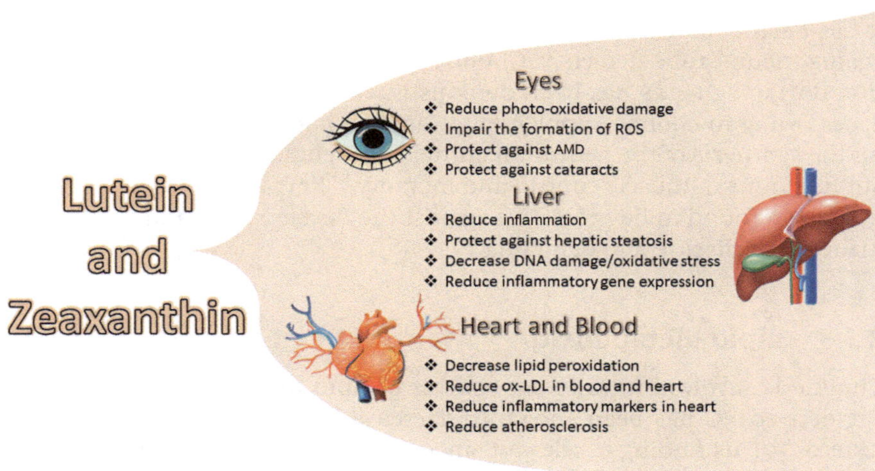

Figure 2.1 Potential effects of lutein and zeaxanthin. Lutein and zeaxanthin have been shown to protect: the eyes by reducing photo-oxidative damage,[35] impairing the formation of reactive oxygen species (ROS),[36] protecting against age-related macular degeneration (AMD) and cataracts;[41,44] the liver by reducing inflammation,[27] protecting against hepatic steatosis,[47] decreasing DNA damage[30] and reducing inflammatory gene expression;[48] the heart and blood by reducing lipid peroxidation,[26] oxidized LDL (ox-LDL) in the blood and heart,[28] and atherosclerosis.[29]

2.3 Eggs and Choline

2.3.1 Introduction

Choline is recognized as an essential nutrient for health owing to its many functions in growth and development, as well as neurological function and formation of membrane phospholipids, including phosphatidylcholine (PC) and sphingomyelin.[52] A great number of adults and children fail to meet their daily adequate intakes (AI) for choline in the US,[53] which may increase the risk of adverse effects including cognitive impairment, neural tube defects, muscle damage and fatty liver.[54] Owing to the impact of choline deficiency on health issues, consumption of dietary sources of choline is very important in protecting against these diseases.

Eggs have been documented as one of the best sources of choline in the diet, in the form of PC, found in the egg yolk.[55,56] Thus, egg intake provides dietary choline, which is essential to the optimization of health and prevention of disease throughout the lifespan.

2.3.2 Neurological Function

The essential role of choline in neurological functions, neurotransmitter synthesis and protection against cognitive impairment is well recognized.[57] It has been demonstrated that diets rich in choline exert a protective effect against neural tube defects.[58] Choline can also promote neurological function during aging as has been demonstrated by the formation of new synapses owing to choline supplementation.[59] In addition, choline is essential for the synthesis of the neurotransmitter acetylcholine, which serves important functions in muscle control and memory.[60] Further, diets rich in choline have been found to be protective against the development and treatment of Alzheimer's disease and dementia.[61]

2.3.3 Lipid Metabolism

Choline is involved in different aspects of lipid metabolism. For example, egg-derived PC has been shown to decrease lymphatic absorption of cholesterol.[62] This finding is relevant since a component present in eggs serves to decrease the absorption of cholesterol, another egg component. Choline stimulates hepatic secretion of very-low-density lipoprotein (VLDL) and protects against hepatic steatosis.[63,64] Further, intake of three eggs for 12 weeks has been shown to alter the phospholipid composition of HDL by increasing PC in men and women with metabolic syndrome,[22] leading to an increased cholesterol-accepting capacity, a key component of reverse cholesterol transport, which protects against the severity and risk of CHD.[65] Other studies have also observed a cardioprotective role of choline in which subjects consuming choline-rich diets have lower levels of plasma homocysteine owing to its role in methyl-group metabolism.[66] However, it is important to note recent studies that have found that choline intake could be associated with an increased risk of major adverse cardiovascular events owing to the role of gut microflora-mediated metabolism of choline to trimethylamine *N*-oxide (TMAO).[67]

2.3.4 Choline and TMAO

The metabolism of choline is crucial owing to the various metabolites that are formed inside the body. Lecithin, or PC, once ingested can be broken down into choline by phospholipase D[68] to form free choline. Choline can be metabolized to betaine by choline dehydrogenase and betaine aldehyde dehydrogenase, and/or trimethylamine (TMA). The reaction to form the metabolite TMA is mediated by the gut microbiota, *Firmicutes* and *Bacteroidetes*[69]. Importantly, modulation of the gut microbiota is mediated by diet.[70] Therefore, inter-individual variability can be found owing to differences in diet composition.[71] For instance, omnivores have a different microbiota flora to vegetarians and vegans.[72] Nevertheless, TMA is absorbed and circulates in plasma until it reaches the liver, where it is further oxidized by flavin monooxygenases (FMO) to TMAO.[73] There are various isoforms of FMO, but the most predominant is FMO3 in the hepatic tissue.[73] TMAO has been the major concern in cardiovascular disease owing to elevated fasting TMAO observed in patients at risk for cardiovascular disease (CVD).[74] Importantly, about 90% of phospholipids are absorbed in the ileum[52] *via* micelle formation and incorporation into chylomicrons before reaching the gut microbiota. Therefore, phosphatidylcholine from eggs is believed to follow the phospholipid route and not be further metabolized to TMA in the large intestine. This will eventually result in previously observed increased bioavailability of plasma choline,[75] which can further contribute to ameliorating the functions of this essential nutrient. The different proposed fates of choline *versus* PC are depicted in Figure 2.2.

Emerging studies are exploring the metabolism of different forms of choline and its contribution to CVD risk, if any. Animal models have shown that high plasma TMAO is associated with increased atherosclerosis progression.[74] TMAO can induce expression of two major scavenger receptors, cluster of differentiation-36 (CD36) and steroid receptor-A1 (SR-A1), in mice.[74] These receptors are present in macrophages residing in the intima, with the main function of recognizing modified LDL particles, which can trigger the formation of foam cells and further aggravate atherosclerotic lesions.[76] Since eggs are a great source of dietary choline, a TMAO precursor, they have been targeted because TMAO increases the risk of cardiovascular disease. Clinical trials have evaluated the effects of increasing the dosage of eggs,[71,77] egg intake in comparison to an oatmeal breakfast,[78] and an intake of three eggs per day in comparison to another choline source (choline bitartrate supplement) without observing increases in fasting plasma TMAO[75] nor other association to CVD risk. In fact, these trials have all observed an increase

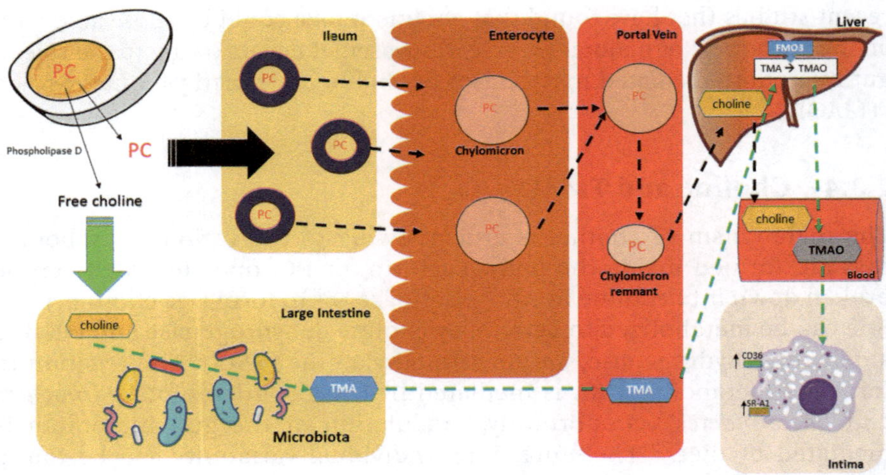

Figure 2.2 Postulated pathways for phosphatidylcholine (PC) and free choline. PC, as is found in eggs, is absorbed in the small intestine and incorporated into the chylomicron and delivered to the liver through the chylomicron remnant to be later secreted into circulation (black arrows). Free choline is not so readily absorbed in the small intestine, and a large portion of this choline will be converted by microbiota into trimethylamine (TMA); this metabolite will go to the liver and be converted into trimethylamine-*N*-oxide (TMAO) by flavin monooxygenase 3 (FMO3). TMAO increases the expression of the macrophage scavenger receptors cluster of differentiation 36 (CD36) and scavenger receptor-A1 (SR-A1) (green arrows), which can remove modified cholesterol from circulation and increase development of atherosclerosis and the risk for heart disease.

in fasting plasma choline, which helps prove that choline present in eggs is more bioavailable and can further contribute to ameliorating the current choline deficiency in American children and adults.

2.4 Eggs and Protein

2.4.1 Introduction

Egg protein, in both the white and the yolk, has a high biological value. Eggs contain a variety of proteins that have been shown to have bioactive properties, including promotion of immunity, antimicrobial activity, and exerting protection against cancer and hypertension.[79] Because egg protein contains all the essential amino acids, it has been shown to contribute to the maintenance of skeletal muscle,[80] and it has been suggested to reduce sarcopenia in the elderly[81] as well as protecting against protein malnutrition in children.[82] Furthermore, egg protein has also been shown to decrease glycemic index and to be effective in weight control.[83] All these beneficial effects will be discussed in the following paragraphs.

2.4.2 Egg Protein and Skeletal Muscle Health

Healthy skeletal muscle is essential throughout the lifespan owing to its key function in maintaining body shape and providing strength for physical activity;[69] this is the reason why dietary sources of high biological value protein become essential.[84] The high biological value of eggs has been long recognized as well as the fact that they provide all essential amino acids, which are efficiently utilized by the body.[85]

In children from underdeveloped countries, eggs or other high protein sources are not introduced early on in life, which can lead to kwashiorkor, marasmus and other forms of protein malnutrition.[86] Studies have demonstrated that introduction of eggs after weaning leads to fewer cases of kwashiorkor.[87] Other studies have demonstrated improvement in physical growth with egg supplementation in children.[88] In healthy young males, egg protein has been shown to improve muscle protein synthesis after resistance exercise.[89] In older populations, suboptimal intake in terms of protein quality and quantity increases the risk of sarcopenia.[90] In a recent study, egg white supplementation increased muscle mass in the elderly.[91] In contrast, high protein diets with eggs being the major protein source did not additionally affect skeletal muscle fiber size or body composition in 36 older individuals who were undergoing a program of resistance training.[92] For the most part, these studies support that egg protein is beneficial for healthy muscle across the life spectrum.

2.4.3 Egg Proteins, Immunity and Other Protective Effects

Eggs contain numerous proteins with antimicrobial and immunoprotective properties, which serve as a natural defense for the egg; however, they have demonstrated potential for therapeutic applications.[68] Lysozyme, for example, hydrolyzes structural peptidoglycans in bacterial cell walls[93] and ovotransferrin inhibits microbial infection by preventing the microorganisms from utilizing iron *via* its iron-scavenging property,[94] while avidin binds to biotin and prevents bacteria from accessing this vitamin.[95] All these proteins are present in egg white.

In egg yolk, there is immunoglobulin Y, which has been reported to protect against numerous pathogens by preventing growth and colonization[68] of bacteria, including *Escherichia Coli*[96] and *Staphylococcus aureus*.[97] Additionally, the phosphoprotein phosvitin has been shown to possess antimicrobial activity.[98]

Egg proteins have also been shown to protect against chronic disease. A hypotensive activity has been shown with peptides derived from ovalbumin in rats.[99] To further confirm these observations seen in animals, in a recent study conducted in a young healthy population, one egg per day resulted in a decrease in blood pressure compared to no egg intake.[21] Lysozyme from egg white has also been shown to exert anti-cancer activity in both *in vitro* and *in vivo* conditions.[100,101] To summarize, the proteins in eggs not only protect against skeletal muscle loss and protein-related malnutrition, but they are also a source of biologically active components, which protect against hypertension and cancer.

2.4.4 Egg Protein, Satiety and Weight Loss

Obesity costs will increase to 900 billion US dollars annually by the year 2030;[102] therefore, high protein foods that have been shown to decrease appetite deserve serious consideration. For example, foods with a high satiety index (SI) have been shown to reduce energy intake in the following meal.[103] In addition, foods that suppress ghrelin, a hormone associated with appetite,[104] may be another important way of controlling obesity through a possible decrease in hunger.

Eggs have been shown to suppress appetite and decrease plasma ghrelin levels.[7] In a randomized crossover study, 25 men aged 20–70 years were given either eggs or bagel-based isocaloric breakfasts to determine the effects of egg protein on postprandial appetite hormones, plasma insulin and glucose. After 7 days, subjects were switched to the alternate breakfast.[7] Blood was taken every hour for a total of 5 hours in order to measure all the mentioned biomarkers following each breakfast food. All 25 subjects had greater decreases in appetite following the egg breakfast using a measurement of visual scales. In addition, these individuals consumed less kcal both in their next meal and in the next 24 hours with egg intake, using dietary records for assessment, in comparison to the bagel-based breakfast.[94] The decreases in appetite were correlated with lower plasma glucose, insulin and ghrelin, based on areas under the curve, suggesting potential mechanisms through which eggs have a high SI. The lowering of plasma ghrelin levels could be related to the high protein from eggs.[105] Similar to this study, Vander Wal *et al.*[106] also reported greater satiety following an egg breakfast when compared to a non-egg breakfast.

When eggs are incorporated into meal plans, they can enhance weight loss.[72] In a weight loss study with 152 men and women, an egg and a bagel breakfast were compared.[6] With the egg breakfast, greater weight loss (65%), greater reduction in waist circumference (34%) and greater reduction in body fat (10%) were observed. Additionally, there were no significant changes in blood cholesterol between groups. However, in a recent study, no differences in weight were observed for college students consuming an egg *versus* a non-egg breakfast, although eggs, in spite of an additional 400 mg of dietary cholesterol, did not result in any blood cholesterol changes when compared to a non-egg breakfast.[107]

The effects of egg proteins on satiety, malnutrition, muscle mass, hypertension, cancer and immunity are summarized in Table 2.1.

Table 2.1 Effects of egg proteins or peptides on health.

Effect	Egg component	Reference
Protection against malnutrition	Whole eggs	(87)
Improvement of physical growth	Whole eggs	(88)
Increased protein synthesis during resistance training	Whole eggs	(89)
Muscle maintenance in elderly	Whole eggs	(90), (91)
Antimicrobial	Egg white	(93), (94), (95)
Antimicrobial	Egg yolk	(93), (96)
Hypotensive agent	Whole eggs	(21), (99)
Anti-cancer	Egg white	(100), (101)
Reduction of appetite	Whole eggs	(7), (106)
Weight loss	Whole eggs	(6)

2.5 Conclusions

Numerous health benefits are derived from eggs. The purpose of this chapter was to emphasize components of eggs that provide protection that goes beyond nutrition with the main focus on carotenoids, choline and proteins. It is clear that once the concern for dietary cholesterol is removed, in agreement with our dietary guidelines, the importance of the health effects of eggs becomes evident. Eggs, as we have described in this chapter, can exert protection against heart disease thanks to the antioxidant and anti-inflammatory properties of egg carotenoids, and improve cognitive function owing to choline effects. In addition, they can also contribute to preserving muscle mass and be a good choice for weight loss interventions owing to the high quality and satiety properties of egg protein. Overall, eggs can be considered as a natural nutraceutical to be incorporated in the diet.

References

1. US Department of Health and Human Services and US Department of Agriculture, http://health.gov/dieataryguidelines/2015/ (accessed on April 2018).
2. M. L. Fernandez and M. C. Calle, Revisiting dietary cholesterol recommendations: does the evidence support a 300 mg/d limit?, *Curr. Atheroscler. Rep.*, 2010, **12**, 377–383.
3. M. L. Fernandez and C. J. Andersen, Eggs, Composition and Health, in *Encyclopedia of Food and Health*, ed. B. Caballero, P. M. Finglas and F. Toldra, 2014, vol. 201, pp. 470–475.
4. G. J. Handelman, A. J. Ningthingale and A. H. Lichesnstein, Lutein and zeaxanthin concentrations in plasma after dietary supplementation with egg yolk, *Am. J. Clin. Nutr.*, 1999, **70**, 247–251.
5. S. H. Zeisel and K. A. da Costa, Choline: an essential nutrient for public health, *Nutr. Rev.*, 2009, **67**, 615–623.

6. J. S. Vander Wal, A. Gupta, P. Khosla and N. V. Dhurandhar, Egg breakfast enhances weight loss, *Int. J. Obes.*, 2008, **32**, 1545–1551.
7. J. Ratliff, J. O. Leite, R. de Ogburn, M. J. Puglisi, J. VanHeest and M. L. Fernandez, Consuming eggs for breakfast influences plasma glucose and ghrelin, while reducing energy intake during the next 24 hours in adult men, *Nutr. Res.*, 2010, **30**, 96–103.
8. F. B. Hu, M. J. Stampfer, E. B. Rimm, J. E. Manson, A. Ascherio and G. A. Colditz, *et al.* A prospective study of egg consumption and risk of cardiovascular disease in men and women, *JAMA*, 1999, **281**, 1387–1394.
9. A. I. Qureshi, F. K. Suri, S. Ahmed, A. Nasar, A. A. Divani and J. F. Kirmani, Regular egg consumption does not increase the risk of stroke and cardiovascular diseases, *Med. Sci. Monit.*, 2007, **13**, CR1–8.
10. K. L. Herron, I. E. Lofgren, M. Sharma, J. S. Volek and M. L. Fernandez, A high intake of dietary cholesterol does not result in more atherogenic LDL particles in men and women independent of response classification, *Metab., Clin. Exp.*, 2004, **53**, 823–830.
11. B. S. Lemos, I. Medina-Vera, C. N. Blesso and M. L. Fernandez, Intake of 3 eggs per day when compared to a choline bitartrate supplement, downregulates cholesterol synthesis without changing the LDL/HDL ratio, *Nutrients*, 2018, **10**(2), 258.
12. G. Mutungi, J. Ratliff, M. Puglisi, M. Torres-Gonzalez, U. Vaishnav, J. O. Leite, E. Quann, J. S. Volek and M. L. Fernandez, Dietary cholesterol from eggs increases HDL cholesterol in overweight men consuming a carbohydrate restricted diet, *J. Nutr.*, 2008, **138**, 272–276.
13. C. N. Blesso, C. J. Andersen, J. Barona, B. Volk, J. S. Volek and M. L. Fernandez, Effects of carbohydrate restriction and dietary cholesterol provided by eggs on clinical risk factors of metabolic syndrome, *J. Clin. Lipidol.*, 2013, **7**, 463–471.
14. M. N. Ballesteros, F. Valenzuela, A. E. Robles, E. Artalejo, D. Aguilar, C. J. Andersen, H. Valdez and M. L. Fernandez, One egg per day improves inflammation when compared to an oatmeal-based breakfast without increasing other cardiometabolic risk factors in diabetic patients, *Nutrients*, 2015, **7**, 3449–3463.
15. M. L. Fernandez, Effects of eggs on plasma lipoproteins in healthy populations, *Food Funct.*, 2010, **1**, 156–160.
16. Transport, Uptake and Target Tissue of Carotenoids, in *Carotenoids in Health and Disease*, ed. H. C. Furr and R. M. Clark, CRC Press, Boca Raton, Florida, USA, 2004, p. 576.
17. H. Y. Chung, H. M. Rasmussen and E. J. Johnson, Lutein bioavailability is higher from lutein-enriched eggs than from supplements or spinach in men, *J. Nutr.*, 2004, **134**, 1887–1893.
18. M. N. Ballesteros, R. M. Cabrera, M. S. Saucedo and M. L. Fernandez, Dietary cholesterol does not increase biomarkers for chronic disease in a pediatric population at risk from Northern Mexico, *Am. J. Clin. Nutr.*, 2004, **80**, 855–861.

19. G. Mutungi, D. Waters, J. Ratliff, M. J. Puglisi, R. M. Clark, J. S. Volek and M. L. Fernandez, Eggs distinctly modulate plasma carotenoid and lipoprotein subclasses in adult men following a carbohydrate restricted diet, *J. Nutr. Biochem.*, 2010, **21**, 261–267.
20. C. M. Greene, D. Waters, R. M. Clark, J. H. Contois and M. L. Fernandez, Plasma LDL and HDL characteristics and carotenoid content are positively influenced by egg consumption in an elderly population, *Nutr. Metab.*, 2006, **3**, 6.
21. D. M. DiMarco, G. H. Norris, C. Millar, C. N. Blesso and M. L. Fernandez, Intake of up to 3 eggs per day is associated with changes in HDL function and increased plasma antioxidants in healthy young adults, *J. Nutr.*, 2017, **147**, 323–339.
22. C. J. Andersen, C. N. Blesso, J. Lee, J. Barona, D. Shah, M. J. Thomas and M. L. Fernandez, Egg Consumption Modulates HDL Lipid Composition and Increases the Cholesterol-Accepting Capacity of Serum in Metabolic Syndrome, *Lipids*, 2013, **48**, 557–567.
23. C. N. Blesso, C. J. Andersen, B. W. Bolling and M. L. Fernandez, Egg intake improves carotenoid status by increasing plasma HDL cholesterol in adults with metabolic syndrome, *Food Funct.*, 2013, **4**, 213–221.
24. G. J. McKay, E. Loane, J. M. Nolan, C. C. Patterson, K. J. Meyers and J. A. Mares, *et al.* Investigation of genetic variation in scavenger receptor class B, member 1 (SCARB1) and association with serum carotenoids, *Ophthalmology*, 2013, **120**, 1632–1640.
25. W. E. Connor, P. B. Duell, R. Kean and Y. Wang, The prime role of HDL to transport lutein into the retina: evidence from HDL-deficient WHAM chicks having a mutant ABCA1 transporter, *Invest. Ophthalmol. Visual Sci.*, 2007, **48**, 4226–4231.
26. P. Fernandez-Robredo, J. A. Rodriguez, L. M. Sadaba, S. Recalde and A. Garcia-Layana, Egg yolk improves lipid profile, lipid peroxidation and retinal abnormalities in a murine model of genetic hypercholesterolemia, *J. Nutr. Biochem.*, 2008, **19**, 40–48.
27. J. E. Kim, R. M. Clark, Y. Park, J. Lee and M. L. Fernandez, Lutein decreases oxidative stress and inflammation in liver and eyes of guinea pigs fed a hypercholesterolemic diet, *Nutr. Res. Pract.*, 2012, **6**, 113–119.
28. J. E. Kim, J. O. Leite, R. DeOgburn, J. A. Smyth, R. M. Clark and M. L. Fernandez, A lutein-enriched diet prevents cholesterol accumulation and decreases oxidized LDL and inflammatory cytokines in the aorta of guinea pigs, *J. Nutr.*, 2011, **141**, 1458–1463.
29. R. Shanmugasundaram and R. K. Selvaraj, Dietary lutein and fish oil interact to alter atherosclerotic lesions in a Japanese quail model of atherosclerosis, *J. Anim. Physiol. Anim. Nutr.*, 2011, **95**, 762–770.
30. J. M. Serpeloni, I. M. Colus, F. S. de Oliveira, A. F. Aissa, A. Z. Mercadante, M. L. Bianchi and L. M. Antunes, Dietary carotenoid lutein modulates the expression of genes related to oxygen transporters and decreases DNA damage and oxidative stress in mice, *Food Chem. Toxicol.*, 2014, **70C**, 205–213.

31. P. V. Algvere, J. Marshall and S. Seregard, Age-related maculopathy and the impact of blue light hazard, *Acta Ophthalmol. Scand.*, 2006, **84**, 4–15.
32. S. Foran, J. J. Wang and P. Mitchell, Causes of visual impairment in two older population cross-sections: the Blue Mountains Eye Study, *Ophthalmic Epidemiol.*, 2003, **10**, 215–225.
33. L. Hyman, A. P. Schachat, Q. He and M. C. Leske, Hypertension, cardiovascular disease, and age-related macular degeneration. Age-Related Macular Degeneration Risk Factors Study Group, *Arch. Ophthalmol.*, 2000, **118**, 351–358.
34. S. C. Tomany, R. Klein, B. E. Klein and S. Beaver Dam Eye, The relationship between iris color, hair color, and skin sun sensitivity and the 10-year incidence of age-related maculopathy: the Beaver Dam Eye Study, *Ophthalmology*, 2003, **110**, 1526–1533.
35. J. M. Sedon, U. A. Ajani, R. D. Sperduto, N. Hitler and T. C. Blair, *et al.* Dietary carotenoids, vitamins A, C and E and advanced age-related macular degeneration. Eye Disease Case-Control Study Group, *JAMA*, 1994, **272**, 1413–1420.
36. P. Morganti, G. Fabrizi and C. Bruno, Protective effects of oral antioxidants on skin and eye function, *SKINmed*, 2004, **3**, 310–316.
37. S. M. Abdel-Aal el, H. Akhtar, K. Zaheer and R. Ali, Dietary sources of lutein and zeaxanthin carotenoids and their role in eye health, *Nutrients*, 2013, **5**, 1169–1185.
38. R. K. Murthy, K. Ravi, S. Balaiya, V. S. Brar and K. V. Chalam, Lutein protects retinal pigment epithelium from cytotoxic oxidative stress, *Cutaneous Ocul. Toxicol.*, 2014, **33**, 132–137.
39. R. Vishwanathan, E. F. Goodrow-Kotyla, B. R. Wooten, T. A. Wilson and R. J. Nicolosi, Consumption of 2 and 4 egg yolks/d for 5 wk increases macular pigment concentrations in older adults with low macular pigment taking cholesterol-lowering statins, *Am. J. Clin. Nutr.*, 2009, **90**, 1272–1279.
40. A. J. Wenzel, C. Gerweck, D. Barbato, R. J. Nicolosi, G. J. Handelman and J. Curran-Celentano, A 12-wk egg intervention increases serum zeaxanthin and macular pigment optical density in women, *J. Nutr.*, 2006, **136**, 2568–2573.
41. E. R. Kelly, J. Plat, G. R. Haenen, A. Kijlstra and T. T. Berendschot, The effect of modified eggs and an egg-yolk based beverage on serum lutein and zeaxanthin concentrations and macular pigment optical density: results from a randomized trial, *PLoS One*, 2014, **9**, e92659.
42. S. Sabour-Pickett, S. Beatty, E. Connolly, J. Loughman, J. Stack, A. Howard and R. Klein, *et al.* Supplementation with Three Different Macular Carotenoid Formulations in Patients with Early Age-Related Macular Degeneration, *Retina*, 2014, **34**, 1757–1766.
43. M. E. Aronow and E. Y. Chew, Age-related Eye Disease Study 2: perspectives, recommendations, and unanswered questions, *Curr. Opin. Ophtalmol.*, 2014, **25**, 186–190.

44. J. Wu, E. Cho, W. C. Willett, S. M. Sastry and D. A. Schaumberg, During 2 decades of prospective follow-up, *JAMA Ophthalmol.*, 2015, **133**, 1415–1424.
45. Q. Bian, S. Gao, J. Zhou, J. Qin, A. Taylor and E. J. Johnson, *et al.* Lutein and zeaxanthin supplementation reduces photooxidative damage and modulates the expression of inflammation-related genes in retinal pigment epithelial cells, *Free Radical Biol. Med.*, 2012, **53**, 1298–1307.
46. A. P. Firdouos, G. Kuttan and R. Kuttan, Anti-inflammatory potential of carotenoid meso-zeaxanthin and its mode of action, *Pharm. Biol.*, 2015, **53**, 961–967.
47. A. G. Murillo, D. Aguilar, G. H. Norris, D. M. DiMarco, A. Missimer, S. Hu, J. A. Smyth, S. Gannon, C. N. Blesso, Y. Luo and M. L. Fernandez, Compared to powdered lutein, a lutein nanoemulsion increases plasma and liver lutein, protects against hepatic steatosis and affects lipoprotein Metabolism in guinea pigs, *J. Nutr.*, 2016, **146**, 1961–1969.
48. J. H. Kim, H. J. Na, C. K. Kim, J. Y. Kim, K. S. Ha and H. Lee, *et al.* The non-provitamin a carotenoid, lutein, inhibits NF-κB-dependent gene expression through redox-based regulation of the phosphatidylinositol 3-kinase/pten/akt and nf-kappab-inducing kinase pathways: Role of H2O2 in NF-κB activation, *Free Radical Biol. Med.*, 2008, **45**, 885–896.
49. J. C. Ratliff, G. Mutungi, M. J. Puglisi, J. S. Volek and M. L. Fernandez, Eggs modulate the inflammatory response to carbohydrate restricted diets in overweight men, *Nutr. Metab.*, 2008, **5**, 6.
50. S. M. Grundy, Metabolic syndrome: a multiplex cardiovascular risk factor, *J. Clin. Endocrinol. Metab.*, 2007, **92**, 399–404.
51. K. Kontoangelos, C. C. Papageorgiuo, A. E. Raptis, P. Tsiotra, E. Boutati and V. Lambadiari, *et al.* Cytokines, diabetes mellitus and psychopathology: A challenging combination, *Neuroendocrinol. Lett.*, 2014, **35**, 159–169.
52. C. N. Blesso, Egg, phospholipids and cardiovascular health, *Nutrients*, 2015, **7**, 2731–2747.
53. T. C. Wallace and V. L. Fulgoni, 3rd. Assessment of total choline intakes in the United States, *J. Am. Coll. Nutr.*, 2016, **35**, 108–112.
54. S. H. Zeisel and K. A. da Costa, Choline: an essential nutrient for public health, *Nutr. Rev.*, 2009, **67**, 615–623.
55. J. Weihrauch and Y.-S. Son, The phospholipid content of foods, *J. Am. Oil Chem. Soc.*, 1983, **60**, 1971–1978.
56. J. S. Cohn, A. Kamili, E. Wat, R. W. Chung and S. Tandy, Dietary phospholipids and intestinal cholesterol absorption, *Nutrients*, 2010, **2**, 116–127.
57. S. H. Zeisel, A brief history of choline, *Ann. Nutr. Metab.*, 2012, **6**, 254–258.
58. G. M. Shaw, R. H. Finnell, H. J. Blom, S. L. Carmichael, S. E. Volset, W. Yang and P. M. Ueland, *Epidemiology*, 2009, **20**, 714–719.
59. R. J. Wurtman, A nutrient combination that can affect synapse formation, *Nutrients*, 2014, **6**, 1701–1710.

60. J. H. Ulus, R. J. Wurtman, C. Mauron and J. K. Bluztajn, Choline increases acetylcholine and protects against the stimulation-induced decrease in phosphatide levels within membranes of rat corpus striatum, *Brain Res.*, 1989, **484**, 217–227.
61. M. De Jesus Moreno Moreno, Cognitive improvement in mild to moderate Alzheimer's dementia after treatment with the acetylcholine precursor choline alfoscerate: a multicenter, double-blind, randomized, placebo-controlled trial, *Clin. Ther.*, 2003, **25**, 178–193.
62. Y. Jiang, S. K. Noh and S. I. Koo, Egg phosphatidylcholine decreases the lymphatic absorption of cholesterol in rats, *J. Nutr.*, 2001, **131**, 2358–2363.
63. D. Kullenger, L. A. Taylor, M. Schneider and U. Massing, Health effects of dietary phospholipids, *Lipids Health Dis.*, 2012, **11**, 3.
64. M. E. Rinella, M. S. Elias, R. R. Smolak, T. Fu, J. Borensztjan and R. M. Green, Mechanisms of hepatic steatosis in mice fed a lipogenic methionine choline-deficient diet, *J. Lipid Res.*, 2008, **49**, 1068–1076.
65. A. V. Khera, M. Cuchel, M. de la Llera-Moya, A. Rodrigues, M. F. Burke and K. Jafri, *et al.* Cholesterol efflux capacity, high-density lipoprotein function, and atherosclerosis, *N. Engl. J. Med.*, 2011, **364**, 127–135.
66. K. A. Da costa, C. E. Gaffney, L. M. Fisher and S. H. Zeisel, Choline deficiency in mice and humans is associated with increased plasma homocysteine concentration after a methionine load, *Am. J. Clin. Nutr.*, 2005, **8**, 440–444.
67. W. H. Tang, Z. Wang, B. S. Levison, R. A. Koeth, E. B. Britt, X. Fu, Y. Wu and S. L. Hazen, Intestinal microbial metabolism of phosphatidylcholine and cardiovascular risk, *N. Engl. J. Med.*, 2013, **368**, 1575–1584.
68. D. Fennema, I. R. Phillips and E. A. Shephard, Minireview Trimethylamine and Trimethylamine N -Oxide, a Flavin-Containing Axis Implicated in Health and Disease, *Drug Metab. Dispos.*, 2016, 70615.
69. K. A. Romano, E. I. Vivas, D. Amador-noguez and F. E. Rey, Intestinal Microbiota Composition Modulates Choline Bioavailability, *mBio*, 2015, **6**, 1–8.
70. J. M. Brown and S. L. Hazen, Meta-Organismal Nutrient Metabolism as a Basis of Cardiovascular Disease, *Curr. Opin. Lipidol.*, 2015, **25**, 48–53.
71. C. A. Miller, K. D. Corbin, K. Costa, S. Zhang, X. Zhao, J. A. Galanko, T. Blevins, B. J. Bennett, A. O. Connor and S. H. Zeisel, Effect of egg ingestion on trimethylamine- *N*-oxide production in humans: a randomized, controlled, dose-response study, *Am. J. Clin. Nutr.*, 2014, **100**, 778–786.
72. W. H. W. Tang and S. L. Hazen, The contributory role of gut microbiota in cardiovascular disease, *J. Clin. Invest.*, 2014, **124**, 4204–4211.
73. M. Warrier, D. M. Shih, R. E. Temel, J. M. Brown, M. Warrier and D. M. Shih, *et al.* The TMAO-Generating Enzyme Flavin Monooxygenase 3 Is a Central Regulator of Report The TMAO-Generating Enzyme Flavin Monooxygenase 3 Is a Central Regulator of Cholesterol Balance, *Cell Rep.*, 2015, **10**, 326–338.

74. Z. Wang, E. Klipfell, B. J. Bennett, R. Koeth, S. Bruce and B. Dugar, *et al.* Gut flora metabolism of phosphatidylcholine promotes cardiovascular disease, *Nature*, 2011, **472**, 57–63.
75. B. S. Lemos, I. Medina-Vera, O. V. Malysheva, M. A. Caudil and M. L. Fernandez, Effect of egg consumption and choline supplementation on plasma choline and trimethylamine-*N*-oxide in a young population, *J. Am. Coll. Nutr.*, 2018, **37**, 716–723.
76. M. Ufnal, A. Zadlo and R. Ostaszewski, TMAO: A small molecule of great expectations, *Nutrition*, 2015, **31**, 1317–1323.
77. D. M. DiMarco, A. Missimer, A. G. Murillo, B. Lemos, C. N. Blesso and M. L. Fernandez, Intake of up to 3 eggs per day increases HDL cholesterol and plasma choline while plasma trimethylamine-N-Oxide is unchanged in a healthy population, *Lipids*, 2017, **52**, 255–263.
78. A. Missimer, M. L. Fernandez, D. M. DiMarco, G. H. Norris and C. N. Blesso, *et al.* Compared to an oatmeal breakfast, two eggs/day increased plasma carotenoids and choline without increasing trimethyl amine-oxide concentrations, *J. Am. Coll. Nutr.*, 2018, **37**, 140–148.
79. J. Kovacs-Nolan and Y. Mine, Egg yolk antibodies for passive immunity, *Annu. Rev. Food Sci. Technol.*, 2012, **3**, 163–182.
80. R. R. Wolfe, The underappreciated role of muscle in health and disease, *Am. J. Clin. Nutr.*, 2006, **84**, 475–482.
81. A. Smith and J. Gray, Considering the benefit of egg consumption for older people at risk of sarcopenia, *Br. J. Community Nurs.*, 2016, **21**, 305–309.
82. K. Mayurasakorn, P. Siphauli and P. O. Hongto, Supplement of three eggs a week improves protein malnutrition in Thai children from rural areas, *J. Med. Assoc. Thailand*, 2010, **93**, 301–309.
83. C. J. Rebello, A. G. Liu, F. L. Greenway and N. V. Dhurandhar, 2013. Dietary strategies to increase satiety, *Adv. Food Nutr. Res.*, 2013, **69**, 105–182.
84. D. Paddon-Jones, M. Sheffield-Moore, R. J. Urban, A. P. Sanford, A. Aarsland, R. R. Wolfe and A. Ferrando, AEssential amino acid and carbohydrate supplementation ameliorates muscle protein loss in humans during 28 days bedrest, *J. Clin. Endocrinol. Metab.*, 2004, **89**, 4351–4358.
85. J. R. Hoffman and M. J. Falvo, Protein - Which is Best?, *J. Sports Sci. Med.*, 2004, **3**, 118–130.
86. M. K. Jinadu, E. O. Ojofeitimi and E. O. Sifor, Feeding patterns of children with protein-energy malnutrition in Nigeria, *Trop. Doct.*, 1986, **16**, 82–85.
87. J. Sullivan, M. Ndekha, D. Maker, C. Hotz and M. J. Manary, The quality of the diet in Malawian children with kwashiorkor and marasmus, *Matern Child Nutr.*, 2006, **2**, 114–122.
88. J. Cao, X. Wei, X. Tang, H. Jiang, Z. Fan, Q. Yu, J. Chen, Y. Liu and T. Li, Effects of egg and Vitamin A supplementation on hemoglobin, retinol status and physical growth of primary and middle school students in Chongqing, China, *Asia Pac. J. Clin. Nutr.*, 2013, **22**, 214–221.

89. D. R. Moore, M. J. Robinson, J. L. Fry, J. E. Tang, E. I. Glover, S. B. Wilkinson, T. Prior, M. A. Tarnopolsky and S. M. Phillips, Ingested protein dose response of muscle and albumin protein synthesis after resistance exercise in young men, *Am. J. Clin. Nutr.*, 2009, **89**, 161–168.
90. L. Breen and S. M. Phillips, Skeletal muscle protein metabolism in the elderly: Interventions to counteract the 'anabolic resistance' of ageing, *Nutr. Metab.*, 2011, **8**, 68.
91. M. Teland, L. de Groot and L. van Loon, Recent Research: egg shite supplementation during longterm resistance training increases muscle mass in the frail elderly, *Tijdschr. Gerontol. Geriatr.*, 2013, **44**, 90–91.
92. H. B. Iglay, J. E. Apoizan, D. E. Gerrard, J. K. Eash, J. C. Anderson and W. W. Campbell, Moderately increased protein intake predominantly from egg sources does not influence whole body, regional, or muscle composition responses to resistance training in older people, *J. Nutr., Health Aging*, 2009, **13**, 108–114.
93. H. R. Ibrahim, T. Aoki and A. Pellegrini, Strategies for new antimicrobial proteins and peptides: lysozyme and aprotinin as model molecules, *Curr. Pharm. Des.*, 2002, **8**, 671–693.
94. F. Giansanti, L. Leboffe, G. Pitari, R. Ippoliti and G. Antonini, Physiological roles of ovotransferrin, *Biochim. Biophys. Acta*, 2012, **1820**, 218–225.
95. J. G. Banks, R. G. Board and N. H. Sparks, Natural antimicrobial systems and their potential in food preservation of the future, *Biotechnol. Appl. Biochem.*, 1986, **8**, 103–147.
96. Q. Wang, X. J. Hou, K. Cai, T. Li, Y. N. Liu, W. Tu, L. Xiao, S. Z. Bao, J. Shi, X. Gao, H. Liu, R. M. Tian and H. Wang, Passive protection of purified yolk immunoglobulin administered against Shiga toxin 1 in mouse models, *Can. J. Microbiol.*, 2010, **56**, 1003–1010.
97. R. D. LeClaire, R. E. Hunt and S. Bavari, Protection against bacterial superantigen staphylococcal enterotoxin B by passive vaccination, *Infect. Immun.*, 2002, **70**, 2278–2281.
98. D. Brady, S. Gaines and J. Fenelon, A Lipoprotein-derived Antimicrobial Factor from Hen-egg Yolk is Active Against Streptococcus Species, *J. Food Sci.*, 2002, **67**, 3096–3103.
99. H. Fujita, R. Sasaki and M. Yoshikawa, Potentiation of the antihypertensive activity of orally administered ovokinin, a vasorelaxing peptide derived from ovalbumin, by emulsification in egg phosphatidylcholine, *Biosci., Biotechnol., Biochem.*, 1995, **59**, 2344–2345.
100. S. Das, S. Banerjee and J. D. Gupta, Experimental evaluation of preventive and therapeutic potentials of lysozyme, *Chemotherapy*, 1992, **38**, 350–357.
101. G. Sava, A. Benetti, V. Ceschia and S. Pacor, Lysozyme and cancer: role of exogenous lysozyme as anticancer agent (review), *Anticancer Res.*, 1989, **9**, 583–591.
102. Y. Wang, M. A. Beydoun, L. Liang, B. Caballero and S. K. Kumanyika, Will all Americans become overweight or obese? estimating the progression and cost of the US obesity epidemic, *Obesity*, 2008, **16**, 2323–2330.

103. S. H. Holt, J. C. Miller, P. Petocz and E. Farmakalidis, A satiety index of common foods, *Eur. J. Clin. Nutr.*, 1995, **49**, 675–690.
104. D. E. Cummings, J. Q. Purnell, R. S. Frayo, K. Schmidova, B. E. Wisse and D. S. Weigle, A preprandial rise in plasma ghrelin levels suggests a role in meal initiation in humans, *Diabetes*, 2001, **50**, 1714–1719.
105. K. E. Foster-Schubert, J. Overduin, C. E. Prudom, J. Liu, H. S. Callahan, B. D. Gaylinn, M. O. Thorner and D. E. Cummings, Acyl and total ghrelin are suppressed strongly by ingested proteins, weakly by lipids, and biphasically by carbohydrates, *J. Clin. Endocrinol. Metab.*, 2008, **93**, 1971–1979.
106. J. S. Vander Wal, J. S. Vander Wal, J. M. Marth, P. Khosla, K. L. Jen and N. V. Dhurandhar, Short-term effect of eggs on satiety in overweight and obese subjects, *J. Am. Coll. Nutr.*, 2005, **24**, 510–515.
107. J. M. Rueda and P. Khosla, Impact of breakfasts (with or without Eggs) on body weight regulation and blood lipids in university students over a 14-week semester, *Nutrients*, 2013, **5**, 5097–5113.

CHAPTER 3

Egg Consumption for Appetite Control and Body Weight Regulation

MYOUNGJIN SON[a], XIAOFENG WANG[a] AND JIANPING WU*[a,b]

[a]Department of Agricultural, Food and Nutritional Science, 4-10 Agriculture/Forestry Centre, University of Alberta, Edmonton, Alberta, T6G 2P5, Canada; [b]Cardiovascular Research Centre, University of Alberta, Edmonton, AB, Canada
*E-mail: jwu3@ualberta.ca

3.1 Introduction

The prevalence of obesity is dramatically increasing worldwide. Obesity results in a number of adverse health conditions, including hypertension, type 2 diabetes, coronary heart disease, and osteoarthritis.[1–4] In addition, obesity is associated with negative social and psychological consequences, such as discrimination and depression.[5,6] In addition to genetics, excessive calorie intake and inactive lifestyle are the major contributing factors. One major approach to cope with obesity is to decrease energy intake; thus, dietary interventions that modulate satiety and food consumption may offer positive approaches for reducing energy intake.[7] Therefore, understanding factors affecting appetite, satiety, and food selection is critically important to develop more effective strategies for obesity management.

Food Chemistry, Function and Analysis No.14
Eggs as Functional Foods and Nutraceuticals for Human Health
Edited by Jianping Wu

Published by the Royal Society of Chemistry, www.rsc.org

One promising food that can be incorporated into the diet to achieve this goal is eggs. Eggs are affordable and provide high-quality protein and other valuable nutrients. Whole eggs also contain antioxidants, such as lutein and choline, which protect against various inflammatory processes.[8] Additionally, including egg in the diet is reported to enhance satiety and reduce energy intake.[82] Thus, eggs might represent an ideal food to be included as part of dietary interventions designed to reduce obesity. The aim of this chapter is to review existing evidence on the effects of egg consumption on appetite regulation, body weight, and body composition. The second aim of this chapter is to elucidate the potential mechanism underlying the regulatory effect of egg on appetite.

3.2 Appetite Regulation

The control of energy intake is vital to maintain energy balance.[9] Satiety is the feeling of fullness and the suppression of hunger for a period of time after a meal.[10] Satiety plays a key role in controlling the amount of energy consumed at each of these eating occasions. Furthermore, it affects the period of time between eating and potentially how much we eat in the next meal. Thus, it is important to consider the impact of satiety on energy balance and whether it can be enhanced in order to facilitate the reduction of energy intake and weight control. An ideal weight loss strategy would promote satiety and maintain basal metabolic rates despite a negative energy balance and reduction in fat-mass.

3.2.1 Gut–Brain Axis and Appetite

Our understanding of the importance of the gut–brain axis for appetite regulation has improved considerably over the last few decades. It is becoming increasingly evident that direct signaling between the gastrointestinal (GI) tract and the brain regulates appetite.[11] Various sensors in the gut respond to mechanical stimuli (contraction and distention), chemicals, including nutrients in the gut lumen, hormonal stimuli, such as gut hormones, neurotransmitters, as well as cytokines and inflammatory mediators produced by microbes in the gut.[12] These homeostatic signals arise from the gut sensors and are transmitted to the central nervous system (CNS) through vagal nerves and regulate hunger or satiety. Thus, understanding these signals and augmenting them pharmacologically may provide an important strategy to treat obesity.

3.2.1.1 Central Nervous System

3.2.1.1.1 Hypothalamus. The hypothalamus plays a predominant role in the control of the central appetite system.[13] The nutrients from food and hormonal signals are integrated in the hypothalamus, generating communications between the hypothalamus and the other organs, such as the gut, pancreas, adipose tissue and liver. In response to peripheral signals from organs, the hypothalamus modulates appetite and food memory *via* the corticolimbic system, which ultimately influences gastric motility and hormone secretion to maintain energy homeostasis.

Within the hypothalamus, the arcuate nucleus (ARC), known as the infundibular nucleus in humans, is one of the main nuclei regulating appetite.[13] The ARC expresses the receptors for many of the hormones and neuropeptides that are known to regulate food intake. Moreover, the ARC communicates with other hypothalamic nuclei involved in appetite control, such as the paraventricular nucleus, the dorsomedial nucleus, the lateral hypothalamus, and the ventromedial nucleus.[14]

3.2.1.1.2 The Brainstem. Recently, the importance of the brainstem, which is located outside of the hypothalamus as a secondary homeostatic integrator in appetite control, has been demonstrated.[15] The dosal vagal complex in the brainstem mediates communication between the peripheral tissues and the hypothalamus in regard to food intake regulation. Thus, nutrients and hormonal signals from the gastrointestinal tract are sensed in the brainstem, and further delivered to the hypothalamus.[16] Consequently, the hypothalamus generates an efferent signal modulating appetite and gastrointestinal function.[17]

3.2.1.1.3 Corticolimbic System. Food intake is also influenced by non-homeostatic factors from the environment, such as pleasure, reward, and food experience. Recent studies suggest that homeostatic appetite control system in the hypothalamus is modulated by non-homeostatic factors from the corticolimbic system, indicating the importance of the connection between the hypothalamus and the corticolimbic system.[18] Interestingly, recent data indicates that the non-homeostatic system is also affected by gut hormones, which suggests the possibility that altering the homeostatic signaling, such as from gut hormones, may be effective for modulating the motivation to consume foods.[19]

3.2.1.2 Adiposity Signal that Modulates Appetite Behavior

The leptin in adipose tissue has been well demonstrated to influence appetite.[20] Leptin is primarily produced in adipose tissue and its level in circulation is directly proportional to whole body adiposity.[21] The binding of leptin to its receptor in the hypothalamus, LepR, controls food intake as well as various metabolic activities, including thermogenesis.[22] Central and peripheral administration of leptin in rodents results in a profound decrease in food intake and thus weight loss.[23] In obesity, the circulating leptin level is increased with impaired hypothalamic leptin signaling. The resistance to leptin signaling may contribute to the increased food intake, resulting in impaired homeostatic feedback for weight gain and hunger.[24] Thus, leptin treatment appears to have a limited benefit in treating obesity.

3.2.1.3 Gut Hormones in the Control of Appetite Behavior

There are a number of gut hormones that have been identified as regulating appetite in the gastrointestinal system (Table 3.1). Some of the key hormones and their role in food intake are reviewed in the following sections.

3.2.1.3.1 Cholecystokinin (CCK). CCK is the first gut hormone found to have a role in appetite control.[25] CCK is secreted from the endocrine cells of the small intestine in response to food consumption. It binds to its receptor, CCK_A, on vagal afferent neurons and consequently reduces food intake.[26] Although acute administration of CCK has been shown to inhibit food consumption in animal and human studies,[27,28] prolonged treatment with CCK was reported to induce tolerances in either total food consumption or body weight.[29,30] However, CCK may play a role in long-term energy regulation by synergistically interacting with leptin. Significant reduction in daily calorie intake was detected after the administration of leptin and CCK together over 24 hours compared to leptin alone.[31]

3.2.1.3.2 Ghrelin. Ghrelin is famously known as the "hunger hormone" that stimulates food intake by acting on the growth hormone secretagogue receptor on afferent and hypothalamic neurons.[32] It is secreted by the stomach in fasted condition, explaining that it transmits a hunger signal

Table 3.1 Major appetite-regulating GI hormones.

Hormone/signaling molecule	Location	Effect on appetite	Mechanism
Amylin[45]	Pancreas	Satiety	Not known
Apolipoprotein A-IV (Apo-A-IV)[46]	Jejunum	Satiety	Indirect activation of the vagus nerve *via* CCK
CCK[47]	Duodenum and jejunum	Satiety	Direct activation of the vagus nerve
Ghrelin[48]	Stomach	Hunger	*Via* ghrelin receptors in the brain
GLP-1[49]	Ileum and colon	Satiety	*Via* GLP-1 receptor in the brain
Leptin[50]	Stomach	Satiety	*Via* leptin receptor in the brain
Oxyntomodulin[51]	Ileum and colon	Satiety	Not known
Pancreatic polypeptide[52]	Pancreas	Satiety	*Via* Y5 receptors in the brain
Peptide tyrosine tyrosine (PYY)[53]	Ileum and colon	Satiety	Direct activation of vagus nerve

to the CNS. In addition, ghrelin stimulates the release of growth hormone and is the only circulatory hormone known to potently enhance feeding and weight gain.[33] Therapeutic administration of ghrelin may induce food intake, gastric emptying, nutrient storage, and fat deposition.[34] These actions of ghrelin suggest that it may have a therapeutic value in treating malnutrition during acute and chronic disorders. In contrast, the inhibition of ghrelin may be a useful strategy for the prevention of obesity and metabolic syndrome. The discovery of ghrelin *O*-acyltransferase, an enzyme that enables the binding of ghrelin to the growth hormone secretagogue receptor, has provided a new opportunity to utilize ghrelin.[35] In particular, targeting the inhibition of ghrelin *O*-acyltransferase has been researched as an anti-obesity strategy.

3.2.1.3.3 Glucagon-like Peptide-1(GLP-1). GLP-1 is derived from the proglucagon gene,[36] which is expressed in the α-cells of the pancreas, the L-cells of the intestine, and neurons located in the caudal brainstem and hypothalamus.[37] GLP-1 is primarily synthesized and secreted by the mucosal endocrine L-cells of the small intestine in response to an oral nutrient load.[38] The action of GLP-1 is *via* GLP-1 receptors in the ARC, paraventricular nucleus and optic nuclei of the hypothalamus, and the area postrema of the brainstem and vagus.[39] GLP-1 potentiates glucose disposal by stimulating insulin secretion, which accounts for at least 50% of the total postprandial insulin release.[40] Besides its insulinotropic action, GLP-1 inhibits glucagon secretion in a glucose-dependent manner, diminishing post-prandial glucose rise.[41] In addition, GLP-1 suppresses gastrointestinal motility, appetite, and food intake.[42,43] A recent meta-analysis provides various evidence showing that GLP-1 receptor agonists are effective for weight loss in obese patients.[44] In addition, this report also highlighted that GLP-1 receptor agonists were beneficial to blood pressure and circulating cholesterol concentration.

3.2.2 Current Treatments for Appetite

Although a number of potential targets modulating appetite and energy expenditure have been identified, developing a safe and effective drug for weight loss remains a big challenge. It is not surprising that altering appetite signaling by a neurotransmitter may result in unwanted side effects. For example, rimonabant, a selective CB1 receptor antagonist, was withdrawn from the European market in 2009 after resulting in psychiatric adverse effects such as depression and suicide.[54] Another example is sibutramine, a serotonin and noradrenalin reuptake inhibitor, which was licensed for the treatment of obesity in 1997. However, increased blood pressure and serious cardiovascular side effects, such as stroke and myocardial infarction, led to the withdrawal of this drug from both European and US markets.[55] These examples illustrate the potential of adverse events from anti-obesity drugs modulating neurotransmission and appetite. Numerous studies have suggested the efficacy of using a high-protein diet as an alternative method of controlling appetite and weight.[56] Thus, dietary food protein might be a promising tool for the treatment of obesity without adverse effects.

3.3 Protein Diet and Satiety

Different foods and food constituents are known to affect satiation, with protein being the most satiety-inducing macronutrient. It is well established that protein is more satiating than the isoenergetic ingestion of carbohydrate or fat.[57–59] In a study that investigated the satiating properties of different lunches that contained the same amount of calories but different compositions of protein and carbohydrates, people who consumed the carbohydrate-dominant lunch ingested more calories than the high-protein lunch group. Significantly higher pre-dinner hunger and eating desire were reported in the high-carbohydrate lunch group.[60] With respect to the difference between protein and fat in terms of the feeling of satiety, it was reported that the consumption of high-protein yogurt as an afternoon snack led to greater reductions in afternoon hunger compared to isoenergetic ingestion of high-fat chocolate in young healthy women (< 30 years old). The yogurt snack also led to delayed eating initiation and lower dinner calorie consumption than the high-fat chocolate and high-fat cracker snacks.[61]

High-protein foods are believed to exert a higher effect on both inter-meal satiation and post-ingestive satiety than low-protein foods.[62,63] A strawberry yogurt with added whey-protein consumed in the meal was shown to have a greater hunger-decreasing effect than a regular strawberry yogurt.[62] In addition, whey was shown to have a greater hunger-decreasing effect than casein and soy protein when protein accounts for 10% of total calories, while the difference was gone when 25% of calories were from protein.[64] However, there is also evidence showing that casein and pea protein resulted in stronger feelings of satiety compared to whey when consumed 30 min before the meal, which was abolished when consuming the protein as a starter to a meal,[65] suggesting the time of consumption is also critical for the satiating properties of protein. Some studies showed that vegetable protein (fava beans/split peas) and animal protein (veal, pork or eggs) have similar effects on satiety sensation when the meals are isocaloric, macronutrient-balanced, and fiber-matched.[66]

The mechanisms of protein's satiating power are largely unknown. However, current evidence suggests that the potential mechanisms may include: (1) Altering the production and secretion of satiety-modulating gastrointestinal hormones. Protein-induced satiety seems to be associated with a higher increase in the production and secretion of anorexigenic hormones along with a greater decrease in orexigenic hormones. In a study that involved 15 healthy men, a high-protein breakfast produced greater satiety than a high-carbohydrate breakfast, which was accompanied by a lower postprandial blood ghrelin concentration than the high-carbohydrate breakfast.[11] Ghrelin is an appetite-increasing hormone that is produced and released mainly by the stomach with small amounts released by the small intestine, pancreas and brain.[68] Furthermore, the high-protein breakfast increased the secretion of CCK and GLP-1,[67] which are both hormones produced in the gastrointestinal tract and function to reduce gastric emptying.[69] (2) Enhancing energy expenditure. A high-protein diet is connected to higher diet-induced thermogenesis, thus promoting energy expenditure. Higher thermogenesis may increase oxygen consumption and body temperature, which may result in a greater feeling of oxygen depletion and satiety.[70,71] (3) Stimulating gluconeogenesis. A high-protein diet was shown to promote hepatic gluconeogenesis in rats,[72] which may contribute to enhancing the satiety signal to the brain through the vagal nerve.[73,74] (4) Inducing higher blood concentration of amino acids. The correlation between higher blood amino acid concentration and satiety has long been established in the 1950s.[75] It has been shown that amino acids such as Arg, Lys, and Ala can be detected by hypothalamic tanycytes, which are glial cells lining the wall of the third ventricle and bridging the cerebrospinal fluid to the portal capillaries.[76] In addition, some dietary amino acids, such as glutamate, may function as neural transmitters modulating satiety through the glutamatergic arcuate nucleus–paraventricular hypothalamus circuit.[77]

3.4 High-egg-protein Diet and Satiety

3.4.1 Effect of High-egg-protein Diet on Appetite Control

Egg protein is considered to be complete or high quality because it contains all nine essential amino acids.[78] In several studies, when compared to other protein-containing food, an egg-based meal was shown to increase satiety and decrease energy intake using a visual analogue scale (VAS) and *ad libitum* energy intake, which is typically accompanied by altered postprandial GI hormone responses.[79,80]

Evidence showed that egg has more satiating power than carbohydrate with equal calories (Table 3.2). Thirty obese women were recruited to participate in a randomized crossover study to investigate the difference in satiety for an isocaloric equal-weight bagel-based breakfast and an egg breakfast. The results showed that the egg breakfast induced greater satiety and significantly reduced energy intake for up to 36 hours.[81] In a study that involved 156 obese Chinese adolescents (14–17 years), the subjects received one of two isoenergetic breakfasts, either with egg or steamed bread. The food intake at lunch was lower while satiety was higher with the egg breakfast group, which was associated with increased serum concentrations of two anorexigenic hormones, peptide YY (PYY) and GLP-1.[82] In a long-term study with 50 healthy young subjects, eating two eggs for breakfast for 4 weeks was reported to increase satiety compared to oatmeal breakfast, which was accompanied by a lower plasma orexigenic hormone ghrelin concentration.[83] However, there was also a report showing that isocaloric

Table 3.2 Comparison of the satiating properties of egg *versus* other protein sources.

Meals	Subjects	Time of consumption	Study Design	Satiety determination	Results
Meat/fiber, bean/pea, egg/fiber, egg[66]	35 men (18–50 years, BMI: 18.5–30 kg m^{-2})	Breakfast	Crossover	VAS	There was no difference between meals in hunger, satiety, fullness, prospective food consumption and composite appetite score.
Egg, cereal, croissant[79]	30 men (20–23 years; BMI: 20.4–25.8 kg m^{-2})	Breakfast	Crossover	VAS	Participants consuming egg-based meal had increased satiety, less hunger, and lower energy intake in the subsequent meals.
Egg or bagel[81]	30 women (25–60 years, BMI: 25–35 kg m^{-2})	Breakfast	Crossover	Fullness questionnaire	Egg-based breakfast resulted in a greater feeling of satiety before lunch and significantly less energy in lunch.
Egg or steamed bread[82]	156 obese adolescents (14–17 years)	Breakfast	Randomized	VAS	1. Subjects on the egg-based breakfast had a lower lunchtime food intake and higher satiety. 2. Egg-based breakfast led to increased serum PYY and GLP-1.
Two eggs per day or one packet of oatmeal per day[83]	26 women and 24 men (age of 18–30 years; BMI: 18.5–29.9 kg m^{-2})	First meal of the day	Randomized, crossover	VAS	Higher satiety and lower plasma ghrelin concentration in subjects consuming egg.

(continued)

Table 3.2 (*continued*)

Meals	Subjects	Time of consumption	Study Design	Satiety determination	Results
Egg or bagel[84]	13 children (6 males and 7 females, 4–6 years) and 15 adolescents (6 males and 9 females, 14–17 years)	Breakfast	Randomized, crossover	VAS	1. Lunchtime food intake and satiety were not different between the two meals. 2. Egg breakfast resulted in a higher serum PYY level in adolescents.
Egg albumin, casein, gelatin, soy protein, pea protein, and wheat gluten[86]	12 men (22–23 years, BMI: 21.4–22.4 kg m^{-2})	Lunch	Crossover	VAS	All meals had no effect on satiety.
Whey, soy protein, or egg albumen containing beverages[87]	13 men (19–28 years, BMI: 21.4–22.4 kg m^{-2})	1 h before a pizza meal	Repeated measures design	N/A	1. Whey and soy protein, but not egg albumen, suppressed subsequent food intake. 2. Meal energy intake was higher when egg albumen and soy were preloaded in the late morning (11:00 am) than earlier (08:30–09:10 am).
Preload containing 20 g of casein, whey, pea protein, egg albumin or maltodextrin[88]	32 men (25 ± 4 years, BMI: 24 ± 0.4 kg m^{-2})	Breakfast	Randomized, single-blind, crossover	VAS	Although albumin load increased the feeling of satiety, the effect of casein or pea protein on satiety was higher than that of albumin.

egg and bagel breakfasts had comparable impacts on satiety and lunchtime food intake in both children (age 4–6 years) and adolescents, although the serum PYY level was significantly higher in adolescents consuming an egg breakfast than adolescents who took the bagel breakfasts.[84] The inconsistency may be caused by a number of reasons, including: (1) the relatively small sample size in this study, which included 25 children and 16 adolescents; (2) the lack of ability to self-regulate food intake in children; (3) less sensitivity of children to alterations in appetite hormone levels compared to adults.[85] Thus, these results indicate that egg may influence satiety differently in people in different age groups.

Research on the differences between the satiating properties of egg and other sources of protein is limited and contradictory so far. Isocaloric meals based on egg, meat, and fava beans/split peas produced similar satiety in an acute study that involved 35 healthy men.[66] Similarly, in another study, six protein meals containing egg albumin, casein, gelatin, soy protein, pea protein, and wheat gluten were shown to have comparable satiating effects in 12 healthy young subjects.[86] However, casein and pea protein were shown to have a stronger effect on satiety compared to egg albumin when they were consumed 30 min before the meal. The effect was gone when a different protein was ingested as a starter of the meal.[65] In a study conducted in healthy young men, subjects were provided whey, soy protein, or egg albumen in sweet and flavored beverages as a preload followed by a pizza meal 1 h later. The results showed that the whey and soy protein preloads resulted in higher satiety than egg albumen.[87]

Likewise, the effect of albumin on food intake was compared to other proteins (casein, whey, pea protein) in 32 healthy male volunteers. Subjective appetite was assessed using a VAS at 10 min intervals after the protein preload. Although the feelings of satiety were significantly higher after the albumin preload in comparison with maltodextrin or water, casein and pea protein showed stronger effects compared to albumin.[88] Although egg albumin suppresses food intake and leads to activation of cholecystokinin-A (CCKA) receptors,[89] egg albumin, in contrast to whole egg or egg yolk, does not raise the blood concentration of CCK in humans.[90] Thus, satiety hormones might appear to be stimulated less by egg albumin compared to whole egg or other egg white protein.

3.4.2 Effect of High-egg-protein Diet on the Regulation of Body Weight and Body Composition

The effects of a high-protein diet and the protein source of the diet on regulation of body weight and body composition are well investigated.[91–94] High-protein diets have been a key component of most weight loss programs. Diets high in protein reduce dietary intake as well as calorie intake while supporting lean body mass by increasing protein synthesis. The mechanism of this regulatory effect of high-protein diets includes their thermogenic effect, inhibition of food intake as well as promotion of protein synthesis.

However, only a few studies have investigated the effects of egg diets or egg protein on body weight. In an animal model, treatment with egg white protein or egg white protein hydrolysates for 8 weeks resulted in inhibited food intake, body weight gain and fat accumulation in the liver and adipose tissue, while muscle weight was increased. In addition, dietary egg white protein and its hydrolysates decreased stearoyl-CoA desaturase and glucose-6-phosphate dehydrogenase activity in the liver and gastrocnemius muscle, indicating its modulatory effect on fat synthesis in the liver and muscle.[95] Another animal study conducted by Saande *et al.* also showed consistent results in reducing weight gain.[96] Body weight gain and body fat were significantly reduced by whole egg consumption compared to a casein-based diet in Zucker diabetic fatty rats.

In a human study, overweight or obese participants were assigned to either an egg breakfast containing two eggs (340 kcal) or a breakfast containing bagels matched for energy density. After 8 weeks, in comparison to the bagel diet group, the egg breakfast group showed a greater reduction in BMI, body weight, and waist circumference.[97] In another recent human study, a total of 140 participants were randomly assigned to two groups and both groups were matched for protein intake. The high egg group was instructed to eat two eggs per day at breakfast for 6 days per week for 3 months. As a result, the high egg group reported less hunger and greater satiety post-breakfast. However, there were no significant differences in weight change over the 3 month period between groups. Furthermore, no between-group differences were detected for total cholesterol, low-density lipoprotein cholesterol, triglycerides, and glucose in blood.[98]

By contrast, a recent health examinee study using Korean adults (aged 40–69, a total of 130 420 subjects; 43 682 men and 86 738 women) showed that consumption of more than seven eggs per week was associated with lower metabolic syndrome risk compared to those who consumed less than one egg per week in women.[99] Higher egg consumption was inversely associated with the metabolic syndrome risk factors, including waist circumference, blood triglyceride, and high-density lipoprotein cholesterol.

Until now, the associations between egg consumption and body weight/composition changes are still controversial. Further research is warranted to establish the role of eggs in regulating body composition using a longitudinal study with a more precise diet-assessment method.

3.5 Conclusion and Future Research

This chapter provides a literature review on the beneficial properties of eggs for appetite control and weight management. The current evidence was mostly obtained from human studies. Although contradictions exist, the literature suggests that eggs might have promising satiating properties, which seems to be dependent on the time of consumption and age of the subjects. However, further research is needed to understand the effects of long-term consumption and the comparison of egg protein with other types of proteins. In addition, a more precise diet-assessment method is needed. In a comparison study with a meal including six different protein sources, Lang *et al.* suggested that including a protein source in a meal mixed with carbohydrate and fat in a study to assess the food behavior of protein is not appropriate because the carbohydrate and fat might buffer the physiological mechanisms implicated in postprandial satiety after protein consumption.[86]

Moreover, a more accurate index for assessing obesity should be used in the future research. Most of the previous research used BMI as an indication of obesity. The calculation of the BMI scale is based on height and weight alone; however, it does not take into account differences in bone, muscle, and fat. For example, muscle is heavier than fat tissue. Thus, alternative methods, such as dual energy X-ray absorptiometry and imaging techniques for detecting fat distribution, should be selected to demonstrate the effects of egg protein on body composition and obesity.

In addition, the mechanism related to appetite control still largely remains to be elucidated, which may require further *in vivo* studies in animals and *in vitro* experiments. The model suggested in this chapter is based mainly on gut–brain signaling and energy homeostasis. The recent alternative model involving gut microbiota and host communication might suggest the direction of future research. The role of gut microbiota in the regulation of health and disease is increasingly becoming recognized.[100] Mechanisms in which the gut microbiota influence the host's appetite and metabolism are being investigated at a rapid rate, providing the potential for targeting the gut microbiota as an effective therapeutic option for obesity and appetite control.[101,102] It has been reported that the diet plays a fundamental role in microbiome profiles and function.[103] As such, further research regarding egg protein and gut microbiota with respect to appetite control would be helpful to address the mechanism.

References

1. C. D. Brown, M. Higgins, K. A. Donato, F. C. Rohde, R. Garrison, E. Obarzanek, N. D. Ernst and M. Horan, Body mass index and the prevalence of hypertension and dyslipidemia, *Obes. Res.*, 2000, **8e**, 605–619.
2. D. P. Guh, W. Zhang, N. Bansback, Z. Amarsi, C. L. Birmingham and A. H. Anis, The incidence of co-morbidities related to obesity and overweight: A systematic review and meta-analysis, *BMC Public Health*, 2009, **9**, 88.
3. S. Lamon-Fava, P. W. Wilson and E. J. Schaefer, Impact of body mass index on coronary heart disease risk factors in men and women, The Framingham Offspring Study, *Arterioscler., Thromb., Vasc. Biol.*, 1996, **16**, 1509–1515.

4. P. Wilson, R. D'Agostino, L. Sullivan, H. Parise and W. Kannel, Overweight and obesity as determinants of cardiovascular risk: the Framingham experience, *Arch. Intern. Med.*, 2002, **162**, 1867–1872.
5. R. L. Kolotkin, K. Meter and G. R. Williams, Quality of life and obesity, *Obes. Rev.*, 2001, **2**, 219–229.
6. R. Puhl and K. D. Brownell, Bias, discrimination, and obesity, *Obes. Res.*, 2001, **9**, 788–805.
7. T. Amin and J. G. Mercer, Hunger and Satiety Mechanisms and Their Potential Exploitation in the Regulation of Food Intake, *Curr. Obes. Rep.*, 2016, **5**(1), 106–112.
8. C. Nimalaratne and J. Wu, Hen Egg as an Antioxidant Food Commodity: A Review, *Nutrients*, 2015, **7**(10), 8274–8293.
9. J. O. Hill, H. R. Wyatt and J. C. Peters, The Importance of Energy Balance, *Eur. Endocrinol*, 2013, **9**, 111–115.
10. B. Benelam, Satiation, satiety and their effects on eating behaviour, *Nutr. Bull.*, 2009, **34**, 126–173.
11. C. Clemmensen, T. D. Müller, S. C. Woods, H. R. Berthoud, R. J. Seeley and M. H. Tschöp, Gut–Brain Cross-Talk in Metabolic Control, *Cell*, 2017, **168**(5), 758–774.
12. S. S. Hussain and S. R. Bloom, The regulation of food intake by the gut-brain axis: implications for obesity, *Int. J. Obes.*, 2013, **37**, 625–633.
13. A. C Konner, T. Klockener and J. C. Bruning, Control of energy homeostasis by insulin and leptin: targeting the arcuate nucleus and beyond, *Physiol. Behav.*, 2009, **97**, 632–638.
14. S. G. Bouret, S. J. Draper and R. B. Simerly, Formation of projection pathways from the arcuate nucleus of the hypothalamus to hypothalamic regions implicated in the neural control of feeding behavior in mice, *J. Neurosci.*, 2004, **24**, 2797–2805.
15. H. J. Grill and J. M. Kaplan, The neuroanatomical axis for control of energy balance, *Front. Neuroendocrinol.*, 2002, **23**, 2–40.
16. J. E. Blevins and D. G. Baskin, Hypothalamic-brainstem circuits controlling eating, *Forum Nutr.*, 2010, **63**, 133–140.
17. G. J. Schwartz, The role of gastrointestinal vagal afferents in the control of food intake: current prospects, *Nutrition*, 2000, **16**, 866–873.
18. H. R. Berthoud, Homeostatic and non-homeostatic pathways involved in the control of food intake and energy balance, *Obesity*, 2006, **14**, 197S–200S.
19. K. A. Page, D. Seo, R. Belfort-DeAguiar, C. Lacadie, J. Dzuira, S. Naik, S. Amarnath, R. T. Constable, R. S Sherwin and R. Sinha, Circulating glucose levels modulate neural control of desire for high-calorie foods in humans, *J. Clin. Invest.*, 2011, **121**, 4161–4169.
20. L. A. Velloso and M. W. Schwartz, Altered hypothalamic function in diet-induced obesity, *Int. J. Obes.*, 2011, **35**, 1455–1465.
21. L. A. Tartaglia, M. Dembski, X. Weng, N. Deng, J. Culpepper, R. Devos, G. J. Richards, L. A. Campfield, F. T. Clark, J. Deeds, C. Muir, S. Sanker, A.

Moriarty, K. J. Moore, J. S. Smutko, G. G. Mays, E. A. Wool, C. A. Monroe and R. I. Tepper, Identification and expression cloning of a leptin receptor, OB-R, *Cell*, 1995, **83**(7), 1263–1271.

22. S. C. Chua Jr, D. W. White, X. S. Wu-Peng, S. M. Liu, N. Okada, E. E. Kershaw, W. K. Chung, L. Power-Kehoe, M. Chua, L. A. Tartaglia and R. L. Leibel, Phenotype of fatty due to Gln269Pro mutation in the leptin receptor (Lepr), *Diabetes*, 1996, **45**(8), 1141–1143.
23. M. D. Klok, S. Jakobsdottir and M. L. Drent, The role of leptin and ghrelin in the regulation of food intake and body weight in humans: a review, *Obes. Rev.*, 2007, **8**(1), 21–34.
24. A. Raben and A. Astrup, Leptin is influenced both by predisposition to obesity and diet composition, *Int. J. Obes. Relat. Metab. Disord.*, 2000, **24**, 450–459.
25. J. Gibbs, R. C. Young and G. P. Smith, Cholecystokinin decreases food intake in rats, *J. Comp. Physiol. Psychol.*, 1973, **84**, 488–495.
26. J. E. Blevins, B. G. Stanley and R. D. Reidelberger, Brain regions where cholecystokinin suppresses feeding in rats, *Brain Res.*, 2000, **860**, 1–10.
27. R. A. Gibbs, C. Young and G. P. J. Smith, Cholecystokinin decreases food intake in rats, *Physiol. Psychol.*, 1973, **84**, 488–495.
28. R. A. L. Sturdevant and H. Goetz, Cholecystokinin both stimulates and inhibits human food intake, *Nature*, 1976, **261**, 713–715.
29. J. N. Crawley and M. C. Beinfeld, Rapid development of tolerance to the behavioural actions of cholecystokinin, *Nature*, 1983, **302**, 703–706.
30. D. B. West, M. R. Greenwood, A. C. Sullivan, L. Prescod, L. R. Marzullo and J. Triscari, Infusion of cholecystokinin between meals into free-feeding rats fails to prolong the intermeal interval, *Physiol. Behav.*, 1987, **39**, 111–115.
31. C. A. Matson, M. F. Wiater, J. L. Kuijper and D. S. Weigle, Synergy between leptin and cholecystokinin (CCK) to control daily caloric intake, *Peptides*, 1997, **18**(8), 1275–1278.
32. G. Pradhan, S. L. Samson and Y. Sun, Ghrelin: much more than a hunger hormone, *Curr. Opin. Clin. Nutr. Metab. Care*, 2013, **16**(6), 619–624.
33. M. Kojima and K. Kanagawa, Ghrelin: structure and function, *Physiol. Rev.*, 2005, **85**(2), 495–522.
34. M. Patterson, S. R. Bloom and J. V. Gardiner, Ghrelin and appetite control in humans-Potential application in the treatment of obesity, *Peptides*, 2011, **32**, 2290–2294.
35. T. R. Castaneda, J. Tong, R. Datta, M. Culler and M. H. Tschop, Ghrelin in the regulation of body weight and metabolism, *Front. Neuroendocrinol.*, 2010, **31**, 44–60.
36. J. J. Holst, The physiology of glucagon-like peptide 1, *Physiol. Rev.*, 2007, **87**(4), 1409–1439.

37. L. L. Baggio and D. J. Drucker, Biology of incretins: GLP-1 and GIP, *Gastroenterology*, 2007, **132**(6), 2131–2157.
38. T. P. Vahl, D. L. Drazen, R. J. Seeley, D. A. D'Alessio and S. C. Woods, Meal-anticipatory glucagon-like peptide-1 secretion in rats, *Endocrinology*, 2010, **151**(2), 569–575.
39. J. R. Parkinson, O. B. Chaudhri, Y. T. Kuo, B. C. Field, A. H. Herlihy, W. S. Dhillo, M. A. Ghatei, S. R. Bloom and J. D. Bell, Differential patterns of neuronal activation in the brainstem and hypothalamus following peripheral injection of GLP-1, oxyntomodulin and lithium chloride in mice detected by manganese-enhanced magnetic resonance imaging (MEMRI), *NeuroImage*, 2009, **44**, 1022–1031.
40. B. Kreymann, G. Williams, M. A. Ghatei and S. R. Bloom, Glucagon-like peptide-1 7-36: a physiological incretin in man, *Lancet*, 1987, **2**(8571), 1300–1304.
41. W. O. Creutzfeldt, N. Kleine, B. Willms, C. Orskov, J. J. Holst and M. A. Nauck, Glucagonostatic actions and reduction of fasting hyperglycemia by exogenous glucagon-like peptide I(7-36) amide in type I diabetic patients, *Diabetes Care*, 1996, **19**(6), 580–586.
42. T. Edholm, M. Degerblad, P. Grybäck, L. Hilsted, J. J. Holst, H. Jacobsson, S. Efendic, P. T. Schmidt and P. M. Hellström, Differential incretin effects of GIP and GLP-1 on gastric emptying, appetite, and insulin-glucose homeostasis, *Neurogastroenterol. Motil.*, 2010, **22**(11), 1191–1200.
43. D. J. Drucker and C. F. Rosen, Glucagon-like peptide-1 (GLP-1) receptor agonists, obesity and psoriasis: diabetes meets dermatology, *Diabetologia*, 2011, **54**(11), 2741–2744.
44. T. Vilsboll, M. Christensen, A. E. Junker, F. K. Knop and L. L. Gluud, Effects of glucagon-like peptide-1 receptor agonists on weight loss: systematic review and meta-analyses of randomised controlled trials, *BMJ*, 2012, **344**, d7771.
45. T. A. Lutz, N. Geary, M. M. Szabady, E. Del Prete and E. Scharrer, Amylin decreases meal size in rats, *Physiol. Behav.*, 1995, **58**(6), 1197–1202.
46. K. Fujimoto, H. Machidori, R. Y. Iwakiri, K. Yamamoto, J. Fujisaki, T. Sakata and P. Tso, Effect of intravenous administration of apolipoprotein A-IV on patterns of feeding, drinking and ambulatory activity of rats, *Brain Res.*, 1993, **608**(2), 233–237.
47. J. Gibbs, R. C. Young and G. P. Smith, Cholecystokinin decreases food intake in rats, *J. Comp. Physiol. Psychol*, 1973, **84**, 488–495.
48. M. Tschop, D. L. Smiley and M. L. Heiman, Ghrelin induces adiposity in rodents, *Nature*, 2000, **407**, 908–913.
49. M. D. Turton, D. O'Shea, I. Gunn, S. A. Beak, C. M. Edwards, K. Meeran, S. J. Choi, G. M. Taylor, M. M. Heath, P. D. Lambert, J. P Wilding, D. M. Smith, M. A. Ghatei, J. Herbert and S. R. Bloom, A role for glucagon-like peptide-1 in the central regulation of feeding, *Nature*, 1996, **379**, 69–72.

50. Y. Zhang, R. Proenca, M. Maffei, M. Barone, L. Leopold and J. M. Friedman, Positional cloning of the mouse obese gene and its human homologue, *Nature*, 1994, **372**, 425–432.
51. C. L. Dakin, I. Gunn, C. J. Small, C. M. Edwards, D. L. Hay, D. M. Smith, M. A. Ghatei and S. R. Bloom, Oxyntomodulin inhibits food intake in the rat, *Endocrinology*, 2001, **142**, 4244–4250.
52. A. Asakawa, A. Inui, H. Yuzuriha, N. Ueno, G. Katsuura, M. Fujimiya, M. A. Fujino, A. Niijima, M. M. Meguid and M. Kasuga, Characterization of the effects of pancreatic polypeptide in the regulation of energy balance, *Gastroenterology*, 2003, **124**(5), 1325–1336.
53. R. L. Batterham, M. A. Cowley, C. J. Small, H. Herzog, M. A. Cohen, C. L. Dakin, A. M. Wren, A. E. Brynes, M. J. Low, M. A Ghatei, R. D. Cone and S. R. Bloom, Gut hormone PYY(3-36) physiologically inhibits food intake, *Nature*, 2002, **418**, 650–654.
54. R. Christensen, P. K. Kristensen, E. M. Bartels, H. Bliddal and A. Astrup, Efficacy and safety of the weight-loss drug rimonabant: a meta-analysis of randomised trials, *Lancet*, 2007, **370**, 1706–1713.
55. W. P. T. James, I. D. Caterson, W. Coutinho, N. Finer, L. F. Van Gaal, A. P. Maggioni, C. Torp-Pedersen, A. M. Sharma, G. M. Shepherd, R. A. Rode, C. L. Renz and SCOUT Investigators, Effect of Sibutramine on Cardiovascular Outcomes in Overweight and Obese Subjects, *N. Engl. J. Med.*, 2010, **363**, 905–917.
56. D. S. Weigle, P. A. Breen, C. C. Matthys, H. S. Callahan, K. E. Meeuws, V. R. Burden and J. Q. Purnell, A high-protein diet induces sustained reductions in appetite, ad libitum caloric intake, and body weight despite compensatory changes in diurnal plasma leptin and ghrelin concentrations, *Am. J. Clin. Nutr.*, 2005, **82**(1), 41–48.
57. D. A. Schoeller and A. C. Buchholz, Energetics of obesity and weight control: does diet composition matter?, *J. Am. Diet. Assoc.*, 2005, **105**, S24–S28.
58. B. L. Luhovyy, T. Akhavan and G. H. Anderson, Whey proteins in the regulation of food intake and satiety, *J. Am. Coll. Nutr.*, 2007, **26**, 704S–7012S.
59. A. Bensaid, D. Tome, D. Gietzen, P. Even, C. Morens, N. Gausseres and G. Fromentin, Protein is more potent than carbohydrate for reducing appetite in rats, *Physiol. Behav.*, 2002, **75**, 577–582.
60. J. D. Latner and M. Schwartz, The effects of a high-carbohydrate, high-protein or balanced lunch upon later food intake and hunger ratings, *Appetite*, 1999, **33**, 119–128.
61. L. C. Ortinau, H. A. Hoertel, S. M. Douglas and H. J. Leidy, Effects of high-protein vs. high- fat snacks on appetite control, satiety, and eating initiation in healthy women, *Nutr. J.*, 2014, **13**, 97.
62. K. Vandewater and Z. Vickers, Higher-protein foods produce greater sensory-specific satiety, *Physiol. Behav.*, 1996, **59**, 579–583.

63. J. Johnson and Z. Vickers, Factors influencing sensory-specific satiety, *Appetite*, 1992, **19**, 15–31.
64. M. A. Veldhorst, A. G. Nieuwenhuizen, A. Hochstenbach-Waelen, A. J. van Vught, K. R. Westerterp, M. P. Engelen, R. J. Brummer, N. E. Deutz and M. S. Westerterp-Plantenga, Dose-dependent satiating effect of whey relative to casein or soy, *Physiol. Behav.*, 2009, **96**, 675–682.
65. R. Abou-Samra, L. Keersmaekers, D. Brienza, R. Mukherjee and K. Mace, Effect of different protein sources on satiation and short-term satiety when consumed as a starter, *Nutr. J.*, 2011, **10**, 139.
66. L. V. Nielsen, M. D. Kristensen, L. Klingenberg, C. Ritz, A. Belza, A. Astrup and A. Raben, Protein from Meat or Vegetable Sources in Meals Matched for Fiber Content has Similar Effects on Subjective Appetite Sensations and Energy Intake-A Randomized Acute Cross-Over Meal Test Study, *Nutrients*, 2018, **10**(1), E96.
67. W. A. Blom, A. Lluch, A. Stafleu, S. Vinoy, J. J. Holst, G. Schaafsma and H. F. Hendriks, Effect of a high-protein breakfast on the postprandial ghrelin response, *Am. J. Clin. Nutr.*, 2006, **83**, 211–220.
68. G. Pradhan, S. L. Samson and Y. Sun, Ghrelin: much more than a hunger hormone, *Curr. Opin. Clin. Nutr. Metab. Care*, 2013, **16**, 619–624.
69. R. E. Steinert, C. Feinle-Bisset, L. Asarian, M. Horowitz, C. Beglinger and N. Geary, Ghrelin, CCK, GLP-1, and PYY(3-36): Secretory Controls and Physiological Roles in Eating and Glycemia in Health, Obesity, and After RYGB, *Physiol. Rev.*, 2017, **97**, 411–463.
70. T. L. Halton and F. B. Hu, The effects of high protein diets on thermogenesis, satiety and weight loss: a critical review, *J. Am. Coll. Nutr.*, 2004, **23**, 373–385.
71. D. H. Pesta and V. T. Samuel, A high-protein diet for reducing body fat: mechanisms and possible caveats, *Nutr. Metab.*, 2014, **11**, 53.
72. D. Azzout-Marniche, C. Gaudichon, C. Blouet, C. Bos, V. Mathe, J. F. Huneau and D. Tomé, Liver glyconeogenesis: a pathway to cope with postprandial amino acid excess in high-protein fed rats?, *Am. J. Physiol.: Regul., Integr. Comp. Physiol.*, 2007, **292**, R1400–R1407.
73. H. R. Berthoud, The vagus nerve, food intake and obesity, *Regul. Pept.*, 2008, **149**, 15–25.
74. G. H. Anderson and D. Woodend, Consumption of sugars and the regulation of short-term satiety and food intake, *Am. J. Clin. Nutr.*, 2003, **78**, 843S–849S.
75. S. M. Mellinkoff, M. Frankland, D. Boyle and M. Greipel, Relationship between serum amino acid concentration and fluctuations in appetite, *J. Appl. Physiol.*, 1956, **8**, 535–538.
76. G. Lazutkaite, A. Solda, K. Lossow, W. Meyerhof and N. Dale, Amino acid sensing in hypothalamic tanycytes via umami taste receptors, *Mol. Metab.*, 2017, **6**, 1480–1492.

77. H. Fenselau, J. N. Campbell, A. M. Verstegen, J. C. Madara, J. Xu, B. P. Shah, J. M. Resch, Z. Yang, Y. Mandelblat-Cerf, Y. Livneh and B. B. Lowell, A rapidly acting glutamatergic ARC-->PVH satiety circuit postsynaptically regulated by alpha-MSH, *Nat. Neurosci.*, 2017, **20**, 42–51.
78. P. B. Pencharz, R. Elango and R. R. Wolfe, Recent developments in understanding protein needs - How much and what kind should we eat?, *Appl. Physiol., Nutr., Metab.*, 2016, **41**, 577–580.
79. R. Fallaize, L. Wilson, J. Gray, L. M. Morgan and B. A. Griffin, Variation in the effects of three different breakfast meals on subjective satiety and subsequent intake of energy at lunch and evening meal, *Eur. J. Nutr.*, 2013, **52**, 1353–1359.
80. C. K. Rayner and M. Horowitz, Gastrointestinal motility and glycemic control in diabetes: the chicken and the egg revisited?, *J. Clin. Invest.*, 2006, **116**, 299–302.
81. J. S. Vander Wal, J. M. Marth, P. Khosla, K. L. Jen and N. V. Dhurandhar, Short-term effect of eggs on satiety in overweight and obese subjects, *J. Am. Coll. Nutr.*, 2005, **24**, 510–515.
82. S. Wang, L. Yang, J. Lu and Y. Mu, High-protein breakfast promotes weight loss by suppressing subsequent food intake and regulating appetite hormones in obese Chinese adolescents, *Horm. Res. Paediatr.*, 2015, **83**, 19–25.
83. A. Missimer, D. M. DiMarco, C. J. Andersen, A. G. Murillo, M. Vergara-Jimenez and M. L. Fernandez, Consuming Two Eggs per Day, as Compared to an Oatmeal Breakfast, Decreases Plasma Ghrelin while Maintaining the LDL/HDL Ratio, *Nutrients*, 2017, **9**(2), E89.
84. A. G. Liu, R. S. Puyau, H. Han, W. D. Johnson, F. L. Greenway and N. V. Dhurandhar, The effect of an egg breakfast on satiety in children and adolescents: a randomized crossover trial, *J. Am. Coll. Nutr.*, 2015, **34**, 185–190.
85. J. P. Lomenick, M. S. Melguizo, S. L. Mitchell, M. L. Summar and J. W. Anderson, Effects of meals high in carbohydrate, protein, and fat on ghrelin and peptide YY secretion in prepubertal children, *J. Clin. Endocrinol. Metab.*, 2009, **94**, 4463–4471.
86. V. Lang, F. Bellisle, J. M. Oppert, C. Craplet, F. R. Bornet, G. Slama and B. Guy-Grand, Satiating effect of proteins in healthy subjects: a comparison of egg albumin, casein, gelatin, soy protein, pea protein, and wheat gluten, *Am. J. Clin. Nutr.*, 1998, **67**, 1197–1204.
87. G. H. Anderson, S. N. Tecimer, D. Shah and T. A. Zafar, Protein source, quantity, and time of consumption determine the effect of proteins on short-term food intake in young men, *J. Nutr.*, 2004, **134**, 3011–3015.
88. R. Abou-Samra, L. Keersmaekers, D. Brienza, R. Mukherjee and K. Macé, Effect of different protein sources on satiation and short-term satiety when consumed as a starter, *Nutr. J.*, 2011, **10**, 139.

89. L. Trigazis, A. Orttmann and G. H. Anderson, Effect of a cholecystokinin-a receptor blocker on protein-induced food intake suppression in rats, *Am. J. Physiol.*, 1997, **272**, 1826–1833.
90. X. Pelletier, P. Thouvenot, S. Belbraouet, J. A. Chayvialle, B. Hanesse, D. Mayeux and G. Debry, Effect of egg consumption in healthy volunteers: influence of yolk, white or whole-egg on gastric emptying and on glycemic and hormonal responses, *Ann. Nutr. Metab.*, 1996, **40**, 109–115.
91. P. Deibert, D. König, A. Schmidt-Trucksaess, K. S. Zaenker, I. Frey, U. Landmann and A. Berg, Weight loss without losing muscle mass in pre-obese and obese subjects induced by a high-soy-protein diet, *Int. J. Obes.*, 2004, **28**(10), 1349–1352.
92. T. P. Wycherley, L. J. Moran, P. M. Clifton, M. Noakes and G. D. Brinkworth, Effects of energy-restricted high-protein, low-fat compared with standard-protein, low-fat diets: a meta-analysis of randomized controlled trials, *Am. J. Clin. Nutr.*, 2012, **96**(6), 1281–1298.
93. D. J. Baer, K. S. Stote, D. R. Paul, G. K. Harris, W. V. Rumpler and B. A. Clevidence, Whey protein but not soy protein supplementation alters body weight and composition in free-living overweight and obese adults, *J. Nutr.*, 2011, **141**(8), 1489–1494.
94. D. P. Belobrajdic, G. H. McIntosh and J. A. Owens, A high-whey-protein diet reduces body weight gain and alters insulin sensitivity relative to red meat in wistar rats, *J. Nutr.*, 2004, **134**(6), 1454–1458.
95. M. Garcés-Rimón, C. González, J. A. Uranga, V. López-Miranda, R. López-Fandiño and M. Miguel, Pepsin Egg White Hydrolysate Ameliorates Obesity-Related Oxidative Stress, Inflammation and Steatosis in Zucker Fatty Rats, *PLoS One*, 2016, **11**(3), e0151193.
96. C. J. Saande, S. K. Jones, K. E. Hahn, C. H. Reed, M. J. Rowling and K. L. Schalinske, Dietary Whole Egg Consumption Attenuates Body Weight Gain and Is More Effective than Supplemental Cholecalciferol in Maintaining Vitamin D Balance in Type 2 Diabetic Rats, *J. Nutr.*, 2017, **147**(9), 1715–1721.
97. J. S. Vander Wal, A. Gupta, P. Khosla and N. V. Dhurandhar, Egg breakfast enhances weight loss, *Int. J. Obes.*, 2008, **32**(10), 1545–1551.
98. N. R. Fuller, I. D. Caterson, A. Sainsbury, G. Denyer, M. Fong, J. Gerofi, K. Baqleh, K. H. Williams, N. S. Lau and T. P. Markovic, The effect of a high-egg diet on cardiovascular risk factors in people with type 2 diabetes: the Diabetes and Egg (DIABEGG) study-a 3-mo randomized controlled trial, *Am. J. Clin. Nutr.*, 2015, **101**(4), 705–713.
99. S. Shin, H. W. Lee, C. E. Kim, J. Lim, J. K. Lee, S. A. Lee and D. Kang, Egg Consumption and Risk of Metabolic Syndrome in Korean Adults: Results from the Health Examinees Study, *Nutrients*, 2017, **9**(7), E687.

100. J. R. Marchesi, D. H. Adams, F. Fava, G. D. Hermes, G. M. Hirschfield, G. Hold, M. N. Quraishi, J. Kinross, H. Smidt, K. M. Tuohy, L. V. Thomas, E. G. Zoetendal and A. Hart, The gut microbiota and host health: a new clinical frontier, *Gut*, 2016, **65**, 330–339.
101. R. E. Ley, P. J. Turnbaugh, S. Klein and J. I. Gordon, Microbial ecology: human gut microbes associated with obesity, *Nature*, 2006, **444**, 1022–1023.
102. P. V. Bauer, S. C. Hamr and F. A. Duca, Regulation of energy balance by a gut-brain axis and involvement of the gut microbiota, *Cell. Mol. Life Sci.*, 2016, **73**(4), 737–755.
103. A. C. Michael and R. B. Anthony, The Impact of Diet and Lifestyle on Gut Microbiota and Human Health, *Nutrients*, 2015, **7**(1), 17–44.

CHAPTER 4

Egg Consumption and Cardiometabolic Health

JESSY AZARCOYA-BARRERA, CATHERINE J. FIELD, RENE L. JACOBS AND CAROLINE RICHARD*

Department of Agricultural, Food and Nutritional Sciences, 4-002G Li Ka Shing Centre for Health Innovation, University of Alberta, Edmonton, Alberta, T6G 2E1, Canada
*E-mail: cr5@ualberta.ca

4.1 Introduction

Cardiovascular disease (CVD) is currently the leading cause of death worldwide. It is estimated that 17 million people die from CVD per year, representing 31% of all global deaths.[1] Dietary egg consumption is traditionally related to the development of CVD owing to their high cholesterol content. However, dietary cholesterol itself is only a minor determinant of plasma cholesterol concentrations.[2] As such, the new Dietary Guidelines for Americans along with several other worldwide organizations, including the British Heart Foundation and the National Heart Foundation of Australia, no longer emphasize reducing egg consumption.[3–5] Recent systematic reviews and meta-analyses of prospective cohort studies have

Food Chemistry, Function and Analysis No.14
Eggs as Functional Foods and Nutraceuticals for Human Health
Edited by Jianping Wu

Published by the Royal Society of Chemistry, www.rsc.org

reported, for the most part, no association between dietary cholesterol or egg intake and the risk of developing CVD.[6–11] Some meta-analyses of prospective cohort studies have observed a positive association between egg consumption and the risk of developing diabetes.[8,11] However, observational studies are unable to determine cause and effect relationship. Furthermore, eggs are an excellent source of several essential nutrients, including choline, lutein and vitamin B12, as well as high-quality protein.[12]

This book chapter will provide an overview of the literature regarding the impact of egg consumption on traditional and non-traditional cardiovascular risk factors in healthy individuals and in individuals with or at risk of CVD (*i.e.* those with metabolic syndrome (MetS) or type 2 diabetes). A systematic search was performed in the PubMed database in June 2018. Only randomized intervention studies in human (>18 years old) that manipulated the amount of egg consumed and that were published in English were considered. Acute short-term studies (<1 week intervention) and postprandial studies were excluded from the search.

4.2 Egg Consumption, Traditional CVD Risk Factors and Atherogenic LDL Particles

Common traditional CVD risk factors include low levels of circulating high-density lipoprotein-cholesterol (HDL-C), high plasma triglyceride (TG) and glucose/insulin concentrations, elevated systolic (SBP) and diastolic blood pressure (DBP), and obesity.[13] An elevated plasma concentration of LDL-C is one of the main risk factors that contribute to the development of CVD.[14] However, small dense LDL particles have been shown to be more atherogenic than normal-size LDL particles.[15–17] This is due in part to a lower catabolic rate of small dense LDL particles increasing their residence time and susceptibility to oxidation in circulation.[15,18] The number of small dense LDL particles and oxidized LDL particles (ox-LDL) both play an important role in the development of atherosclerosis since they easily cross the endothelial wall and favor the recruitment of macrophages and subsequently the formation of foam cells, contributing to atherosclerotic plaque.[19–21]

We have recently performed a systematic review on the effect of egg consumption on major CVD risk factors in individuals with type 2 diabetes or at risk of CVD (*i.e.* insulin resistance or MetS).[22] Overall, we found that consuming between six to 12 eggs per week as part of a healthy diet has no adverse effect on CVD risk factors (total-C, LDL-C, HDL-C, TG, glucose and insulin) in individuals at risk of developing diabetes or with type 2 diabetes.[23–32] In this book chapter, we have extended the search to include healthy individuals as well as LDL particle phenotype and ox-LDL. A summary of the effects of egg consumption on traditional CVD risk factors, LDL particle size and ox-LDL is provided in Table 4.1.

Table 4.1 Effects of egg consumption on traditional CVD risk factors, LDL particle size and oxidized LDL.[a]

Study	No. of individuals enrolled, sex and age	Population characteristics	Design	Intervention	Duration	Results[b]
Healthy individuals						
Missimer *et al.*, 2017[35] Missimer *et al.*, 2018[34]	$n = 50$ allocated ($n = 48$ completed) 24F/26M 18–30 years	Healthy and young individuals with a BMI between 18.5–29.9 kg m^{-2}, TG < 500 mg dL^{-1}, total-C < 240 mg dL^{-1}, glucose < 126 mg dL^{-1}	Randomized, single-blind, crossover	Participants were assigned to consume 2 eggs (370 mg cholesterol) or 1 packet of oatmeal per day for 4 weeks, followed by a 3 week washout period and then allocated to the alternate breakfast	11 weeks	Between groups: ↔ BMI, WC, SBP, DBP. ↑ total-C, LDL-C, HDL-C in EGG group Between groups: ↑ large LDL conc. in EGG group ↔ small LDL conc. ↔ ApoB
DiMarco *et al.*, 2017[36] DiMarco *et al.*, 2017[64]	$n = 40$ Recruited ($n = 37$ completed) 20F/20M 18–30 years	Healthy and young subjects with a BMI between 18.5–29.9 kg m^{-2}, BP < 140/90 mm Hg, glucose < 126 mg dL^{-1}, total-C < 240 mg dL^{-1}, TG < 500 mg dL^{-1}	Crossover	Began with a 2 week wash-out period (no eggs). Then, subjects were fed with 1 egg per day for 4 weeks, 2 eggs per day for 4 weeks and 3 eggs per day for 4 weeks	14 weeks	Between groups: ↔ BMI, WC, SBP, TG, total-C, glucose ↓ DBP with 1, 2 and 3 egg d^{-1} *vs.* 0 egg d^{-1} ↓ LDL-C with 1 egg d^{-1} *vs.* 0 and 3 egg d^{-1} ↑ HDL-C with 1, 2 and 3 egg d^{-1} *vs.* 0 egg d^{-1} ↑ large LDL conc. with 1, 2 and 3 egg d^{-1} ↔ Mean particle size

Lemos *et al.*, 2018[37]	$n = 30$ recruited ($n = 29$ completed) 16F/14M 18–30 years	Healthy and young subjects with a BMI 18.5–29.9 kg m^{-2}, BP < 140/90 mm Hg, glucose < 126 mg dL^{-1}, total-C < 240 mg dL^{-1}, TG < 500 mg dL^{-1}	Randomized, crossover	2 week run-in period (no egg). Subjects allocated to 1 of the 2 breakfasts: EGG group: 3 eggs per day; choline group: 1.5 tablets of choline Bitartrate for 4 weeks with a 3 week washout	13 weeks	Between groups: ↔ BMI, SBP, DBP, glucose, TG, ApoB ↑ total-C, HDL-C, LDL-C with EGG
Harman *et al.*, 2008[33]	$n = 67$ recruited ($n = 45$ completed) 32F/14M 18–55 years	Healthy subjects with BMI < 35 kg m^{-2}, total-C < 6.5 mmol L^{-1}, TG < 3 mmol L^{-1}	Randomized, parallel	Individuals were randomized to 1 of the 2 energy-restricted diets: 2 eggs per day ($n = 24$) or 0 eggs per day ($n = 21$) Blood samples collected at 0, 6 and 12 weeks	12 weeks	From baseline: ↓ BW in both groups ↓ LDL-C at 6 weeks in no-egg group only Between groups: ↔ BW, total-C, HDL-C, TG, ApoB, LDL peak density and % of sdLDL particles

(continued)

Table 4.1 (*continued*)

Study	No. of individuals enrolled, sex and age	Population characteristics	Design	Intervention	Duration	Results[b]
Individuals at risk of CVD or with type 2 diabetes[c]						
Mutungi *et al.*, 2010[29]	$n = 31$ men recruited (n = 28 completed) 40–70 years	Men with a BMI between 26 and 37 kg m^{-2} Subjects on lipid-lowering medications were excluded 18 subjects had MetS based on NCEP ATP III	Randomized, placebo-controlled, single-blinded, parallel	Participants followed a carbohydrate-restricted diet (10–15% energy from carbohydrates) and were randomized in 2 groups: EGG group: 3 liquid eggs per day ($n = 15$); egg-substitute group (SUB, $n = 13$)	12 weeks	From baseline: ↑ mean LDL diameter in both groups ↓ small LDL conc. in both groups Between groups: ↑ large LDL conc. in EGG group
Blesso *et al.*, 2013[24]	$n = 40$ recruited ($n = 37$ completed) 12M/25F 30–70 years	Participants were included if they met the MetS criteria from the NCEP ATP III No significant difference between groups at baseline	Randomized, single-blind, parallel	Participants followed a moderate carbohydrate-restricted diet (25–30% of energy from carbohydrates) and were randomly assign to 2 groups: EGG: 3 whole eggs per day ($n = 20$) or egg substitute (SUB, n = 17)	12 weeks	From baseline: ↑ mean LDL particle size and large LDL conc. in egg group only ↓ small and medium LDL conc. in egg group only. ↓ ox-LDL in SUB group only No difference between group

Ballesteros *et al.*, 2015[23]	33 recruited (n = 29 completed) 19F/10M 35–65 years	Subjects with controlled type 2 diabetes (HbA1c < 9%) All subjects were on glucose-lowering medication, blood pressure medication ($n = 19$) and reductase inhibitors ($n = 9$)	Randomized, single-blind, crossover	Two isocaloric breakfast options: 1 egg per day or 40 g of oatmeal with 2 cups per day lactose-free milk. Individuals were allocated to 1 of the 2 breakfasts for 5 weeks followed by a 3 week washout and then to the alternate breakfast	13 weeks	Between groups: ↔ ox-LDL, small, medium and large LDL particles

[a]Abbreviations: Apo, apolipoprotein; BW, body weight; BMI, body mass index; BP, blood pressure; C, cholesterol; conc., concentration; CVD, cardiovascular disease; d, day; DBP, diastolic blood pressure; F, female; HDL-C, high-density lipoprotein-cholesterol; LDL-C, low-density lipoprotein-cholesterol; ox-LDL, oxidized low-density lipoprotein; M, Male; MetS, metabolic syndrome; NCEP ATP III, National Cholesterol Education Program Adult Treatment Panel III; SBP, systolic blood pressure; TG, triglycerides; WC, waist circumference.

[b]↓ indicates a decrease, ↑ indicates an increase, ↔ indicates no effect.

[c]The effect of egg consumption on major CVD risk factors in individuals at risk of CVD or with type 2 diabetes has been recently reviewed in.[22]

4.2.1 Egg Consumption in Individuals with MetS or Type 2 Diabetes

In a randomized crossover trial, Ballesteros *et al.*[23] reported no significant difference in plasma ox-LDL concentrations in the EGG group (1 egg d^{-1} for 5 weeks) when compared to the oatmeal group in diabetic individuals. Major CVD risk factors (total cholesterol (total-C), LDL-C, HDL-C, TG and insulin) and the number of small, medium and large LDL particles also remained unchanged after both phases of the trial. Blesso *et al.*[24] conducted a randomized parallel study, in which individuals with MetS consumed either, as part of a moderate carbohydrate-restricted diet (25–30% energy from carbohydrates), 3 eggs d^{-1} (EGG group) or the equivalent of yolk-free egg substitute (SUB group) for 12 weeks. They reported a decrease in the number of small and medium LDL particles along with an increase in the number of large and mean diameter LDL particles in all participants. Even though these improvements were greater in the EGG group than in the SUB group, the difference did not reach significance. A reduction in ox-LDL concentrations was also observed in the SUB group only. Improvement in plasma TG concentrations and the HOMA-IR index (an index of insulin resistance) was observed in all participants, which is most likely attributable to the body weight (BW) reduction following the intervention. A significantly greater increase in HDL-C was observed in the EGG group as compared to the SUB group. No changes were observed in SBP, DBP, total-C, LDL-C, fasting glucose and apolipoprotein B (ApoB) during the intervention in both groups. Similar results were reported by Mutungi *et al.*[28] In this randomized single-blinded parallel study, overweight/obese men consumed either three liquids eggs per day (n = 15) or egg substitute (n = 13) for 12 weeks while following a carbohydrate-restricted diet (10–15% energy from carbohydrates). Significant reductions in BW and waist circumference (WC) were observed in both groups as well as improvement in other CVD risk factors (SBP, DBP, ApoB, TG and fasting insulin).[28,31] Increased HDL-C concentrations were only observed in the EGG group. An increase in mean LDL diameter and a reduction in the number of small LDL particles was noted in both groups. However, the increase in the number of large LDL particles was significantly greater in the EGG group than in the SUB group.[29]

4.2.2 Egg Consumption in Healthy Individuals

Recent studies have investigated the impact of consuming egg on LDL particles in a healthy young population. Harman *et al.*[33] conducted a randomized parallel study in which 45 healthy overweight/obese individuals were assigned to consume either 2 eggs d^{-1} (EGG group; n = 24) or 0 egg d^{-1} (no-EGG group; n = 21) for 12 weeks as part of an energy-restricted diet. A reduction in BW was observed in both groups at the end of the 12 weeks. At 6 weeks, LDL-C concentrations were lower from baseline in the no-EGG group only. No differences from baseline or between groups were observed in total-C, HDL-C, ApoB, TG and LDL peak particle size, as well as the relative proportion of small, dense LDL particles. Missimer *et al.*[34] reported, in a randomized single-blinded crossover study, that consumption of 2 eggs d^{-1} for 4 weeks increased the number of large LDL particles as compared to an oatmeal breakfast, whereas no significant differences were reported in the number of small LDL particles and ApoB concentrations between groups. BW, WC, SBP and DBP were unchanged during both phases. Egg consumption led to an increase in total-C, LDL-C and HDL-C concentrations compared to the oatmeal breakfast.[34,35] In a crossover trial, DiMarco *et al.*[36] examined the effect of gradually increasing egg intake in a healthy population (n = 37). The trial began with a 2 week run-in period (0 egg d^{-1}) followed by 4-week interventions of increased egg consumption (1, 2 and 3 eggs d^{-1}). Body mass index (BMI), WC, SBP and TG, fasting glucose and total-C concentrations all remained stable during the course of the intervention. Egg consumption (1, 2 and 3 eggs d^{-1}) decrease DBP compared to the 0 egg d^{-1} phase (baseline). LDL-C concentrations were lower with 1 egg d^{-1} compared to 0 and 3 eggs d^{-1} whereas HLD-C concentrations increased with egg intake (1, 2 and 3 eggs d^{-1}) compared to the 0 egg d^{-1} phase. Although no change in the mean LDL particle size was observed, the number of large LDL particles increased with egg consumption. Lemos *et al.*[37] conducted a randomized crossover study, in which healthy individuals consumed in random order 3 eggs d^{-1} and a choline supplement (1.5 tablets of choline bitartrate) for 4 weeks. Although there were no changes in BMI, SBP, DBP, the LDL-C/HDL-C ratio, fasting glucose, TG and ApoB concentrations after both phases, egg consumption led to an increase in total-C, LDL-C and HDL-C concentrations compared to the choline group.

In summary, egg consumption appears to have an overall neutral effect on most traditional CVD risk factors in both healthy individuals and those at high risk of CVD. In healthy individuals, an increase in LDL-C concentrations was observed in some but not all studies (2/4 studies) while most studies reported an increased in HDL-C concentrations (3/4 studies). Improvement in LDL particle phenotype was also reported in most of these studies with an increase in the number of large LDL particles (2/3 studies). In individuals at high risk of CVD, improvements in most CVD risk factors were attributed to weight loss rather than egg consumption *per se*, except for HDL-C concentrations, which were increased to a greater extent in the EGG group (2/3 studies). However, most studies reported an increase in the number of large LDL particles with egg consumption (2/3 studies). Ox-LDL concentrations were only measured in two studies in individuals at high risk of CVD and both reported no effect of egg consumption on ox-LDL. Altogether, the evidence suggests that egg consumption may improve LDL particle phenotype while having little effect on other traditional CVD risk factors. More studies are required before one can conclude about the effects of egg on ox-LDL particles, especially in healthy individuals.

4.3 Egg Consumption and Endothelial Function

Vascular endothelial dysfunction is an important predictor of early atherosclerosis leading to CVD.[38,39] Endothelial dysfunction can be assessed using different surrogate markers of atherosclerosis, including plasma levels of cell adhesion molecules and the percentage of flow-mediated dilatation (FMD). For instance, vascular cell adhesion molecule-1 (VCAM-1), intercellular adhesion molecule-1 (ICAM-1), E-selectin and P-selectin are cell adhesion molecules involved in leukocyte recruitment and infiltration into arteries when there is an accumulation of LDL particles. Several studies have reported an increased risk of CVD events with elevated circulating levels of cell adhesion molecules.[40–43] FMD is a non-invasive method that assesses the vasodilation function of an artery (normally the brachial artery) in response to stress and correlates well with coronary atherosclerosis.[44] A summary of the effects of egg consumption on endothelial function is provided in Table 4.2.

4.3.1 Egg Consumption in Individuals with or at Risk of CVD

In a randomized single-blinded crossover study, Katz *et al.*[45] compared the impact of three 6 week dietary interventions in adults with clinically established coronary artery disease (n = 30) on FMD. Subjects consumed in random order three different breakfasts: (1) EGG: 2 eggs d^{-1}; (2) egg substitute: 1/2 cup of Egg Beaters; (3) high-carbohydrate: bagel, waffles, pancakes, or cereal and skim milk. No changes in BW or WC were observed during the intervention. Consumption of the egg substitute and high-carbohydrate breakfasts led to an increase in FMD when compared to the baseline value. However, no differences were observed between groups. In a randomized single-blinded parallel trial, Blesso *et al.*[25] assessed the impact of consuming 3 eggs d^{-1} (EGG group; n = 20) or egg substitute (SUB group; n = 17) as part of a carbohydrate-restricted diet (25–30% energy from carbohydrates) for 12 weeks in individuals with MetS. While BW and WC were reduced in both groups, no changes in plasma VCAM-1 and ICAM-1 concentrations were observed. The effect of egg consumption on endothelial function has also been assessed in hyperlipidemic adults (n = 40).[46] In this randomized placebo-controlled crossover study, the acute (*i.e.* postprandial) and the sustained (6 weeks) effects of consuming egg on FMD were assessed. During the acute phase, subjects consumed in random order three medium hardboiled eggs and a sausage/cheese breakfast sandwich; the FMD was measured at baseline and in the postprandial state. Both breakfasts had no effect on postprandial FMD. In the sustained phase, participants consumed in random order 2 medium hardboiled eggs per day and 1/2 cup of egg substitute per day for 6 weeks. Although no change in FMD from baseline was observed with the egg phase, an increase in FMD occurred during the egg-substitute phase, which was significantly different from the egg phase.

Table 4.2 Effect of egg consumption on endothelial function and vascular adhesion molecules.[a]

Study	No. of individuals enrolled, sex and age	Population characteristics	Design	Intervention	Duration	Results[b]
Healthy individuals						
Ratliff *et al.*, 2009[31]	$n = 31$ men recruited ($n = 28$ completed) 40–70 years	Healthy overweight men with a BMI between 26 and 37 kg m^{-2}	Randomized, single-blind, parallel	Participants followed a carbohydrate-restricted diet (17% energy from carbohydrates) and were randomly assigned to egg group ($n = 15$) or egg-substitute group (SUB, $n = 13$)	12 weeks	From baseline: ↓ BW and WC in both groups ↔ ICAM-1, VCAM-1 in both groups No difference between groups
Individuals at risk of CVD or with CVD						
Blesso *et al.*, 2013[25]	$n = 40$ recruited ($n = 37$ completed) 25F/12M 30–70 years	Participants with MetS based on the NCEP ATP III No significant difference between groups at baseline	Randomized, single-blind, parallel	Participants followed a moderate carbohydrate-restricted diet and were randomly assign to: EGG: 3 whole eggs d^{-1} ($n = 20$) or egg SUB ($n = 17$) groups	12 weeks	From baseline: ↓ BW and WC in both groups ↔ ICAM-1 and VCAM-1 No difference between groups
Katz *et al.*, 2015[45]	$n = 32$ recruited ($n = 30$ completed) 6F/26M Age mean 67 years	Individuals with clinically established coronary artery disease, non-smokers Excluded subjects using lipid-lowering or antihypertensive medications	Randomized, single-blind, crossover	Randomly assigned to 1 of 3 dietary interventions EGG: 2 eggs d^{-1}; egg substitute (SUB): 1/2 cup of Egg Beaters; high-carbohydrate (CHO): Bagel, waffles, pancakes, or cereal and skim milk Three 6 week treatment phases interrupted by a 4 week washout period	26 weeks	From baseline: ↔ In BW and BMI. ↑ FMD in egg SUB and CHO groups No difference between groups

(*continued*)

Table 4.2 (*continued*)

Study	No. of individuals enrolled, sex and age	Population characteristics	Design	Intervention	Duration	Results[b]
Njike *et al.*, 2010[46]	n = 40 recruited (n = 36 completed) 24F/16M ≥35 years	Hyperlipidemic men and post-menopausal women Excluded subjects On lipid-lowering medication, insulin or glucose-sensitizing medication, vaso-active medication	Randomized, placebo-controlled, crossover	Consisted of 2 phases: Acute phase (1 day): Participants assigned to 1 of the 2 breakfast options: 3 eggs or a sausage/cheese sandwich for a day Sustained phase (6 weeks): Participants assigned to 1 of the 2 breakfast options: 2 eggs d^{-1} or 1/2 cup of egg substitute d^{-1} for 6 weeks. Each treatment separated by a 4 week washout period	20 weeks	Acute phase: ↔ FMD in both groups from baseline and between groups Sustained phase: ↔ BMI in both groups ↔ FMD in EGG group from baseline ↑ FMD in SUB group *vs.* EGG group

[a]Abbreviations: FMD, flow-mediated dilatation; VCAM-1, vascular cell adhesion protein 1; ICAM-1, intracellular adhesion molecule; BW, body weight; WC, waist circumference; F, female; M, male; NCEP ATP III, National Cholesterol Education Program Adult Treatment Panel III; MetS, metabolic syndrome.
[b]↓ indicates a decrease, ↑ indicates an increase, ↔ indicates no effect.

4.3.2 Egg Consumption in Healthy Individuals

A few interventions have assessed the impact of egg consumption on endothelial function in healthy individuals. Ratliff *et al.*[31] assessed the effect of consuming 3 liquid whole eggs d^{-1} (EGG group; n = 15) or a liquid cholesterol- and fat-free egg substitute (SUB group; n = 13), purchased from the Vistar Corporation (Windsor, CT, USA) as part of a carbohydrate-restricted diet (25–30% energy from carbohydrates) for 12 weeks in overweight/obese healthy men on cell adhesion molecules. Although both groups experienced a significant reduction in BW and WC, no changes in plasma ICAM-1 and VCAM-1 concentrations were observed.

In summary, more studies assessing the effect of egg consumption on endothelial function are needed before we can draw firm conclusions. The available evidence so far suggests a neutral effect of egg consumption on circulating cell adhesion molecule concentrations in both healthy individuals and those at risk of CVD. Egg consumption also appears to have a neutral effect on FMD in individuals with CVD while an improvement in FMD has been observed with egg-substitute intake.

4.4 Egg Consumption and Inflammation

Many studies have established the role of inflammation in the development of chronic diseases, including CVD and type 2 diabetes.[47,48] CVD and type 2 diabetes are associated with a state of chronic low-grade systemic inflammation characterized, among others, by elevated plasma concentration of C-reactive protein (CRP), interleukin-6 (IL-6), tumor necrosis factor-a (TNF-α), IL-1β and IL-18.[48–52] CRP in particular has emerged as a powerful clinical predictor of cardiovascular events independently of other CVD risk factors.[49,53,54] Serum amyloid A (SAA) is another acute-phase protein that has been associated with an increased risk of CVD.[55,56]

4.4.1 Egg Consumption in Individuals at Risk of CVD or with Type 2 Diabetes

Blesso *et al.*[25] reported in their randomized single-blinded parallel study that consumption of 3 eggs d^{-1} (EGG group) or egg substitute for 12 weeks in conjunction with a carbohydrate-restricted diet (25–30% energy from carbohydrates) had no effect on plasma CRP, IL-6 and IL-10 concentrations despite a significant reduction in BW. Although reductions in TNF-α and SAA levels were noted in the EGG group only, no significant differences were observed between groups. In a randomized crossover trial, Ballesteros *et al.*[23] investigated the effect of consuming 1 egg d^{-1} or 40 g of oatmeal with 2 cups of lactose-free milk for 5 weeks on inflammation in individuals with type 2 diabetes. A reduction in plasma TNF-α concentrations along with a trend toward a reduction in IL-6 concentrations was observed with egg consumption. No change in CRP concentrations was observed following both phases. The effect of egg consumption on inflammation in individuals with prediabetes or type 2 diabetes was also reported by Fuller *et al.*[26] In their randomized parallel study, participants consumed either a high-egg diet (2 eggs per day on 6 days per week) or a low-egg diet (<2 eggs per week + 10 g of lean animal protein) for 12 weeks. A slight but significant reduction in BW was observed in the low-egg group whereas no change in plasma CRP levels was observed in both groups.

4.4.2 Egg Consumption in Healthy Individuals

Recently, Missimer *et al.*[34] examined markers of inflammation in healthy young individuals who were assigned to consume either 2 eggs d^{-1} or one package of oatmeal for 4 weeks in a crossover design. Egg consumption was associated with a reduction in plasma TNF-α levels compared to the oatmeal phase. No differences were found in plasma levels of IL-6 and CRP.

In contrast, Ratliff *et al.*[31] reported a significant reduction in plasma concentrations of CRP in overweight/obese participants consuming 3 eggs d^{-1} as part of a carbohydrate-restricted diet (17% energy from carbohydrates) for 12 weeks compared to participants who consumed an egg substitute. Although a reduction in BW and WC was observed in both groups, no effect on plasma TNF-α and IL-8 concentrations was observed. A reduction in MCP-1(monocyte chemoattractant protein 1) concentrations was also observed in the egg-substitute group compared to the egg group. The impact of egg consumption on systemic inflammation was investigated in a subgroup of subjects who had completed the 4 eggs d^{-1} intervention in the randomized double-blinded crossover study published by Knopp *et al.*[27] In this study, healthy subjects were separated based on their insulin sensibility level and presence of obesity and consumed in random order a NCET step 1 diet containing 0 egg d^{-1} or 4 eggs d^{-1} for 4 weeks. Consumption of 4 eggs d^{-1} led to increased plasma CRP and SAA concentrations only in the lean insulin-sensitive group; no changes were observed in the lean insulin-resistant and obese insulin-resistant groups.

Overall, conflicting results have been reported regarding the effect of egg consumption on markers of inflammation. In healthy individuals, a reduction, no change and an increase in plasma CRP concentrations have been reported so far. Of note, the increase in plasma levels of CRP was only observed with the 4 eggs d^{-1} intervention, which is an unusually high consumption of eggs. In individual at risk of CVD, most studies showed no change in CRP concentrations with egg intake (3/3 studies) while most studies reported a beneficial effect of egg consumption on TNF-α concentrations (2/2 studies). Altogether, egg consumption seems to have little effect on markers of inflammation in healthy individuals whereas, in individuals at risk of CVD with chronic low-grade systemic inflammation, egg consumption may improve a specific marker of inflammation (TNF-α). However, considering the inconsistency of results, further investigations are required (Table 4.3).

Table 4.3 Effect of egg consumption on inflammatory markers.[a]

Study	No. of individuals enrolled, sex and age	Population characteristics	Design	Intervention	Duration	Results[b]
Healthy individuals						
Missimer *et al.*, 2018[34]	$n = 50$ recruited ($n = 48$ completed) 24F/26M 18–30 years	Healthy and young individuals with a BMI between 18.5 and 29.9 kg m^{-2}	Randomized, single-blind, crossover	Participants were assigned to consume 2 eggs or 1 packet of oatmeal per day for 4 weeks with a 3-week washout period	11 weeks	Between groups ↓ TNF-α with egg ↔ CRP and IL-6
Ratliff *et al.*, 2009[31]	$n = 31$ men ($n = 28$ completed) 40–70 years	Healthy overweight men with a BMI between 26 and 37 kg m^{-2}	Randomized, single-blind, parallel	Participants followed a carbohydrate-restricted diet (17% energy from carbohydrates) and were randomly assigned to egg group ($n = 15$) or egg substitute group (SUB, $n = 13$)	12 weeks	From baseline: ↓ BW and WC in both groups ↔ TNF-α, IL-8 in both groups Between groups: ↓ CRP with egg ↓ MCP-1 in SUB group
Tannock *et al.*, 2005[32] Subanalysis of Knopp's 2003 study[27]	$n = 221$ recruited ($n = 201$ completed the 4 egg phase)	Healthy individuals separated based on insulin sensitivity index and BMI: Lean (BMI < 27.5 kg m^{-2}) or Obese (BMI ≥ 27.5 kg m^{-2})	Randomized, double-blinded, crossover	Subjects consumed NCEP step 1 diet with 4 week periods of 0 and 4 eggs d^{-1} with a 4 week washout 3 groups: Lean insulin-sensitive Lean insulin-resistant Obese insulin-resistant	20 weeks	From baseline: ↑ CRP and SAA in lean insulin-sensitive group only with 4 eggs d^{-1}

(continued)

Table 4.3 (*continued*)

Study	No. of individuals enrolled, sex and age	Population characteristics	Design	Intervention	Duration	Results[b]
Individuals at risk of CVD or with type 2 diabetes						
Blesso *et al.*, 2013[25]	$n = 40$ recruited ($n = 37$ completed) 25F/12M 30–70 years	Participants with MetS based on the NCEP ATP III No significant difference between groups at baseline	Randomized, single-blind, parallel	Participants followed a moderate carbohydrate-restricted diet and were randomly assign to: EGG: 3 whole eggs d^{-1} ($n = 20$) or egg SUB ($n = 17$) groups	12 weeks	From baseline: ↓ BW in both groups ↓ SAA and TNF-α in EGG group only ↔ CRP, IL-6, IL-10 in both groups No difference between groups
Fuller *et al.*, 2015[26]	$n = 140$ recruited ($n = 121$ completed) 77F/63M ≥18 years	Individuals with prediabetes or type 2 diabetes (BMI ≥ 25 kg m^{-2} and HbA1C < 9.5%)	Randomized, parallel	Participants followed an isocaloric diet and were assigned to: high-egg diet (2 eggs d^{-1}; 6 d $week^{-1}$; $n = 60$) or low-egg diet (<2 eggs $week^{-1}$ + 10 g animal protein; $n = 61$)	12 weeks	From baseline: ↔ CRP in both groups No difference between groups
Ballesteros *et al.*, 2015[23]	$n = 33$ recruited ($n = 29$ completed) 19F/10M 35–65 years	Subjects with controlled type 2 diabetes (HbA1c <9%). All subjects were on glucose-lowering medication	Randomized, single-blind, crossover	2 isocaloric breakfasts: 1 egg d^{-1} or 40 g of oatmeal with 2 cups d^{-1} lactose-free milk. Subjects allocated to 1 of the 2 breakfasts for 5 weeks with a 3-week washout	13 weeks	Between groups: ↔ BW and BMI ↓ TNF-α and a trend to ↓ IL-6 ($p = 0.051$) with egg ↔ CR

[a]Abbreviations: BMI, body mass index; BW, body weight; BP, blood pressure; WC, waist circumference; CRP, C-reactive protein; F, female; M, male; IL, interleukin; SAA, serum amyloid A; TNF-α, tumor necrosis factor alpha; MetS, metabolic syndrome; NCEP ATP III, National Cholesterol Education Program Adult Treatment Panel III.
[b]↓ indicates a decrease, ↑ indicates an increase, ↔ indicates no effect.

4.5 Egg Consumption and TMAO

Choline metabolites have recently gained attention in relation to atherosclerosis development.[57] Trimethylamine-*N*-oxide (TMAO) is an oxidation product of trimethylamine (TMA) produced endogenously by phosphatidylcholine metabolism by the microbiome.[58] Some studies have observed a positive relationship between plasma TMAO levels and CVD.[59–62] Furthermore, dietary choline, as well as TMAO supplementation, in mice has been shown to promote atherosclerosis.[61] Major dietary sources of phosphatidylcholine include eggs, milk, red meat and fish.[63] Therefore, we reviewed the literature regarding the impact of egg consumption on this emerging CVD risk factor.

Three randomized crossover intervention studies in healthy individuals have investigated the impact of egg consumption on plasma TMAO concentrations. DiMarco *et al.*[64] examined the effect of consuming 1, 2 and 3 eggs per day for 4 weeks compared to a no-egg 2 week run-in period. No change in plasma TMAO concentrations was observed with egg consumption. However, plasma choline concentrations increased along with the increase in egg intake. Similarly, Missimer *et al.*[34] demonstrated that consumption of 2 eggs per day for 4 weeks had no effect on plasma TMAO levels but increased plasma choline concentrations when compared to an oatmeal breakfast. Finally, Lemos *et al.*[57] also reported no change in plasma TMAO concentrations with the consumption of 3 eggs per day for 4 weeks compared to a 2 week run-in period with no egg. They also reported a greater increase in plasma choline concentrations compared to the choline supplementation phase (1.5 tablets of choline bitartrate).

Despite the recent concern about egg intake and its phosphatidylcholine content, evidence does not support the association between egg consumption and increased plasma levels of TMAO, at least in healthy individuals. Nevertheless, the number of interventions that have assessed the impact of egg consumption on plasma TMAO is limited. Further studies in individuals at high risk of CVD are needed before we can conclude on the effects of egg consumption on plasma TMAO levels in this population. This is particularly important since TMAO is produced by the gut microbiota and differences in microbiota species have been reported between healthy lean individuals and overweight/obese individuals (Table 4.4).

4.6 Conclusions

Although egg consumption has been a health concern owing to their high dietary cholesterol content, to date randomized intervention studies have failed to demonstrate an adverse effect of egg consumption on traditional and non-traditional CVD risk factors. Data reported in this chapter suggest that intake of up to 3 eggs d^{-1} does not increase clinical biomarkers of CVD, including markers of inflammation, endothelial function and plasma TMAO concentrations. Moreover, egg consumption seems to improve LDL

Table 4.4 Effects of egg consumption on TMAO.[a]

Study	No. of individuals enrolled, sex and age	Population characteristics	Design	Intervention	Duration	Results[b]
DiMarco *et al.*, 2017[64]	n = 40 recruited (n = 37 completed) 20F/20M 18–30 years	Healthy and young subjects with a BMI between 18.5 and 29.9 kg m^{-2}	Crossover	Began with a 2 week washout period (no eggs). Then, subjects were fed with 1 egg d^{-1} for 4 weeks, 2 eggs d^{-1} for 4 weeks and 3 eggs d^{-1} for 4 weeks	14 weeks	Between groups: ↔ BMI and W ↔ TMAO ↑ Plasma choline with egg intake
Missimer *et al.*, 2018[34]	n = 50 recruited (n = 48 completed) 24F/26M 18–30 years	Healthy and young individuals with a BMI between 18.5 and 29.9 kg m^{-2}	Randomized, single-blind, crossover	Participants were assigned to consume 2 eggs or 1 packet of oatmeal per day for 4 weeks with a 3 week washout period	11 weeks	Between groups: ↔ In BW and BMI ↔ TMAO ↑ Plasma choline with egg
Lemos *et al.*, 2018[57]	n = 30 recruited (n = 29 completed) 16F/14M 18–30 years	Healthy and young subjects with a BMI of 18.5–29.9 kg m^{-2}.	Randomized, crossover	2 week run-in period (no egg). Subjects allocated to 1 of the 2 breakfasts: EGG group: 3 eggs d^{-1}; choline group: 1.5 tablets of choline Bitartrate for 4 weeks with a 3 week washout	13 weeks	From baseline: ↔ BMI ↔ TMAO ↑ Plasma choline in EGG group and *vs.* choline group

[a]Abbreviations: BMI, body mass index; BW, body weight; WC, waist circumference; F, female; M, male; TMAO, trimethylamine *N*-oxide.
[b]↓ indicates a decrease, ↑ indicates an increase, ↔ indicates no effect.

particle phenotype by increasing the number of large LDL particles and improving HDL-C concentrations in both healthy individuals and those at risk of CVD. It is important to stress that most of these interventions have increased egg intake as part of a healthy diet and often promote weight loss in obese individuals. Therefore, we can conclude that, based on the available evidence, egg consumption, as part of a healthy diet, has no adverse effect on the cardiometabolic health of healthy individuals and those at risk of CVD.

Summary

- Egg intake between 1 and 3 eggs d^{-1} as part of a healthy diet has little effect on major traditional CVD risk factors.
- Egg consumption improves LDL particle phenotype with larger LDL particles.
- Egg consumption increases HDL-C concentrations in both healthy individuals and those at risk of CVD.
- In healthy individuals, egg intake appears to have no effect on emerging CVD risk factors, including plasma TMAO.

Acknowledgements

This book chapter was supported by CR's discovery grant from the Natural Sciences and Engineering Research Council of Canada (NSERC). Outside the submitted work, CR also reports grants from the Canadian Institutes of Health Research (CIHR) and Dairy Farmers of Canada (DFC); CJF reports grants from NSERC, CIHR, Canadian Foundation for Dietetic Research and DFC; RLJ reports grants from NSERC and CIHR. JAB is a graduate student funded by the Consejo Nacional de Ciencia y Tecnología (CONACYT).

References

1. World Health Organization, *Global Status Report on Noncommunicable Diseases 2010*, World Health Organization, Geneva, Switzerland, 2011.
2. J. D. Griffin and A. H. Lichtenstein, Dietary Cholesterol and Plasma Lipoprotein Profiles: Randomized-Controlled Trials, *Curr. Nutr. Rep.*, 2013, 2(4), 274–282.
3. US Department of Health and Human Services and US Department of Agriculture, *2015–2020 Dietary Guidelines for Americans*, Washington, DC, 8th edn, December 2015.
4. National Heart Foundation of Australia, *Dietary fats and dietary cholesterol for cardiovascular health*, http://heartfoundation.org.au/images/uploads/publications/Dietary-fats-summary-evidence.pdf, accessed July 10 2018.

5. British Heart Foundation, https://www.bhf.org.uk/heart-health/preventing-heart-disease/healthy-eating, accessed July 9 2018.
6. S. Berger, G. Raman, R. Vishwanathan, P. F. Jacques and E. J. Johnson, Dietary cholesterol and cardiovascular disease: a systematic review and meta-analysis, *Am. J. Clin. Nutr.*, 2015, **102**(2), 276–294.
7. N. R. Fuller, A. Sainsbury, I. D. Caterson and T. P. Markovic, Egg Consumption and Human Cardio-Metabolic Health in People with and without Diabetes, *Nutrients*, 2015, **7**(9), 7399–7420.
8. Y. Li, C. Zhou, X. Zhou and L. Li, Egg consumption and risk of cardiovascular diseases and diabetes: a meta-analysis, *Atherosclerosis*, 2013, **229**(2), 524–530.
9. Y. Rong, L. Chen, T. Zhu, Y. Song, M. Yu and Z. Shan, *et al.*, Egg consumption and risk of coronary heart disease and stroke: dose-response meta-analysis of prospective cohort studies, *BMJ*, 2013, **346**, e8539.
10. N. L. Tran, L. M. Barraj, J. M. Heilman and C. G. Scrafford, Egg consumption and cardiovascular disease among diabetic individuals: a systematic review of the literature, *Diabetes, Metab. Syndr. Obes.*, 2014, **7**, 121–137.
11. J. Y. Shin, P. Xun, Y. Nakamura and K. He, Egg consumption in relation to risk of cardiovascular disease and diabetes: a systematic review and meta-analysis, *Am. J. Clin. Nutr.*, 2013, **98**(1), 146–159.
12. E. Applegate, Introduction: nutritional and functional roles of eggs in the diet, *J. Am. Coll. Nutr.*, 2000, **19**(5 Suppl), 495S–498S.
13. S. M. Grundy, J. I. Cleeman, S. R. Daniels, K. A. Donato, R. H. Eckel and B. A. Franklin, *et al.*, Diagnosis and management of the metabolic syndrome: an American Heart Association/National Heart, Lung, and Blood Institute Scientific Statement, *Circulation*, 2005, **112**(17), 2735–2752.
14. S. M. Grundy, J. I. Cleeman, C. N. Merz, H. B. Brewer Jr, L. T. Clark and D. B. Hunninghake, *et al.*, Implications of recent clinical trials for the National Cholesterol Education Program Adult Treatment Panel III guidelines, *Circulation*, 2004, **110**(2), 227–239.
15. K. K. Berneis and R. M. Krauss, Metabolic origins and clinical significance of LDL heterogeneity, *J. Lipid Res.*, 2002, **43**(9), 1363–1379.
16. N. F. Galeano, M. Al-Haideri, F. Keyserman, S. C. Rumsey and R. J. Deckelbaum, Small dense low density lipoprotein has increased affinity for LDL receptor-independent cell surface binding sites: a potential mechanism for increased atherogenicity, *J. Lipid Res.*, 1998, **39**(6), 1263–1273.
17. P. Tornvall, F. Karpe, L. A. Carlson and A. Hamsten, Relationships of low density lipoprotein subfractions to angiographically defined coronary artery disease in young survivors of myocardial infarction, *Atherosclerosis*, 1991, **90**(1), 67–80.
18. D. C. Chan, P. H. Barrett and G. F. Watts, Lipoprotein transport in the metabolic syndrome: pathophysiological and interventional studies employing stable isotopy and modelling methods, *Clin. Sci.*, 2004, **107**(3), 233–249.

19. F. M. Sacks and H. Campos, Clinical review 163: Cardiovascular endocrinology: Low-density lipoprotein size and cardiovascular disease: a reappraisal, *J. Clin. Endocrinol. Metab.*, 2003, **88**(10), 4525–4532.
20. T. Kita, N. Kume, M. Minami, K. Hayashida, T. Murayama and H. Sano, *et al.*, Role of oxidized LDL in atherosclerosis, *Ann. N. Y. Acad. Sci.*, 2001, **947**, 199–205; discussion -6.
21. S. Parthasarathy, A. Raghavamenon, M. O. Garelnabi and N. Santanam, Oxidized low-density lipoprotein, *Methods Mol. Biol.*, 2010, **610**, 403–417.
22. C. Richard, L. Cristall, E. Fleming, E. D. Lewis, M. Ricupero and R. L. Jacobs, *et al.*, Impact of Egg Consumption on Cardiovascular Risk Factors in Individuals with Type 2 Diabetes and at Risk for Developing Diabetes: A Systematic Review of Randomized Nutritional Intervention Studies, *Can. J. Diabetes*, 2017, **41**, 453–463.
23. M. N. Ballesteros, F. Valenzuela, A. E. Robles, E. Artalejo, D. Aguilar and C. J. Andersen, *et al.*, One Egg per Day Improves Inflammation when Compared to an Oatmeal-Based Breakfast without Increasing Other Cardiometabolic Risk Factors in Diabetic Patients, *Nutrients*, 2015, **7**(5), 3449–3463.
24. C. N. Blesso, C. J. Andersen, J. Barona, J. S. Volek and M. L. Fernandez, Whole egg consumption improves lipoprotein profiles and insulin sensitivity to a greater extent than yolk-free egg substitute in individuals with metabolic syndrome, *Metabolism*, 2013, **62**(3), 400–410.
25. C. N. Blesso, C. J. Andersen, J. Barona, B. Volk, J. S. Volek and M. L. Fernandez, Effects of carbohydrate restriction and dietary cholesterol provided by eggs on clinical risk factors in metabolic syndrome, *J. Clin. Lipidol.*, 2013, **7**(5), 463–471.
26. N. R. Fuller, I. D. Caterson, A. Sainsbury, G. Denyer, M. Fong and J. Gerofi, *et al.*, The effect of a high-egg diet on cardiovascular risk factors in people with type 2 diabetes: the Diabetes and Egg (DIABEGG) study-a 3-mo randomized controlled trial, *Am. J. Clin. Nutr.*, 2015, **101**(4), 705–713.
27. R. H. Knopp, B. Retzlaff, B. Fish, C. Walden, S. Wallick and M. Anderson, *et al.*, Effects of insulin resistance and obesity on lipoproteins and sensitivity to egg feeding, *Arterioscler., Thromb., Vasc. Biol.*, 2003, **23**(8), 1437–1443.
28. G. Mutungi, J. Ratliff, M. Puglisi, M. Torres-Gonzalez, U. Vaishnav and J. O. Leite, *et al.*, Dietary cholesterol from eggs increases plasma HDL cholesterol in overweight men consuming a carbohydrate-restricted diet, *J. Nutr.*, 2008, **138**(2), 272–276.
29. G. Mutungi, D. Waters, J. Ratliff, M. Puglisi, R. M. Clark and J. S. Volek, *et al.*, Eggs distinctly modulate plasma carotenoid and lipoprotein subclasses in adult men following a carbohydrate-restricted diet, *J. Nutr. Biochem.*, 2010, **21**(4), 261–267.
30. K. L. Pearce, P. M. Clifton and M. Noakes, Egg consumption as part of an energy-restricted high-protein diet improves blood lipid and blood glucose profiles in individuals with type 2 diabetes, *Br. J. Nutr.*, 2011, **105**(4), 584–592.

31. J. Ratliff, G. Mutungi, M. J. Puglisi, J. S. Volek and M. L. Fernandez, Carbohydrate restriction (with or without additional dietary cholesterol provided by eggs) reduces insulin resistance and plasma leptin without modifying appetite hormones in adult men, *Nutr. Res.*, 2009, **29**(4), 262–268.
32. L. R. Tannock, K. D. O'Brien, R. H. Knopp, B. Retzlaff, B. Fish and M. H. Wener, *et al.*, Cholesterol feeding increases C-reactive protein and serum amyloid A levels in lean insulin-sensitive subjects, *Circulation*, 2005, **111**(23), 3058–3062.
33. N. L. Harman, A. R. Leeds and B. A. Griffin, Increased dietary cholesterol does not increase plasma low density lipoprotein when accompanied by an energy-restricted diet and weight loss, *Eur. J. Nutr.*, 2008, **47**(6), 287–293.
34. A. Missimer, M. L. Fernandez, D. M. DiMarco, G. H. Norris, C. N. Blesso and A. G. Murillo, *et al.*, Compared to an Oatmeal Breakfast, Two Eggs/Day Increased Plasma Carotenoids and Choline without Increasing Trimethyl Amine *N*-Oxide Concentrations, *J. Am. Coll. Nutr.*, 2018, **37**(2), 140–148.
35. A. Missimer, D. M. DiMarco, C. J. Andersen, A. G. Murillo, M. Vergara-Jimenez and M. L. Fernandez, Consuming Two Eggs per Day, as Compared to an Oatmeal Breakfast, Decreases Plasma Ghrelin while Maintaining the LDL/HDL Ratio, *Nutrients*, 2017, **9**(2), 89.
36. D. M. DiMarco, G. H. Norris, C. L. Millar, C. N. Blesso and M. L. Fernandez, Intake of up to 3 Eggs per Day Is Associated with Changes in HDL Function and Increased Plasma Antioxidants in Healthy, Young Adults, *J. Nutr.*, 2017, **147**(3), 323–329.
37. B. S. Lemos, I. Medina-Vera, C. N. Blesso and M. L. Fernandez, Intake of 3 Eggs per Day When Compared to a Choline Bitartrate Supplement, Downregulates Cholesterol Synthesis without Changing the LDL/HDL Ratio, *Nutrients*, 2018, **10**(2), 258.
38. J. Davignon and P. Ganz, Role of endothelial dysfunction in atherosclerosis, *Circulation*, 2004, **109**(23 Suppl 1), III27–III32.
39. H. A. Hadi, C. S. Carr and J. Al Suwaidi, Endothelial dysfunction: cardiovascular risk factors, therapy, and outcome, *Vasc. Health Risk Manage.*, 2005, **1**(3), 183–198.
40. E. Bonora, S. Kiechl, J. Willeit, F. Oberhollenzer, G. Egger and R. C. Bonadonna, *et al.*, Metabolic syndrome: epidemiology and more extensive phenotypic description. Cross-sectional data from the Bruneck Study, *Int. J. Obes. Relat. Metab. Disord.*, 2003, **27**(10), 1283–1289.
41. A. Fornoni and L. Raij, Metabolic syndrome and endothelial dysfunction, *Curr. Hypertens. Rep.*, 2005, **7**(2), 88–95.
42. S. J. Hwang, C. M. Ballantyne, A. R. Sharrett, L. C. Smith, C. E. Davis and A. M. Gotto Jr, *et al.*, Circulating adhesion molecules VCAM-1, ICAM-1, and E-selectin in carotid atherosclerosis and incident coronary heart disease cases: the Atherosclerosis Risk In Communities (ARIC) study, *Circulation*, 1997, **96**(12), 4219–4225.

43. P. M. Ridker, J. E. Buring and N. Rifai, Soluble P-selectin and the risk of future cardiovascular events, *Circulation*, 2001, **103**(4), 491–495.
44. O. T. Raitakari and D. S. Celermajer, Flow-mediated dilatation, *Br. J. Clin. Pharmacol.*, 2000, **50**(5), 397–404.
45. D. L. Katz, J. Gnanaraj, J. A. Treu, Y. Ma, Y. Kavak and V. Y. Njike, Effects of egg ingestion on endothelial function in adults with coronary artery disease: a randomized, controlled, crossover trial, *Am. Heart J.*, 2015, **169**(1), 162–169.
46. V. Njike, Z. Faridi, S. Dutta, A. L. Gonzalez-Simon and D. L. Katz, Daily egg consumption in hyperlipidemic adults – effects on endothelial function and cardiovascular risk, *Nutr. J.*, 2010, **9**, 28.
47. J. T. Willerson and P. M. Ridker, Inflammation as a cardiovascular risk factor, *Circulation*, 2004, **109**(21 Suppl 1), II2–II10.
48. G. J. Blake and P. M. Ridker, Novel clinical markers of vascular wall inflammation, *Circ. Res.*, 2001, **89**(9), 763–771.
49. A. H. Berg and P. E. Scherer, Adipose tissue, inflammation, and cardiovascular disease, *Circ. Res.*, 2005, **96**(9), 939–949.
50. E. Golia, G. Limongelli, F. Natale, F. Fimiani, V. Maddaloni and I. Pariggiano, *et al.*, Inflammation and cardiovascular disease: from pathogenesis to therapeutic target, *Curr. Atheroscler. Rep.*, 2014, **16**(9), 435.
51. P. Libby, P. M. Ridker and A. Maseri, Inflammation and atherosclerosis, *Circulation*, 2002, **105**(9), 1135–1143.
52. B. B. Duncan, M. I. Schmidt, J. S. Pankow, C. M. Ballantyne, D. Couper and A. Vigo, *et al.*, Low-grade systemic inflammation and the development of type 2 diabetes: the atherosclerosis risk in communities study, *Diabetes*, 2003, **52**(7), 1799–1805.
53. T. A. Pearson, G. A. Mensah, R. W. Alexander, J. L. Anderson, R. O. Cannon 3rd and M. Criqui, *et al.*, Markers of inflammation and cardiovascular disease: application to clinical and public health practice: A statement for healthcare professionals from the Centers for Disease Control and Prevention and the American Heart Association, *Circulation*, 2003, **107**(3), 499–511.
54. P. M. Ridker, N. Rifai, L. Rose, J. E. Buring and N. R. Cook, Comparison of C-reactive protein and low-density lipoprotein cholesterol levels in the prediction of first cardiovascular events, *N. Engl. J. Med.*, 2002, **347**(20), 1557–1565.
55. B. D. Johnson, K. E. Kip, O. C. Marroquin, P. M. Ridker, S. F. Kelsey and L. J. Shaw, *et al.*, Serum amyloid A as a predictor of coronary artery disease and cardiovascular outcome in women: the National Heart, Lung, and Blood Institute-Sponsored Women's Ischemia Syndrome Evaluation (WISE), *Circulation*, 2004, **109**(6), 726–732.
56. R. Z. Yang, M. J. Lee, H. Hu, T. I. Pollin, A. S. Ryan and B. J. Nicklas, *et al.*, Acute-phase serum amyloid A: an inflammatory adipokine and potential link between obesity and its metabolic complications, *PLoS Med.*, 2006, **3**(6), e287.

57. B. S. Lemos, I. Medina-Vera, O. V. Malysheva, M. A. Caudill and M. L. Fernandez, Effects of Egg Consumption and Choline Supplementation on Plasma Choline and Trimethylamine-*N*-Oxide in a Young Population, *J. Am. Coll. Nutr.*, 2018, 1–8.
58. S. L. Hazen and J. M. Brown, Eggs as a dietary source for gut microbial production of trimethylamine-*N*-oxide, *Am. J. Clin. Nutr.*, 2014, **100**(3), 741–743.
59. R. A. Koeth, Z. Wang, B. S. Levison, J. A. Buffa, E. Org and B. T. Sheehy, *et al.*, Intestinal microbiota metabolism of L-carnitine, a nutrient in red meat, promotes atherosclerosis, *Nat. Med.*, 2013, **19**(5), 576–585.
60. W. H. Tang, Z. Wang, B. S. Levison, R. A. Koeth, E. B. Britt and X. Fu, *et al.*, Intestinal microbial metabolism of phosphatidylcholine and cardiovascular risk, *N. Engl. J. Med.*, 2013, **368**(17), 1575–1584.
61. Z. Wang, E. Klipfell, B. J. Bennett, R. Koeth, B. S. Levison and B. Dugar, *et al.*, Gut flora metabolism of phosphatidylcholine promotes cardiovascular disease, *Nature*, 2011, **472**(7341), 57–63.
62. A. Mente, K. Chalcraft, H. Ak, A. D. Davis, E. Lonn and R. Miller, *et al.*, The Relationship Between Trimethylamine-*N*-Oxide and Prevalent Cardiovascular Disease in a Multiethnic Population Living in Canada, *Can. J. Cardiol.*, 2015, **31**(9), 1189–1194.
63. S. H. Zeisel, M. H. Mar, J. C. Howe and J. M. Holden, Concentrations of choline-containing compounds and betaine in common foods, *J. Nutr.*, 2003, **133**(5), 1302–1307.
64. D. M. DiMarco, A. Missimer, A. G. Murillo, B. S. Lemos, O. V. Malysheva and M. A. Caudill, *et al.*, Intake of up to 3 Eggs/Day Increases HDL Cholesterol and Plasma Choline While Plasma Trimethylamine-*N*-oxide is Unchanged in a Healthy Population, *Lipids*, 2017, **52**(3), 255–263.

CHAPTER 5

Food for Thought – Eggs and Neurocognition

NICOLE SEKEL[a], RAFIA VIRK[a] AND TAYLOR C. WALLACE*[a,b]

[a]Department of Nutrition and Food Studies, George Mason University, MS: 1F7, 4400 University Drive, Fairfax, VA 22030, USA; [b]Think Healthy Group, Inc., 127 U Street NW, Washington, DC 20001, USA
*E-mail: taylor.wallace@me.com

5.1 Nutrition and Cognitive Neuroscience

Nutrition plays a vital role in brain function throughout the life cycle, with profound implications for mental health and degenerative disease. The role of nutrition in cognitive neuroscience is complex because, as with all aspects of nutrition, it is multifactorial. Many aspects of nutrition, from entire diets to individual nutrients, have been associated with cognition, mental health, dysfunction, and disease.[1–5] It is not surprising that nutrition affects cognition across the lifespan because brain structure and function are ultimately dependent on nutritional input. However, it is difficult to assess the precise actions of specific foods and dietary components because individuals consume whole diets, have genetic variations, and differ in baseline status of each individual nutrient.[6] In recent years, advances have been made in several key areas of nutrition and cognitive neuroscience. Two key factors are of particular importance: early environment and

Food Chemistry, Function and Analysis No.14
Eggs as Functional Foods and Nutraceuticals for Human Health
Edited by Jianping Wu

Published by the Royal Society of Chemistry, www.rsc.org

genetic variability. Early nutrition profoundly influences mental health later in life, and multiple gene variants markedly alter the cognitive response to nutrition.

Cognition is key to sustaining quality of life and refers to the mental processes involved in acquiring knowledge and the integration of these processes into responses such as learning, attention, memory, intelligence, and consciousness. Suboptimal cognitive development during the first 1000 days post-conception, owing to macronutrient and micronutrient deficiencies, is prevalent at high rates in the developing world and is certainly not absent in developed countries. Research suggests a direct relationship between maternal and early childhood nutrition and cognitive function across the lifespan.[7] The American Academy of Pediatrics (AAP) advocates that protein, zinc, iron, choline, folate, iodine, vitamin A, vitamin D, vitamin B_6, vitamin B_{12}, and long-chain polyunsaturated fatty acids are of particular importance during the first 1000 days in order to support child development and prevent lifelong deficits in brain function.[8] Even past the first 1000 days of life, a handful of studies suggest that mental development in preschoolers is predictive of later academic achievement.[9]

Cognition in the aging population is also of particular interest because older individuals often experience cognitive decline and may develop dementia and/or Alzheimer's disease.[10–12] An increasing body of research suggests a relationship between nutritional status during adolescence to middle/older adulthood and the speed of cognitive decline later in life;[7] however, critical windows during which optimal nutrition may have the greatest impact, if present, have yet to be identified in the peer-reviewed literature. Over the last 100 years, the human lifespan has increased exponentially and with that, there are more elderly people now than ever before. Virtually every country in the world is experiencing growth in the number and proportion of older people in their population. Between 2015 and 2030, the number of people aged ≥ 60 years worldwide is projected to grow by 56%, from 901 million to 1.4 billion; by 2050, the global population of older people is projected to more than double its size in 2015, reaching nearly 2.1 billion.[13] As the elderly population increases, so too does the incidence of people with cognitive impairment. The ability to carry out complex thought processes is the basis for maintaining quality of life; elderly individuals with cognitive impairment may have few alternatives to entering assisted living facilities.[10–12] Therefore, the goal is to slow this inevitable cognitive decline so that individuals can maintain quality of life as they age. To accomplish this, health systems should prepare now to address cognitive impairment and other specific health concerns of older people.

5.2 Current Research on Whole Eggs and Cognition

Considering the rapidly growing body of evidence, nutritional strategies should be employed to achieve and maintain substantial cognitive development across the lifespan. Emerging evidence suggests that eggs might play an important role in promoting and maintaining cognitive function throughout life. Eggs contain many of the essential nutrients that the AAP has highlighted for their importance in brain development. Whole eggs are a rich source of complete protein, essential fatty acids, B vitamins (including choline), vitamins A and D, iron, and selenium. They are particularly rich in the xanthophyll carotenoid lutein, which has recently been shown to have consistent and strong associations with cognitive development and maintenance.[14] Although more lutein is found in dark green leafy vegetables than in eggs, the lipid-rich matrix of the egg increases its bioavailability threefold in comparison.[15] Eggs are also a primary contributor of choline to the diet and are a source of docosahexaenoic acid (DHA).[16] The nutrient package present in eggs, with particular emphasis on lutein and choline, has been distinctively associated with brain development as well as a reduced risk of cognitive decline.[17,18] The egg yolk composition is primarily nutritive, whereas the egg white serves mainly as a defense mechanism against pathogens.

Large regional differences in egg consumption exist. The prevalence of egg consumption among African children is less than half that of most other world regions and is threefold less than in Latin America and the Caribbean. The general U.S. population consumes approximately 24 g d^{-1} of whole eggs (approximately half an egg), either as whole eggs or as part of prepared foods.[19] Among women of reproductive age, egg consumption is strongly associated with socioeconomic status in a dose–response fashion, with women in the lowest wealth quintile consuming the fewest eggs and those in the highest wealth quintile consuming the most. Cultural factors likely play a role in worldwide consumption of eggs during early childhood and across the lifespan; however, economic barriers that limit access are likely to be far more important than cultural ones in explaining low consumption.[20] Owing to their increasing availability around the world, eggs have the potential to act as a nutrition vehicle from which individuals can more easily obtain nutrients known to promote cognitive development and maintenance.

There is a limited but emerging scientific body of evidence suggesting that adequate consumption of whole eggs promotes higher cognitive processes.[21–25] A landmark randomized controlled trial, the "Lulun Project" in Ecuador, recently suggested that egg nutrition could improve the nutrient status associated with healthy brain development and function in a rural population of Andean children who were enrolled at age 6–9 months at the initiation of the study.[21] Biomarkers previously associated with improved child development and important physiological processes in the brain showed increased concentrations in the egg group compared to the control. Blood concentrations increased by effect sizes of 0.35 for choline and 0.43 for DHA.[26] Overall, Ecuadorian children that consumed approximately one egg per day for 6 months experienced a 47% reduced rate of stunting, a strong indicator of lifelong cognition.[21] A similar observational study of infants enrolled in the U.S. National Health and Nutrition Examination

Survey (NHANES) showed similar results, with egg consumption increasing intakes of several nutrients, including protein, lutein plus zeaxanthin, choline, DHA, vitamin B_{12}, selenium, and phosphorus.[27] Another study examined the role of egg intake with incidence of dementia, Alzheimer's disease, and cognitive ability in 2427 middle-aged men at baseline. After a 21.9 year follow-up, increased egg intake was beneficially associated with enhanced performance on both neuropsychological and verbal frequency tests. The researchers concluded that each additional 0.5 egg per day was related to a decrease in the incidence of dementia.[22] Other observational studies on the elderly population also show inverse associations between egg consumption and mild cognitive decline.[23–25] One cross-sectional analysis of 178 elderly institutionalized individuals (aged ≥ 65 years) found that those with a higher egg intake did not make as many mistakes on the Short Portable Mental Status Questionnaire.[23] Together, these studies suggest that egg consumption in early and mid-life may be linked to cognitive decline later in life; however, additional studies are needed as evidence is emerging. These studies do not show eggs to help improve cognitive function in those with current cognitive impairment, which is yet another important research gap.

5.3 The Incredible, Edible Choline Powerhouse

Choline's role in human health begins prenatally and extends into adulthood and old age. Choline status is especially important to the mother and child during lactation since human milk is rich in choline. The functions of choline related to cognition are complex and include, but are not limited to, neurotransmitter synthesis (acetylcholine), cell membrane signaling (phospholipids), lipid transport (lipoproteins), and methyl-group metabolism (homocysteine conversion to methionine).

5.3.1 Choline in Placental Health

Emerging evidence supports the need for an adequate choline supply for proper placenta function throughout pregnancy. To sustain both maternal and fetal health, the placenta must function optimally; impaired placental function can lead to maternal disease (*e.g.*, pre-eclampsia) or hinder fetal development and growth. A randomized controlled trial found significant changes in the expression of genes regulating placental vascularization, angiogenesis, and stress reactivity when women in their third trimester were supplemented with 930 mg d^{-1} of choline compared with the control (480 mg d^{-1}). Placental expression of antiangiogenic factor Fms-like tyrosine kinase-1 (sFLT1) is decreased with higher maternal choline intake.[28,29] This decrease was previously shown to result in a reduced risk for developing preeclampsia and stress disorders later in life. *In vitro* analyses suggest that lower choline availability induces inflammation,[30] which may negatively interfere with early placental development and the arterial remodeling necessary for proper placental perfusion and nutrient transfer to the fetus. These results have been replicated in rodent models, whereby higher dietary choline decreases markers of inflammation and angiogenesis and enhances nutrient transfer (particularly DHA) across the placenta to the fetus.[31,32]

5.3.2 Neurological Birth Defects

A small number of human studies have assessed maternal choline intake or status and illustrated a potential association with neurological birth defects in offspring, as recently reviewed by Wallace.[14] Research suggests an inverse relationship between higher maternal choline intakes (estimated using food frequency questionnaires) and spina bifida.[33–36] A case-controlled retrospective study (440 neural defect cases and 440 controls) found an inverse relationship between dietary choline intake and incidence of spina bifida.[36] On the contrary, a longitudinal study of 955 infants found that there was an insignificant decline in the incidence of spina bifida.[33] Differences in these studies could be due to common single nucleotide polymorphisms (SNPs) that alter the choline and/or folate requirements. For instance, approximately 15–30% of humans possess genetic polymorphisms that alter the activity of methylenetetrahydrofolate dehydrogenase 1 (MTHFD1), resulting in a greater requirement for folate or potentially for choline, even when dietary intake of folate is high.[37]

5.3.3 Prenatal and Child Cognitive Development

Both animal and human studies have shown that higher choline intakes during the perinatal period have a lasting neuroprotective effect. Caudill *et al.*[38] reported effects of human maternal choline supplementation (480 or 930 mg d^{-1}) during the third trimester on infant processing speed and visuospatial memory at 4, 7, 10, and 13 months of age ($n = 24$). This controlled feeding study found that maternal consumption of approximately twice the adequate intake (AI) for choline during the third trimester (*i.e.*, 930 *vs.* 480 mg d^{-1}) improved infant information processing speed. There was also a linear effect of exposure duration (*i.e.*, infants exposed longer showed faster reaction times) in the lower intake group (*i.e.*, 480 mg d^{-1}), suggesting that even modest increases in prenatal choline intake may produce cognitive benefits in humans.[38] To evaluate the persistence of the cognitive benefits observed by Caudill *et al.*, investigators recently conducted a follow-up study of the children in this cohort at 7 years of age.[39] Results of the cognitive assessment revealed lasting benefits of the higher maternal choline intake on child attention, memory, and problem-solving areas of cognition previously shown to be sensitive to maternal choline supplementation.[39] Although these findings must be confirmed in a larger sample, they provide compelling evidence that maternal choline intake during pregnancy has lasting effects on a child's cognitive function. A randomized controlled trial found null effects of 750 mg d^{-1}

of choline supplementation (as phosphatidylcholine) on infant cognitive function[39] from 18 weeks of gestation to 90 days postpartum. It is unclear why the investigators did not observe cognitive effects similar to those reported by Caudill *et al.*;[38] however, poor participant adherence and/or uncontrolled variations in intake of choline and other nutrients were suggested to play a role.[14] Data from observational studies are somewhat mixed but tend to also support that higher choline intakes during pregnancy enhance cognitive outcomes of offspring.[14] Consistent with the findings of Caudill *et al.*, data obtained from Project Viva in Massachusetts demonstrated that maternal choline intake within the AI range during pregnancy was associated with better memory function in children 7 years of age compared with children of mothers whose consumption was approximately 50% of the AI.[40]

A narrative review by McCann *et al.*[41] highlighted 34 rodent studies that examined choline during early development. The authors suggested that supplementation during pregnancy may strongly contribute to changes in neurological function in the fetus as well as improvement in postnatal cognitive behavioral tests across the lifespan. In rats, high maternal choline intake at specific times during the pregnancy and lactation periods enhances the cognitive ability of the offspring throughout life. Studies on rats suggest that there are two critical periods of brain development during which treatment with choline may result in lifelong enhancement of spatial memory. The first stage is during embryonic days 12–17 (rats give birth on day 21) and the second is during postnatal days 16–30.[17,42–51] A previous study showed that supplementation with choline in rats results in enhancement of memory performance on a 12 arm radial maze.[47] The improvement in spatial memory is directly related to cellular growth in the rat hippocampus during fetal brain development and to neuron growth for memory storage.[46,49] Considering these findings, it seems practical that consuming an egg-rich diet during pregnancy may have beneficial effects on infant brain development. Free choline concentrations have been used to assess choline status; however, concentrations are homeostatically regulated and plasma concentrations are rarely below 50% of the normal fasting concentration range (7–20 mmol L^{-1}), making it a poor indicator of status.[52]

5.3.4 The Relation of Choline Intake or Status to Cognition During Adulthood

Whether choline has immediate effects on cognition during early- to mid-adulthood is still relatively unknown; however, several short-duration challenge studies have evaluated choline intake and its relation to enhanced cognition.[53–63] A recent double-blind, placebo-controlled study showed supplementation with 2 g of choline bitartrate to have positive effects on action coordination in humans. 70 minutes post-ingestion, 28 participants performed a visuomotor aiming task in which they had to rapidly hit centers of targets. Participants hit targets more centrally after the choline treatment. Pupil size (a cognition-sensitive biomarker) also significantly decreased after choline intake and correlated positively with the hit distance to the targets and number of targets missed and negatively with reaction times. These findings suggest that choline uptake alters cholinergic functions in the nervous system.[59] Other challenge studies by Knott *et al.* have also suggested immediate benefits of choline bitartrate supplementation on multiple cognitive measures in young males with low baseline performance, as well as in those with increased P50 expression.[57,58,64] Studies using various cognitive battery assessments have shown mixed results. A 6 week interventional study of 65 individuals found that the group supplemented with phosphatidylcholine exhibited higher test scores pertinent to concentration and attention.[61] Conversely, a double-blind crossover study found no significant memory enhancement in the lecithin-supplemented group compared with a placebo group.[56]

5.3.5 Cognitive Maintenance During the Elderly Years

Blusztajn *et al.*[65] recently reviewed the mechanisms and clinical evidence in regard to neurodevelopmental and neuroprotective actions of choline. A recent Cochrane systematic review and meta-analysis of cytidinediphosphocholine (CDP choline) supplementation reported short-term improvements in memory and behavior deficits among elderly subjects with chronic cerebral disorders, although only one study lasted longer than 3 months. Evidence on global impression was also strong but limited by the duration of studies.[66] Higher choline intake has been inversely correlated with white-matter hyperintensity volume, a fairly well-accepted marker for Alzheimer's disease and age-related cognitive decline, among participants in the Framingham Offspring Cohort (average baseline intake, approximately 320 mg d^{-1}).[67] The strongest evidence for neuroprotection in humans stems from a case-controlled study of individuals with diagnosed cognitive decline, in which patients with Alzheimer's disease exhibited lower levels of eight choline-containing phospholipids (and two non-choline-containing species) compared with healthy controls. It should be noted that other causes may have been responsible for the disease state and this study was not designed to assess causality. These 10 lipids derived from peripheral blood have been validated to predict mild cognitive impairment or Alzheimer's disease within a 2 to 3 year timeframe with >90% accuracy.[68] Although no animal model of age-related cognitive decline fully imitates the human disease state, supplementation has been shown to influence Alzheimer's disease through modulation of the accumulation of amyloid plaques in mice.[65]

5.4 The Egg: An Excellent Bioavailable Source of Lutein

Carotenoids are naturally occurring pigments that are commonly found in the diet. Of the 40 carotenoids found commonly in foods, approximately 25 are measurable in human serum, tissues, and milk but only two (lutein and zeaxanthin) cross the blood–retina barrier to form macular pigment in the human retina. The preferential accumulation of these two carotenoids, also known as "xanthophylls", in the human retina can be explained by three retinal carotenoid-binding proteins: (1) a lutein-binding protein, steroidogenic acute regulatory protein-related lipid transfer domain-3 (StARD3); (2) a zeaxanthin-binding protein, glutathione *S*-transferase P1; and (3) tubulin, which serves as a site for high-capacity deposition of carotenoids in the retina with less specificity than the other two binding proteins.[69–71] The eye is an extension of the brain, with nerve tissue contained in the retina.[69–71] Subsequently, it is not surprising that a growing body of research collectively demonstrates that lutein has "vitamin-like" effects not only in the eye but also with respect to brain development and cognitive maintenance. StARD3 is an integral membrane protein that is proposed to be involved in intracellular lipid (*e.g.*, cholesterol) trafficking. This may be important in relation to cognitive function given that aberrations of cholesterol transport in the brain are often linked to suboptimal cognitive development as well as processes of aging and onset of neurological disorders, including Alzheimer's disease.[72] Similar to the retina, lutein is also the predominant carotenoid in human brain tissue both in early and late life.[73–75] Lutein accounts for 31% and 59% of total brain carotenoids in adults and infants, respectively[75,76] (Figure 5.1).

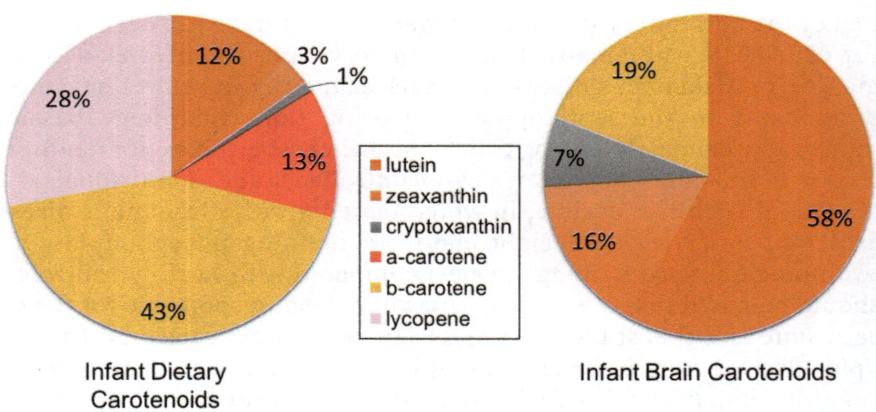

Figure 5.1 Dietary intake *vs.* brain uptake of carotenoids in infants. Data from ref. 73.

5.4.1 Macular Pigment Optical Density and Its Relationship to Cognition

Lutein and zeaxanthin intakes are highly correlated with their concentrations in the brain,[75,76] which makes macular pigment optical density (MPOD) a reflective marker of brain lutein and zeaxanthin. Cross-sectional studies show significant relationships between MPOD and cognitive health.[77–79] The ability to directly measure macular pigments provides the advantage of being able to monitor the results of an intervention. One can recommend foods rich in lutein or dietary supplements and then measure changes in MPOD, while assessing possible functional changes that result (and how those changes relate to an actual change in tissue levels). A number of studies have shown that higher intakes of lutein increase MPOD and alter behaviors that are thought to be mediated by the brain. For example, a diet high in lutein-rich avocados has been shown to increase MPOD and spatial working memory.[80] Young subjects supplemented with lutein showed improvements in visual temporal processing speed when MPOD increased by 0.1 log units of optical density or more, using a placebo-controlled design.[81,82] MPOD has also been linked to numerous measures that are mediated by the brain, including cognition, auditory thresholds, balance time, reaction time, and temporal vision.[14]

5.4.2 Prenatal and Child Cognitive Development

Emerging evidence supports the hypothesis that lutein plays an important role in early human development. Lutein is the most abundant carotenoid in the umbilical cord plasma and its concentration has been strongly correlated with maternal plasma lutein, suggesting a possible role of lutein in the neonatal period.[83] Preferential accumulation in the infant brain again implies a possible role in central nervous system development[18] (Figure 5.1). In a metabolomic study, lutein concentrations were significantly correlated with neurotransmitters that are involved with neuronal proliferation and maturation, neurite outgrowth, and synapse formation.[47] Lutein supplementation in the first postnatal hours of life increases antioxidant potential and decreases oxidative stress.[84] Thus, lutein may be crucial in the development of the infant brain since it requires a higher amount of antioxidants owing to the higher metabolic rate.[85] Bioaccumulation of lutein during the early postnatal months is not fully understood owing to the lack of human infant tissue samples and because lutein is poorly absorbed and in negligible levels in the retina and brain of most experimental animal models, aside from primates.

5.4.3 The Relation of Choline Intake or Status to Cognition During Adulthood

Cognition studies in younger adults are scarce, given that they are less likely to experience changes in status with a nutritional intervention. However, studies by Bovier *et al.* found improvements in visual temporal processing speed that are correlated with changes in MPOD owing to increased dietary intake of lutein in young adults.[81,82] Visual processing speed is unique because although it is a lower-level visual function (basically, the fusion of square- and sine-wave modulated light), it is thought to be mediated by central brain mechanisms. Processing speed, in general, underlies many other complex cognitive traits that many have argued should be considered fundamental to cognition.[86] Daily supplementation with lutein (and zeaxanthin) increased MPOD and resulted in significant improvements in spatial memory, reasoning ability, and complex attention in a recent randomized, double-blind, placebo-controlled trial of younger healthy adults (aged 18–30 years; $n = 51$).[87] Two other cross-sectional studies report similar effects of lutein intake, status, or MPOD during young adulthood.[88,89] A 2017 study of healthy subjects ($n = 60$) by Walk *et al.* found that cognitive control was subsequently increased during cognitive control tasks designed to assess different aspects of attentional control. The authors found a relationship between MPOD and neuroelectric indices underlying cognitive control, suggesting that lutein may have a protective role in the central nervous system, prior to the onset of disease.[88] MPOD was also "significantly related" to reaction time and high-speed coincidence anticipation errors in younger adults, suggesting that it plays a critical role in visual and motor behavior and integration.[89] It is plausible that lutein may benefit neurocognitive function owing to some type of local, neural cell interaction, otherwise referred to as the neural efficiency hypothesis,[90] and is likely due to, at least in part, its antioxidant functions.[73]

5.4.4 Cognitive Maintenance During the Elderly Years

Although evidence is accumulating for the role of lutein in cognitive function among older adults, the majority of studies to date are correlative and thus cannot establish causation. However, a 4 month double-blinded, placebo-controlled trial of older women revealed that those who were supplemented with lutein (12 mg d^{-1}), DHA (800 mg d^{-1}), or a combination of both had improved verbal frequency scores compared with the placebo group. Memory scores and rate of learning improved significantly in the treatment group, which also trended toward more efficient learning.[91] A large, population-based prospective investigation of the Irish Longitudinal Study on Aging found a significant association between older adults with higher MPOD performing better than their lower MPOD counterparts on various indices of cognitive function, including cognitive assessment and prospective memory.[68] Examining the regional and subcellular membrane distribution of lutein (and zeaxanthin) in the brain will provide a critical starting point for understanding its role in the maintenance of cognition in older adulthood. Lutein, as stated previously, is likely neuroprotective through its role as an antioxidant, an effect that may apply globally and is not limited to specific regions of the brain or cognitive domains. The aging brain is especially vulnerable to free radical attack owing to its high polyunsaturated fatty acid content and high metabolic activity, as previously discussed. Since lutein is differentially localized to membrane domains rich in polyunsaturated fatty acids, including DHA, it is therefore well positioned to block oxidation of these vulnerable lipids.[92]

Elevated DHA oxidation has been observed in the brains of patients with Alzheimer's disease and in those with mild cognitive impairment;[93] therefore, this potential lipid-protective action by lutein may, in part, explain the inverse correlation between MPOD and Alzheimer's disease. Cognitive decline has been shown to be related to age-related eye diseases, suggesting that similar risk factors might be involved in their etiologies.[93] Dietary intake of lutein, as well as blood measures, have been frequently, but not always consistently, correlated with improved cognitive performance and functionality among middle-aged to older adults. MPOD has been steadily correlated with better global cognition in this group, including beneficial effects on balance ability, reaction time, verbal learning, and recall.[77–79,89,90,94,95] A randomized, double-blind intervention study of patients with Alzheimer's disease (n = 31) *versus* healthy control subjects (n = 31) found significant benefit in four of five spatial frequencies tested, resulting from supplementation with 10 mg d^{-1} of lutein and 2 mg d^{-1} of zeaxanthin in the Alzheimer's group.[96] Longitudinal evidence from the Three-City Bordeaux prospective cohort, in which nondemented elderly participants were followed for 10 years, found beneficial effects of five plasma carotenoids (beta-carotene, alpha-carotene, lycopene, lutein, zeaxanthin, and beta-cryptoxanthin) on the risk of developing dementia. However, lutein was the only plasma carotenoid that showed a decrease in the subsequent risk of all-cause dementia and Alzheimer's disease by 19% and 24%, respectively.[97]

There is also evidence to support that elevated serum cholesterol concentrations in mid-life increase the subsequent risk for the development of Alzheimer's disease. Lower concentrations of high-density lipoprotein (HDL) and its principal apolipoprotein A1 (ApoA1) have been associated with an increased risk of Alzheimer's disease. A primary role of HDL is to efficiently transport oxocarotenoids, which are scavengers of peroxynitrite. A recent study suggests that lower levels of oxocarotenoids during Alzheimer's disease may inadvertently render HDL susceptible to nitration and oxidation and, in turn, reduce its competency to reverse cholesterol transport from lipid-laden cells.[98] At least three other studies assessed patients with Alzheimer's disease and found significant beneficial effects of higher lutein intake on blood or tissue levels in this regard.[96,99,100]

5.5 Conclusion

The amount of research supporting a positive relationship between egg and two of its innate essential nutrients (choline and lutein) and cognition has grown exponentially over the last decade. Therefore, it is plausible that egg intake may be more critical during certain stages of the life cycle, particularly within the first 1000 days post-conception as well as in older adulthood. Future clinical and longitudinal studies assessing egg intake and cognitive outcomes are greatly needed as the majority of studies assess nutrients such as choline and lutein in isolation. Eggs may very well provide a unique matrix in which nutrients such as choline and lutein act synergistically to enhance brain development and optimize cognitive function throughout the lifespan.

Acknowledgements

TCW has received consulting fees and research support from the Egg Nutrition Center. NS and RV report no conflicts.

References

1. P. Barberger-Gateau, C. Raffaitin, L. Letenneur, C. Berr, C. Tzourio, J. F. Dartigues and A. Alperovitch, Dietary patterns and risk of dementia: the Three-City cohort study, *Neurology*, 2007, **69**(20), 1921–1930.
2. J. A. Luchsinger, J. M. Noble and N. Scarmeas, Diet and Alzheimer's disease, *Curr. Neurol. Neurosci. Rep.*, 2007, **7**(5), 366–372.
3. Associate Parliamentary Food and Health Forum, The Links Between Diet and Behaviour: The Influence of Nutrition on Mental Health, 2008, Available from: http://www.fhf.org.uk/meetings/inquiry2007/FHF_inquiry_report_diet_and_behaviour.pdf.
4. C. S. Stokes, Foods for the brain–can they make you smarter?, *Nutr. Bull.*, 2008, **33**(3), 221–223.
5. E. M. van der Beek and P. J. Kamphuis, The potential role of nutritional components in the management of Alzheimer's disease, *Eur. J. Pharmacol.*, 2008, **585**(1), 197–207.
6. J. Blumberg, R. P. Heaney, M. Huncharek, T. Scholl, M. Stampfer, R. Vieth, C. M. Weaver and S. H. Zeisel, Evidence-based criteria in the nutritional context, *Nutr. Rev.*, 2010, **68**(8), 478–484.
7. A. Nyaradi, J. Li, S. Hickling, J. Foster and W. H. Oddy, The role of nutrition in children's neurocognitive development, from pregnancy through childhood, *Front. Hum. Neurosci.*, 2013, **7**, 97.
8. S. J. Schwarzenberg and M. K. Georgieff, Advocacy for improving nutrition in the first 1000 days to support childhood development and adult health, *Pediatrics*, 2018, **141**(2), e20173716.
9. P. L. Engle and P. D. Fernandez, INCAP studies of malnutrition and cognitive behavior, *Food Nutr. Bull.*, 2010, **31**(1), 83–94.

10. M. Tomiak, J. M. Berthelot, E. Guimond and C. A. Mustard, Factors associated with nursing-home entry for elders in Manitoba, Canada, *J. Gerontol., Ser. A*, 2000, **55**(5), M279–M287.
11. D. H. Thom, M. N. Haan and S. K. Van Den Eeden, Medically recognized urinary incontinence and risks of hospitalization, nursing home admission and mortality, *Age Ageing*, 1997, **26**(5), 367–374.
12. B. S. Black, P. V. Rabins and P. S. German, Predictors of nursing home placement among elderly public housing residents, *Gerontologist*, 1999, **39**(5), 559–568.
13. United Nations, *World Population Ageing 2015 (ST/ESA/SER.A/390)*, 2015, Available from: http://www.un.org/en/development/desa/population/publications/pdf/ageing/WPA2015_Report.pdf.
14. T. C. Wallace, A comprehensive review of eggs, choline, and lutein on cognition across the life-span, *J. Am. Coll. Nutr.*, 2018, **37**(4), 269–285.
15. H. Y. Chung, H. M. Rasmussen and E. J. Johnson, Lutein bioavailability is higher from lutein-enriched eggs than from supplements and spinach in men, *J. Nutr.*, 2004, **134**(8), 1887–1893.
16. T. C. Wallace and V. L. Fulgoni, Usual choline intakes are associated with egg and protein food consumption in the United States, *Nutrients*, 2017, **9**(8), 839.
17. S. H. Zeisel, Choline: an essential nutrient for humans, *Nutrition*, 2000, **16**(7–8), 669–671.
18. E. J. Johnson, Role of lutein and zeaxanthin in visual and cognitive function throughout the lifespan, *Nutr. Rev.*, 2014, **72**(9), 605–612.
19. Z. Conrad, L. K. Johnson, J. N. Roemmich, W. Juan and L. Jahns, Time trends and patterns of reported egg consumption in the U.S. by sociodemographic characteristics, *Nutrients*, 2017, **9**(4), 333.
20. C. K. Lutter, L. L. Iannotti and C. P. Stewart, The potential of a simple egg to improve maternal and child nutrition, *Matern. Child Nutr.*, 2018, **14**(Suppl. 3), e12678.
21. L. L. Iannotti, C. K. Lutter, C. P. Stewart, C. A. Gallegos Riofrio, C. Malo, G. Reinhart, A. Palacios, C. Karp, M. Chapnick, K. Cox and W. F. Waters, Eggs in early complementary feeding and child growth: a randomized controlled trial, *Pediatrics*, 2017, **140**(1), e20163459.
22. M. P. Ylilauri, S. Voutilainen, E. Lonnroos, J. Mursu, H. E. Virtanen, T. T. Koskinen, J. T. Salonen, T. P. Tuomainen and J. K. Virtanen, Association of dietary cholesterol and egg intakes with the risk of incident dementia or Alzheimer disease: the Kuopio Ischaemic Heart Disease Risk Factor Study, *Am. J. Clin. Nutr.*, 2017, **105**(2), 476–484.
23. A. Aparicio Vizuete, F. Robles, E. Rodriguez-Rodriguez, A. M. Lopez-Sobaler and R. M. Ortega, Association between food and nutrient intakes and cognitive capacity in a group of institutionalized elderly people, *Eur. J. Nutr.*, 2010, **49**(5), 293–300.
24. X. Chen, Y. Huang and H. G. Cheng, Lower intake of vegetables and legumes associated with cognitive decline among illiterate elderly Chinese: a 3-year cohort study, *J. Nutr., Health Aging*, 2012, **16**(6), 549–552.

25. X. Zhao, L. Yuan, L. Feng, Y. Xi, H. Yu, W. Ma, D. Zhang and R. Xiao, Association of dietary intake and lifestyle pattern with mild cognitive impairment in the elderly, *J. Nutr., Health Aging*, 2015, **19**(2), 164–168.
26. L. L. Iannotti, C. K. Lutter, W. F. Waters, C. A. Gallegos Riofrio, C. Malo, G. Reinhart, A. Palacios, C. Karp, M. Chapnick, K. Cox, S. Aguirre, L. Narvaez, F. Lopez, R. Sidhu, P. Kell, X. Jiang, H. Fujiwara, D. S. Ory, R. Young and C. P. Stewart, Eggs early in complementary feeding increase choline pathway biomarkers and DHA: a randomized controlled trial in Ecuador, *Am. J. Clin. Nutr.*, 2017, **106**(6), 1482–1489.
27. Y. Papanikolaou and V. L. Fulgoni 3rd, Egg consumption in infants is associated with longer recumbent length and greater intake of several nutrients essential in growth and development, *Nutrients*, 2018, **10**(6), E719.
28. X. Jiang, H. Y. Bar, J. Yan, S. Jones, P. M. Brannon, A. A. West, C. A. Perry, A. Ganti, E. Pressman, S. Devapatla, F. Vermeylen, M. T. Wells and M. A. Caudill, A higher maternal choline intake among third-trimester pregnant women lowers placental and circulating concentrations of the antiangiogenic factor fms-like tyrosine kinase-1 (sFLT1), *FASEB J.*, 2013, **27**(3), 1245–1253.
29. X. Jiang, J. Yan, A. A. West, C. A. Perry, O. V. Malysheva, S. Devapatla, E. Pressman, F. Vermeylen and M. A. Caudill, Maternal choline intake alters the epigenetic state of fetal cortisol-regulating genes in humans, *FASEB J.*, 2012, **26**(8), 3563–3574.
30. X. Jiang, S. Jones, B. Y. Andrew, A. Ganti, O. V. Malysheva, N. Giallourou, P. M. Brannon, M. S. Roberson and M. A. Caudill, Choline inadequacy impairs trophoblast function and vascularization in cultured human placental trophoblasts, *J. Cell. Physiol.*, 2014, **229**(8), 1016–1027.
31. S. T. C. Kwan, J. H. King, J. Yan, X. Jiang, E. Wei, V. G. Fomin, M. S. Roberson and M. A. Caudill, Maternal choline supplementation during murine pregnancy modulates placental markers of inflammation, apoptosis and vascularization in a fetal sex-dependent manner, *Placenta*, 2017, **53**, 57–65.
32. S. T. C. Kwan, J. H. King, J. Yan, Z. Wang, X. Jiang, J. S. Hutzler, H. R. Klein, J. T. Brenna, M. S. Roberson and M. A. Caudill, Maternal choline supplementation modulates placental nutrient transport and metabolism in late gestation of mouse pregnancy, *J. Nutr.*, 2017, **147**(11), 2083–2092.
33. S. L. Carmichael, W. Yang and G. M. Shaw, Periconceptional nutrient intakes and risks of neural tube defects in California, *Birth Defects Res., Part A*, 2010, **88**(8), 670–678.
34. A. M. Lavery, J. D. Brender, H. Zhao, A. Sweeney, M. Felkner, L. Suarez and M. A. Canfield, Dietary intake of choline and neural tube defects in Mexican Americans, *Birth Defects Res., Part A*, 2014, **100**(6), 463–471.
35. G. M. Shaw, S. L. Carmichael, C. Laurent and S. A. Rasmussen, Maternal nutrient intakes and risk of orofacial clefts, *Epidemiology*, 2006, **17**(3), 285–291.

36. G. M. Shaw, S. L. Carmichael, W. Yang, S. Selvin and D. M. Schaffer, Periconceptional dietary intake of choline and betaine and neural tube defects in offspring, *Am. J. Epidemiol.*, 2004, **160**(2), 102–109.
37. A. B. Ganz, K. C. Klatt and M. A. Caudill, Common genetic variants alter metabolism and influence dietary choline requirements, *Nutrients*, 2017, **9**(8), E837.
38. M. A. Caudill, B. J. Strupp, L. Muscalu, J. E. H. Nevins and R. L. Canfield, Maternal choline supplementation during the third trimester of pregnancy improves infant information processing speed: a randomized, double-blind, controlled feeding study, *FASEB J.*, 2018, **32**(4), 2172–2180.
39. C. L. Cheatham, B. D. Goldman, L. M. Fischer, K. A. da Costa, J. S. Reznick and S. H. Zeisel, Phosphatidylcholine supplementation in pregnant women consuming moderate-choline diets does not enhance infant cognitive function: a randomized, double-blind, placebo-controlled trial, *Am. J. Clin. Nutr.*, 2012, **96**(6), 1465–1472.
40. C. E. Boeke, M. W. Gillman, M. D. Hughes, S. L. Rifas-Shiman, E. Villamor and E. Oken, Choline intake during pregnancy and child cognition at age 7 years, *Am. J. Epidemiol.*, 2013, **177**(12), 1338–1347.
41. J. C. McCann, M. Hudes and B. N. Ames, An overview of evidence for a causal relationship between dietary availability of choline during development and cognitive function in offspring, *Neurosci. Biobehav. Rev.*, 2006, **30**(5), 696–712.
42. J. M. Cermak, J. K. Blusztajn, W. H. Meck, C. L. Williams, C. M. Fitzgerald, D. L. Rosene and R. Loy, Prenatal availability of choline alters the development of acetylcholinesterase in the rat hippocampus, *Dev. Neurosci.*, 1999, **21**(2), 94–104.
43. R. Loy, D. Heyer, C. L. Williams and W. H. Meck, Choline-induced spatial memory facilitation correlates with altered distribution and morphology of septal neurons, *Adv. Exp. Med. Biol.*, 1991, **295**, 373–382.
44. W. H. Meck and C. L. Williams, Perinatal choline supplementation increases the threshold for chunking in spatial memory, *NeuroReport*, 1997, **8**(14), 3053–3059.
45. W. H. Meck and C. L. Williams, Characterization of the facilitative effects of perinatal choline supplementation on timing and temporal memory, *NeuroReport*, 1997, **8**(13), 2831–2835.
46. W. H. Meck and C. L. Williams, Simultaneous temporal processing is sensitive to prenatal choline availability in mature and aged rats, *NeuroReport*, 1997, **8**(14), 3045–3051.
47. G. K. Pyapali, D. A. Turner, C. L. Williams, W. H. Meck and H. S. Swartzwelder, Prenatal dietary choline supplementation decreases the threshold for induction of long-term potentiation in young adult rats, *J. Neurophysiol.*, 1998, **79**(4), 1790–1796.
48. C. L. Williams, W. H. Meck, D. D. Heyer and R. Loy, Hypertrophy of basal forebrain neurons and enhanced visuospatial memory in perinatally choline-supplemented rats, *Brain Res.*, 1998, **794**(2), 225–238.

49. W. H. Meck and C. L. Williams, Choline supplementation during prenatal development reduces proactive interference in spatial memory, *Brain Res. Dev. Brain Res.*, 1999, **118**(1–2), 51–59.
50. R. C. Tees, The influences of rearing environment and neonatal choline dietary supplementation on spatial learning and memory in adult rats, *Behav. Brain Res.*, 1999, **105**(2), 173–188.
51. R. C. Tees, The influences of sex, rearing environment, and neonatal choline dietary supplementation on spatial and nonspatial learning and memory in adult rats, *Dev. Psychobiol.*, 1999, **35**(4), 328–342.
52. E. D. Lewis, C. J. Field and R. L. Jacobs, Should the forms of dietary choline also be considered when estimating dietary intake and the implications for health?, *Lipid Technol.*, 2015, **27**(10), 227–230.
53. D. Benton and R. T. Donohoe, The influence on cognition of the interactions between lecithin, carnitine and carbohydrate, *Psychopharmacology*, 2004, **175**(1), 84–91.
54. K. L. Davis, R. C. Mohs, J. R. Tinklenberg, L. E. Hollister, A. Pfefferbaum and B. S. Kopell, Cholinomimetics and memory. The effect of choline chloride, *Arch. Neurol.*, 1980, **37**(1), 49–52.
55. P. A. Deuster, A. Singh, R. Coll, D. E. Hyde and W. J. Becker, Choline ingestion does not modify physical or cognitive performance, *Mil. Med.*, 2002, **167**(12), 1020–1025.
56. C. M. Harris, M. W. Dysken, P. Fovall and J. M. Davis, Effect of lecithin on memory in normal adults, *Am. J. Psychiatry*, 1983, **140**(8), 1010–1012.
57. V. Knott, S. de la Salle, J. Choueiry, D. Impey, D. Smith, M. Smith, E. Beaudry, S. Saghir, V. Ilivitsky and A. Labelle, Neurocognitive effects of acute choline supplementation in low, medium and high performer healthy volunteers, *Pharmacol., Biochem. Behav.*, 2015, **131**, 119–129.
58. V. Knott, S. de la Salle, D. Smith, J. Choueiry, D. Impey, M. Smith, E. Beaudry, S. Saghir, V. Ilivitsky and A. Labelle, Effects of acute CDP-choline treatment on resting state brain oscillations in healthy volunteers, *Neurosci. Lett.*, 2015, **591**, 121–125.
59. M. Naber, B. Hommel and L. S. Colzato, Improved human visuomotor performance and pupil constriction after choline supplementation in a placebo-controlled double-blind study, *Sci. Rep.*, 2015, **5**, 13188.
60. D. P. Lippelt, S. van der Kint, K. van Herk and M. Naber, No acute effects of choline bitartrate food supplements on memory in healthy, young, human adults, *PLoS One*, 2016, **11**(6), e0157714.
61. H. Sorgatz, The effect of lecithin on the state of health and concentration in healthy adults, *Fortschr. Med.*, 1988, **106**, 233–236.
62. N. Sitaram, H. Weingartner, E. D. Caine and J. C. Gillin, Choline: Selective enhancement of serial learning and encoding of low imagery words in man, *Life Sci.*, 1978, **22**(17), 1555–1560.
63. S. L. Ladd, S. A. Sommer, S. LaBerge and W. Toscano, Effect of phosphatidylcholine on explicit memory, *Clin. Neuropharmacol.*, 1993, **16**(6), 540–549.
64. V. Knott, D. Smith, S. de la Salle, D. Impey, J. Choueiry, E. Beaudry, M. Smith, S. Saghir, V. Ilivitsky and A. Labelle, CDP-choline: effects of the

procholine supplement on sensory gating and executive function in healthy volunteers stratified for low, medium and high P50 suppression, *J. Psychopharmacol.*, 2014, **28**(12), 1095–1108.
65. J. K. Blusztajn, B. E. Slack and T. J. Mellott, Neuroprotective actions of dietary choline, *Nutrients*, 2017, **9**(8), 815.
66. M. Fioravanti and M. Yanagi, Cytidinediphosphocholine (CDP-choline) for cognitive and behavioural disturbances associated with chronic cerebral disorders in the elderly, *Cochrane Database Syst. Rev.*, 2005, (2), CD000269.
67. C. Poly, J. M. Massaro, S. Seshadri, P. A. Wolf, E. Cho, E. Krall, P. F. Jacques and R. Au, The relation of dietary choline to cognitive performance and white-matter hyperintensity in the Framingham Offspring Cohort, *Am. J. Clin. Nutr.*, 2011, **94**(6), 1584–1591.
68. M. Mapstone, A. K. Cheema, M. S. Fiandaca, X. Zhong, T. R. Mhyre, L. H. MacArthur, W. J. Hall, S. G. Fisher, D. R. Peterson, J. M. Haley, M. D. Nazar, S. A. Rich, D. J. Berlau, C. B. Peltz, M. T. Tan, C. H. Kawas and H. J. Federoff, Plasma phospholipids identify antecedent memory impairment in older adults, *Nat. Med.*, 2014, **20**(4), 415–418.
69. P. Bhosale, B. Li, M. Sharifzadeh, W. Gellermann, J. M. Frederick, K. Tsuchida and P. S. Bernstein, Purification and partial characterization of a lutein-binding protein from human retina, *Biochemistry*, 2009, **48**(22), 4798–4807.
70. P. Bhosale and P. S. Bernstein, Synergistic effects of zeaxanthin and its binding protein in the prevention of lipid membrane oxidation, *Biochim. Biophys. Acta*, 2005, **1740**(2), 116–121.
71. B. Li, P. Vachali, J. M. Frederick and P. S. Bernstein, Identification of StARD3 as a lutein-binding protein in the macula of the primate retina, *Biochemistry*, 2011, **50**(13), 2541–2549.
72. J. E. Vance, Dysregulation of cholesterol balance in the brain: contribution to neurodegenerative diseases, *Dis. Models Mech.*, 2012, **5**(6), 746–755.
73. R. Vishwanathan, M. J. Kuchan, S. Sen and E. J. Johnson, Lutein and preterm infants with decreased concentrations of brain carotenoids, *J. Pediatr. Gastroenterol. Nutr.*, 2014, **59**(5), 659–665.
74. E. J. Johnson, R. Vishwanathan, M. A. Johnson, D. B. Hausman, A. Davey, T. M. Scott, R. C. Green, L. S. Miller, M. Gearing, J. Woodard, P. T. Nelson, H. Y. Chung, W. Schalch, J. Wittwer and L. W. Poon, Relationship between serum and brain carotenoids, alpha-tocopherol, and retinol concentrations and cognitive performance in the oldest old from the Georgia Centenarian Study, *J. Aging Res.*, 2013, **2013**, 951786.
75. R. Vishwanathan, W. Schalch and E. J. Johnson, Macular pigment carotenoids in the retina and occipital cortex are related in humans, *Nutr. Neurosci.*, 2016, **19**(3), 95–101.
76. R. Vishwanathan, M. Neuringer, D. M. Snodderly, W. Schalch and E. J. Johnson, Macular lutein and zeaxanthin are related to brain lutein and zeaxanthin in primates, *Nutr. Neurosci.*, 2013, **16**(1), 21–29.

77. R. Vishwanathan, A. Iannaccone, T. M. Scott, S. B. Kritchevsky, B. J. Jennings, G. Carboni, G. Forma, S. Satterfield, T. Harris, K. C. Johnson, W. Schalch, L. M. Renzi, C. Rosano and E. J. Johnson, Macular pigment optical density is related to cognitive function in older people, *Age Ageing*, 2014, **43**(2), 271–275.
78. J. Feeney, C. Finucane, G. M. Savva, H. Cronin, S. Beatty, J. M. Nolan and R. A. Kenny, Low macular pigment optical density is associated with lower cognitive performance in a large, population-based sample of older adults, *Neurobiol. Aging*, 2013, **34**(11), 2449–2456.
79. L. M. Renzi, M. J. Dengler, A. Puente, L. S. Miller and B. R. Hammond Jr, Relationships between macular pigment optical density and cognitive function in unimpaired and mildly cognitively impaired older adults, *Neurobiol. Aging*, 2014, **35**(7), 1695–1699.
80. E. Johnson, R. Vishwanathan, E. Mohn, J. Haddock, H. Rasmussen and T. Scott, Avocado consumption increases neural lutein and improves cognitive function, *FASEB J.*, 2015, **29**(1 suppl), 32.38.
81. E. R. Bovier, L. M. Renzi and B. R. Hammond, A double-blind, placebo-controlled study on the effects of lutein and zeaxanthin on neural processing speed and efficiency, *PLoS One*, 2014, **9**(9), e108178.
82. E. R. Bovier and B. R. Hammond, A randomized placebo-controlled study on the effects of lutein and zeaxanthin on visual processing speed in young healthy subjects, *Arch. Biochem. Biophys.*, 2015, **572**, 54–57.
83. K. J. Yeum, G. Ferland, J. Patry and R. M. Russell, Relationship of plasma carotenoids, retinol and tocopherols in mothers and newborn infants, *J. Am. Coll. Nutr.*, 1998, **17**(5), 442–447.
84. S. Perrone, M. Tei, M. Longini, A. Santacroce, G. Turrisi, F. Proietti, C. Felici, A. Picardi, F. Bazzini, P. Vasarri and G. Buonocore, Lipid and protein oxidation in newborn infants after lutein administration, *Oxid. Med. Cell. Longevity*, 2014, **2014**, 781454.
85. G. Buonocore, S. Perrone and R. Bracci, Free radicals and brain damage in the newborn, *Biol. Neonate*, 2001, **79**(3–4), 180–186.
86. R. L. Zlody, The relationship between critical flicker frequency (CFF) and several intellectual measures, *Am. J. Psychol.*, 1965, **78**(4), 596–602.
87. L. M. Renzi-Hammond, E. R. Bovier, L. M. Fletcher, L. S. Miller, C. M. Mewborn, C. A. Lindbergh, J. H. Baxter and B. R. Hammond, Effects of a lutein and zeaxanthin intervention on cognitive function: a randomized, double-masked, placebo-controlled trial of younger healthy adults, *Nutrients*, 2017, **9**(11), E1246.
88. A. M. Walk, C. G. Edwards, N. W. Baumgartner, M. R. Chojnacki, A. R. Covello, G. E. Reeser, B. R. Hammond, L. M. Renzi-Hammond and N. A. Khan, The role of retinal carotenoids and age on neuroelectric indices of attentional control among early to middle-aged adults, *Front. Aging Neurosci.*, 2017, **9**, 183.
89. L. M. Renzi, E. R. Bovier and B. R. Hammond Jr, A role for the macular carotenoids in visual motor response, *Nutr. Neurosci.*, 2013, **16**(6), 262–268.

90. C. A. Lindbergh, L. M. Renzi-Hammond, B. R. Hammond, D. P. Terry, C. M. Mewborn, A. N. Puente and L. S. Miller, Lutein and zeaxanthin influence brain function in older adults: a randomized controlled trial, *J. Int. Neuropsychol. Soc.*, 2018, **24**(1), 77–90.
91. E. J. Johnson, K. McDonald, S. M. Caldarella, H. Y. Chung, A. M. Troen and D. M. Snodderly, Cognitive findings of an exploratory trial of docosahexaenoic acid and lutein supplementation in older women, *Nutr. Neurosci.*, 2008, **11**(2), 75–83.
92. J. Widomska and W. K. Subczynski, Why has nature chosen lutein and zeaxanthin to protect the retina?, *J. Clin. Exp. Ophthalmol.*, 2014, **5**(1), 326.
93. S. J. Woo, K. H. Park, J. Ahn, J. Y. Choe, H. Jeong, J. W. Han, T. H. Kim and K. W. Kim, Cognitive impairment in age-related macular degeneration and geographic atrophy, *Ophthalmology*, 2012, **119**(10), 2094–2101.
94. C. A. Lindbergh, C. M. Mewborn, B. R. Hammond, L. M. Renzi-Hammond, J. M. Curran-Celentano and L. S. Miller, Relationship of lutein and zeaxanthin levels to neurocognitive functioning: an fMRI study of older adults, *J. Int. Neuropsychol. Soc.*, 2017, **23**(1), 11–22.
95. D. Kelly, R. F. Coen, K. O. Akuffo, S. Beatty, J. Dennison, R. Moran, J. Stack, A. N. Howard, R. Mulcahy and J. M. Nolan, Cognitive function and its relationship with macular pigment optical density and serum concentrations of its constituent carotenoids, *J. Alzheimer's Dis.*, 2015, **48**(1), 261–277.
96. J. M. Nolan, E. Loskutova, A. Howard, R. Mulcahy, R. Moran, J. Stack, M. Bolger, R. F. Coen, J. Dennison, K. O. Akuffo, N. Owens, R. Power, D. Thurnham and S. Beatty, The impact of supplemental macular carotenoids in Alzheimer's disease: a randomized clinical trial, *J. Alzheimer's Dis.*, 2015, **44**(4), 1157–1169.
97. C. Feart, L. Letenneur, C. Helmer, C. Samieri, W. Schalch, S. Etheve, C. Delcourt, J. F. Dartigues and P. Barberger-Gateau, Plasma carotenoids are inversely associated with dementia risk in an elderly French cohort, *J. Gerontol., Ser. A*, 2016, **71**(5), 683–688.
98. I. H. Dias, M. C. Polidori, L. Li, D. Weber, W. Stahl, G. Nelles, T. Grune and H. R. Griffiths, Plasma levels of HDL and carotenoids are lower in dementia patients with vascular comorbidities, *J. Alzheimer's Dis.*, 2014, **40**(2), 399–408.
99. W. Wang, L. Shinto, W. E. Connor and J. F. Quinn, Nutritional biomarkers in Alzheimer's disease: the association between carotenoids, n-3 fatty acids, and dementia severity, *J. Alzheimer's Dis.*, 2008, **13**(1), 31–38.
100. P. Rinaldi, M. C. Polidori, A. Metastasio, E. Mariani, P. Mattioli, A. Cherubini, M. Catani, R. Cecchetti, U. Senin and P. Mecocci, Plasma antioxidants are similarly depleted in mild cognitive impairment and in Alzheimer's disease, *Neurobiol. Aging*, 2003, **24**(7), 915–919.

CHAPTER 6

Egg Protein in Sports Nutrition

I. G. MARTINEZ[a], C. F. MCKENNA[b] AND N. A. BURD*[a,b]

[a]University of Illinois at Urbana – Champaign, Department of Kinesiology and Community Health, 906 South Goodwin Avenue, Urbana, IL, USA 61801; [b]University of Illinois at Urbana – Champaign, Division of Nutritional Sciences, 449 Bevier Hall, 905 South Goodwin Avenue, Urbana, IL, USA 61801
*E-mail: naburd@illinois.edu

6.1 Introduction

Eggs, being a nutritious and versatile food, have been part of the diets of humans throughout history. Chicken egg – the most commonly consumed egg today, is commonly eaten not only by itself but also as part of other food products, such as baked goods and noodles. In the United States alone, there has been a recent increase of about 3% in egg production.[1] Along with this, compared to the late 1990s, an increasing trend in *per capita* consumption – a measure of total egg production, less exports, plus imports, divided by the total population[2] – has also been observed. Despite the misconceptions surrounding egg intake and its implications on health, it is still routinely incorporated in the diets of many people because of the wide array of benefits that egg offers (cost,[3] culinary versatility[4] and nutrient density[5]). In fact, around 21% to 22% of the US population are egg consumers.[5–7] Specifically, athletes may benefit from consuming egg as part of a healthy diet as these individuals require optimal nutrition to support the demands of high-intensity training and sports competition. Therefore, the aim of this chapter is to highlight

Food Chemistry, Function and Analysis No.14
Eggs as Functional Foods and Nutraceuticals for Human Health
Edited by Jianping Wu

Published by the Royal Society of Chemistry, www.rsc.org

the nutritional value of eggs within a sports nutrition context; specifically, in terms of supporting training adaptations and optimizing recovery and performance.

6.2 Nutritional Profile of Eggs

The unique nutritional properties of egg can be attributed to its complex biological and chemical structure. A whole egg is a mixture of water (75%), proteins (12%), lipids (12%), vitamins, minerals and other compounds[8] (Figure 6.1), and consists of approximately 10% shell, 58% white and 32% yolk.[1] A medium-size whole chicken egg weighs around 44 grams (g) and has 63 kilocalories (kcal), 5.53 g of protein, 4.18 g of fat and 0.3 g of carbohydrates.[9] Table 6.1 summarizes the nutrient composition of various edible forms of whole egg.

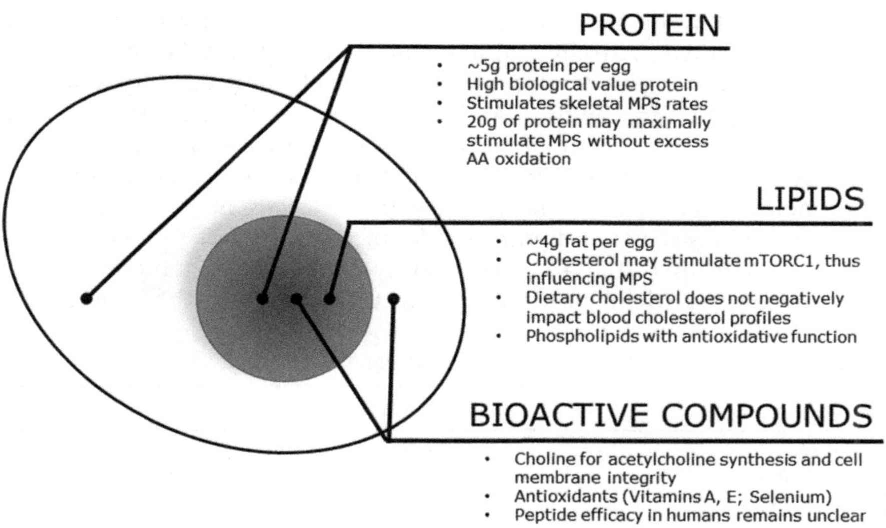

Figure 6.1 Nutrients in egg. MPS, muscle protein synthesis; AA, amino acid.

Table 6.1 Nutrient composition of whole eggs based on cooking method, per 100 g.[a]

Nutrient	Hard-boiled	Fried	Poached	Scrambled
Energy (kcal)	155	196	143	149
Protein (g)	12.58	13.61	12.51	9.99
Fat (g)	10.61	14.84	9.47	10.98
Carbohydrate (g)[b]	1.12	0.83	0.71	1.61
Water (g)	74.62	69.47	78.85	76.40

[a]Data from USDA National Nutrient Database for Standard Reference, Release 28 (slightly revised).[73]
[b]By difference.

The majority of an egg's total protein content (60%) is contained in the white, while the remaining 40% is in the yolk.[10] A common notion about the consumption of egg is its negative implications for cardiometabolic health owing to the cholesterol and saturated fat found in the yolk. As such, removal of the nutrient-dense yolk is often encouraged for health benefits when multiple eggs are consumed;[11] however, recent evidence[7,12] has shown the disparity between dietary cholesterol intake and serum cholesterol levels. Table 6.2 outlines the fatty acid profile of egg.

The fatty acid and micronutrient profiles of eggs vary depending on the source and feed composition[13] or living conditions[14] of the hens. In fact, production of "specialty eggs" *via* fortification of the feed of hens is a recent trend that has emerged in the food industry. As an example, omega-3 bio-fortified eggs are now available in the market—especially in populations where egg is identified as an ideal food item to be value-added from a public health perspective.[15] The ratio of omega-3 and omega-6 fatty acid intake has been an area of concern, especially considering that the typical Western diet, which consists of high intakes of saturated fat, sodium and sugar, is also usually short of omega-3 fatty acids but high in omega-6 fatty acids.[16] As for athletes, supplementation of omega-3 fatty acids has been shown to attenuate muscle soreness,[17,18] but does not modulate post-exercise skeletal muscle protein remodeling.[19] Nonetheless, opting for omega-3 bio-fortified eggs may be a consideration, especially if usual dietary intake of omega-3 fatty acids is low. It must be underlined that all three healthy eating patterns recommended in the recent US Dietary Guidelines for Americans (DGA)[20] include eggs

Table 6.2 Fatty acid content of hard-boiled egg, per 100 grams.[a]

Lipid	Amount (mg)
Saturated	**3267**
14:0 Myristic	35
16:0 Palmitic	2349
16:0 Stearic	828
Monounsaturated	**4077**
16:1 Palmitoleic	310
18:1 Oleic	3725
20:1 Eicosenoic	30
Polyunsaturated	**1414**
18:2 Linoleic	1888
18:3 Linolenic	35
18:4 Morocitic	0
20:4 Apachidonic	149
20:5 EPA	5
22:6 DHA	38
Trans fat	**54**
Cholesterol	**373**

[a]Data from USDA National Nutrient Database for Standard Reference, Release 28 (slightly revised).[73]

as they contribute to protein intake and improve the bioavailability of certain antioxidants found in other food.[21] In addition to this, the food matrix of whole egg and its constituent macro- and micro-nutrients seem to synergistically facilitate various aspects of the muscle remodeling process. Specifically, cholesterol has been shown to exert a stimulatory effect on the mechanistic target of rapamycin complex 1 (mTORC1)[22] – the complex primarily responsible for regulating protein synthesis to anabolic stimuli.[23] Specifically, cholesterol serves as a nutrient cue for the recruitment of mTORC1 to the lysosomes to initiate the protein synthetic machinery signaling.[22] In addition, there is evidence of fatty acids, specifically, saturated fatty acids, enhancing the translocation of mTORC1 to the lysosome.[24] It is then important to highlight that the lipid content of egg exerts an influence on muscle protein synthesis rates synergistically, or even independently, of the amino acid profile of egg protein and also offers additional nutrients to improve diet quality. Table 6.3 shows the micronutrient content of egg.

One large egg is packed with 13 essential vitamins and minerals. Consumption of eggs is associated with improved nutritional quality of one's diet – egg consumers have better diet quality than non-consumers,[5] which may contribute to health promotion and athletic performance. Specifically, naturally found micronutrients, such as vitamins A, D and E, choline and antioxidants, such as lutein and zeaxanthin, in egg are most relevant for the athletic population and will be discussed further in a section of this chapter. The nutrient density of eggs and other whole food protein sources is unquestionably an advantage over isolated protein supplements.

Table 6.3 Micronutrient profile of hard-boiled egg, per 100 grams.[a]

Vitamin	Amount	Mineral	Amount
Thiamin (mg)	0.066	Calcium (mg)	50
Riboflavin (mg)	0.513	Copper (mg)	0.013
Niacin (mg)	0.064	Fluoride (mcg)	4.8
Pantothenic acid (mg)	1.398	Iron (mg)	1.19
Pyridoxine (mg)	0.121	Magnesium (mg)	10
Folate (mcg)	44	Manganese (mg)	0.026
Vitamin B12 (mcg)	1.11	Phosphorus (mg)	126
Vitamin A (IU)	520	Potassium (mg)	126
Vitamin D (IU)	87	Selenium (mcg)	30.8
Vitamin E (mg)	1.03	Sodium (mg)	124
Vitamin K (mcg)	0.3	Zinc (mg)	1.05
Choline (mg)	293.8		
Lutein + zeaxanthin (mcg)	353		

[a]Data from USDA National Nutrient Database for Standard Reference, Release 28 (slightly revised).[73]

6.3 Protein Quality of Egg

Egg protein's quality makes it valuable in sports nutrition. Traditionally, dietary protein quality is defined as the ability of a food source to provide essential amino acids (EAA) in specific proportions necessary for the formation of new proteins to support growth.[25] Alternatively, it can also be defined as the capacity of a protein source to stimulate muscle protein synthesis rates in order to support exercise-induced adaptations to training to help optimize performance.[26] Stable isotope amino acid tracer methods are most commonly applied to directly assess the anabolic potential of dietary proteins within skeletal muscle tissue; however, the use of metabolic tracers requires expertise in the technique and a decent amount of resources, as well as a specialized research infrastructure. As such, it is quite common that alternative measures are used to define dietary protein quality, and it is generally determined on the whole-body level.

Prior to the development of amino acid scoring, protein quality was assessed using indices such as Protein Efficiency Ratio (PER) and NPU (Net Protein Utilization) in growth experiments with rats. PER is derived by feeding a standardized diet and assessing weight gain against the amount of protein consumed over a period of time.[27] NPU represents the percentage of protein retained compared to the amount of protein consumed. Additionally, Biological Value (BV) is a similar measure to NPU but represents the amount of utilized nitrogen *versus* the amount of absorbed nitrogen. The Protein Digestibility Corrected Amino Acid Score (PDCAAS)[28] and the more recent Digestible Indispensable Amino Acid Score (DIAAS)[29] are perhaps the most widely used indices to assess protein quality in recent years. PDCAAS is derived by comparing the concentration of the limiting EAA of a protein food to the amount of EAA in a given reference protein, which is then corrected for true fecal digestibility.[28] By taking into consideration digestibility factors, PDCAAS provides more information compared to just examining the amino acid profile of a protein food. One major issue noted with this method is that scores that exceed 100% are truncated. Along with this, the validity of the amino acid requirements of a preschool-aged child and the true fecal digestibility correction have been recognized as limitations of this method; as such, PDCAAS has been replaced by DIAAS. DIAAS evaluates protein quality based on the digestibility of individual dietary amino acid and is defined as the amount of digestible dietary amino acid in a gram of dietary protein compared to the amount of the same dietary indispensable amino acid in a reference protein.[29] Unfortunately, a DIAAS has yet to be established for egg. The different protein quality scores of egg are highlighted in Table 6.4.

It is evident that egg protein is of high quality based on the different protein quality scores, but perhaps a common pitfall for these protein quality assessment methods is their relevance to humans, as these indices are determined through animal models (*e.g.*, rats, pigs). Moreover, these ranking

Table 6.4 Protein quality scores of whole egg.[a,c]

Protein quality indices	PDCAAS[b]	PER	NPU	BV
Egg	1.18	3.8	94	93.7

[a]Based on data from ref. 28,86,87.
[b]Non-truncated PDCAAS for egg based on true fecal digestibility value of 98%.[28]
[c]PDCAAS, Protein Digestibility Corrected Amino Acid Score; PER, Protein Efficiency Ratio; NPU, Net Protein Utilization; BV, Biological Value.

methods do not reflect the actual capacity of a protein source to stimulate skeletal muscle protein synthesis rates but instead only provide information on the minimum amount of nitrogen and amino acid necessary to prevent deficiency on a whole-body level. From a sports nutrition perspective, it is useful to combine protein digestibility data with relevant metabolic outputs (*e.g.*, measurements of protein synthesis, oxidation) to better elucidate how nutrition and training are facilitating muscle repair and recovery. It has been shown that dietary proteins may have different stimulatory effects on muscle protein synthesis rates during resting or post-exercise conditions despite having similar protein quality scores[30,31] and this is highly dependent on the digestion and absorption kinetics of amino acids, especially when consuming isolated protein sources.

Egg protein contains the complete array of EAA that are readily digested and become highly bioavailable in the body, and has been used in the past as a standard to assess protein quality.[32] The amino acid concentrations of egg and egg fractions compared to human skeletal muscle are outlined in Table 6.5.

Eggs offer the complete array of EAA, and it is often assumed that a high-quality protein source to stimulate skeletal muscle protein synthesis rates has a similar amino acid composition to that of human body protein.[33,34] This is important as an unbalanced ratio of essential to non-EAA within a protein food source may lead to greater splanchnic sequestration (namely in the gut and liver) of amino acids and/or increase irreversible loss to oxidation.[35] While no data is available for the amount of the EAA tryptophan in human muscle protein, estimates of EAA concentrations suggest that egg fractions contain a comparable ratio to human protein. Moreover, leucine is an essential amino acid and is of particular importance when it comes to stimulating muscle protein synthesis (MPS) rates owing to its role as an anabolic signaling molecule.[36] It is generally thought that the leucine content of a dietary protein predicts its ability to stimulate postprandial MPS, at least when ingesting isolated protein sources.[37–39] In fact, an enhanced muscle protein synthetic response has been observed with leucine supplementation.[40–42] Around 9% of an egg's protein content is leucine, but it also contains other specific amino acids (*e.g.*, alanine, glutamate, isoleucine) that have additional roles in supporting exercise performance, aside from a muscle health perspective.

Table 6.5 Amino acid profile of egg fractions *versus* human muscle, mg per g.[a]

Amino acid	Human muscle[a]	Whole egg[b]	Egg yolk[b]	Egg white[b]
Alanine	41.52	56.3	52.1	63.2
Arginine	43.90	63.9	69.5	57.2
Aspartic acid	66.29	104.5	98.4	86.7
Cystine		22.3	17.5	24.3
Glutamic acid	129.92	132.9	126.8	136.7
Glycine	30.70	33.8	31.0	36.7
Histidine	28.08	25.0	25.6	22.3
Isoleucine	33.45	50.7	50.6	59.7
Leucine	63.36	86.4	86.5	85.3
Lysine	65.64	69.5	78.8	60.4
Methionine	16.86	31.1	25.5	38.1
Phenylalanine	38.16	52.7	43.8	61.6
Proline		38.1	39.4	36.8
Serine	22.59	78.5	83.7	72.3
Threonine	29.18	44.3	45.9	43.6
Tryptophan		16.1	11.6	15.1
Tyrosine	20.29	41.2	42.3	39.4
Valine	42.76	62.2	57.5	73.4
% EAA	31.7%[c]	37.9%	38.3%	38.3%

[a]Data from healthy older men (n = 8); Cys, Pro, Trp were not measured.[88]
[b]Data for dried product, from USDA National Nutrient Database for Standard Reference, Release 28 (Slightly revised).[73]
[c]Value likely underestimates EAA concentration of human muscle as Trp not measured.

6.4 Dietary Protein Contributions to Skeletal Muscle

6.4.1 Skeletal Muscle Remodeling

Skeletal muscle is a major physiological determinant of sports performance and health. It is vital for movement and function and is also highly involved in the metabolism of substrates in the human body (*i.e.*, lipid and blood glucose regulation). These tissues are highly plastic and, in fact, training can modify their metabolic, physiological and contractile properties.[43,44] This is achieved through muscle protein remodeling wherein nutrition plays a key a role in maximizing the exercise-adaptive response.

Muscle protein remodeling, or turnover, is mainly regulated by fluctuations between MPS and muscle protein breakdown rates (MPB) (Figure 6.2). The synchronized and counterbalanced nature of these two processes defines net protein balance (NPB = MPS − MPB).

Shifting NPB to a more positive state (*i.e.*, feeding and exercise) occurs *via* increasing MPS and, to a lesser extent, decreasing MPB. Hence, the whole-body and muscle protein synthetic responses to dietary protein-derived amino acids support the maintenance of a positive net protein balance[45] and can offset the increase in MPB rates during fasted states, thus maintaining protein balance. The latter paradigm is dependent on the notion that an individual is consuming adequate protein and energy throughout the day.

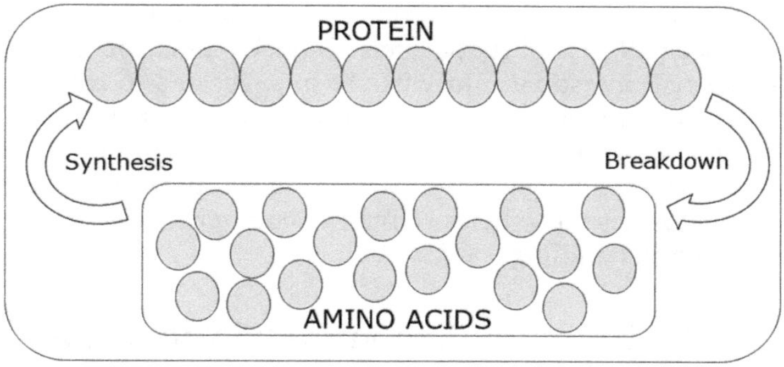

Figure 6.2 Overview of regulation of protein balance.

Similarly, exercise is capable of inducing a protein synthetic response and promoting a positive net protein balance;[46] however, post-exercise protein ingestion is necessary in order to facilitate the desired adaptive response to training, as well as promote recovery and long-term physical performance. It is important to note that muscle protein remodeling can be either hypertrophic or non-hypertrophic in nature.[47] Moreover, the interaction between dietary protein and exercise can enhance the structural changes in non-muscle tissue, which is beneficial for injury prevention.[48,49]

6.5 Metabolism of Dietary Proteins

As previously mentioned, dietary protein ingestion is a potent anabolic stimulus for skeletal MPS – especially when coupled with the recovery phase after an exercise bout. Conversely, it is not the preferred fuel source of the body during exercise. It is interesting to note, however, that the deamination and intermediary metabolism of certain amino acids (*e.g.*, glutamate, alanine, leucine, isoleucine and valine) contribute vital substrates to the tricarboxylic acid (TCA) cycle,[50,51] resulting in a significant impact on the adenosine triphosphate (ATP)-producing processes in the body. The contribution of whole-body amino acid oxidation rates during short-term high-intensity exercise is often considered negligible as it only accounts for 3–6% of the total ATP resources during prolonged exercise;[50] still, the concentration of these TCA cycle intermediates has been linked to other factors that may affect exercise performance (*i.e.*, muscle fatigue). During sustained submaximal exercise, muscle glycogen stores are diminished,[52] causing an increase in oxidation and inefficient recycling of amino acids.[53] However, the mechanisms driving these observations remain unclear.[54–57] As an example, it has been demonstrated that leucine can be oxidized at a rate of ~8 mg^{-1} kg body $weight^{-1}$ h^{-1} during moderate intensity endurance exercise (~60% VO_2 max).[58] Thus, depending on the intensity and duration of the endurance exercise bout, the extent of exercise-induced amino acid oxidative loss may place substantially more stress on the ingested post-exercise nutrition to support a positive whole-body leucine balance when compared to the resting state.[59] In addition, it has been suggested that exercise induces transient small intestinal injury. This small intestinal injury has been suggested to result in impairments in dietary protein digestion and absorption kinetics, limiting the amount of dietary protein-derived amino acids available in circulation to stimulate MPS rates.[60,61] Given all this, increased intake of protein during recovery from exercise may be warranted to counter these exercise-induced changes in protein handling.

6.6 Sports Nutrition: Recommendations and Applications

6.6.1 Dietary Protein Recommendations

In the United States, the current Recommended Dietary Allowance (RDA) of protein is 0.8 g^{-1} kg body $weight^{-1}$ day^{-1} for healthy adults.[62] However, this amount may only be sufficient to prevent protein deficiency and a higher intake may be required to optimize recovery from exercise and facilitate training adaptations. Therefore, the American College of Sports Medicine (ACSM) and the Academy of Nutrition and Dietetics (AND)[63] have established supplemental nutrient recommendations for exercise and athletics. Generally, protein intake ranging from 1.2 to 2.0 g^{-1} kg body $weight^{-1}$ day^{-1} will be sufficient to support adequate recovery from, and adaptation to, exercise training. Specific dosing is influenced by various factors, including, but not limited to: training modality, exercise intensity and duration, and performance goals. However, strategic timing of protein consumption may be a more efficient practice than meeting total daily intake targets. Thus, there is a shift to provide protein guidelines on a per meal basis as opposed to daily recommendations. The oxidative loss of amino acids experienced during endurance exercise[64] and the contribution of dietary-derived amino acids to muscle fiber remodeling necessitate adequate protein ingestion specifically in the recovery period. It is often not recognized that the post-exercise recovery window is quite prolonged in nature, lasting 2–3 days, depending on the intensity and volume of exercise.[46] As such, ACSM currently recommends 20–30 g total protein, with 10 g from EAA,[63] and a targeted nutritional strategy should persist beyond the immediate post-exercise meal. Additionally, co-ingestion of carbohydrates in the post-exercise meal may improve net whole-body protein balance,[63] but not at the muscle level.[65] It is worth noting, however, that current guidelines are based on maximal dosing of isolated protein sources for maximal MPS responses and are often taken as a proxy for optimal protein intake. Conversely, optimal protein intake would be an amount that elicits maximal MPS with minimal amino acid oxidation. An optimal ingested protein dose–response curve on MPS has not been defined, but may depend on the ingestion of nutrient-rich and protein-dense foods to potentiate the anabolic action of dietary amino acids on MPS.[66]

6.6.2 Egg Protein: Applications for Athletes

Egg- and egg protein-specific influences on various indices of skeletal muscle function and athletic performance have been examined. A dose–response study conducted by Moore and colleagues[67] utilized a post-exercise drink containing egg protein isolate in graded amounts (*i.e.*, 0, 5, 10, 20 and 40 g) to assess its effect on the simulation of MPS after a bout of resistance exercise. Stimulation of albumin protein synthesis (APS) and MPS responded in a dose-dependent manner and it was found that the post-exercise ingestion of 20 g of protein was able to maximally stimulate both APS and MPS, but higher doses resulted in a marked increase in whole-body leucine oxidation rates.[67] It was unclear what form of egg protein was used in this study (*i.e.*, egg white protein or whole egg protein isolate) but it is evident that it was able to induce an increase in the mixed muscle fractional synthetic rate (FSR) compared to fasted state when ingested after exercise. More researchers are acknowledging the fact that the majority of individuals acquire their dietary protein from whole food sources; it is then highly relevant to examine the effects of ingesting protein-rich whole foods such as eggs in supporting adaptations to training and optimizing performance.

A recent study published by our group[66] assessed the post-exercise effects of ingesting intrinsically labelled whole egg *versus* an isonitrogenous amount of egg white among healthy young men. A greater postprandial myofibrillar protein synthesis rate was observed with the post-exercise ingestion of whole eggs *versus* egg whites, despite having the same amount of protein. Interestingly, a 12-week resistance training study done by Iglay and colleagues,[68] wherein they mainly utilized eggs to achieve a moderate intake of protein (1.2 g^{-1} kg body $weight^{-1}$ day^{-1}) found no differential effects on whole-body and muscle composition response to training. It is important to note though that this study was done among older people (average age: 61 ± 1 year), which could have added another layer of complexity owing to the postulated age-related anabolic resistance.[69,70] Nonetheless, results from the comparison of whole egg *versus* egg whites provide evidence to dismiss the common practice of disposing of the egg yolk among athletes and fitness professionals and highlights that other nutrients and bioactive compounds found in the yolk matrix may play a role in stimulating MPS. Furthermore, a study among healthy, sedentary adults that aimed to determine how endurance training would impact blood lipid metabolism with habitual consumption of eggs providing dietary cholesterol above the upper limits.[71] It was demonstrated that the benefits of short-term aerobic exercise training (*i.e.*, improved lipoprotein profile independent of weight loss or body composition changes) were not altered with daily egg consumption. Another 12 week resistance training study that involved consumption of an egg-based breakfast compared with a more carbohydrate-based breakfast showed no adverse effects on lipid profiles and glucose handling among healthy young men and women.[72] This emphasizes the role of exercise in maintaining health and implies that eggs may be regularly consumed within a healthy diet for most individuals, including athletes.

6.7 Micronutrient Implications for Exercise and Athletics

Whole chicken eggs are not only a protein-dense food with high indices of protein quality, they also include other bioactive constituents that may beneficially influence sports performance and skeletal muscle health.

6.7.1 Choline

Whole eggs are the food source with the highest amount of the micronutrient choline.[73] Choline is a component of cell membranes and a substrate for acetylcholine synthesis.[74] Endogenous production is limited, so it is essential for humans to consume foods containing choline in order to prevent deficiency. Choline deficiency impairs the integrity of cell membranes, increasing the risk of intracellular components leaking out into extracellular spaces.[74] This is of particular concern for the proper functioning of skeletal muscle because, for example, the intracellular enzyme that propels ATP production from adenosine diphosphate (ADP) and phosphocreatine, allowing for energy utilization when mitochondrial-sourced ATP is unable to meet energy demands of an exercising muscle if intracellular levels are insufficient. Additionally, structural impairments of cellular membranes may reduce capacity for mechanical stress and it is speculated that choline deficiency may increase the onset of muscular fatigue owing to cellular damage.[74] Acetylcholine, derived from choline, is a neurotransmitter acting at the neuromuscular junction to initiate myofibrillar contraction. Endurance and high-intensity exercise have been associated with a decrease in serum concentrations of choline.[75–78] Speculations have been made, but mechanisms driving this reduction remain unclear. Interestingly, oral choline supplementation to supraphysiological concentrations does not elicit superior athletic performance (*e.g.*, time to exhaustion, maximal oxygen consumption, VO_2 max).[74] While supplementation seems unnecessary, habitual consumption of whole eggs would be adequate to prevent deficiency and replace exercise-induced losses.

6.7.2 Antioxidants

Whole eggs are abundant in micronutrients with antioxidation capacity. Exercise substantially increases oxygen consumption, with estimates projected up to 15-fold.[63] Elevated reactive oxygen species (ROS) can cause cellular damage and are linked with various unfavorable pathologies, including fatigue, muscle damage and reduced immune function, as well as chronic diseases.[79] While acute exercise may transiently increase ROS production, upregulation of antioxidant pathways is observed with chronic training. Watson *et al.* examined peroxidation and antioxidation markers in trained athletes *versus* age- and sex-matched sedentary controls.[79] There were no differences in plasma free F_2-isoprotane (lipid peroxidation marker in bodily fluids) and total antioxidant capacity (remaining H_2O_2 after a defined quantity reacts with serum constituents) across groups. This supports that endogenous and exogenous systems adapt appropriately to accommodate exercise-induced ROS production. Furthermore, there is minimal reliable evidence advocating for antioxidant supplementation in athletes. However, a diet adequate in antioxidative nutrients will help to maintain exogenous oxidation defense systems to combat exercise-induced ROS production. Whole chicken eggs contain a plethora of antioxidants. Bioactive compounds include phospholipids, vitamin A, vitamin E and carotenoids.[80] It is interesting to note that egg-specific protein has antioxidative capacity as well, specifically peptides derived from ovalbumin, ovotransferrin and ovomucin.[80]

6.8 Protein Derivatives: Bioactive Peptides

Egg protein derivatives, peptides, may provide functional benefits for sport. As previously mentioned, egg white proteins like ovalbumin, ovotransferrin and ovomucin may exhibit antioxidative properties. Additionally, the egg-specific peptide ovotransferrin can function as a metal chelator. As such, the peptide binds to iron ions, inhibiting iron-induced oxidative damage and microbial growth.[81] Egg white ovomucin and yolk protein fractions have been observed to have angiotensin-converting enzyme (ACE)-inhibitory activity.[82,83] Yousr and colleagues[82] enzymatically digested and filtered chicken egg yolk protein to assess its bioactivity. A gel-filtered fraction containing ~21% leucine, ~16% arginine and ~14% tryptophan elicited an ACE-inhibitory capacity comparable to that of the antihypertensive medication captopril. Low angiotensin II concentrations, a potent vasoconstrictor, may provide a favorable environment for athletes. A rodent model investigating skeletal muscle adaptation and performance in response to ACE-inhibitor (ACEI) drug use found that ACEI use coupled with exercise training resulted in higher capillary density in the soleus muscle compared to exercise alone.[84] However, angiogenesis is only observed in non-sulfhydryl ACEIs and it is unknown if egg bioactive peptides possess the same capacity within the human body. Egg-specific bioactive peptides have not only been identified in the white and yolk, but also the shell and membrane as well. It has been suggested that chicken egg membrane constituents can help treat connective tissue disorders. However, research investigating oral ingestion of egg membrane supplements for treating chronic joint pain found no functional advantages of egg membrane supplementation *versus* a microcrystalline cellulose placebo in terms of range of motion.[85] While current evidence shows a high potential for bioactive peptides, it is unclear if these constituents remain stable throughout *in vivo* digestion and absorption, and if observed *in vitro* activities occur within the human body, resulting in functional benefits.

6.9 Conclusion

Protein is a nutrient of particular importance for athletes given its contribution to skeletal muscle remodeling, glycogen repletion when sub-optimal amounts of carbohydrates are consumed and tissue repair during post-exercise recovery. Egg protein is a highly digestible whole food source of all EAA and it is sufficient in augmenting post-exercise MPS. However, the athletic advantage of egg consumption is not limited to its proteins. The food matrix of whole eggs (white and yolk) may synergistically improve physiological function and performance. Whole egg consumption does not negatively impact lipid or carbohydrate metabolism or blood cholesterol levels, and even elicits increased myofibrillar protein synthesis rates compared to isonitrogenous egg white protein alone in healthy young adults. Furthermore, egg-derived peptides may induce angiogenesis through ACE inhibition. Other whole egg constituents, including vitamins and minerals, help to maintain adequate levels of enzymes and co-enzymes for proper physiological functioning. Overall, whole chicken eggs serve as a cost-effective, versatile, protein-dense functional food to meet the increased protein needs of athletes.

References

1. United States Department of Agriculture, *Chickens and Eggs*, 2017.
2. United States Department of Agriculture, *World Agricultural Supply and Demand Estimates*, 2017.
3. United States Department of Agriculture, *Egg Markets Overview*, 2017.
4. J. M. Miranda, X. Anton, C. Redondo-Valbuena, P. Roca-Saavedra, J. A. Rodriguez, A. Lamas, C. M. Franco and A. Cepeda, *Nutrients*, 2015, **7**, 706–729.
5. W. O. Song and J. M. Kerver, *J. Am. Coll. Nutr.*, 2000, **19**, 556S–562S.
6. Z. Conrad, L. K. Johnson, J. N. Roemmich, W. Juan and L. Jahns, *Nutrients*, 2017, **9**(4), 333.
7. T. A. Nicklas, C. E. O'Neil and V. L. Fulgoni, *J. Nutr.*, 2015, **145**, 170S–176S.
8. J. Kovacs-Nolan, M. Phillips and Y. Mine, *J. Agric. Food Chem.*, 2005, **53**, 8421–8431.
9. United States Department of Agriculture, *National Nutrient Database for Standard Reference Release 28-Egg, whole, raw, fresh*, 2016.
10. United States Department of Agriculture, *Biology of Eggs*, 2000, vol. 2, pp. 1–14.
11. M. M. Kanter, P. M. Kris-Etherton, M. L. Fernandez, K. C. Vickers and D. L. Katz, *Adv. Nutr.*, 2012, **3**, 711–717.
12. D. D. Alexander, P. E. Miller, A. J. Vargas, D. L. Weed and S. S. Cohen, *J. Am. Coll. Nutr.*, 2016, **35**, 704–716.
13. D. J. Farrell, *Am. J. Clin. Nutr.*, 1998, **68**, 538–544.
14. K. E. Anderson, *Poult. Sci.*, 2011, **90**, 1600–1608.

15. G. Cherian, T. B. Holsonbake and M. P. Goeger, *Poult. Sci.*, 2002, **81**, 30–33.
16. A. P. Simopoulos, *Biomed. Pharmacother.*, 2002, **56**, 365–379.
17. K. B. Jouris, J. L. McDaniel and E. P. Weiss, *J Sports Sci. Med.*, 2011, **10**, 432–438.
18. P. Lembke, J. Capodice, K. Hebert and T. Swenson, *J. Sports Sci. Med.*, 2014, **13**, 151–156.
19. C. Mcglory, S. L. Wardle, L. S. Macnaughton, O. C. Witard, F. Scott, J. Dick, J. G. Bell, S. M. Phillips, S. D. R. Galloway, D. L. Hamilton and K. D. Tipton, *Physiol. Rep.*, 2016, **4**, 1–11.
20. National Health and Medical Research Council, *Dietary Guidelines*, 2013.
21. J. E. Kim, M. G. Ferruzzi and W. W. Campbell, *J. Nutr.*, 2016, **146**, 2199–2205.
22. B. M. Castellano, A. M. Thelen, O. Moldavski, M. Feltes, R. E. N. Van Der Welle, L. Mydock-McGrane, X. Jiang, R. J. Van Eijkeren, O. B. Davis, S. M. Louie, R. M. Perera, D. F. Covey, D. K. Nomura, D. S. Ory and R. Zoncu, *Science*, 2017, **355**, 1306–1311.
23. N. Hodson, C. McGlory, S. Y. Oikawa, S. Jeromson, Z. Song, M. A. Rüegg, D. L. Hamilton, S. M. Phillips and A. Philp, *Am J Physiol. Cell Physiol.*, 2017, **313**, C604–C611.
24. M. Yasuda, Y. Tanaka, S. Kume, Y. Morita, M. Chin-Kanasaki, H. Araki, K. Isshiki, S. Araki, D. Koya, M. Haneda, A. Kashiwagi, H. Maegawa and T. Uzu, *Biochim Biophys Acta*, 2014, **1842**, 1097–1108.
25. D. J. Millward, D. K. Layman, D. Tomé and G. Schaafsma, *Am. J. Clin. Nutr.*, 2008, **87**, 1576S–1581S.
26. S. M. Phillips and L. J. C. Van Loon, *J. Sport Sci.*, 2011, **29**, S29–S38.
27. G. V. Mitchell, M. Young Jenkins and E. Grundel, *Plant Foods Hum. Nutr.*, 1989, **39**, 53–58.
28. G. Schaafsma, *J. Nutr.*, 2000, **130**, 1865S–1867S.
29. FAO, *Dietary Protein Quality Evaluation in Human Nutrition: Report of an FAO Expert Consultation*, Rome, Italy, 2013.
30. S. M. Phillips, *Meat Sci.*, 2012, **92**, 174–178.
31. J. E. Tang, D. R. Moore, G. W. Kujbida, M. A. Tarnopolsky and S. M. Phillips, *J. Appl. Physiol.*, 2009, **107**, 987–992.
32. Food and Agriculture Organization of the United Nations, World Health Organization and The United Nations University, in *Joint FAO/WHO/UNU Expert Consultation on Energy and Protein Requirements*, ed. S. Srikantia, Rome, 1981.
33. P. J. Reeds and P. J. Garlick, *J. Nutr.*, 2003, **133**, 2953S–2961S.
34. Y. Yang, T. A. Churchward-Venne, N. A. Burd, L. Breen, M. A. Tarnopolsky and S. M. Phillips, *Nutr. Metab.*, 2012, **9**, 57.
35. S. H. Gorissen, A. M. Horstman, R. Franssen, J. J. Crombag, H. Langer, J. Bierau, F. Respondek and L. J. van Loon, *J. Nutr.*, 2016, **146**, 1651–1659.
36. P. J. Atherton, K. Smith, T. Etheridge, D. Rankin and M. J. Rennie, *Amino Acids*, 2010, **38**, 1533–1539.
37. P. Garlick, *J. Nutr.*, 2005, **135**, 1553S–1556S.

38. L. J. C. van Loon, *Curr. Opin. Clin. Nutr. Metab. Care*, 2012, **15**, 71–77.
39. C. S. Katsanos, H. Kobayashi, M. Sheffield-Moore, A. Aarsland and R. R. Wolfe, *Am. J. Clin. Nutr.*, 2006, **291**, E381–E387.
40. T. A. Churchward-Venne, N. A. Burd, C. J. Mitchell, D. W. D. West, A. Philp, G. R. Marcotte, S. K. Baker, K. Baar and S. M. Phillips, *J. Physiol.*, 2012, **590**, 2751–2765.
41. T. A. Churchward-Venne, L. Breen, D. M. Di Donato, A. J. Hector, C. J. Mitchell, D. R. Moore, T. Stellingwerff, D. Breuille, E. A. Offord, S. K. Baker and S. M. Phillips, *Am. J. Clin. Nutr.*, 2014, **99**, 276–286.
42. S. M. Pasiakos, T. M. McLellan and H. R. Lieberman, *Sports Med.*, 2014, **45**, 111–131.
43. J. M. Wilson, J. P. Loenneke, E. Jo, G. J. Wilson, M. C. Zourdos and J. S. Kim, *J. Strength Cond. Res.*, 2012, **26**, 1724–1729.
44. E. Ferraro, A. M. Giammarioli, S. Chiandotto, I. Spoletini and G. Rosano, *Antioxid. Redox Signaling*, 2014, **21**, 154–176.
45. G. Biolo, K. D. Tipton, S. Klein and R. R. Wolfe, *Am. J. Clin. Nutr.*, 1997, **273**, E122–E129.
46. S. M. Phillips, K. D. Tipton, A. Aarsland, S. E. Wolf and R. R. Wolfe, *Am. J. Physiol.*, 1997, **273**, 99–107.
47. N. A. Burd and M. De Lisio, *Exercise Sport Sci. Rev.*, 2017, **45**, 187–191.
48. J. Farup, S. K. Rahbek, M. H. Vendelbo, A. Matzon, J. Hindhede, A. Bejder, S. Ringgard and K. Vissing, *Scand. J. Med. Sci. Sports*, 2014, **24**, 788–798.
49. D. R. Moore, *Curr. Sports Med. Rep.*, 2015, **14**, 294–300.
50. M. J. Gibala, *Int. J. Sport Nutr. Exercise Metab.*, 2001, **11**, 87–108.
51. G. Van Hall, B. Saltin, G. J. Van Der Vusse, K. Soderlund and A. J. M. Wagenmakers, *J. Physiol.*, 1995, **489**, 251–261.
52. M. Hargreaves, G. McConell and J. Proietto, *J. Appl. Physiol.*, 1995, **78**, 288–292.
53. E. Blomstrand and B. Saltin, *J. Physiol.*, 1999, **514**, 293–302.
54. A. C. Brown, H. S. H. Macrae and N. S. Turner, *Int. J. Sport Nutr. Exercise Metab.*, 2004, **14**, 720–729.
55. K. D. Dawson, D. J. Baker, P. L. Greenhaff and M. J. Gibala, *J. Physiol.*, 2005, **565**, 637–643.
56. G. H. Koo, J. Woo, S. Kang and K. O. Shin, *J. Phys. Ther. Sci.*, 2014, **26**, 1241–1246.
57. T. Sugino, S. Aoyagi, T. Shirai, Y. Kajimoto and O. Kajimoto, *J. Clin. Biochem. Nutr.*, 2007, **41**, 224–230.
58. J. L. Bowtell, G. P. Leese, K. Smith, P. W. Watt, A. Nevill, O. Rooyackers, A. J. M. Wagenmakers and M. J. Rennie, *J. Appl. Physiol.*, 1998, **85**, 1744–1752.
59. M. Mazzulla, J. T. Parel, J. W. Beals, S. van Vliet, S. Abou Sawan, D. W. D. West, S. A. Paluska, A. V. Ulanov, D. R. Moore and N. A. Burd, *Med. Sci. Sports Exercise*, 2017, 1.
60. K. Van Wijck, K. Lenaerts, J. Grootjans, K. A. P. Wijnands, M. Poeze, L. J. C. Van Loon, C. H. C. Dejong and W. A. Buurman, *Am. J. Physiol.: Gastrointest. Liver Physiol.*, 2012, **303**, 155–168.

61. K. van Wijck, K. Lenaerts, L. J. C. van Loon, W. H. M. Peters, W. A. Buurman and C. H. C. Dejong, *PLoS One*, 2011, **6**, e22366.
62. Institute of Medicine, *Dietary Reference Intakes for Energy, Carbohydrate, Fiber, Fat, Fatty Acids, Cholesterol, Protein, and Amino Acids (Macronutrients)*, National Academies Press, Washington, D.C., 2005.
63. D. T. Thomas, K. A. Erdman and L. M. Burke, *J. Acad. Nutr. Diet.*, 2016, **116**, 501–528.
64. S. A. Sawan, S. Van Vliet, J. T. Parel, J. W. Beals, M. Mazzulla, D. W. D. West, A. Philp, Z. Li, S. A. Paluska, N. A. Burd and D. R. Moore, *Physiol. Rep.*, 2018, **6**, 1–14.
65. A. W. Staples, N. A. Burd, D. W. D. West, K. D. Currie, P. J. Atherton, D. R. Moore, M. J. Rennie, M. J. Macdonald, S. K. Baker and S. M. Phillips, *Med. Sci. Sports Exercise*, 2011, **43**, 1154–1161.
66. S. van Vliet, E. L. Shy, S. Abou Sawan, J. W. Beals, D. W. West, S. K. Skinner, A. V. Ulanov, Z. Li, S. A. Paluska, C. M. Parsons, D. R. Moore and N. A. Burd, *Am. J. Clin. Nutr.*, 2017, **106**, 1401–1412.
67. D. R. Moore, M. J. Robinson, J. L. Fry, J. E. Tang, E. I. Glover, S. B. Wilkinson, T. Prior, M. A. Tarnopolsky and S. M. Phillips, *Am. J. Clin. Nutr.*, 2008, **89**, 161–168.
68. H. B. Iglay, J. W. Apolzan, D. E. Gerrard, J. K. Eash, J. C. Anderson and W. W. Campbell, *J. Nutr., Health Aging*, 2009, **13**, 108–114.
69. V. Kumar, A. Selby, D. Rankin, R. Patel, P. Atherton, W. Hildebrandt, J. Williams, K. Smith, O. Seynnes, N. Hiscock and M. J. Rennie, *J. Physiol.*, 2009, **587**, 211–217.
70. W. W. Campbell, T. A. Trappe, R. R. Wolfe and W. J. Evans, *J. Gerontol.*, 2001, **56**, M373–M380.
71. L. M. Vislocky, M. A. Pikosky, K. H. Rubin, S. Vega-López, P. C. Gaine, W. F. Martin, T. L. Zern, I. E. Lofgren, M. L. Fernandez and N. R. Rodriguez, *J. Nutr. Biochem.*, 2009, **20**, 26–34.
72. Z. S. Clayton, K. R. Scholar, M. Shelechi, L. M. Hernandez, A. M. Barber, Y. J. Petrisko, S. Hooshmand and M. Kern, *J. Am. Coll. Nutr.*, 2015, **34**, 113–119.
73. United States Department of Agriculture, USDA National Nutrient Database for Standard Reference, release 28, https://ndb.nal.usda.gov/ndb/, accessed 25 August 2017.
74. J. T. Penry and M. M. Manore, *Int. J. Sport Nutr. Exercise Metab.*, 2008, **18**, 191–203.
75. A. L. Buchman, D. Jenden and M. Roch, *J. Am. Coll. Nutr.*, 1999, **18**, 598–601.
76. L. Conlay, L. Sabounjian and R. Wurtman, *Int. J. Sports Med.*, 1992, **13**, S141–S142.
77. H. N. von Allwörden, S. Horn, J. Kahl and W. Feldheim, *Eur. J. Appl. Physiol. Occup. Physiol.*, 1993, **67**, 87–91.
78. C. Piérard, D. Béracochéa, M. Pérès, J.-C. Jouanin, P. Liscia, P. Satabin, S. Martin, G. Testylier, C. Y. Guézennec and M. Beaumont, *Neuropsychobiology*, 2004, **49**, 210–217.

79. T. A. Watson, L. K. Macdonald-Wicks and M. L. Garg, *Int. J. Sport Nutr. Exercise Metab.*, 2005, **15**, 131–146.
80. C. Nimalaratne and J. Wu, *Nutrients*, 2015, **7**, 8274–8293.
81. J. Wu and A. Acero-Lopez, *Food Res. Int.*, 2012, **46**, 480–487.
82. M. Yousr and N. Howell, *Int. J. Mol. Sci.*, 2015, **16**, 29161–29178.
83. E. D. N. S. Abeyrathne, X. Huang and D. U. Ahn, *Poult. Sci.*, 2018, **97**, 1462–1468.
84. N. Minami, Y. Li, Q. Guo, T. Kawamura, N. Mori, M. Nagasaka, M. Ogawa, O. Ito, H. Kurosawa, M. Kanazawa and M. Kohzuki, *J. Hypertens.*, 2007, **25**, 1241–1248.
85. G. S. Jensen, M. R. Lenninger, J. L. Beaman, R. Taylor and K. F. Benson, *J. Med. Food*, 2015, **18**, 1042–1048.
86. FAO, *Amino-acid Content of Foods and Biological Data on Proteins*, FAO, 1970.
87. E. E. Sumner and J. R. Murlin, *J. Nutr.*, 1938, **16**, 141–152.
88. N. A. Burd, H. M. Hamer, B. Pennings, W. F. Pellikaan, J. M. G. Senden, A. P. Gijsen and L. J. C. van Loon, *PLoS One*, 2013, **8**(6), e68109.

CHAPTER 7

Egg Carotenoids for Eye Health

GARRY HANDELMAN*

University of Massachusetts, Lowell, USA
*E-mail: Garry_Handelman@uml.edu

7.1 Introduction

The eggs of the domestic chicken, *Gallus domesticus*, typically contain an abundance of two polar carotenoids, lutein and zeaxanthin (L and Z) (Figures 7.1 and 7.2).[1–3] If these two carotenoids are provided in the diet of the chicken, the hen will preferentially deposit these carotenoids in the yolk. Chickens raised in North America are usually supplied with corn (*Zea maize*) as a major dietary component and yellow corn is an important contributor of L and Z to the diet of the chicken.[4]

In humans, these carotenoids accumulate in the center of the human retina, called the macula lutea[5–7] (Figure 7.3). Specific retinal transport mechanisms have evolved that selectively deposit zeaxanthin at the center of the macula and lutein at the periphery of the macula.[8] There is ample evidence that macular carotenoids contribute to improved visual acuity,[9,10] and these carotenoids may also provide protection against some diseases of the macula, such as age-related macular degeneration (AMD).

There is some evidence for additional physiological roles for L and Z, including cognitive function.[11,12] Efforts are underway to collect further data about these proposed mechanisms.

Food Chemistry, Function and Analysis No.14
Eggs as Functional Foods and Nutraceuticals for Human Health
Edited by Jianping Wu

Published by the Royal Society of Chemistry, www.rsc.org

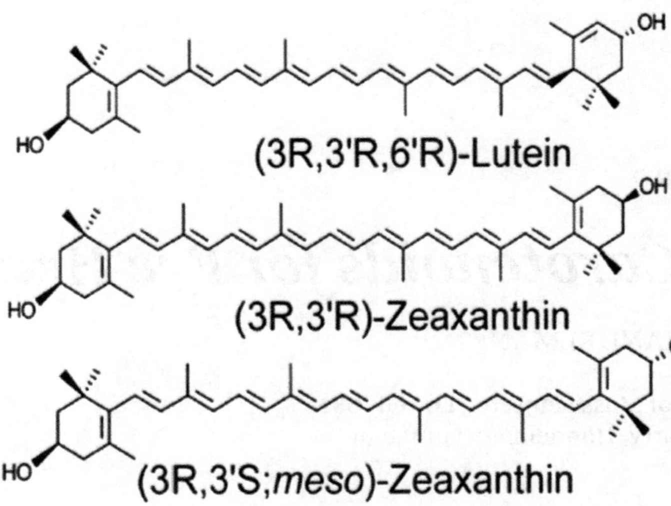

Figure 7.1 Carotenoids in the macula. The first two compounds are present in chicken eggs and other foods. The last compound appears to be formed by *in vivo* modification of lutein.

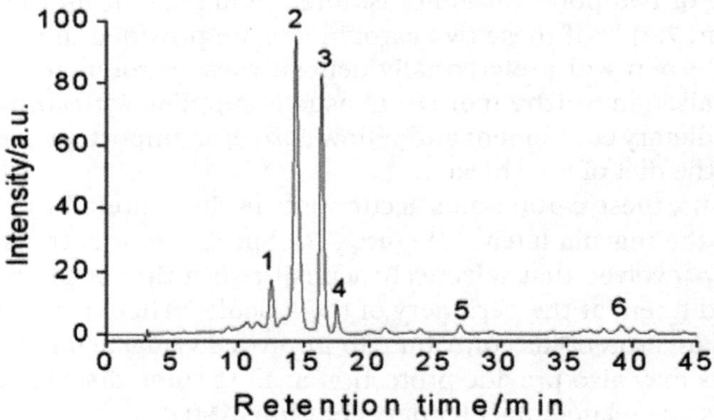

Figure 7.2 HPLC analysis of carotenoids in chicken egg yolk: Unknown, peak 1; lutein, peak 2; zeaxanthin, peak 3; apo-8-carotenal, peak 4; beta-cryptoxanthin, peak 5; beta-carotene, peak 6. Reproduced from ref. 3 with permission from Springer Nature, Copyright 2012.

Since the L and Z in the egg yolk are absorbed into the human bloodstream more efficiently than these carotenoids present in most other foods and dietary sources,[13–17] it is relevant to examine chicken eggs as a source of L and Z for human nutrition, and to consider the potential impact of human visual function and health from these egg carotenoids in the diet.

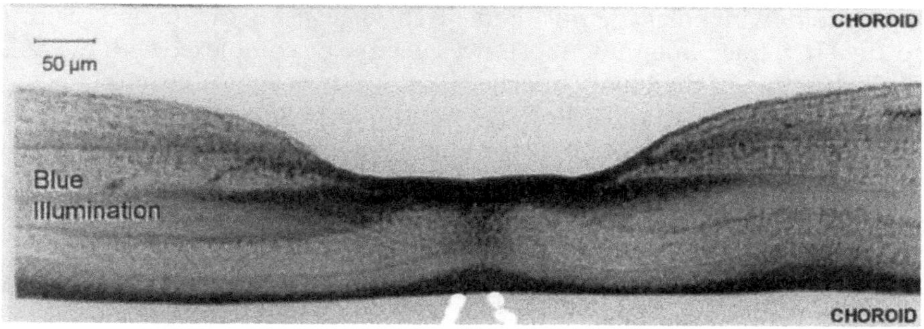

Figure 7.3 Cross-section of the macula, photographed in blue light. The carotenoids are concentrated in the macular region. Reproduced from ref. 69 with permission from Oxford University Press, Copyright 1995.

7.2 Accumulation of Polar Carotenoids in Egg Yolk, and Enhanced Nutritional Bioavailability of Lutein and Zeaxanthin from this Dietary Source

Lutein and zeaxanthin are utilized by chickens and other birds for coloration, and to provide carotenoids for specific oil droplets in the retina of birds and some other vertebrates.[18] The carotenoids in the oil droplets enhance color perception in these species; the role of carotenoids in vision therefore has a long evolutionary history. The accumulation in the yolk of the chicken egg is highly specific; although yellow corn also contains an abundance of the polar carotenoid beta-cryptoxanthin,[4] the hen oviduct discriminates in favor of L and Z, depositing very little beta-cryptoxanthin in the yolk[3] (Figure 7.2). Some species of wild birds also show preferential deposition of L and Z in the yolk,[19] suggesting a general avian preference for these polar carotenoids. The biochemical pathways that lead to this accumulation have not been clearly defined, and specific transport proteins might play a role during maturation of the egg in the oviduct. It is therefore appropriate to conclude that many birds are accumulator species for both L and Z, with selective deposition in egg yolk.[3,20]

To ensure an abundance of L + Z in hen's eggs, yellow maize will provide high levels of both carotenoids in the chicken diet. Modified poultry diets have led to the production of special eggs with as much as 400% higher amounts of L and Z than conventional eggs,[21,22] and these eggs have been used in some human intervention trials. In the future, the L + Z content of eggs may be a component of food analysis, listed as part of the nutritional analysis on the container that holds the eggs.

The nutritional bioavailability to humans of L + Z in egg yolk is considerably higher than the same carotenoids provided in plant foods and the effectiveness of L + Z from egg yolk has been extensively documented.[13–17] This favorable effect on absorption is caused by the physical association of the egg carotenoids with polar egg yolk lipids. To be digested in the human gastrointestinal (GI) tract, lipophilic substances need to be complexed with the polar lipid structure of the biliary micelle.[23] The lipids of egg yolk contain a large fraction of the polar lipids cholesterol and phosphatidylcholine, along with neutral triglycerides,[20] similar to the lipids of the biliary micelle.[23] L + Z in the yolk has formed an association with polar lipids before the food is ingested, which accomplishes a portion of the task that is required for lipid absorption in the small intestine.

By contrast, L + Z from most plant sources requires more complex processes within the GI tract to transfer L + Z to the polar lipid micelles. This difference, at the level of the egg yolk, would largely explain why L + Z in eggs is generally three to four times more bioavailable than these carotenoids provided with plant dietary components or supplements. The bioavailability index can be described as the relative change in plasma concentration of a nutrient, at a similar dose, based on dietary source. For example, 0.6 mg of zeaxanthin day^{-1} from eggs in the diet leads to 3–4× higher plasma increases than a similar amount from a food source. As a general rule, higher amounts of L + Z from plant foods and supplements are needed to achieve a similar response to L + Z from egg yolks.[13–16]

7.3 Selective Accumulation in the Human Macula: Biochemical Mechanisms

The macula of higher primates (humans, apes, and monkeys) has developed specific mechanisms to accumulate L + Z.[24–26] The pigment density is very low at birth[7,27] but may reach adult values by the age of 3 years.[24,27] The accumulation is in photoreceptor axons that overlay the region of the retina responsible for central vision[28] (Figure 7.3); when a person reads a stop sign or looks for a baseball thrown by the pitcher, the image of the object will generally fall directly on the macula, and those photons pass through macular carotenoids before reaching the photoreceptors. Some L + Z is found in photoreceptor membranes in the peripheral retina, but at levels much lower than in the macular region.[29] The critical role of the macular region in human visual function has led to a great deal of interest in the function of the macular pigment.

The accumulation in the macula is highly selective; although L + Z account for 25% of total plasma carotenoids, these molecules constitute >90% of the carotenoids in the macula,[7,30] and traces of beta-carotene and lycopene detected in autopsy specimens may reflect small amounts of blood in the sample.[30] Recent investigations have identified certain proteins in the retina that lead to the selective accumulation of L and Z in the photoreceptor axons. The protein that binds lutein may be StARD3, a member of the steroidogenic acute regulatory domain (StARD) protein family,[8] which performs many functions in lipid transfer across membranes. StARD3 is present in photoreceptor axons and can function as a lutein-binding protein and lead to lutein accumulation in the axon cell bodies. The protein that binds zeaxanthin may be an isomer of glutathione-*S*-transferase, GST-P1,[31] and this protein would function to accumulate zeaxanthin in the axons at the center of the macula.

Some of the zeaxanthin in the retina is in the form of a different geometrical isomer, called *meso*-zeaxanthin (Figure 7.1), which is found at very low levels in the diet. It is proposed that *meso*-zeaxanthin is produced within the retina by biochemical modification of lutein, through migration of a double bond to a different position on the molecule. A candidate protein, RPE-65, has been described that carries out this transformation.[32] RPE-65 was previously shown to function in the vitamin A cycle needed for visual perception. Therefore, dietary lutein may also serve as a source for macular *meso*-zeaxanthin.

Further progress on the biochemical regulation of macular carotenoids levels may include studies of genetic variations in human populations. In twin studies, closer agreement between identical twins was seen in macular carotenoids levels than was observed without genetic concordance,[33] indicating some effects of genetic factors. However, efforts to define how genotype affects phenotype are very challenging, requiring large cohorts and analysis of many genes, and this needs to be considered in studies of the genetics of macular carotenoid accumulation.[34] Studies of single-nucleotide-polymorphisms[35–37] have indicated some possible associations, but data so far is not consistent between studies. The ability to screen large numbers of individuals for macular carotenoids should allow this effort to move forward in the future.

7.4 Dietary Modification of Macular Carotenoids

The levels of macular carotenoids can be affected by dietary intake; increases have been consistently obtained with large supplements of L + Z.[38,39] Recent findings indicate that consumption of eggs containing L and Z may increase the carotenoid levels.[40,41] The change may be most prominent in subjects with below-average levels of macular carotenoids at baseline and may require high consumption of eggs (4 day^{-1}) for several months. The effect on subjects with low baseline levels is typical in nutrition research, where individuals with low levels of a nutrient show a more robust response to increased dietary intake than is observed in replete individuals. This change has not been observed in other short-duration studies[42] and the effect of increased egg intake on macular carotenoids levels requires further controlled investigation.

In the rhesus monkey, about 6 months was needed to restore macular carotenoid levels in animals given carotenoid-free diets for an extended period.[43] High-dose supplements of L + Z can produce effects more rapidly than a dietary modification and the effects of increased egg intake should be considered in view of the time needed to show changes, which could be 1 year or longer. As non-invasive macular carotenoid screening becomes a more common research and clinical tool, data may become available at the population level on egg consumption and macular carotenoids. As a precaution, changes in macular carotenoids following increased consumption of eggs in the diet cannot be expected to show the same more rapid changes that can be obtained with large dietary supplements of L + Z.

Although some individuals have levels of macular L + Z that reach 90% attenuation of blue light (1 absorbance unit at 450 nm),[44] it cannot be assumed that such levels will be consistently achieved even on a diet very high in L + Z since other factors in physiology and genetics play a role in controlling the accumulation of the carotenoids in the macula. The reliance on dietary intake has been demonstrated in controlled trials with rhesus monkeys, where several years on a low L + Z diet led to almost complete disappearance of the macular carotenoids;[43,45] as to be expected with changes in the biochemistry of CNS components, the rate of change is very gradual and these effects only occurred after a very extended experimental period. Recently, several genetic factors that control macular carotenoid levels have been reported,[35–37] although this research is very preliminary.

7.5 Comparison of Dietary Supplements and Eggs as Sources of Lutein and Zeaxanthin

Eggs and dietary supplements are both effective strategies for increasing levels of these carotenoids in the plasma, and potentially increasing provision of L and Z to other tissues, including the macula. The bioavailable matrix of the egg carotenoids provides certain advantages, especially at the level of nutrient competition in the GI tract. High levels of one carotenoid in the diet can suppress the absorption of other carotenoids because some of the mechanisms are saturable. Typical L + Z supplement formulations contain 10 mg of L and 2 mg of Z,[46] and those levels might interfere with absorption of other carotenoids. By contrast, consumption of two standard eggs day^{-1} in the US can provide about 800 µg of L and 600 µg of Z, depending on the source of the eggs, in a bioavailable form that will lead to increases in plasma levels within a month.[13] Special eggs from chickens provided with increased dietary L + Z contain higher levels, and have a larger effect on plasma levels;[21,22] because the L and Z in the egg lipid matrix is highly bioavailable, this should be considered as a more appropriate strategy for increasing intake.

7.6 Role of Polar Carotenoids in the Human Eye: Visual Acuity

High optical resolution in the macular region of the retina is critical for visual acuity. The carotenoids L and Z are present in the peripheral retina, but at much lower levels.[7,30] The macular carotenoids, L and Z, are deposited in the cellular axons in front of the macular photoreceptors (Figure 7.3). Because of

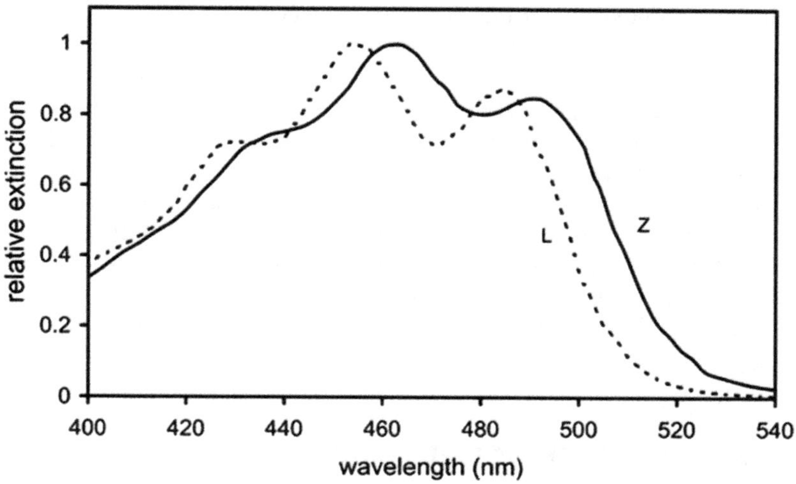

Figure 7.4 Absorption spectra of lutein (L) and zeaxanthin (Z).

retinal anatomy, light will pass through these carotenoids before it reaches the photoreceptors and certain wavelengths will be attenuated (Figure 7.4). The spectrum of these carotenoids (Figure 7.4) is selective for the absorbance of blue light in the region of 425–500 nm and in some individuals the intensity of these wavelengths reaching the macular photoreceptors may be attenuated by 50–90%.[47]

In general terms, the effect of these pigments is that the macula receives less blue light (425–500 nm) than the other regions of the retina, a phenomenon sometimes referred to as the "inner sunglass effect". However, the level of macular carotenoids is not the same between different individuals, and attenuation of blue light transmittance to the photoreceptors can be as low as 10% and as high as 90%.[47]

The selective attenuation of blue light can minimize a phenomenon known as chromatic aberration. Color "fringes" can occur when light over the complete visible spectrum is refracted by a lens because of the differential refraction of different wavelengths of visible light passing through the lens and cornea. Blue wavelengths can be bent considerably more than wavelengths in the other regions of the spectrum. There are some adaptations in the cornea and lens for this, but removing much of the blue light at the macula provides even better acuity by diminishing blue light fringes.

This selective attenuation of blue light reaching the macular photoreceptors can have several visual benefits. Visual acuity with intense blue light is improved with increased macular carotenoids.[9] The threshold for photophobia is increased with higher levels of macular carotenoid[48] and the recovery time after photostress is decreased.[10] Measurements of a variety of different indicators of visual acuity and light stress are consistent with improved function, especially when there are high levels of blue ambient light.[49]

Variation in macular carotenoid levels between different individuals is an important biological question. A portion of the data on macular carotenoid density has been obtained with autopsy specimens,[6,7,24] but this is a limited resource. The majority of current data has been obtained by the indirect measurement of these carotenoids in the retina using several devices that focus a weak-intensity beam of blue light on the macula and make measurements that indicate how much of this light reaches the photoreceptors.[50–53] These devices can be used in a local clinician's office, or in a large population study, and have enabled a great deal of data to be obtained on macular carotenoid density. Further wide-scale use of these devices is expected in the future and a very large database of macular carotenoid levels may be developed in the coming years.

7.7 Role of Macular Carotenoids for the Health of Retina

The region of the retina that contains the macular carotenoids is vulnerable to AMD, a common age-related condition.[54] This disorder, which appears in some individuals by age 60 and shows high prevalence (>20%) after age 75,[54] is accompanied by loss of central vision, and can lead to considerable disability. In the United States, as many as 15 000 000 individuals may be affected.[53] Prevention and treatment are important public health objectives, and the role of macular carotenoids has received considerable attention. A protective role for the pigment has been hypothesized because it can absorb blue light, which is more harmful to the macular region of the retina than other wavelengths. This may be linked to a greater susceptibility to the harmful effects of blue light on cells in the pigment epithelium, which nourishes and maintains the photoreceptors[55] because cytochromes strongly absorb these wavelengths. Other proposed mechanisms include production of singlet oxygen from melanosomes or lipofuscin in the pigment epithelium.[56,57] Following cataract surgery, patients are often advised to use yellow sunglasses to reduce blue light reaching the retina because the lens of older individuals plays a role in decreasing blue light transmittance.[58]

Earlier research on dietary constituents[59] identified carotenoid-rich foods, especially foods that contain abundant lutein, as protective against AMD, and research on this hypothesis has intensified in recent years.[60] In the year 1994, an antioxidant intervention for individuals with early AMD, called the Age-Related Eye Disease Study (AREDS), was launched by the US National Institutes of Health and the results were released in 2001.[61] The intervention consisted of a supplement with vitamin E, selenium, vitamin C, zinc, and beta-carotene; it was not possible at that time to obtain L + Z suitable for a dietary intervention. The supplements in AREDS were effective at decreasing long-term development of AMD by 20%,[61] highlighting the importance of nutrition for visual health.

As commercial sources of L + Z become available in quantity, the AREDS working group modified the supplement formulation away from beta-carotene, and new subjects recruited to the trial were given supplements containing lutein (10 mg) and zeaxanthin (2 mg). The second trial was called AREDS-2.[46] Although the study design is complex, the general conclusion is that the inclusion of L + Z led to a more effective formulation. It must be emphasized that the dietary intervention contained several components and synergistic actions at macular tissues must be considered when evaluating the effectiveness in this study of L + Z for macular health.

Observational studies of macular carotenoids and AMD have shown some positive results, although findings have not been consistent. Following the identification of the macular carotenoids as L and Z, there were investigations of plasma levels of these carotenoids and their relation to the optical density of macular carotenoids,[62] and positive trends were observed, including early associations between plasma carotenoid levels and AMD risk. However, the emphasis in the popular literature on the protective role of these carotenoids has led to many at-risk individuals taking L + Z supplements, and in some studies subjects with early AMD have higher plasma levels.[63] The utility of plasma measurements will likely decrease with changes in nutrient supplement intake, especially as L + Z dietary supplements become more prevalent. As a further precaution, associations of macular carotenoids levels with AMD can be confounded by the effects of smoking.[64] Individuals who smoke have a clearly increased risk of AMD and macular carotenoids levels are also lower in this group.[64]

Since the incidence of macular degeneration typically increases sharply after age 70 as a result of slowly progressing changes in retinal physiology, an appropriate research model would evaluate AMD incidence and macular carotenoid density in a long-term longitudinal study over a 10–20 year period, and compare that to plasma levels. Several trial designs of this kind are underway. As a general rule, research to examine how diet affects the incidence of diseases with a lengthy development phase has to address major difficulties in experimental design. Research designs to examine the interaction between L + Z intake from various sources and AMD incidence and severity will need to develop strategies that allow longitudinal tracking and correction for confounders. Increased use of non-invasive screening for macular carotenoids[50–53] should allow better testing of the hypothesis that egg consumption is associated with macular carotenoids levels.

The similarity of macular carotenoid distribution in humans and several other primates[25,26,28] enables useful studies of the effects of deficiency and supplementation to be done using primate models. The rhesus monkey has been used effectively for this purpose[43,45,65] since its diet can be controlled for extended periods of time. Certain retinal changes suggestive of macular degeneration were observed in monkeys maintained on a (L + Z)-deficient diet for >10 years,[65] but it is not likely that humans would experience a diet completely lacking these carotenoids, and therefore this result must be interpreted with caution.

7.8 Antioxidant Properties of Polar Carotenoids

Some *in vitro* studies have shown that many kinds of carotenoids, including L and Z, can function as free-radical scavengers, which suggests an antioxidant role for these molecules *in vivo*.[66] This hypothesis is appealing because retinal tissues contain an abundance of certain polyunsaturated fatty acids, 20 : 6n3 and 22 : 5n3, which are highly vulnerable to peroxidative damage. The best-established antioxidant effects for carotenoids arise from their ability to scavenge singlet oxygen, which is one of several different forms of active oxygen than that may lead to free-radical damage. Singlet oxygen is often a consequence of chemical processes initiated by photons,[67] acting through a class of molecules known as photosensitizers. Since a large amount of light can reach the retina, damage from photosensitizers is considered as a potential cause of retinal aging.

If it was established that blue light in the foveal region was producing singlet oxygen by reaction with a photosensitizer in the cell, this would support a proposed antioxidant function for macular carotenoids by attenuation of photochemically active blue-wavelength photons reaching the photoreceptors, and several hypotheses have been proposed for this mechanism.[55–57] The damaging light-driven processes might also occur directly in the cellular axons where carotenoids are deposited, although AMD generally occurs in the pigment epithelium cell layer behind the photoreceptors.

Other forms of antioxidant function for carotenoids, including scavenging of peroxyl radicals and chain termination, have been reported for high levels of these carotenoids in organic solvents.[66] The amount of L + Z in the axons overlying the photoreceptors may reach 1 mMole kg tissue^{-1}, or 10 mMole (kg of lipid component)$^{-1}$, since neural tissue is typically 10% lipid by weight.[68] Direct free-radical scavenging is possible for carotenoids that reach those concentrations in tissues. However, the most vulnerable tissue in the retina, the pigment epithelium (the RPE), contains very little carotenoid, and a direct free-radical scavenging mechanism is not consistent with the concentrations of carotenoids in the pigment epithelial cells. The axons that contain the macular carotenoid are 40–60 μm distant from the pigment epithelium cells. An effect of macular carotenoids as protective blue light filters would be consistent with protection at the level of the RPE.

Appropriate experimental designs, which examine alternative hypotheses, are needed to fully address these proposed mechanisms for protection against active oxygen species, which currently await experimental confirmation.

7.9 Conclusions

The eggs of domestic chickens in the US are an established dietary source of the carotenoids of the macula. These carotenoids (lutein and zeaxanthin) have enhanced bioavailability from egg yolk, compared to other dietary sources, and increased egg intake in controlled trials reliably leads to increased plasma levels. Increased macular carotenoids may also result from this dietary change.

Since eggs consistently contribute to the circulating plasma pool of L + Z, this dietary source provides carotenoids to the macula. Individuals who consume eggs in the American diet are utilizing a good source of these carotenoids and elevated egg consumption should increase plasma levels, and possibly levels in the macula. Data on this hypothesis may be gained with increased use of non-invasive measurement of macular carotenoids.

Visual acuity responds well to increased macular carotenoids owing to complex interactions between blue light and these pigments in the retina. Screening for the level of macular carotenoids is recommended for use in clinical practice[60] and may become more prevalent with wider adoption of non-invasive technology for screening. Some individuals have low levels of macular pigment, and the optical density for blue-wavelength light is less than 0.1 AU; in practice this means that most of the blue light reaches the macula. For those individuals, consumption of eggs would be a reasonable strategy to increase macular carotenoids levels; changes may require 1 year or longer to be seen since response to increased dietary intake occurs slowly.

References

1. S. M. Abdel-Aal el, H. Akhtar, K. Zaheer and R. Ali, Dietary sources of lutein and zeaxanthin carotenoids and their role in eye health, *Nutrients*, 2013, **5**, 1169–1185.
2. K. Zaheer, Hen egg carotenoids (lutein and zeaxanthin) and nutritional impacts on human health: a review, *CyTA--J. Food*, 2017, **15**, 474–487.
3. A. Pintea, F. Dulf, A. Bunea, C. Matea and S. Andrei, Comparative analysis of lipophilic compounds in eggs of organically raised ISA Brown and Araucana hens, *Chem. Pap.*, 2012, **66**, 955–963.
4. C. O. Grogan and C. W. Blessin, Characterization of major carotenoids in yellow maize lines of differing pigment concentration, *Crop Sci.*, 1968, **8**, 730–732.
5. R. A. Bone, J. T. Landrum and L. M. Friedes, *et al.* Distribution of lutein and zeaxanthin stereoisomers in the human retina, *Exp. Eye Res.*, 1997, **64**, 211–218.
6. R. A. Bone, J. T. Landrum and S. L. Tarsis, Preliminary identification of the human macular pigment, *Vision Res.*, 1985, **25**, 1531–1535.
7. G. J. Handelman, E. A. Dratz, C. C. Reay and F. J. G. M. van Kuijk, Carotenoids in the human macula and whole retina, *Invest. Ophthalmol. Visual Sci.*, 1988, **29**, 850–855.
8. B. Li, P. Vachali, J. M. Frederick and P. S. Bernstein, Identification of StARD3 as a lutein-binding protein in the macula of the primate retina, *Biochemistry*, 2011, **50**(13), 2541–2549.
9. B. R. Hammond Jr, L. M. Fletcher and J. G. Elliott, Glare disability, photostress recovery, and chromatic contrast: relation to macular pigment and serum lutein and zeaxanthin, *Invest. Ophthalmol. Visual Sci.*, 2013, **54**, 476–481.

10. J. M. Stringham, K. J. O'Brien and N. T. Stringham, Contrast Sensitivity and Lateral Inhibition Are Enhanced With Macular Carotenoid Supplementation, *Invest. Ophthalmol. Visual Sci.*, 2017, **58**, 2291–2295.
11. R. Vishwanathan, W. Schalch and E. J. Johnson, Macular pigment carotenoids in the retina and occipital cortex are related in humans, *Nutr. Neurosci.*, 2015, **19**, 95–101.
12. L. Renzi-Hammond, E. Bovier and L. Fletcher, *et al.* Effects of a Lutein and Zeaxanthin Intervention on Cognitive Function: A Randomized, Double-Masked, Placebo-Controlled Trial of Younger Healthy Adults, *Nutrients*, 2017, **9**(11), 1246.
13. G. J. Handelman, Z. D. Nightingale, A. Lichtenstein, E. J. Schaefer and J. B. Blumberg, Plasma lutein and zeaxanthin after dietary egg yolk supplementation, *Am. J. Clin. Nutr.*, 1999, **70**, 247–251.
14. H. Y. Chung, H. M. Rasmussen and E. J. Johnson, Lutein bioavailability is higher from lutein-enriched eggs than from supplements and spinach in men, *J. Nutr.*, 2004, **134**, 1887–1893.
15. E. F. Goodrow, T. A. Wilson and S. C. Houde, *et al.* Consumption of one egg per day increases serum lutein and zeaxanthin concentrations in older adults without altering serum lipid and lipoprotein cholesterol concentrations, *J. Nutr.*, 2006, **136**, 2519–2524.
16. N. Severins, R. P. Mensink and J. Plat, Effects of lutein-enriched egg yolk in buttermilk or skimmed milk on serum lipids & lipoproteins of mildly hypercholesterolemic subjects, *Nutr., Metab. Cardiovasc. Dis.*, 2015, **25**, 210–217.
17. A. Missimer, M. L. Fernandez and D. M. DiMarco, *et al.* Compared to an Oatmeal Breakfast, Two Eggs/Day Increased Plasma Carotenoids and Choline without Increasing Trimethyl Amine N-Oxide Concentrations, *J. Am. Coll. Nutr.*, 2018, **37**, 140–148.
18. N. S. Hart, T. J. Lisney and S. P. Collin, Cone photoreceptor oil droplet pigmentation is affected by ambient light intensity, *J. Exp. Biol.*, 2006, **209**, 4776–4787.
19. C. Isaksson, A. Johansson and S. Andersson, Egg yolk carotenoids in relation to habitat and reproductive investment in Parus major, *Physiol. Biochem. Zool.*, 2008, **81**, 112–118.
20. V. Sinanoglou, I. Strati and S. Miniadis-Meimaroglou, Lipid, fatty acid and carotenoid content of edible egg yolks from avian species: A comparative study, *Food Chem.*, 2011, **124**, 971–977.
21. P. F. Surai, A. MacPherson, B. K. Speake and N. H. Sparks, Designer egg evaluation in a controlled trial, *Eur. J. Clin. Nutr.*, 2000, **54**, 298–305.
22. S. Fredriksson, K. Elwingerb and J. Pickovaa, Fatty acid and carotenoid composition of egg yolk as an effect of microalgae addition to feed formula for laying hens, *Food Chem.*, 2006, **99**, 530–537.
23. M. C. Carey, D. M. Small and C. M. Bliss, Lipid Digestion and Absorption, *Annu. Rev. Physiol.*, 1983, **45**, 651–677.

24. R. A. Bone, J. T. Landrum, Z. Dixon, Y. Chen and C. M. Llerena, Lutein and zeaxanthin in the eyes, serum and diet of human subjects, *Exp. Eye Res.*, 2000, **71**, 239–245.
25. G. J. Handelman, D. M. Snodderly, N. I. Krinsky, M. D. Russett and A. J. Adler, Biological control of primate macular pigment. Biochemical and densitometric studies, *Invest. Ophthalmol. Visual Sci.*, 1991, **32**, 257–267.
26. D. M. Snodderly, G. J. Handelman and A. J. Adler, Distribution of individual macular pigment carotenoids in central retina of macaque and squirrel monkeys, *Invest. Ophthalmol. Visual Sci.*, 1991, **32**, 268–279.
27. R. A. Bone, J. T. Landrum, L. Fernandez and S. L. Tarsis, Analysis of the macular pigment by HPLC: retinal distribution and age study, *Invest. Ophthalmol. Visual Sci.*, 1988, **29**, 843–849.
28. D. M. Snodderly, J. D. Auran and F. C. Delori, The macular pigment. II. Spatial distribution in primate retinas, *Invest. Ophthalmol. Visual Sci.*, 1984, **25**, 674–685.
29. L. M. Rapp, S. S. Maple and J. H. Choi, Lutein and zeaxanthin concentrations in rod outer segment membranes from perifoveal and peripheral human retina, *Invest. Ophthalmol. Visual Sci.*, 2000, **41**, 1200–1209.
30. G. J. Handelman, D. M. Snodderly, A. J. Adler, M. D. Russett and E. A. Dratz, Measurement of carotenoids in human and monkey retinas, *Methods Enzymol.*, 1992, **213**, 220–230.
31. P. Bhosale, A. J. Larson, J. M. Frederick, K. Southwick, C. D. Thulin and P. S. Bernstein, Identification and characterization of a Pi isoform of glutathione S-transferase (GSTP1) as a zeaxanthin-binding protein in the macula of the human eye, *J. Biol. Chem.*, 2004, **279**, 49447–49454.
32. R. Shyam, A. Gorusupudi, K. Nelson, M. P. Horvath and P. S. Bernstein, RPE65 has an additional function as the lutein to meso-zeaxanthin isomerase in the vertebrate eye, *Proc. Natl. Acad. Sci. U. S. A.*, 2017, **114**, 10882–10887.
33. C. Hammond, S. Liew and F. Van Kuijk, *et al.* The Heritability of Macular Response to Supplemental Lutein and Zeaxanthin: A Classic Twin Study, *Invest. Ophthalmol. Visual Sci.*, 2012, **53**(8), 4963.
34. K. Koo, M. Neuringer and J. SanGiovanni, Macular xanthophylls, lipoprotein-related genes, and age-related macular degeneration, *Am. J. Clin. Nutr.*, 2014, **100**(supp), 336S–346S.
35. B. Feigl, C. Morris, J. Voisey, A. Kwan and A. J. Zele, The relationship between BCMO1 gene variants and macular pigment optical density in persons with and without age-related macular degeneration, *PLoS One*, 2014, **9**, e89069.
36. Z. Kyle-Little, A. Zele, P. Morris and B. Feigl, The effect of BCMO1 gene variants on macular pigment optical density in young healthy Caucasians, *Front. Nutr.*, 2014, **1**, 1–5.
37. E. Yonova-Doing, P. G. Hysi and C. Venturini, *et al.* Candidate gene study of macular response to supplemental lutein and zeaxanthin, *Exp. Eye Res.*, 2013, **115**, 172–177.

38. J. T. Landrum, R. A. Bone, H. Joa, M. D. Kilburn, L. L. Moore and K. E. Sprague, A one year study of the macular pigment: the effect of 140 days of a lutein supplement, *Exp. Eye Res.*, 1997, **65**, 57–62.
39. H. H. Koh, I. J. Murray, D. Nolan, D. Carden, J. Feather and S. Beatty, Plasma and macular responses to lutein supplement in subjects with and without age-related maculopathy: a pilot study, *Exp. Eye Res.*, 2004, **79**, 21–27.
40. A. J. Wenzel, C. Gerweck, D. Barbato, R. J. Nicolosi, G. J. Handelman and J. A. Curran-Celentano, 12-wk egg intervention increases serum zeaxanthin and macular pigment optical density in women, *J. Nutr.*, 2006, **136**, 2568–2573.
41. R. Vishwanathan, E. F. Goodrow-Kotyla, B. R. Wooten, T. A. Wilson and R. J. Nicolosi, Consumption of 2 and 4 egg yolks/d for 5 wk increases macular pigment concentrations in older adults with low macular pigment taking cholesterol-lowering statins, *Am. J. Clin. Nutr.*, 2009, **90**, 1272–1279.
42. D. Kelly, J. M. Nolan and A. N. Howard, *et al.* Serum and macular response to carotenoid-enriched egg supplementation in human subjects: the Egg Xanthophyll Intervention clinical Trial (EXIT), *Br. J. Nutr.*, 2017, **117**, 108–123.
43. M. Neuringer, M. M. Sandstrom, E. J. Johnson and D. M. Snodderly, Nutritional manipulation of primate retinas, I: effects of lutein or zeaxanthin supplements on serum and macular pigment in xanthophyll-free rhesus monkeys, *Invest. Ophthalmol. Visual Sci.*, 2004, **45**, 3234–3243.
44. B. R. Hammond Jr, E. J. Johnson and R. M. Russell, *et al.* Dietary modification of human macular pigment density, *Invest. Ophthalmol. Visual Sci.*, 1997, **38**, 1795–1801.
45. E. J. Johnson, M. Neuringer, R. M. Russell, W. Schalch and D. M. Snodderly, Nutritional manipulation of primate retinas, III: Effects of lutein or zeaxanthin supplementation on adipose tissue and retina of xanthophyll-free monkeys, *Invest. Ophthalmol. Visual Sci.*, 2005, **46**, 692–702.
46. AREDS-2 Study Group, Lutein + zeaxanthin and omega-3 fatty acids for age-related macular degeneration: the Age-Related Eye Disease Study 2 (AREDS2) randomized clinical trial, *JAMA*, 2013, **309**, 2005–2015.
47. B. R. Hammond Jr, B. R. Wooten and J. Curran-Celentano, Carotenoids in the retina and lens: possible acute and chronic effects on human visual performance, *Arch. Biochem. Biophys.*, 2001, **385**, 41–46.
48. A. J. Wenzel, K. Fuld, J. M. Stringham and J. Curran-Celentano, Macular pigment optical density and photophobia light threshold, *Vision Res.*, 2006, **46**, 4615–4622.
49. J. M. Stringham, E. R. Bovier, J. C. Wong and B. R. Hammond Jr, The influence of dietary lutein and zeaxanthin on visual performance, *J. Food Sci.*, 2010, **75**, R24–R29.
50. J. Curran Celentano, J. D. Burke and B. R. Hammond Jr, *In vivo* assessment of retinal carotenoids: macular pigment detection techniques and their impact on monitoring pigment status, *J. Nutr.*, 2002, **132**, 535S–539S.

51. R. A. Bone and J. T. Landrum, Heterochromatic flicker photometry, *Arch. Biochem. Biophys.*, 2004, **430**, 137–142.
52. I. Y.-F. Leung, Macular pigment: New clinical methods of detection and the role of carotenoids in age-related macular degeneration, *Optometry*, 2008, **79**, 266–272.
53. P. S. Bernstein, F. C. Delori, S. Richer, F. J. van Kuijk and A. J. Wenzel, The value of measurement of macular carotenoid pigment optical densities and distributions in age-related macular degeneration and other retinal disorders, *Vision Res.*, 2009, **50**, 716–728.
54. Eye Disease Research Study Group, Prevalence of Age-Related Macular Degeneration in the United States, *JAMA*, 2004, **122**, 564–572.
55. J. Wu, S. Seregard and P. Algvere, Photochemical damage of the retina, *Surv. Ophthalmol.*, 2006, **51**, 461–481.
56. M. Rozanowska, W. Korytowski and B. Rozanowski, *et al.* Photoreactivity of aged human RPE melanosomes: a comparison with lipofuscin, *Invest. Ophthalmol. Visual Sci.*, 2002, **43**, 2088–2096.
57. J. R. Sparrow, J. Zhou, S. Ben-Shabat, H. Vollmer, Y. Itagaki and K. Nakanishi, Involvement of oxidative mechanisms in blue-light-induced damage to A2E-laden RPE, *Invest. Ophthalmol. Visual Sci.*, 2002, **43**, 1222–1227.
58. S. Meyers, M. Ostrovsky and R. Bonner, A model of spectral filtering to reduce photochemical damage in age-related macular degeneration, *Trans. Am. Ophthalmol. Soc.*, 2004, **102**, 83–93.
59. J. M. Seddon, U. A. Ajani and R. D. Sperduto, *et al.* Dietary carotenoids, vitamins A, C, and E, and advanced age-related macular degeneration. Eye Disease Case-Control Study Group, *JAMA*, 1994, **272**, 1413–1420.
60. R. Arunkumar, C. Calvo, C. Conrady and P. Bernstein, What do we know about the macular pigment in AMD: the past, the present, and the future, *Eye*, 2018, **32**, 992–1004.
61. AREDS Study Group, A randomized, placebo-controlled, clinical trial of high-dose supplementation with vitamins C and E and beta carotene for age-related cataract and vision loss: AREDS report no. 9, *Arch. Ophthalmol.*, 2001, **119**, 1439–1452.
62. S. Beatty, I. J. Murray, D. B. Henson, D. Carden, H. Koh and M. E. Boulton, Macular pigment and risk for age-related macular degeneration in subjects from a Northern European population, *Invest. Ophthalmol. Visual Sci.*, 2001, **42**, 439–446.
63. S. Alassane, C. Binquet and V. Cottet, *et al.* Relationships of Macular Pigment Optical Density With Plasma Lutein, Zeaxanthin, and Diet in an Elderly Population: The Montrachet Study, *Invest. Ophthalmol. Visual Sci.*, 2016, **57**, 1160–1167.
64. B. R. Hammond Jr, B. R. Wooten and D. M. Snodderly, Cigarette smoking and retinal carotenoids: implications for age-related macular degeneration, *Vision Res.*, 1996, **36**, 3003–3009.
65. T. J. McGill, L. M. Renner and M. Neuringer, Elevated Fundus Autofluorescence in Monkeys Deficient in Lutein, Zeaxanthin, and Omega-3 Fatty Acids, *Invest. Ophthalmol. Visual Sci.*, 2016, **57**, 1361–1369.

66. S. Kiokias and M. Gordon, Antioxidant Properties of Carotenoids *In Vitro* and *In Vivo*, *Food Rev. Int.*, 2007, **20**, 99–121.
67. C. Flors, M. Fryer and J. Waring, *et al.* Imaging the production of singlet oxygen *in vivo* using a new fluorescent sensor, Singlet Oxygen Sensor Green, *J. Exp. Bot.*, 2006, **8**, 1725–1734.
68. P. Sastry, Lipids of nervous tissue: composition and metabolism, *Prog. Lipid Res.*, 1985, **24**, 69–176.
69. D. M. Snodderly, Evidence for protection against age-related macular degeneration by carotenoids and antioxidant vitamins, *Am. J. Clin. Nutr.*, 1995, **62**(1), 1448S–1461S.

CHAPTER 8

Eggs and Bone Health

NAN SHANG AND JIANPING WU*

Department of Agricultural, Food and Nutritional Science, 4-10 Agriculture/Forestry Centre, University of Alberta, Edmonton, Alberta, T6G 2P5, Canada
*E-mail: jwu3@ualberta.ca

8.1 Introduction

Bone is a special form of connective tissue providing mobility, flexibility, and mechanical support.[1] Meanwhile, it also protects various organs, stores minerals, and serves as a calcium reservoir to maintain calcium balance.[1] Bone is composed mainly of a mineral phase and an organic phase. The mineral phase consists predominately of mineralized calcium phosphate, also known as hydroxyapatite, which offers strength and rigidity to the bone.[2] The organic phase of bone is made up of type I collagen (90%), noncollagenous protein (5%), and lipids (2%).[3] These components have both mechanical and metabolic functions, and the composition and architectural features vary with age, gender, and species.[3] Throughout life, bone constantly undergoes a cycle of teardown and repair, named remodeling, to remove old, microdamaged bone and replace it with new, mechanically sound bone. During this process, bone can preserve its integrity and strength. Briefly, there are two bone cells involved in the regulation of the remodeling process. Osteoblasts, the bone formation cells, are engaged in producing new bones; osteoclasts, the bone resorption cells, function as the old bone remover.[3] In healthy

Food Chemistry, Function and Analysis No.14
Eggs as Functional Foods and Nutraceuticals for Human Health
Edited by Jianping Wu

Published by the Royal Society of Chemistry, www.rsc.org

individuals, the remodeling cycle is in balance, which means the rate of bone resorption is similar to the rate of bone formation.[3] As part of the aging process, the balance will be disrupted, leading to more bone resorption. This will have serious consequences for the competence of the skeleton and finally leads to osteoporosis and osteoporotic fractures.[3] In addition to age, this imbalance can also be caused by immobilization, estrogen deficiency, secondary hyperparathyroidism, or some medication therapies, such as the side effects of glucocorticoid treatment.

Osteoporosis is the most common bone disorder. According to the World Health Organization, osteoporosis affects more than 75 million people in Europe, Japan, and the USA, causing more than 2.3 million fractures annually in Europe and the USA alone.[4] There were an estimated 9 million osteoporotic fractures worldwide in 2000, of which 1.6 million were hip, 1.7 million forearm, and 1.4 million clinical vertebral fractures.[5] By 2025, the number of hip fractures is expected to increase to almost 3 million worldwide.[4] In general, osteoporosis is three times more prevalent in women than men owing to hormonal changes occurring after the menopause.[6] Aging is recognized as the most common factor leading to poor bone condition.[2] After reaching peak bone mass (usually in the late 20s), both men and women will experience a gradual loss of bone with increasing age.[7] However, dramatic bone loss happens in the case of women after the age of 50 because of postmenopausal-induced low estrogen.[8] Thus, women are more susceptible to suffering from osteoporotic fractures at an earlier age (50–65 years old) compared with men (≥ 70 years old).[5]

Osteoporotic fractures can result in disability, diminished function, loss of independence, and premature death.[1] Hip fractures, the leading cause of osteoporotic-related disability and death, occur predominantly in the older age group and the incidence increases exponentially with age.[9] With the rapid increase in the number of elderly people and the increase in life expectancy worldwide, the estimated number of hip fractures is predicted to rise from 1.7 million in 1990 to 6.3 million in 2025.[9] In addition to making bones more fragile and resulting in fractures of the hips, spine, and wrist, osteoporosis also causes people to become bedridden with secondary complications, such as back pain and loss of height, that may be life-threatening in the elderly.[4] Not surprisingly, bone diseases will take a significant financial toll on both society and individuals who suffer from it. The direct care expenditures for osteoporotic fractures alone range from $12.2 to $17.9 billion each year, measured in 2002 dollars.[1] Recognizing that bone health can have a significant impact on individual health and the whole society, there is a big challenge to extend knowledge of bone pathology, improve diagnosis methods, and develop treatment approaches.

Nutrition and diet are known to play an important role in bone health. Owing to the close relation between nutrition and bone health, dietary intervention represents an effective and safe strategy for bone health management.[1] Several studies have reported the positive relation between dairy food products and bone acquisition.[10] Food proteins can presumably improve bone quality.[11] In addition to the well-known nutrients of calcium and vitamin D, other micronutrients, such as vitamin K, magnesium, and strontium, are increasingly recognized for their roles in bone health management.[12] Unlike dairy products (milk and cheese)[13] and soy foods (soybean, soy drinks, and tofu),[14] little is known about the potential of egg for bone health. As a nutritious food commodity, egg contains all the essential nutrients, such as protein, lipids, vitamins, and minerals, which all play fundamental roles in bone metabolism. Meanwhile, eggs offer a moderate calorie source (about 150 kcal 100 g^{-1}), an excellent quality of protein profile, great culinary versatility, and low cost, which make them suitable for people of all ages and at different stages of life.[15,16] In particular, egg may play a useful role in those who are at risk of low nutrient intakes, such as the elderly, pregnant women, and children.[15] In this chapter, the beneficial potential of egg and egg-derived bioactive compounds for bone health management will be reviewed.

8.2 Egg Nutrients and Bone Health

Bone health is mainly affected by two factors: genes and environment. Although genes largely determine bone quality, environmental factors, such as diet and physical activity, are critically important to bone health because they are modifiable. Nutritional deficiencies, such as in minerals, vitamins, or proteins, can result in the formation of weak, poorly mineralized bone.[1] Thus, adequate dietary intake is essential to maintain bone health.

Mineral, the major constituent of bone tissues, offers strength and rigidity to bone by forming calcium phosphate (hydroxyapatite).[17] Thus, calcium and phosphate are definitely important to bone. In addition, magnesium and selenium also play a critical role in bone health. It has been reported that selenium inadequacy can retard growth and change bone metabolism.[18,19] Meanwhile, the blood selenium concentration is positively correlated with the prevalence of low bone mineral density in humans.[18,20,21] Iron deficiency has also been reported to decrease bone turnover in rats[22] and is thought of as an emerging risk factor for human osteoporosis.[23] In addition, zinc is another key mineral for bone health. Bone growth retardation is a common finding in various conditions associated with dietary zinc deficiency.[24] Bone zinc content has also been shown to be decreased in aging, skeletal unloading, and postmenopausal conditions,[24] suggesting the physiological role of zinc in the growth of bone tissue. Supplements of calcium and phosphate are easily obtained in the market; however, it is also important to ensure adequate intake of other minerals, especially trace elements. Eggs are considered a good source of minerals. Phosphorus (~16%), selenium (~29%), iron (~9%), and zinc (~9%) in eggs show the highest proportion of the recommended daily intake.[25] In addition, egg contains almost all minerals and trace elements in small amounts,[25] which could provide a good mineral profile. More importantly, since the mineral content of eggs varies with the laying hen's diet, manipulation of the mineral concentration in eggs is possible and has already been applied in the production of fortified eggs, such as for selenium or iodine.[25]

In addition to minerals, protein makes up a third of the bone mass and undergoes continuous formation and resorption. Type I collagen is the major part of the organic matrix (~98% of total bone protein), providing the basic structure of bone for binding with mineral crystals and offering flexibility and resilience.[1] Other main non-collagenous proteins including osteocalcin, osteopontin, sialoprotein, and osteonectin can help to strengthen the collagen matrix, and further regulate its ability to bind mineral crystals.[1] Thus, dietary protein represents a key nutrient for bone health as a "brick supplier". High protein intake, particularly when associated with physical activity, favors healthy development and peak bone mass acquisition, enabling individuals to reach their genetic potential.[11] Meanwhile, resistance exercise and high protein supplementation have been considered as preventive therapy for osteoporosis associated with aging.[26] A positive correlation between protein intake and bone mass has also been found in premenopausal women.[27] Eggs have been widely accepted as a high-quality food protein source. A medium-sized egg contains 6.5 g of protein as well as a great amino acid profile and higher bioavailability and digestibility compared to other protein sources.[28] Thus, egg consumption could benefit bone health by providing high-quality protein. Furthermore, since bone health is a multifactorial musculoskeletal issue, muscle mass and strength are also important to the development and maintenance of bone health. The loss of bone mass (osteopenia) and loss of muscle mass (sarcopenia) that occur with age are closely related.[17] Several studies have confirmed the positive effects of egg consumption on sarcopenia prevention.[29] Thus, egg might also improve bone health by affecting muscle synthesis. Although some reports still claim that high dietary proteins may be a risk factor for bone health,[30] a large number of studies suggest the positive influence of protein on bone health management and its potential in preventing osteoporosis.

Eggs are also recognized as a major source of vitamins in the diet.[25] One egg provides more than 10% of the recommended daily intake of various vitamins.[25] The fat-soluble vitamins are found almost exclusively in the egg yolk and most of the water-soluble vitamins as well.[25] Vitamins, ranking only behind minerals, are also key nutrients for bone health, especially vitamin D. Thus, egg may also enhance bone health by providing vitamins. A greater intake of vitamin A is associated with reduced bone density and increased risk of hip fractures.[31] Ascorbic acid, known as vitamin C, which is the only vitamin absent from egg, is also an essential vitamin required for the formation of stable collagen, which is important for bone formation.[32] Vitamin E supplementation is reported to protect bones from oxidative damage and maintain the bone matrix.[33] It is interesting to note that the vitamin content can also be manipulated by suitably changing the composition of the hen feed.[25] With this capacity, eggs could have broadened applications by fortifying specific nutrients.

Epidemiological evidence shows an inconsistent trend between the consumption of red meat, poultry, or eggs and the risk of hip fractures. Zeng *et al.* evaluated the association between the consumption of red meat, poultry, or eggs and the risk of hip fracture in elderly Chinese.[9] In their study, the risk of hip fracture was found to be positively associated with total red meat consumption, but not with total poultry or egg consumption.[9] Meanwhile, Inose *et al.* also reported a greater cortical strength found in mothers who consumed more milk, dairy products, and eggs.[34] Although whole eggs have been examined in prior studies with respect to their beneficial effects on bone and fracture outcomes, egg intake was only considered in food groupings and not independently. Recently, Coheley *et al.* studied the relationship between whole egg consumption and cortical bone in healthy children.[35] In this study, 294 9–13 year old black and white males and females were included and offered daily egg consumption. Results showed that egg intake was positively correlated with both radius cortical bone mineral content and osteocalcin, suggesting eggs may represent a viable strategy to promote pediatric bone development and prevent fractures.[35]

8.3 Egg Bioactive Compounds and Bone Health

8.3.1 Eggshell Compounds and Bone Health

Osteoporosis has been linked to insufficient calcium intake. Although calcium supplements are readily available, the best way to meet the daily dietary requirement is through the intake of high-calcium-containing foods.[36] The major component in eggshell powder is calcium carbonate, with 38% of the powder as pure calcium.[37] Thus, calcium fortification with eggshell powder may be an alternative approach for supplying calcium. The ideal dietary calcium : phosphorus ratio is suggested to be between 1 : 1 and 1 : 2.[37] However, studies show that phosphorus intake greatly exceeds that of calcium.[37] This is not only owing to low calcium in the diet but also to the fact that many calcium-fortifying agents, such as fish or animal bones, contain high levels of phosphorus.[37] Fortifying with eggshell powder, which contains only 0.01% phosphorus, would help restore the proper dietary balance between calcium and phosphorus.[37]

Several studies examined the effects of eggshell powder on improving bone quality. Schaafsma and Pakan studied the short-term effects of chicken eggshell powder enriched products on bone mineral density in women and men with osteoporosis or osteopenia.[38] During a study period of 4–8 months, the intervention group consumed twice daily an eggshell powder with vitamin D and magnesium. The study showed that the eggshell powder enriched supplement increased the bone mineral density of individuals within a period of 4 months, but as a consequence delayed bone demineralization for a longer period (over 8 months).[38] This study suggested that eggshell powder is a nice source of bioavailable calcium and has the potential to improve bone mineral density within an adequate treatment period. Following this study, Schaafsma *et al.* further investigated the effects of eggshell powder and purified calcium carbonate on bone mineral density in healthy Caucasian women who had been postmenopausal with low bone quality for at least 5 years.[39] After 12 months of supplementation, both the eggshell powder supplemented group and the calcium carbonate supplemented group showed increased bone mineral density, which indicated a positive correlation between bone mineral density and supplementation of chicken eggshell powder.[39] Interestingly, in this study, no significant difference was found between eggshell powder and purified calcium carbonate. Since calcium carbonate is the most popular calcium supplementation in the market, Hirasawa, Omi and Ezawa further investigated whether eggshell calcium has similar effects to calcium carbonate. In this study, they found that, when supplemented with vitamin D together, both eggshell powder and calcium carbonate increased bone mineral density of the lumbar spine in osteoporotic rats, suggesting that eggshell calcium might be as effective as the commercial calcium supplementation in calcium metabolism.[40] Studies also indicated that nano-sized calcium has greater bioavailability than that of micron-sized calcium.[41] Thus, to improve the bioavailability of eggshell powder, nanopowdered eggshell product has been investigated and its prevention effects on postmenopausal osteoporosis have been studied as well.[42] Ovariectomized rats fed with either nanopowdered eggshell or powdered eggshell showed greater bone mineral density than that of the control group, while the nanopowdered eggshell group exhibited higher bone volume and trabecular number than the powdered eggshell group.[42] This study also confirmed the positive effects of eggshell powder in osteoporosis prevention and suggested that different preparation techniques may also affect the bioactivity of the eggshell powder products.

It is well documented and accepted that calcium plays an important role in maintaining bone health; however, current research has also demonstrated the potential risk of taking excessive calcium. Increasing numbers of studies have indicated that high calcium uptake is associated with the development of urinary stone disease,[43] high blood pressure,[44] and increased breast cancer risk.[45] Compared with commercial calcium supplementation, eggshell powder functions as bone health supplementation by providing other microelements in addition to only calcium. Supplementation of 6 g of eggshell powder per day provides 50% of the daily strontium requirements.[46] Strontium has significant anabolic and antiresorptive effects on bone cells.[46,47] Strontium compounds, such as strontium ranelate, are now being introduced to the market as potential drugs for osteoporosis treatment.[46] Furthermore, small amounts of insulin-like growth factor-1 (12 ng g^{-1}), transforming growth factor-β1 (0.75–7.23 ng g^{-1}), calcitonin (10–25 ng g^{-1}), and progesterone (0.30–0.33 ng g^{-1}) are also found in eggshell.[46] Calcitonin is known for its pharmacologic action as an inhibitor of bone resorption, and it also displays the ability to increase bone formation.[48] Progesterone has also been suggested to prevent bone resorption in women.[49] Thus, eggshell powder may benefit bone health not only by providing calcium, but also with more extensive functions.

Osteoporosis patients treated with a daily dose of 6 g of eggshell powder for 2–6 months showed reduced pain, improved mobility, and increased bone density.[46] After these very promising results, physicians and patients have been slowly becoming aware of the therapeutic effects of eggshell powder.[46] Currently, a chicken eggshell product Biomin H® has already been developed and used in clinical trials.[50]

8.3.2 Egg White Compounds and Bone Health

Egg albumen, also known as egg white, has a very broad molecular mass range of proteins and is considered a good source of protein. The major egg white proteins include ovalbumin, ovotransferrin (conalbumin), ovomucoid, and ovomucin. Other egg proteins include lysozyme, ovoinhibitor, ovomacroglobulin (ovostatin), cystatin, and avidin. Specific binding activities of egg white proteins, such as ovoflavoprotein, thiamin-binding protein, ovoglycoprotein, ovofactor 1, ovoglobulins, and minor glycoproteins have also been identified.[51] Many food proteins, including egg white proteins, play more important roles beyond the nutritional requirements. Thus, there is an increasing commercial interest in the production of bioactive proteins and peptides to enhance activity for therapeutics, functional foods, nutrigenomics, and specific nutraceutical applications.[51] In this section, the bioactivity of egg white proteins for promoting bone health will be discussed.

8.3.2.1 Ovalbumin

Ovalbumin (OVA), which constitutes over half of the total egg white proteins, has been suggested to serve as a source of amino acids for the developing embryo.[51] It may benefit bone health by providing amino acids to develop the organic phase. Meanwhile, ovalbumin has antioxidant and immunomodulatory activity, which can mediate osteoclastogenesis and osteoclastic bone loss.[52,53] Furthermore, ovalbumin has also been used as a bio-based material for bone tissue regeneration.[54] Ovalbumin comprises mainly α-helix and β-sheet structures, but when introduced to an alkaline environment, it transforms into a predominantly β-sheet structure.[54,55] It can be used to create biocompatible scaffolds that aid in osteoblast adhesion and mineralization.[54,56] Farrar, Barone, and Morgan developed an ovalbumin-based scaffold and investigated its application in bone tissue engineering.[54] The confocal images indicated that preosteoblasts responded positively to the scaffold and surrounding environment, and finally reached a proliferative state.[54] Increased alkaline phosphatase (ALP) and osteocalcin (OCN) was also observed when cultured with scaffolds, indicating the potential application of this ovalbumin-based scaffold in bone tissue regeneration.[54]

8.3.2.2 Ovotransferrin

Ovotransferrin is the second major protein in egg white, belonging to the transferrin family and possessing several biological functions. Ovotransferrin has been indicated to play an important role in bone development in chick embryos, suggesting it might be involved in the process of bone formation.[57] Moreover, ovotransferrin possesses immunomodulating activity, which could influence immune system-related bone resorption.[53] More importantly, similar to its homologue lactoferrin, ovotransferrin could directly stimulate osteoblast activity to improve bone formation.[58] In our previous study, osteoblasts treated with ovotransferrin showed significantly increased ALP and type I collagen expression, as well as more calcium nodule formation.[58] At the same time, ovotransferrin mediated the RANKL : OPG ratio, suggesting its possible role in facilitating bone resorption.[58] Following this study, further developed *in vivo* animal work also validated the beneficial effects of ovotransferrin on bone health improvement.

8.3.2.3 Ovomucoid

Ovomucoid is a polymorphic glycoprotein accounting for roughly 10% of egg white protein.[51] Ovomucoid is also one of four egg white proteinase inhibitors, belonging to the group of serine proteinase inhibitors.[51] Ovomucoid has been shown to be particularly useful for the oral delivery of protein/peptide therapeutics.[51] It is helpful in the management of osteoporosis when coadministered with calcitonin.[59] In Shah and Khan's study, turkey ovomucoid, duck ovomucoid, and chicken ovomucoid all showed protection of calcitonin breakdown for oral drug delivery.[59] Furthermore, ovomucoid may benefit bone health alone owing to its homologies with osteonectin.[60] Osteonectin is one of the principle non-collagenous proteins of bone and is a component of osteoid.[60] Meanwhile, osteonectin has a high affinity for collagen, calcium, and hydroxyapatite,[60,61] suggesting its function in bone to link the mineral phase to the collagen matrix.[60,61] The sequence study of osteonectin revealed potential binding regions for calcium and hydroxyapatite and showed homology between osteonectin and serine proteinase inhibitors.[60] Osteonectin shows the highest homology with ovomucoid, suggesting that ovomucoid might have effects helping regulate bone matrix assembly. However, because of its allergenic nature, ovomucoid has limited biological and medical applications.[51]

8.3.2.4 Ovomucin

Ovomucin, which comprises 3.5% of the total egg white protein, is a macromolecular and heavily glycosylated glycoprotein.[51] Similar to ovalbumin, ovomucin has also been used as an implantable biomaterial to create porous scaffolds for tissue engineering.[62] Egg ovomucin-based scaffolds exhibited the ability to support cell adhesion and growth of bone marrow-derived mesenchymal stem cells and allowed cells to infiltrate into the matrix and more readily degrade.[62]

8.3.2.5 Lysozyme

Lysozyme is a ubiquitous enzyme presenting in almost all organisms. The most plentiful source of lysozyme is hen egg white, containing around 0.3–0.4 g of lysozyme per egg.[51] Interestingly, egg white lysozyme was found to inhibit mouse bone collagenase.[63] However, lysozyme is widely distributed in connective tissues and its concentration varies with the rate of tissue remodeling, thus the inhibition of collagenase may not always be negative for bone health. It is possible to regulate collagen degradation during the remodeling, benefitting new bone formation.[63] Furthermore, lysozyme-incorporated bio-based scaffolds stimulated cell differentiation.[64] A chitosan-based scaffold coated with lysozyme-incorporated calcium phosphate provided an improved environment for rat marrow stromal cell differentiation. Meanwhile, increased calcium deposition was also found in this study, indicating that lysozyme incorporation could elevate the production of mineralized extracellular matrix.[64]

8.3.2.6 Cystatin

Hen egg white cystatin is a protein inhibitor of peptidases.[51] It inactivated lysosomal cysteine proteinases, such as cathepsins B, H, and L, as well as several structurally similar plant proteinases.[51] These peptidases play important roles in numerous physiological processes, including bone remodeling.[65] Osteoclastic bone resorption depends on the activity of a group of cysteine proteinases, which could be inhibited by cystatins. Egg white cystatin has been found to inhibit several cysteine proteinases, including papain, cathepsin B, cathepsin H, and cathepsin L.[66] Thus, it is possible that cystatins could be used to protect the bone matrix against degradation, which is induced by cysteine proteinases. Several lines of evidences indicate the crucial role of cysteine proteinases, especially cathepsin K, in osteoclastic bone resorption.[67] Cysteine proteinase inhibitors, for example, E-64 [L-trans-epoxysuccinyl-leucylamido(4-guanidino)butane], leupeptin, and Z-Phe-Ala-CHN_2, reduce osteoclastic pit formation in tissue culture as well as the release of calcium and hydroxyproline into the culture medium.[67] To investigate the effects of egg cystatin in preventing osteoclastic bone resorption, Everts and colleagues studied the bone resorption microscopically and calcium release after treatment with cystatin.[67] Calvarial bone explants were cultured in the presence of cystatin. Both egg white cystatin and human cystatin C decreased calcium release into the medium significantly, suggesting the involvement of cystatins in the modulation of bone degradation. Although the underlying mechanisms still remain unclear, the researchers believe that is because of the inhibition of cathepsin K.[67] In addition, other cysteine proteinases may participate in the degradation of the bone matrix as well, such as cathepsin B, H, L, and S, although they are at a low level compared to cathepsin K.[67] Since egg white cystatin can form complexes with cathepsins B, L, and S,[51] inhibition of these enzymes by cystatin may contribute to the inhibition of bone resorption as well.

8.3.3 Egg Yolk Compounds and Bone Health

Egg yolk consists of nearly 48% water, 32–35% lipids, 15.7–16.6% proteins, 0.2–1.0% carbohydrates, and 1.1% ash content.[68] Since egg yolk provides sufficient amounts of physiologically active substances and nutrients for the hatching and growth of a chick, various functional components have been found in egg yolk.[68] In this section, the benefits of egg yolk protein, lipids, and carotenoids for bone health will be reviewed.

8.3.3.1 Egg Yolk Proteins and Bone Health

Egg yolk can be divided into supernatant (plasma) and precipitate (granules).[68] The major components of plasma are low-density lipoproteins (LDL) and livetin, while the main components of yolk granules are lipovitellins, phosvitin, and LDL.[68] Several experiments have been conducted to investigate the bioactivities of egg yolk proteins, including in bone health management. Leem *et al.* studied the effects of egg yolk proteins on longitudinal bone growth of adolescent male rats.[69] Egg yolk proteins were extracted with ethanol and fractionated into yolk water-soluble protein and yolk water-insoluble protein. Adolescent male rats were fed with whole egg yolk proteins, yolk water-soluble protein, or yolk water-insoluble protein. In this study, all three types of egg yolk protein promoted longitudinal bone growth and the height of growth plates, but the yolk water-soluble protein showed the best promotion effects.[69] This might be owing to the significant induction of bone morphogenetic protein 2 (BMP-2) expression by this yolk water-soluble protein, which can stimulate osteogenic activity.[69] Subsequently, Kim *et al.* further studied the possible mechanisms of egg yolk water-soluble protein promoted bone growth. Egg yolk water-soluble protein stimulated the cell proliferation and differentiation of osteoblasts[70] and inhibited tumor necrosis factor-α (TNF-α)-induced bone resorption.[71] Moreover, they extended the work to examine the bioactive peptide obtained from egg yolk water-soluble protein and found that the peptide has a stronger effect in preventing bone resorption than egg yolk water-soluble protein.[72] Ovariectomized rats supplemented with egg yolk water-soluble peptide showed an increase of bone mineral density and cortical thickness in the tibia, as well as a decrease of ovariectomy-induced bone loss.[72] Other studies also investigated the effects of egg yolk peptide on bone health management. Kobayashi *et al.* investigated the effects of food enriched with egg yolk hydrolysate on bone metabolism in orchidectomized dogs[73] and developed a product called Bonepep® (Pharma Foods International Co., Ltd., Kyoto, Japan), a commercial bone peptide produced by enzymatic treatment of the yolk water-soluble component of defatted chicken eggs. Orchidectomized dogs supplemented with Bonepep® showed significant promotion of bone formation immediately after orchiectomy.[73]

Among all egg yolk proteins, phosvitin is the most promising candidate to maintain bone health because of its strong ability to bind calcium.[68] Phosvitin has been reported to play an important role in bone formation in chicken embryos through dephosphorylation.[74] Liu *et al.* found that phosvitin stimulated osteoblast differentiation in the absence of ascorbic acid,[75] which is known to be essential for bone formation. Although the underlying mechanisms still under remain, it might be because phosvitin has a similar function to that of ascorbic acid in inducing type I collagen and osteocalcin expression during osteoblast differentiation.[75] The bioactivity of phosvitin mirroring the role of ascorbic acid in bone formation has been investigated in live calvarial bone organ culture models.[76] Meanwhile, phosvitin showed inhibition in PTH-induced osteoclastogenesis at the same time, which extended the function of phosvitin in bone health management.[76] Egg yolk phosvitin-derived phosphopeptides are also great candidates to improve bone health. Milk protein casein is currently used to produce phosphopeptides in industry; in comparison, egg yolk phosvitin is considered as the most phosphorylated protein in nature. Two different phosphopeptides derived from hen egg yolk phosvitin were reported to show high binding ability for calcium complex formation and prevent calcium phosphate salt precipitation.[77] Thus, phosvitin phosphopeptides provide a potentially valuable nutraceutical to increase calcium intake.[77] Further study of phosvitin phosphopeptides in bone health management and osteoporosis prevention is now in progress in our laboratory, which will provide more information for the application of phosvitin phosphopeptides.

8.3.3.2 Egg Yolk Lipids and Bone Health

Lipids are one of the major components in egg yolk, comprising nearly 30% of total egg yolk weight.[68] Egg yolk contains ~40% monounsaturated fatty acids (MUFA) [oleic acid and palmitoleic acid] and ~20% polyunsaturated fatty acids (PUFA) [linoleic acid, docosahexaenoic acid (DHA) and arachidonic acid].[78] PUFAs are touted for a wide range of health benefits and are incorporated in infant formula in many countries.[79] They are also recognized for their potential benefits for bone health.[80]

Recently, research has highlighted the potential role of PUFAs in inflammatory regulation of bone remodeling.[81] A protective effect of fish intake and n-3 PUFAs on the loss of femoral neck bone mineral density in the elderly has been reported.[82] Both DHA and eicosapentaenoic acid seem necessary to stimulate osteoblastogenesis and inhibit bone resorption by affecting calcium balance and osteoblast activity, attenuating pro-inflammatory cytokines,[83] such as IL-1, IL-6, and TNF, or modulating peroxisome proliferator active receptor gamma (PPARγ), which is a transcription factor with negative effects on bone homeostasis.[81] n-3 PUFAs may also affect bone *via* several other pathways, such as increasing nitric oxide production[84,85] or promoting osteoblastic differentiation by stimulating production of IGF-1 and PTH.[86] In addition to *in vitro* studies, animal studies and clinical trials also confirmed the role of dietary fatty acids in bone health. Lavado-García *et al.* studied the relationships between dietary intake of n-3 PUFAs and bone mineral density in Spanish women aged 20–79 years old.[87] With a total of 1865 female subjects, they concluded that intake of n-3 PUFAs was positively associated with bone mineral density at both the hips and lumbar spine in normal and osteopenic women, but not in osteoporotic women.[87] Another human study also showed that n-3 PUFAs, especially DHA, were positively associated with bone mineral accrual and thus with peak bone mineral density in young men.[88] Since n-3 PUFAs increase the bone formation rate and bone formation markers both *in vivo* and *in vitro*, consumption of foods enriched with n-3 PUFAs may be a suitable vector to promote bone health and prevent bone disorders, such as osteoporosis. Eggs represent a great candidate to supply n-3 PUFAs as their levels can be further manipulated *via* feed strategy to produce n-3 fatty acid-enriched eggs,[78] although further studies are needed to provide evidence with regard to the effects of consumption of n-3 fatty acid-enriched eggs on bone health.

8.3.3.3 Egg Yolk Carotenoids and Bone Health

Egg yolk is a unique and important carrier of lipid-soluble bioactive carotenoids – lutein and zeaxanthin.[89] It is well accepted that dietary carotenoids play an affirmative role in maintaining ocular health, as well as the prevention of cardiovascular disease, stroke, cancer, and neurodegenerative disorders. Recent evidence showed a positive link between carotenoid consumption and bone health. An Anglo–Celtic Australian population of both men and women was examined with intake of carotenoids. In this study, the bone mass of the total body and the lumbar spine were positively related to lycopene intake in men, and to lycopene and lutein/zeaxanthin intake in premenopausal women.[90] The findings of this study suggested a beneficial effect of dietary carotenoid intake on bone health. Recently, Regu *et al.* published their research about the association between dietary carotenoid intake and bone mineral density by a 4 year examination including more than 8000 subjects.[91] Similarly, in their study, lutein, zeaxanthin, and β-cryptoxanthin intake was positively associated with total hip bone mineral density in males and premenopausal women, while β-carotene intake was positively correlated with femoral neck, total hip, and whole-body bone mineral density in postmenopausal women. These results further confirmed the positive effects of dietary intake of carotenoids on promoting bone health.[91]

Unfortunately, there is no direct evidence indicating the beneficial effect of egg carotenoids intake on bone health. Owing to the high lipid content, the carotenoids present in egg yolk are considered highly bioavailable; furthermore, the type and amount of carotenoids in the yolk can be manipulated through poultry feed strategy. Thus, egg enriched with carotenoids may provide benefits for bone health.

8.4 Summary

Osteoporosis is considered an inevitable consequence of aging.[4] With the increasing of the aging population, bone health is becoming one of the most serious chronic diseases worldwide. Bone health is critically important to overall health, vitality, and quality of life; however, the public awareness of bone health management remains low. Although different pharmaceutical therapies and supplementations have been introduced, dietary intervention remains the most effective long-term approach for bone health management. Emerging evidence suggests the potential of egg application for bone health management because of its high nutritional value and the presence of a variety of bioactive compounds. Eggshell powder has been developed to provide minerals for bone formation, especially for calcium supplementation. Several bioactive proteins have been extracted from both egg white and yolk to investigate their activities in either promoting bone formation or inhibiting bone resorption (Table 8.1). Some egg white proteins have been developed into bio-based materials in bone tissue engineering. Furthermore, egg yolk lipids and carotenoids were also shown to exhibit specific functions in regulating bone health. More importantly, the ability to manipulate the egg nutrient contents, such as vitamins, fatty acids, and carotenoids, *via* feed strategy provides a way to enhance the intake of these nutrients without change of diet habit. Although further animal and human trials are warranted to validate the mechanism of action and efficacy of egg on bone health, egg shows great promise for bone health management.

Table 8.1 The current research on egg protein/peptide and bone health.

Protein/Peptide	Research model	Outcomes	Reference
Egg white protein/peptide			
Ovalbumin	Ovalbumin-based scaffolds	Improved proliferation of MC3T3-E1	54
	In vitro study with MC3T3-E1 cells	Increased expression of alkaline phosphatase (ALP) and osteocalcin	
Ovotransferrin	*In vitro* study with MC3T3-E1	Stimulation of cell proliferation	2
		Increased expression of type I collagen and ALP	
		Promoted cell differentiation	
Ovomucoid	Ovomucoid-based delivery system	Protection of calcitonin breakdown for oral drug delivery	59
	N/A	Homology between ovomucoid and osteonectin	60
		Potential for binding collagen, calcium, and hydroxyapatite	
Ovomucin	Ovomucin-based scaffolds	Supported cell adhesion and growth	62
	In vitro study with bone marrow-derived mesenchymal stem cells		
Lysozyme	N/A	The regulation of collagen degradation during bone remodeling	63
	Lysozyme-incorporated scaffolds	Improved osteogenic activity	64
	In vitro study with rat marrow stromal cells	Increased production of mineralized extracellular matrix	
Cystatin		Inhibited bone matrix degradation	67
		Inhibited osteoclastic bone resorption	

Egg yolk protein/peptide			
Egg yolk proteins	*In vivo* study with adolescent male rats	Promoted longitudinal bone growth and height of growth plates	69
Egg yolk water-soluble protein	*In vitro* study with MC3T3-E1 cells	Promoted cell proliferation and differentiation	92
	In vitro study with bone marrow cells from male ICR (Institute of Cancer Research) mice	Inhibited TNFα-induced osteoclastogenesis	71
Egg yolk water-soluble peptide	*In vivo* study with ovariectomized rats	Increased bone mineral density and cortical thickness in tibia Prevented ovariectomy-induced cancellous bone loss	72
Egg yolk water-soluble peptide product Bonepep®	*In vivo* study with orchidectomized dogs	Promoted bone formation after orchiectomy immediately	73
Phosvitin	*In vitro* study with live calvarial bone organ culture models	Stimulated osteoblast differentiation in the absence of ascorbic acid Inhibited parathyroid hormone-induced osteoclastogenesis	75

References

1. US Department of Health and Human Services, in *US Health and Human Services*, 2004.
2. N. Shang, C. Meram, N. Bandara and J. Wu, *Adv. Protein Chem. Struct. Biol.*, 2018, **112**, 265–308.
3. J. A. Gasser and M. Kneissel, in *Bone Toxicology*, ed. S. Smith, A. Varela and R. Samadfam, Springer, Cham, 2017, pp. 27–94.
4. WHO, Prevention and management of osteoporosis.
5. O. Johnell and J. A. Kanis, *Osteoporosis Int.*, 2006, **17**, 1726–1733.
6. M. X. Ji and Q. Yu, *Chronic Dis. Transl. Med.*, 2015, **1**, 9–13.
7. NIH Consensus Development Panel on Osteoporosis Prevention Diagnosis and Therapy, *JAMA*, 2001, **285**, 785–795.
8. K. N. Tu, J. D. Lie, C. K. V. Wan, M. Cameron, A. G. Austel, J. K. Nguyen, K. Van and D. Hyun, *P T*, 2018, **43**, 92–104.
9. F. Zeng, F. Fan, W. Xue, H. Xie, B. Wu, S. Tu, W. Ouyang and Y. Chen, *Bone*, 2013, **56**, 242–248.
10. R. Rene, *Am. J. Clin. Nutr.*, 2014, **99**, 1256–1262.
11. J. Bonjour, *Nutrition*, 2005, **24**, 526–536.
12. S. J. Whiting, W. M. Kohrt, M. P. Warren, M. I. Kraenzlin and J. P. Bonjour, *Eur. J. Clin. Nutr.*, 2016, **70**, 1099–1105.
13. R. P. Heaney, *J. Am. Coll. Nutr.*, 2009, **28**(Suppl 1), 82S–90S.
14. M. Messina and V. Messina, *J. Renal Nutr.*, 2000, **10**, 63–68.
15. J. M. Miranda, X. Anton, C. Redondo-Valbuena, P. Roca-Saavedra, J. A. Rodriguez, A. Lamas, C. M. Franco and A. Cepeda, *Nutrients*, 2015, **7**, 706–729.
16. K. L. Herron and M. L. Fernandez, *J. Nutr.*, 2004, **134**, 187–190.
17. R. P. Heaney and D. K. Layman, *Am. J. Clin. Nutr.*, 2008, **87**, 1567–1570.
18. H. Zeng, J. J. Cao and G. F. Combs Jr, *Nutrients*, 2013, **5**, 97–110.
19. R. Moreno-Reyes, D. Egrise, J. Nève, J.-L. Pasteels and A. Schoutens, *J. Bone Miner. Res.*, 2001, **16**, 1556–1563.
20. J. J. Cao, B. R. Gregoire and H. Zeng, *J. Nutr.*, 2012, **142**, 1526–1531.
21. A. Hoeg, A. Gogakos, E. Murphy, S. Mueller, J. Köhrle, D. M. Reid, C. C. Glüer, D. Felsenberg, C. Roux, R. Eastell, L. Schomburg and G. R. Williams, *J. Clin. Endocrinol. Metab.*, 2012, **97**, 4061–4070.
22. S. Katsumata, R. Katsumata-Tsuboi, M. Uehara and K. Suzuki, *J. Nutr.*, 2009, **139**, 238–243.
23. L. Toxqui and M. P. Vaquero, *Nutrients*, 2015, **7**, 2324–2344.
24. M. Yamaguchi, *Mol. Cell. Biochem.*, 2010, **338**, 241–254.
25. I. Seuss-Baum, in *Bioactive Egg Compounds*, ed. R. Huopalahti, R. López-Fandiño, M. Anton and R. Schade, Springer Science & Business Media, 2007, pp. 117–144.
26. T. Matsuo, T. Nozaki, K. Okamura, K. Matsumoto, T. Doi, S. Gohtani and M. Suzuki, *Biosci., Biotechnol., Biochem.*, 2003, **67**, 2518–2523.
27. D. Feskanich, W. C. Willett, M. J. Stampfer and G. A. Colditz, *Am. J. Epidemiol.*, 1996, **143**, 472–479.

28. B. A. Griffin, in *Proceedings of the Nutrition Society*, Nottingham, 2016, pp. 259–264.
29. A. Smith and J. Gray, *Br. J. Community Nurs.*, 2016, **21**, 305–309.
30. M. Isanejad, J. Sirola, J. Mursu, H. Kröger, M. Tuppurainen and A. T. Erkkilä, *J. Nutr., Health Aging*, 2017, **21**, 622–630.
31. H. Melhus, K. Michaëlsson, A. Kindmark, R. Bergström, L. Holmberg, H. Mallmin, A. Wolk and S. Ljunghall, *Ann. Intern. Med.*, 1998, **129**, 770–778.
32. P. Aghajanian, S. Hall, M. D. Wongworawat and S. Mohan, *J. Bone Miner. Res.*, 2015, **30**, 1945–1955.
33. R. G. Feresin, S. A. Johnson, M. L. Elam, J.-S. Kim, D. A. Khalil, E. A. Lucas, B. J. Smith, M. E. Payton, M. P. Akhter and B. H. Arjmandi, *J. Osteoporosis*, 2013, **2013**, 825985.
34. T. Inose, T. Takano, K. Nakamura, M. Kizuki and K. Seino, *Acta Paediatr.*, 2007, **95**, 276–282.
35. L. M. Coheley, J. M. Kindler, E. M. Laing, A. Oshri, K. M. Hill Gallant, S. J. Warden, M. Peacock, C. M. Weaver and R. D. Lewis, *Osteoporosis Int.*, 2018, 1–9.
36. J. A. Sunyecz, *Ther. Clin. Risk Manage.*, 2008, **4**, 827–836.
37. Y. Masuda and H. Hiramatsu, in *Egg Bioscience and Biotechnology*, ed. Y. Mine, John Wiley & Sons, Inc., Hoboken, NJ, USA, 2008, pp. 129–140.
38. A. Schaafsma and I. Pakan, *Bratisl. Lek. Listy*, 1999, **100**, 651–656.
39. A. Schaafsma, J. J. van Doormaal, F. A. J. Muskiet, G. J. H. Hofstede, I. Pakan and E. van der Veer, *Br. J. Nutr.*, 2002, **87**, 267–275.
40. T. Hirasawa, N. Omi and I. Ezawa, *J. Bone Miner. Metab.*, 2001, **19**, 84–88.
41. S. Huang, J. C. Chen, C. W. Hsu and W. H. Chang, *Nanotechnology*, 2009, **20**, 375102.
42. M. Al Mijan, Y. K. Lee and H.-S. Kwak, *Food Sci. Biotechnol.*, 2014, **23**, 1667–1676.
43. M. D. Sorensen, *Transl. Androl. Urol.*, 2014, **3**, 235–240.
44. K. L. Margolis, R. M. Ray, L. Van Horn, J. E. Manson, M. A. Allison, H. R. Black, S. A. A. Beresford, S. A. Connelly, J. D. Curb, R. H. Grimm, T. A. Kotchen, L. H. Kuller, S. Wassertheil-Smoller, C. A. Thomson, J. C. Torner and Women's Health Initiative Investigators, *Hypertension*, 2008, **52**, 847–855.
45. Y. Cui and T. E. Rohan, *Cancer Epidemiol., Biomarkers Prev.*, 2006, **15**, 1427–1437.
46. J. Rovenský, M. Stancíková, P. Masaryk, K. Svík and R. Istok, *Int. J. Clin. Pharmacol. Res.*, 2003, **23**, 83–92.
47. P. J. Marie, M. T. Garba, M. Hott and L. Miravet, *Miner. Electrolyte Metab.*, 1985, **11**, 5–13.
48. J. Keller, P. Catala-Lehnen, A. K. Huebner, A. Jeschke, T. Heckt, A. Lueth, M. Krause, T. Koehne, J. Albers, J. Schulze, S. Schilling, M. Haberland, H. Denninger, M. Neven, I. Hermans-Borgmeyer, T. Streichert, S. Breer, F. Barvencik, B. Levkau, B. Rathkolb, E. Wolf, J. Calzada-Wack, F. Neff, V.

Gailus-Durner, H. Fuchs, M. H. de Angelis, S. Klutmann, E. Tsourdi, L. C. Hofbauer, B. Kleuser, J. Chun, T. Schinke and M. Amling, *Nat. Commun.*, 2014, **5**, 5215.
49. V. Seifert-Klauss and J. C. Prior, *J. Osteoporosis*, 2010, **2010**, 845180.
50. M. Stancikova, J. Rovenský, R. Masaryk, K. Svík and R. Istok, *Ces. Revmatol.*, 2009, **17**, 39–48.
51. Y. Mine and I. D'Silva, in *Egg Bioscience and Biotechnology*, ed. Y. Mine, John Wiley & Sons, Inc., Hoboken, NJ, USA, 2008, pp. 141–184.
52. V. Domazetovic, G. Marcucci, T. Iantomasi, M. L. Brandi and M. T. Vincenzini, *Clin. Cases Miner. Bone Metab.*, 2017, **14**, 209–216.
53. J. Zupan, M. Jeras and J. Marc, *Biochem. Med.*, 2013, **23**, 43–63.
54. G. Farrar, J. Barone and A. Morgan, *J. Tissue Eng.*, 2010, **2010**, 209860.
55. H. Y. Hu and H. N. Du, *J. Protein Chem.*, 2000, **19**, 177–183.
56. L. S. Nair and C. T. Laurencin, *Prog. Polym. Sci.*, 2007, **32**, 762–798.
57. C. Gentili, R. Doliana, P. Bet, G. Campanile, A. Colombatti, F. D. Cancedda and R. Cancedda, *J. Cell Biol.*, 1994, **124**, 579–588.
58. N. Shang and J. Wu, *J. Agric. Food Chem.*, 2008, **66**, 2775–2782.
59. R. B. Shah and M. A. Khan, *J. Pharm. Sci.*, 2004, **93**, 392–406.
60. M. E. Bolander, M. F. Youngf, L. W. Fishert, Y. Yamada and J. D. Terminet, *Biochemistry*, 1988, **85**, 2919–2923.
61. J. D. Termine, H. K. Kleinman, S. W. Whitson, K. M. Conn, M. L. McGarvey and G. R. Martin, *Cell*, 1981, **26**, 99–105.
62. N. T. Carpena, C. D. G. Abueva, A. R. Padalhin and B. T. Lee, *J. Biomed. Mater. Res., Part B*, 2017, **105**, 2107–2117.
63. S. Sakamoto, M. Sakamoto, P. Goldhaber and M. J. Glimcher, *Calcif. Tissue Res.*, 1974, **14**, 291–299.
64. A. M. Martins, Q. P. Pham, P. B. Malafaya, R. M. Raphael, F. K. Kasper, R. L. Reis and A. G. Mikos, *Tissue Eng., Part A*, 2009, **15**, 1953–1963.
65. M. Abrahamson, M. Alvarez-Fernandez and C. M. Nathanson, *Biochem. Soc. Symp.*, 2003, **70**, 179–199.
66. A. Anastasi, M. A. Brown, A. A. Kembhavi, M. J. Nicklin, C. A. Sayers, D. C. Sunter and A. J. Barrett, *Biochem. J.*, 1983, **211**, 129–138.
67. H. S. Brand, U. H. Lerner, A. Grubb, W. Beertsen, A. V. Nieuw Amerongen and V. Everts, *Bone*, 2004, **35**, 689–696.
68. H. Hatta, M. P. Kapoor and L. R. Juneja, in *Egg Bioscience and Biotechnology*, ed. Y. Mine, John Wiley & Sons, Inc., Hoboken, NJ, USA, 2008, pp. 185–237.
69. K. H. Leem, M. G. Kim, H. M. Kim, M. Kim, Y. J. Lee and H. K. Kim, *Biosci., Biotechnol., Biochem.*, 2004, **68**, 2388–2390.
70. M. Ji, K. Leem, M. Kim and H. K. Kim, *Biosci., Biotechno., Biochem.*, 2007, **71**, 1327–1329.
71. H. K. Kim, M. G. Kim and K. H. Leem, *Biosci., Biotechnol., Biochem.*, 2008, **72**, 1929–1931.
72. H. K. Kim, S. Lee and K. H. Leem, *Menopause*, 2011, **18**, 307–313.
73. T. Kobayashi, H. Koie, A. Watanabe, A. Ino, K. Watabe, M. Kim, K. Kanayama and K. Otsuji, *J. Vet. Med. Sci.*, 2015, **77**, 503–506.

74. C. Li, F. Geng, X. Huang, M. Ma and X. Zhang, *Poult. Sci.*, 2014, **93**, 3065–3072.
75. Q. Liu, C. Li, F. Geng, X. Huang and M. Ma, *J. Sci. Food Agric.*, 2017, **97**, 4532–4538.
76. J. Liu, D. Czernick, S. C. Lin, A. Alasmari, D. Serge and E. Salih, *Dev. Biol.*, 2013, **381**, 256–275.
77. B. Jiang and Y. Mine, *Biosci., Biotechnol., Biochem.*, 2001, **65**, 1187–1190.
78. A. Gerbi, M. Bernard, B. Gleize, T. C. Coste, J. M. Maixent, C. Lan, F. Paganelli and G. Pieroni, *Cell. Mol. Biol.*, 2004, **50**, 855–860.
79. M. Makrides, J. S. Hawkes, M. A. Neumann and R. A. Gibson, *Am. J. Clin. Nutr.*, 2002, **75**, 1084–1092.
80. R. L. Corwin, *Prostaglandins Leukot. Essent. Fatty Acids*, 2003, **68**, 379–386.
81. K. M. Mangano, S. Sahni, J. E. Kerstetter, A. M. Kenny and M. T. Hannan, *Curr. Osteoporos. Rep.*, 2013, **11**(3), 203–212.
82. E. K. Farina, D. P. Kiel, R. Roubenoff, E. J. Schaefer, L. A. Cupples and K. L. Tucker, *Am. J. Clin. Nutr.*, 2011, **93**, 1142–1151.
83. W. Raphael and L. M. Sordillo, *Int. J. Mol. Sci.*, 2013, **14**, 21167–21188.
84. M. M. Rahman, A. Bhattacharya, J. Banu, J. X. Kang and G. Fernandes, *J. Cell. Mol. Med.*, 2009, **13**, 1833–1844.
85. W. Komatsu, K. Ishihara, M. Murata, H. Saito and K. Shinohara, *Free Radicals Biol. Med.*, 2003, **34**, 1006–1016.
86. B. A. Watkins, Y. Li, H. E. Lippman and S. Feng, *Prostaglandins Leukot. Essent. Fatty Acids*, 2003, **68**, 387–398.
87. J. Lavado-García, R. Roncero-Martin, J. M. Moran, M. Pedrera-Canal, I. Aliaga, O. Leal-Hernandez, S. Rico-Martin and M. L. Canal-Macias, *PLoS One*, 2018, **13**, e0190539.
88. M. Högström, P. Nordström and A. Nordström, *Am. J. Clin. Nutr.*, 2007, **85**, 803–807.
89. K. Zaheer, *J. Food*, 2017, **15**, 474–487.
90. N. Wattanapenpaiboon, W. Lukito, M. L. Wahlqvist and B. J. G. Strauss, *Asia Pac. J. Clin. Nutr.*, 2003, **12**, 467–473.
91. G. Regu, H. Kim, Y. Kim, J. Paek, G. Lee, N. Chang and O. Kwon, *Nutrients*, 2017, **9**, 1025.
92. M. Ji, K. H. Leem, M. Kim and H. K. Kim, *Biosci., Biotechnol., Biochem.*, 2007, **71**, 1327–1329.

CHAPTER 9

Chicken Egg: Wholesome Nutrition Packed with Antioxidants

C. NIMALARATNE AND J. WU*

Department of Agricultural, Food and Nutritional Science, University of Alberta, 4-10 Agriculture/Forestry Centre, Edmonton, Alberta, T6G 2P5, Canada
*E-mail: jwu3@ualberta.ca

9.1 Oxidative Stress and Endogenous Antioxidants

Free radicals include both reactive oxygen species (ROS), such as superoxide anion radical ($O_2^{\bullet -}$), hydrogen peroxide (H_2O_2), singlet oxygen ($^1O_2$) and hydroxyl radical ($OH^{\bullet}$), and reactive nitrogen species (RNS), such as nitric oxide ($NO^{\bullet}$) and nitrogen dioxide radical ($NO_2^{\bullet -}$). Free radicals are generated as a result of normal cellular biochemical conditions and are believed to play an important role in maintaining proper physiological functions, such as in intercellular signalling cascades,[1] wound healing processes[2] and stem cell proliferation,[3] and are also an important part of the body's innate immune system.[4] Cellular redox balance is normally maintained by the action of a complex system of endogenous antioxidant compounds that are capable of breaking down and scavenging radical species, interrupting the

Food Chemistry, Function and Analysis No.14
Eggs as Functional Foods and Nutraceuticals for Human Health
Edited by Jianping Wu

Published by the Royal Society of Chemistry, www.rsc.org

free radical-generating chain reactions, quenching singlet oxygen, decomposing or converting peroxyl radicals, inhibiting pro-oxidative enzymes and acting as metal chelators.[5,6] Major endogenous antioxidants include enzymes such as superoxide dismutase (SOD), catalase (CAT), glutathione peroxidase (GPx), glutathione reductase (GRx) and peroxiredoxins, and also non-enzymatic compounds like vitamin E and C, glutathione, coenzyme Q_{10} and metal-binding proteins (albumin, ferritin, ceruloplasmin, *etc.*).[7,8] Decreased cellular defense capacity owing to natural factors, such as aging or microbial infections, or exposure to pollutants, such as smoking, ionizing radiation and alcohol, can disrupt the cellular redox balance, favouring the oxidants, which is termed as oxidative stress.[9] As a result, the cellular defense system fails to prevent/repair the ROS/RNS-mediated damage to biomolecules such as DNA, proteins and lipids, leading to pathogenesis of various diseases.

9.2 Dietary Antioxidants in Human Health

As suggested by numerous studies, exogenous antioxidants, mainly from dietary sources and also in the form of supplements, can complement the action of the endogenous antioxidant defense system by various means. Commonly consumed foods, including fruits, vegetables, nuts and grains, and beverages (tea, coffee) contain significant amounts of antioxidant compounds, for example, polyphenolic antioxidants, carotenoids, vitamin C, vitamin E, minerals (Zn, Se) and peptides.[10–12] These compounds, upon absorption into the body, can act synergistically with endogenous antioxidants to maintain redox homeostasis and to prevent and/or repair oxidation damage.[13,14] Most of the natural dietary compounds recognized to act as antioxidants in the human body are available in the form of a supplement and may contain several compounds in a single supplement. However, the use of dietary supplements has been a controversial topic owing to conflicting results from clinical trials.[15] Some studies found no effect of antioxidant therapy[16,17] whereas some even found increased mortality rates associated with antioxidant supplementation.[17–19] It has been suggested that supplementation with a higher amount of a single antioxidant compound can alter the endogenous antioxidant defense system, disturbing the cellular signalling system and cell apoptosis pathways.[15] Over-supply of exogenous antioxidants can hinder the synthesis of endogenous antioxidants, thereby leaving the cellular redox status unaffected.[11,15] Consequently, antioxidant supplementation has to be carefully monitored based on individual cases, and a healthy balanced diet is the safest method of taking in exogenous antioxidants.

Most of the well-known antioxidant compounds we consume, such as phenolic compounds (flavonoids, anthocyanins and phenolic acids) and carotenoids, come from plant-based foods, mainly fruits and vegetables. Moreover, spices, grains, pulses, oil seeds and herbs also add significant amounts of antioxidant compounds to our daily diet.[20–22] Methods of extraction and purification of these compounds and their potential antioxidant mechanisms and effects on human health have been extensively explored during the past few decades using various laboratory assays and clinical intervention studies.[6,23–26]

In addition to plant-based antioxidants, animal-derived amino compounds, such as proteins, peptides and amino acids, also make up a significant part of the exogenous antioxidants supplied through daily diet.[27,28] Apart from their essential nutritional value, proteins, peptides and amino acids can exert various beneficial bioactivities, including antioxidant activity.[28–30] The antioxidant activity of proteins and peptides mainly arises through the activities of (radical scavenging, metal chelating and a component of thiol/disulfide equilibrium) thiol-containing amino acids, such as cysteine and methionine.[27,31] The presence of aromatic side chains (tryptophan, tyrosine and phenyl alanine, imidazole ring in histidine) is also considered an important structural feature of antioxidant properties.[32,33] Numerous studies have been reported on the production of antioxidant peptides/protein hydrolysates from different animal proteins and their potential applications in food products. Milk proteins, casein and whey, have been extensively investigated for antioxidant peptides and have been reported to inhibit lipid oxidation in food products.[34–36] Some meat/fish proteins, egg proteins and egg-derived peptides are also reported to have antioxidant properties.[37–41] Other antioxidant compounds such as vitamin E, glutathione, vitamin C and carotenoids (lutein and zeaxanthin in egg yolk, astaxanthin in fish and shrimp) are some of the other well-known antioxidant compounds present in animal tissues.[14,42,43]

9.3 Egg as an Antioxidant Food Commodity

Egg constitutes an important part of the daily diet and contains high-quality proteins, fat and other micronutrients essential to nurture new life. Egg white or the albumen is mainly composed of water (~87%) and proteins (~13%), whereas the egg yolk is made up of ~50% water, lipids (~32–36%), proteins (~15–16%), vitamins and minerals.[44,45] Ovalbumin is the main egg white protein, followed by ovotransferrin, ovomucoid, ovomucin, *etc*. The major constituents of egg proteins are lipoproteins (high-density lipoproteins – HDL; low-density lipoproteins – LDL), phosvitin and livetin. Egg yolk lipids mainly consist of triglycerides, phospholipids (a component of lipoproteins) and cholesterol.[46] A small amount of carbohydrates (~1%) is distributed in both egg white and yolk as oligosaccharides and glycoproteins, respectively.[46] A whole hen egg with the outer shell and membranes is a closed biological system designed to protect and nurture a growing embryo; it is therefore equipped with complete nutritional requirements as well as effective defense mechanisms against pathogens and toxins. Beyond their basic nutritional function, many egg components are known to show biological activities, including antihypertensive, antimicrobial, anticancer, antioxidant, immunomodulatory and antiadhesive.[47–49] Most of the egg white proteins and their derived peptides, egg yolk phospholipids, phosvitin and pigments such as lutein and zeaxanthin are known to possess antioxidant properties.[48] Moreover, the amount of lipophilic antioxidants in egg yolk, such as lutein, zeaxanthin and vitamin E, can be manipulated through hen feed formulation to produce 'antioxidant-enriched eggs'.[50]

9.4 Antioxidant Compounds in Egg

Among egg white proteins, ovalbumin, ovotransferrin, cystatin and ovoinhibitor are reported to show antioxidant properties. Phosvitin, phospholipids, carotenoids and some vitamins and minerals, such as vitamin E and selenium in egg yolk, are also known to have antioxidant properties. In addition to these components, peptides derived from egg proteins are widely investigated for their bioactivities, including antioxidant activity.[51]

9.4.1 Ovalbumin

Ovalbumin is a phosphoglycoprotein composed of three subunits with different phosphate groups and an N-terminal carbohydrate moiety. It makes up around 54% of the egg white proteins[49,51] and plays a key role in egg white's functional properties, such as gelling, foaming and emulsification.[49] Ovalbumin contains six cysteine residues (four of which exist in the reduced state and the other two are involved in disulfide bonds) in its structure and is the only egg white protein with free thiol (-SH) groups. These free thiol groups can play a role in redox regulation and act as metal chelators, and therefore are considered as the main contributing factor to the antioxidant properties of ovalbumin.[31,52] Nakamura *et al.* observed a remarkable increase in the antioxidant activity of ovalbumin when bound with polysaccharides.[53] It was suggested that the increase in antioxidant activity of the conjugate was mainly owing to the effective exposure of the -SH groups of ovalbumin.[53] Heating ovalbumin in a linoleic system was also reported to enhance antioxidant and superoxide radical scavenging activities by increasing the exposure of antioxidant amino acids such as cysteine, histidine and methionine.[54] In another study, a synergistic increase in antioxidant activity was observed when green tea catechins were added to an oil-in-water emulsion with ovalbumin.[55] Ovalbumin contributed to total antioxidant activity and also bound irreversibly to increase the stability of catechins in the emulsion.[56]

9.4.2 Ovotransferrin

Approximately 12–13% of the egg white is ovotransferrin, a member of the transferrin family, which contains a group of proteins with iron-binding capabilities.[49] Ovotransferrin is a glycoprotein that consists of two lobes, the N-lobe and the C-lobe, where each can bind one iron molecule. It can also bind to other heavy metals too. Li-Chan and Kim suggested that the iron-binding ability of ovotransferrin may have an indirect role in preventing iron-induced lipid oxidation.[57] Metal-bound ovotransferrin (Mn^{2+}–Otf, Zn^{2+}–Otf and Cu^{2+}–Otf) was reported to show a dose-dependent SOD-like activity by efficiently quenching superoxide anions.[58] This SOD-like activity was considerably higher than that of well-known antioxidants, such as ascorbate and serum-albumin.

9.4.3 Lysozyme

Lysozyme is an enzyme that belongs to the family of 'defensin proteins', a group of host defense proteins present in all living organisms.[30] Egg white lysozyme is the most abundant source with about 0.3–0.4 g per egg white[30] and accounts for ~3.5% of egg white proteins. As a part of the host defense system, lysozyme has many bioactivities, including antimicrobial, immune-modulatory and antioxidant activities.[49] Lysozyme can bind to advanced glycation end products (compounds formed after protein/lipid and sugar interactions, which can contribute to inflammation, ROS production and increased oxidation stress) *via* its 18 amino acid, cysteine-bound motif, thereby provides protection against potential oxidative injury.[59] Transgenic mice expressing hen egg white lysozyme were resistant to chronic and acute oxidative stress-induced by external factors.[59] In the same study, hepatocytes incubated with lysozyme suppressed oxidative stress response genes and generation of cellular ROS.[59] Another study with lysozyme-deficient mice showed higher susceptibility to oxidant-induced lung injury, indicating the role of lysozyme as an antioxidant.[60]

9.4.4 Cystatin

Cystatins are inhibitors of cysteine proteinases and chicken cystatin (cystatin class B) is the first of its kind to be identified. Cystatin makes up about 0.05% of total egg white proteins.[61] Animal studies performed with cystatin B-deficient mice showed that cystatin B protects cerebellar granule neurons from oxidative stress and the deficiency can increase oxidative damage to the cerebellum.[62] Additionally, all three classes of cystatins (cystatin class A, B and C) were capable of up-regulating NO production by activated murine macrophages. The cellular redox balance is affected by NO levels and cystatin may therefore have an indirect role in cellular antioxidant signalling pathways.[63]

9.4.5 Ovoinhibitor

Ovoinhibitor is a glycoprotein, making up around 1.5% of the egg white protein, and inhibits serine proteases, such as trypsin and chymotrypsin as well as bacterial and fungal proteases.[61] The antioxidant activity of ovoinhibitor is suggested to be exerted through inhibition of ROS formation. Ovoinhibitor suppressed formation of H_2O_2 by activated human polymorphonuclear leukocytes, helping to maintain cell redox balance.[64]

9.4.6 Phosvitin

Phosvitin is a highly phosphorylated protein containing ~80% of yolk phosphorous. More than 50% of its amino acids are serine; most exist as phosphoserines. Owing to the high phosphorous content, it has a strong affinity for metal ions and about 95% of yolk iron is bound to phosvitin. This metal-binding ability serves as the main reason for phosvitin's biological activities, primarily antioxidant activity *via* inhibiting iron-induced oxidation. Iron is an essential nutrient for life; its metabolism in the body is strictly regulated *via* iron-binding proteins, such as ferritin and transferrin, because humans have no efficient mechanism to excrete excess iron.[65,66] Excess Fe^{2+} ions can participate in the Fenton reaction to produce toxic $OH^{\bullet}$ by reacting with H_2O_2 and thus increasing the production of ROS causing oxidative damage to organs and the central nervous system, which could be lethal.[65] Phosvitin can increase autoxidation of Fe^{2+} to Fe^{3+}, thereby limiting the availability of iron (Fe^{2+}) for participating in the Fenton reaction and inhibiting the production of $OH^{\bullet}$.[67] In the presence of excess iron, phosvitin protects DNA against UV-light-induced lipid peroxidation.[68] Studies with human normal and cancer cell lines also indicated that phosvitin protects against oxidative stress-induced DNA damage in normal cells and inhibits the growth of cancer cells, suggesting the potential of phosvitin as an anticancer agent.[69] Furthermore, phosvitin is used to effectively inhibit oxidation of phospholipids in food products.[70]

9.4.7 Phospholipids

Egg yolk phospholipids are a group of lipids including phosphotidylcholine (~73%), phosphatidylethanolamine (~15%), lyso-phosphatidylcholine (~6%), sphingomyelins (2.5%) and minor quantities of other lipids.[71] Phospholipids have been shown to act as natural antioxidants and their antioxidant capacity is closely related to the structural diversity of the fatty acids, especially the degree of unsaturation.[72,73] Moreover, nitrogen-containing phospholipids, such as phosphatidylcholine and phosphatidylethanolamine, tend to show higher antioxidant activity, facilitated by the electron or hydrogen donating ability of their amine group.[73,74]

9.4.8 Carotenoids

Carotenoids are plant-derived, lipid-soluble compounds, which provide the yellow-orange hue of egg yolk.[75] From the large number of carotenoids that have been identified, a few occur in our daily diet and only 14 carotenoids are found in human blood.[76,77] The most studied carotenoids related to health benefits are beta-carotene, lycopene, lutein and zeaxanthin. Most of these are potent antioxidants, while some carotenoids, like beta-carotenoids, can act as vitamin A precursors.[78–80] Carotenoids cannot be synthesized in our body and must be obtained through dietary sources. Because of their lipophilic nature, carotenoids in egg yolk have been proved to have a higher bioavailability compared to those from green leafy vegetables.[81–83] The high lipid content of egg yolk makes it a unique carrier of carotenoids, as well as facilitating its enrichment with beneficial carotenoids. The carotenoid profile of the egg yolk is greatly varied depending on the hen's diet; lutein, zeaxanthin, canthaxanthin, β-apo-8′-carotenal, capsanthin, β-apo-8′-carotenoic acid ethyl ester, β-cryptoxanthin, citranaxanthin and their isomers can be found in egg yolk.[84,85] From these, lutein, zeaxanthin and *meso*-zeaxanthin are the main components in the macular pigment of the eye.[86] The role of lutein and zeaxanthin in age-related macular degeneration has been extensively investigated and is well-documented.[87–89] They may act as direct antioxidants by scavenging singlet oxygen and peroxyl radicals and protecting the eye's macular cells from oxidative damage.[89–91] Based on the number of double bonds in the structure, carotenoids can quench singlet oxygen through direct energy transfer to yield ground state oxygen and an excited carotenoid molecule, which will be neutralized by reacting with the solvent.[92,93] Carotenoids can neutralize peroxyl radicals to form more stable carbon-centred radical adducts. They also absorb high-energy-containing blue light, thereby preventing the generation of free radicals and damage to photoreceptor cells.[94] Studies conducted with human lens epithelial cells showed that pre-incubation with lutein, zeaxanthin and α-tocopherol was reduced hydrogen peroxide-induced Malondialdehyde (MDA) levels and DNA damage, and increased the ratio of GSH : GSSG.[95] In addition to the contribution towards eye health, lutein has been reported to protect against the development of early atherosclerosis, as shown using mouse models.[96] With increasing lutein supplementation, the progression of atherosclerotic lesions in mice declined. Cells supplemented with lutein showed a significant reduction of LDL oxidation and formation of lipid peroxides, suggesting the protective antioxidant role of lutein in early atherosclerotic developments.[96]

9.4.9 Vitamins and Minerals

Among the many vitamins and minerals in egg, vitamin E is the most recognized as exerting antioxidant activity. An average egg contains approximately 1.1 mg of vitamin E, which makes up about 8.5% of the recommended daily intake.[97] Among several forms of vitamin E, α-tocopherol is the most preferred form in our body, acting as a peroxyl radical scavenger and protecting long-chain polyunsaturated fatty acids in cell membranes, maintaining their integrity.[98] The inhibitory role of vitamin E in LDL oxidation is shown to be beneficial in atherosclerotic patients,[99] however routine supplementation with vitamin E did not reduce the risk of cardiovascular diseases in healthy men[100] or women.[101]

Eggs contain minerals with antioxidant properties, such as selenium and iodine. Selenium is a component of many antioxidant enzymes, including glutathione peroxidases, and is also in selenoproteins,[102,103] such as plasma selenoprotein P, which protects LDL from oxidation.[104] Iodine is also believed to play a role in the body's antioxidant defense system.[105] Iodine deficiency is reported to elevate oxidative stress with higher levels of H_2O_2.[106]

9.4.10 Egg-derived Peptides with Antioxidant Properties

Peptides obtained from both egg white and egg yolk, mainly by enzymatic hydrolysis with both gastrointestinal and non-gastrointestinal enzymes, are reported to have antioxidant properties.[107–111] One of the early studies on antioxidant egg peptides reported that egg white albumin hydrolyzed with protease Amano S showed the highest antioxidant activity.[112] Four peptides with high antioxidant activity were purified from the hydrolysate and the peptide Ala-His-Lys was identified to have the strongest activity, His-Lys had no activity, while Ala-His was as potent an antioxidant as the parent peptide.[112] Dávalos *et al.* purified four antioxidant peptides from pepsin-hydrolyzed egg white proteins originated from ovalbumin.[109] Among those, the peptide Tyr-Ala-Glu-Glu-Arg-Tyr-Pro-Ile-Leu had both ACE-inhibitory and radical scavenging properties and showed protective effects against Cu-induced LDL oxidation.[109] Among several enzymatic digests, papain hydrolysate of egg proteins showed the highest radical scavenging activity and two peptides with strong antioxidant activity were purified: Tyr-Leu-Gly-Ala-Lys and Gly-Gly-Leu-Glu-Pro-Ile-Asn-Phe-Gln.[108] Their antioxidant potential was attributed to several structural features, including the presence of terminus Tyr, aromatic amino acids, such as Phe, and hydrophobic amino acids, such as Leu.[108] Among several non-gastric enzymes, protease P-hydrolyzed egg white resulted in higher antioxidant properties, and the purified peptides Ala-Glu-Glu-Arg-Tyr-Pro and Asp-Glu-Asp-Thr-Gln-Ala-Met-Pro both showed similar structural features, such as the presence of aromatic amino acids Tyr and Met in their sequence,[107] indicating the importance of the presence and positioning of certain amino acids in the sequence to exert antioxidant activity. Peptic hydrolysate of egg white-fed (0.5 g kg body weight^{-1} day^{-1}) spontaneously hypertensive rats showed a significant improvement in plasma radical scavenging capacity and decreased MDA concentration in the aorta.[113]

Egg yolk protein hydrolysate also acts as a natural antioxidant, protecting polyunsaturated fatty acids from oxidation, as tested in a linoleic acid system.[110] Two peptides purified from lecithin-free egg yolk hydrolyzed using alcalase significantly lowered lipid peroxidation in normal human liver cells.[111] Peptides derived from tryptic digests of phosvitin, which are known as phosvitin phosphopeptides (PPP), were also reported to exert antioxidant activity similar to that of glutathione and positively correlated with phosphorous content. PPP supressed H_2O_2-induced MDA formation in human intestinal epithelial cells.[114] They also upregulated antioxidant enzymes (glutathione reductase, glutathione *S*-transferase and catalase), supporting the body's natural antioxidant defense system, and were found to be resistant to gastric digestion, suggesting high bioavailability.[115]

The number of amino acids in the peptide and the presence of hydrophobic amino acids in the sequence are suggested as the main features responsible for antioxidant properties.[111] In addition, special structural features, such as the indole ring in Trp, the pyrrolidine ring in Pro, the imidazole ring in His, sulfhydryl groups in Met and Cys, the aromatic ring in Tyr and Phe, and the presence of hydrophobic amino acids are important determinants of the antioxidant potential of a peptide.[28]

9.5 Antioxidant-enriched Eggs

Certain lipid-soluble antioxidant compounds, such as lutein/zeaxanthin, vitamin E, selenium, iodine and lycopene, can be enriched into egg yolk through diet manipulation.[116,117] Omega-3 fatty acids are the most studied compounds in egg enrichment, where feed supplements such as fish oil, flax seed, algae or other ingredients have been used as the source of omega-3 fatty acids.[118,119] However, increasing the levels of omega-3 fatty acids can induce fatty acid oxidation in eggs during storage and processing; therefore, simultaneous enrichment of antioxidant compounds, such as vitamin E or carotenoids, was suggested to decrease fatty acid oxidation while also acting as dietary antioxidants.[117]

The carotenoid content in egg yolk can be varied depending on the hen's feed, where feed fortification with natural marigold (*Tagetes erecta*) or alfalfa (*Medicago sativa*) extracts increased the lutein content in egg yolk, while other natural feed ingredients, such as corn (*Zea mays*) and red pepper (*Capsicum annuum*), provide zeaxanthin and capsanthin, respectively.[120,121] In addition, canthaxanthin, β-apo-8′-carotenal and β-apo-8′-carotenoic acid ethyl ester are some of the chemically synthesized compounds that are used in poultry feed enrichment.[122,123] Following enrichment, the lutein content of the hen's egg can be increased up to 15-fold (~1.9 mg egg^{-1}) compared to the control group.[124] Improved lutein bioavailability observed in lutein-enriched eggs compared to lutein/lutein ester supplements and spinach is one of the key advantages of egg enrichment *via* feed formulations.[125] Among the others, lutein and zeaxanthin are two major carotenoids that are present in human serum, skin and eye macula, and involved in the protective roles against oxidative stress.[126–128] Lycopene is a symmetrical tetraterpene carotenoid that shows strong antioxidant properties and has potential for reducing the risk of human prostate carcinoma.[129,130] However, lycopene is not naturally present in eggs but can be enriched through poultry feed fortification with tomato powder. Reduction of egg yolk lipid peroxidation is an added advantage of lycopene enrichment, in addition to the human health benefits.[131]

Vitamin E is a major antioxidant present in our body, which provides primary protection against free radical-induced lipid peroxidation.[98,132] Setting up a recommended daily requirement for vitamin E has several challenges, but approximately 15 mg of α-tocopherol equivalents per day is considered to be adequate.[133] However, vitamin E is essential in protecting membrane lipids from peroxidation; therefore, the recommended daily intake should be increased along with the increased consumption of polyunsaturated fatty acids.[134,135] Surai *et al.* showed the potential of egg enrichment with up to 20 mg of vitamin E per egg, which is considered to be above the daily requirement of vitamin E.[116] Folate is another water-soluble B-group vitamin that can be enriched into egg yolk *via* feed fortification with a highly bioavailable form of folic acid. Previous studies on egg yolk folic acid fortification resulted in eggs with up to 12.5% of the recommended daily intake of folate.[136,137] In the native state, almost all the folate in eggs exists in the form of 5-methyltetrahydrofolate (5-MTHF), which shows higher stability during cooking and thermal processing. The electron-donating ability of the 5-amino group is considered to be the key contributing factor of the higher antioxidant activity observed in 5-MTHF compared to the other forms of folate.[138] 5-MTHF was reported to improve NO-mediated endothelial function, decrease superoxide production, scavenge peroxynitrite and reverse endothelial nitric oxide synthase (eNOS) uncoupling activities in both *in vivo* and *ex vivo* studies.[139,140] Selenium and iodine are two minerals known to show antioxidant activities, which can also effectively enrich into eggs *via* feed fortification. Researchers were able to enrich egg yolk with selenium and iodine up to 50% and 150% of the daily requirements, respectively.[116,117,141] In summary, eggs enriched with antioxidants *via* hen feed fortification can be used as an excellent dietary source of omega 3, vitamin E, vitamin D, selenium, iodine and lutein while also providing excellent antioxidant activity.

9.6 Effect of Storage, Processing and Gastrointestinal Digestion on Egg Antioxidants

Foods are subjected to a wide array of storage and processing conditions prior to their consumption and gastrointestinal digestion. These conditions may occur consecutively or simultaneously to influence and/or alter the antioxidant capacity of individual food components or the whole food system. Thermal processing conditions are known to create an environment that will favour lipid and protein oxidation, thermal degradation, leaching of nutrients, such as vitamin C and phenolic compounds, and aggregation of protein and other nutrients that can potentially reduce the antioxidant capacity of the food system.[142] In contrast, carotenoids present in the plant and animal food matrix will show improved digestive absorption, bioavailability and increased antioxidant potential owing to dissociation from the food matrix and thermally induced structural changes.[143–145] Other antioxidant compounds present in fruits and vegetables, such as phenolics, carotenoids, and vitamin C, can be affected differently under processing and storage conditions, and subsequently increase[146–148] or decrease[148–151] the total antioxidant activity.

In comparison to plant-based food matrices, the antioxidant capacity of animal-derived food systems is mainly derived from the amino compounds (proteins, peptides, amino acids, *etc.*) and vitamin E. Thermal processing can change the antioxidant capacity of different components present in egg. Egg white proteins such as ovalbumin, lysozyme and ovomucoid can go through the Maillard reaction and produce advanced glycation products with increased radical scavenging capacity.[152,153] In another study, DPPH (1,1-diphenyl-2-picrylhydrazyl) radical scavenging activity, reducing power and lipid peroxidation inhibitory activity did not show a significant difference in the spray dried and freeze dried egg white hydrolysate samples compared to fresh egg white samples.[108] Egg yolk phosvitin shows its antioxidant potential mainly owing to its iron-binding ability; however, heating phosvitin up to 110 °C for 40 min did not change its iron-binding ability or antioxidant potential.[154,155]

During thermal processing, carotenoids and vitamin E present in the egg yolk can be affected in many ways. Especially, carotenoids will undergo *trans–cis* isomerization or degradation in the presence of heat, light and oxygen, thereby changing their bioactivity.[75,156,157] Among different thermal processing methods, pasteurization did not change the carotenoid content of egg yolk,[158] whereas boiling of eggs resulted in a 10–20% loss of carotenoids.[84] Compared to boiling, frying eggs seemed less deleterious to the carotenoid content.[85] Storage temperature can also affect the total carotenoid content and antioxidant activity. The carotenoid content of raw eggs enriched with omega-3 and carophyll (a canthaxanthin preparation) were significantly reduced after 2 weeks at refrigeration temperature, whereas carotenoid loss was significantly higher after 1 week of room temperature storage.[159] In addition, the vitamin E content was also significantly reduced during thermal processing along with increased lipid oxidation products.[160,161] In another study, no significant changes in lutein or zeaxanthin content in egg yolk or in oxygen radical absorbance capacity (ORAC) activity were observed after 6 weeks of refrigerated storage of normal table eggs or omega-3-/lutein-enriched eggs.[162]

In addition to the traditional thermal processing techniques, novel food processing methods, such as ultrasound, high-intensity pulse electric field (PEF) processing and high-pressure processing (HPP), can also affect the antioxidant activity of egg proteins and peptides.[155,163] PEF processing of egg white protein resulted in increased antioxidant activity of the hydrolysate, mainly owing to the release of free amino acids and smaller peptides with high antioxidant properties.[163,164] HPP, sonication or ultrasound pre-treatment also showed an increase in the degree of hydrolysis of egg white proteins, which led to increased antioxidant properties of the hydrolysate.[165,166]

Gastrointestinal digestion involves extreme pH variations, several enzyme cocktails and physical conditions, which may directly or indirectly degrade existing antioxidant compounds or develop novel compounds with improved antioxidant potential. Most of the common food systems, such as wheat,[167] gooseberries,[168] grapes,[169] soy milk,[170] saithe and shrimp,[171] loach protein hydrolysate,[172] eggs,[173] fish[174] and poultry meat,[175] showed improved antioxidant capacity with simulated gastrointestinal digestion using different model systems. The increase in antioxidant activity was mainly attributed to the generation of free amino acids and smaller peptides with higher antioxidant potential.[155] On the other hand, the antioxidant activity of apples[176] and Feijoada whole meal (a traditional Brazilian dish containing vegetables)[177] was significantly reduced after the simulated gastrointestinal digestion.

Simulated gastrointestinal digestion of different egg components has been shown to generate antioxidant peptides in several studies.[164,173,178] A study by Remanan and Wu showed that domestic cooking methods such as boiling and frying can decrease the *in vitro* antioxidant activity of eggs.[164] However, simulated gastrointestinal digestion of cooked eggs with pepsin and pancreatin significantly increased the antioxidant activity of the hydrolysate.[164] Simulated gastrointestinal digestion of egg yolk using the TIM-1 intestinal model showed that the main egg carotenoids lutein and zeaxanthin remained stable during the digestion and showed improved bioaccessibility, probably owing to association with yolk fat.[157] In addition, TIM-1 digestion significantly increased the total antioxidant activity of cooked egg yolk by 5–8-fold, mainly owing to the release of free amino acids and antioxidant peptides.[157] Among several peptides purified from TIM-1-digested eggs, ovalbumin-derived peptides DSTRTQ, DVYSF and ESKPV significantly reduced the superoxide concentration in rat aorta vascular smooth muscle cells compared to the control sample, confirming the generation of antioxidant peptides during digestion.[179]

9.7 Summary

Chicken egg is a nutrient-dense food with highly bioavailable proteins, lipids, vitamins and minerals. In addition to their nutritional role, many egg compounds show different biological activities beneficial for human health, such as antioxidant, antihypertensive and anti-inflammatory activities. It is thought that oxidative stress caused by disturbances to the body's natural cellular redox balance is responsible for the onset and development of various chronic diseases. Dietary antioxidants have been extensively explored over the last few decades owing to their likely beneficial function in maintaining the redox balance. Recent research progress suggests that egg is a rich source of antioxidants, including ovalbumin, ovotransferrin, lysozyme, aromatic amino acids, phosvitin, phospholipids, vitamin E, selenium, carotenoids and bioactive peptides. Thermal processing of eggs can decrease the antioxidant activity depending on the duration and severity of the process; however, gastrointestinal digestion increases the antioxidant activity owing to the release of new antioxidant peptides during gastrointestinal digestion. Furthermore, the antioxidant activity of egg can be enriched with lipid-soluble antioxidants, such as carotenoids and vitamin E.

References

1. M. Schieber and N. S. Chandel, *Curr. Biol.*, 2014, **24**, R453–R462.
2. P. Niethammer, C. Grabher, A. T. Look and T. J. Mitchison, *Nature*, 2009, **459**, 996–999.
3. J. E. Le Belle, N. M. Orozco, A. A. Paucar, J. P. Saxe, J. Mottahedeh, A. D. Pyle, H. Wu and H. I. Kornblum, *Cell Stem Cell*, 2011, **8**, 59–71.
4. C. Kohchi, H. Inagawa, T. Nishizawa and G. I. Soma, *Anticancer Res.*, 2009, **29**, 817–822.
5. S. B. Nimse and D. Pal, *RSC Adv.*, 2015, **5**, 27986–28006.
6. M. S. Brewer, *Compr. Rev. Food Sci. Food Saf.*, 2011, **10**, 221–247.
7. M. C. Linder, *Metallomics*, 2016, **8**, 887–905.
8. A. M. Rizzo, P. Berselli, S. Zava, G. Montorfano, M. Negroni, P. Corsetto and B. Berra, *Adv. Exp. Med. Biol.*, 2010, **698**, 52–67.
9. D. P. Jones, *Antioxid. Redox Signaling*, 2006, **8**, 1865–1879.
10. J. Bouayed and T. Bohn, *Oxid. Med. Cell. Longevity*, 2010, **3**, 228–237.
11. A. M. Pisoschi and A. Pop, *Eur. J. Med. Chem.*, 2015, **97**, 55–74.
12. I. Mirończuk-Chodakowska, A. M. Witkowska and M. E. Zujko, *Adv. Med. Sci.*, 2018, **63**, 68–78.
13. K. B. Pandey and S. I. Rizvi, *Oxid. Med. Cell. Longevity*, 2009, **2**, 270–278.
14. J. Fiedor and K. Burda, *Nutrients*, 2014, **6**, 466–488.
15. B. Poljsak, D. Šuput and I. Milisav, *Oxid. Med. Cell. Longevity*, 2013, **2013**, 956792.
16. S.-K. Myung, Y. Kim, W. Ju, H. J. Choi and W. K. Bae, *Ann. Oncol.*, 2010, **21**, 166–179.
17. A. Bardia, I. M. Tleyjeh, J. R. Cerhan, A. K. Sood, P. J. Limburg, P. J. Erwin and V. M. Montori, *Mayo Clin. Proc.*, 2008, **83**, 23–34.
18. J. Mursu, K. Robien, L. J. Harnack, K. Park and D. R. Jacobs Jr, *Arch. Intern. Med.*, 2011, **171**, 1625–1633.
19. G. Bjelakovic, D. Nikolova, L. L. Gluud, R. G. Simonetti and C. Gluud, in *Cochrane Database of Systematic Reviews*, ed. G. Bjelakovic, John Wiley & Sons, Ltd, Chichester, UK, 2008, p. CD007176.
20. C. Brunetti, M. Di Ferdinando, A. Fini, S. Pollastri and M. Tattini, *Int. J. Mol. Sci.*, 2013, **14**, 3540–3555.
21. P. C. Wootton-Beard and L. Ryan, *Food Res. Int.*, 2011, **44**, 3135–3148.
22. E. Abourashed, *Antioxidants*, 2013, **2**, 309–325.
23. V. Lobo, A. Patil, A. Phatak and N. Chandra, *Pharmacogn. Rev.*, 2010, **4**, 118–126.
24. J. Dai and R. J. Mumper, *Molecules*, 2010, **15**, 7313–7352.
25. M. J. Amiot, C. Riva and A. Vinet, *Obes. Rev.*, 2016, **17**, 573–586.
26. N. Xia, A. Daiber, U. Förstermann and H. Li, *Br. J. Pharmacol.*, 2017, **174**, 1633–1646.
27. E. Sikora, E. Cieślik and K. Topolska, *Acta Sci. Pol., Technol. Aliment.*, 2008, **7**, 5–17.
28. A. G. P. Samaranayaka and E. C. Y. Li-Chan, *J. Funct. Foods*, 2011, **3**, 229–254.
29. B. H. Sarmadi and A. Ismail, *Peptides*, 2010, **31**, 1949–1956.

30. S.-J. You, C. C. Udenigwe, R. E. Aluko and J. Wu, *Food Res. Int.*, 2010, **43**, 848–855.
31. S. M. Deneke, *Curr. Top. Cell. Regul.*, 2001, **36**, 151–180.
32. G. Atmaca, *Yonsei Med. J.*, 2004, **45**, 776–788.
33. T.-B. Zou, T.-P. He, H.-B. Li, H.-W. Tang and E.-Q. Xia, *Molecules*, 2016, **21**, 72.
34. S. Sakanaka, Y. Tachibana, N. Ishihara and L. R. Juneja, *J. Agric. Food Chem.*, 2005, **53**, 464–468.
35. B. Mann, A. Kumari, R. Kumar, R. Sharma, K. Prajapati, S. Mahboob and S. Athira, *J. Food Sci. Technol.*, 2014, **52**, 3235–3241.
36. O. Power, P. Jakeman and R. J. FitzGerald, *Amino Acids*, 2013, **44**, 797–820.
37. M. Chalamaiah, B. Dinesh kumar, R. Hemalatha and T. Jyothirmayi, *Food Chem.*, 2012, **135**, 3020–3038.
38. K. M. Chan and E. A. Decker, *Crit. Rev. Food Sci. Nutr.*, 1994, **34**, 403–426.
39. R. Di Bernardini, P. Harnedy, D. Bolton, J. Kerry, E. O'Neill, A. M. Mullen and M. Hayes, *Food Chem.*, 2011, **124**, 1296–1307.
40. C. Nimalaratne, N. Bandara and J. Wu, *Food Chem.*, 2015, **188**, 467–472.
41. X. Xu, S. Katayama and Y. Mine, *J. Sci. Food Agric.*, 2007, **87**, 2604–2608.
42. W. Miki, *Pure Appl. Chem.*, 1991, **63**, 141–146.
43. D.-H. Ngo, I. Wijesekara, T.-S. Vo, Q. Van Ta and S.-K. Kim, *Food Res. Int.*, 2011, **44**, 523–529.
44. W. Powrie and S. Nakai, in *Egg Science and Technology*, ed. W. J. Stadelman and O. J. Cotterill, Avi Publishing, Westport, CT, 1986, pp. 97–139.
45. H. Sugino, T. Nitoda and L. R. Juneja, in *Hen, Eggs Their Basic and Applied Science*, ed. M. Yamamoto,T. Juneja,L. R. Hatta andH. Kim, CRC Press, New York, 1997, pp. 13–24.
46. T. Yamamoto, L. R. Juneja, H. Hatta and M. Kim, *Hen Eggs: Basic and Applied Science*, CRC Press, 1996.
47. M. Anton, F. Nau and Y. Nys, *World's Poult. Sci. J.*, 2006, **62**, 429–438.
48. J. Kovacs-Nolan, M. Phillips and Y. Mine, *J. Agric. Food Chem.*, 2005, **53**, 8421–8431.
49. Y. Mine and J. Kovacs-Nolan, *J. Poult. Sci.*, 2004, **41**, 1–29.
50. J. S. Sim, in *The Return of Omega 3 Fatty Acids into the Food Supply, 1. Land-Based Animal Food Products and Their Health Effects*, ed. A. P. Simopoulos, Karger, Basel, Switzerland, 1998, pp. 89–101.
51. Y.-F. Liu, I. Oey, P. Bremer, A. Carne and P. Silcock, *Crit. Rev. Food Sci. Nutr.*, 2017, 1–23.
52. R. Requejo, T. R. Hurd, N. J. Costa and M. P. Murphy, *FEBS J.*, 2010, **277**, 1465–1480.
53. S. Nakamura, A. Kato and K. Kobayashi, *J. Agric. Food Chem.*, 1992, **40**, 2033–2037.
54. Y. Yamamoto, E. Kato and A. Ando, *Biosci., Biotechnol., Biochem.*, 1996, **60**, 1430–1433.
55. M. P. Almajano, M. E. Delgado and M. H. Gordon, *Food Chem.*, 2007, **102**, 1375–1382.
56. N. Matoba, Y. Yamada, H. Usui, R. Nakagiri and M. Yoshikawa, *Biosci., Biotechnol., Biochem.*, 2001, **65**, 736–739.

57. E. C. Y. Li-Chan and H. O. Kim, in *Egg Bioscience and Biotechnology*, ed. Y. Mine, John Wiley & Sons, Ltd, Hoboken, NJ, USA, 2008, pp. 1–95.
58. H. R. Ibrahim, M. I. Hoq and T. Aoki, *Int. J. Biol. Macromol.*, 2007, **41**, 631–640.
59. H. Liu, F. Zheng, Q. Cao, B. Ren, L. Zhu, G. Striker and H. Vlassara, *Am. J. Physiol.: Endocrinol. Metab.*, 2006, **290**, E824–E832.
60. J. M. Fritz, M. Ikegami, T. E. Weaver and H. T. Akinbi, *C21. Paths to Lung Injury and Repair*, American Thoracic Society, 2014, p. A4005.
61. S. Réhault, in *Bioactive Egg Compounds*, Springer Berlin Heidelberg, Berlin, Heidelberg, 2007, pp. 85–92.
62. M. K. Lehtinen, S. Tegelberg, H. Schipper, H. Su, H. Zukor, O. Manninen, O. Kopra, T. Joensuu, P. Hakala, A. Bonni and A.-E. Lehesjoki, *J. Neurosci.*, 2009, **29**, 5910–5915.
63. L. Verdot, G. Lalmanach, V. Vercruysse, J. Hoebeke, F. Gauthier and B. Vray, *Eur. J. Biochem.*, 1999, **266**, 1111–1117.
64. K. Frenkel, K. Chrzan, C. A. Ryan, R. Wiesner and W. Troll, *Carcinogenesis*, 1987, **8**, 1207–1212.
65. Y. Kohgo, K. Ikuta, T. Ohtake, Y. Torimoto and J. Kato, *Int. J. Hematol.*, 2008, **88**, 7–15.
66. G. Papanikolaou and K. Pantopoulos, *Toxicol. Appl. Pharmacol.*, 2005, **202**, 199–211.
67. S.-I. Ishikawa, Y. Yano, K. Arihara and M. Itoh, *Biosci., Biotechnol., Biochem.*, 2004, **68**, 1324–1331.
68. S. Ishikawa, S. Ohtsuki, K. Tomita, K. Arihara and M. Itoh, *Biol. Trace Elem. Res.*, 2005, **105**, 249–256.
69. S. H. Moon, J. H. Lee, M. Lee, E. Park, D. U. Ahn and H.-D. Paik, *Poult. Sci.*, 2014, **93**, 2103–2107.
70. S. K. Lee, J. H. Han and E. A. Decker, *J. Food Sci.*, 2002, **67**, 37–41.
71. D. N. Rhodes and C. H. Lea, *Biochem. J.*, 1957, **65**, 526–533.
72. H. Sugino, M. Ishikawa, T. Nitoda, M. Koketsu, L. R. Juneja, M. Kim and T. Yamamoto, *J. Agric. Food Chem.*, 1997, **45**, 551–554.
73. M. F. King, L. C. Boyd and B. W. Sheldon, *J. Am. Oil Chem. Soc.*, 1992, **69**, 545–551.
74. M. Kashima, G.-S. Cha, Y. Isoda, J. Hirano and T. Miyazawa, *J. Am. Oil Chem. Soc.*, 1991, **68**, 119–122.
75. C. Nimalaratne, J. Wu and A. Schieber, *Egg Yolk Carotenoids: Composition, Analysis, and Effects of Processing on Their Stability*, 2013, vol. 1134.
76. N. I. Krinsky, M. D. Russett, G. J. Handelman and D. M. Snodderly, *J. Nutr.*, 1990, **120**, 1654–1662.
77. M. C. Meinke, M. E. Darvin, H. Vollert and J. Lademann, *Eur. J. Pharm. Biopharm.*, 2010, **76**, 269–274.
78. A. V. Rao and L. G. Rao, *Nutr. Pharmacol.*, 2007, **55**, 207–216.
79. L. Ma and X.-M. Lin, *J. Sci. Food Agric.*, 2010, **90**, 2–12.
80. E. J. Johnson, *Nutr. Clin. Care*, 2002, **5**, 56–65.
81. G. J. Handelman, Z. D. Nightingale, A. H. Lichtenstein, E. J. Schaefer and J. B. Blumberg, *Am. J. Clin. Nutr.*, 1999, **70**, 247–251.

82. K. J. Yeum and R. M. Russell, *Annu. Rev. Nutr.*, 2002, **22**, 483–504.
83. K. H. van het Hof, C. E. West, J. A. Weststrate and J. G. A. J. Hautvast, *J. Nutr.*, 2000, **130**, 503–506.
84. J. Schlatterer and D. E. Breithaupt, *J. Agric. Food Chem.*, 2006, **54**, 2267–2273.
85. C. Nimalaratne, D. Lopes-Lutz, A. Schieber and J. Wu, *J. Agric. Food Chem.*, 2012, **60**, 12547–12552.
86. D. I. Thurnham, *Nutr. Res. Rev.*, 2007, **20**, 163–179.
87. S. M. Moeller, N. Parekh, L. Tinker, C. Ritenbaugh, B. Blodi, R. B. Wallace and J. A. Mares, *Arch. Ophthalmol.*, 2006, **124**, 1151–1162.
88. E.-S. Abdel-Aal, H. Akhtar, K. Zaheer and R. Ali, *Nutrients*, 2013, **5**, 1169–1185.
89. J. Wu, E. Cho, W. C. Willett, S. M. Sastry and D. A. Schaumberg, *JAMA Ophthalmol.*, 2015, **133**, 1415.
90. N. I. Krinsky, J. T. Landrum and R. A. Bone, *Annu. Rev. Nutr.*, 2003, **23**, 171–201.
91. S. Carpentier, M. Knaus and M. Suh, *Crit. Rev. Food Sci. Nutr.*, 2009, **49**, 313–326.
92. W. Stahl and H. Sies, *Fat Soluble Vitam. Old Mol. with Nov. Prop.*, 2003, **24**, 345–351.
93. A. Mortensen and L. H. Skibsted, *J. Agric. Food Chem.*, 1997, **45**, 2970–2977.
94. A. Kijlstra, Y. Tian, E. R. Kelly and T. T. J. M. Berendschot, *Prog. Retin. Eye Res.*, 2012, **31**, 303–315.
95. S. Gao, T. Qin, Z. Liu, M. A. Caceres, C. F. Ronchi, C.-Y. O. Chen, K.-J. Yeum, A. Taylor, J. B. Blumberg, Y. Liu and F. Shang, *Mol. Vision*, 2011, **17**, 3180–3190.
96. J. H. Dwyer, M. Navab, K. M. Dwyer, K. Hassan, P. Sun, A. Shircore, S. Hama-Levy, G. Hough, X. Wang, T. Drake, C. N. B. Merz and A. M. Fogelman, *Circulation*, 2001, **103**, 2922–2927.
97. I. Seuss-baum, in *Bioactive Egg Compounds*, Springer, 2007, pp. 117–144.
98. M. G. Traber and J. Atkinson, *Free Radicals Biol. Med.*, 2007, **43**, 4–15.
99. N. Stephens, A. Parsons, M. Brown, P. Schofield, F. Kelly, K. Cheeseman and M. Mitchinson, *Lancet*, 1996, **347**, 781–786.
100. H. D. Sesso, J. E. Buring, W. G. Christen, T. Kurth, C. Belanger, J. MacFadyen, V. Bubes, J. E. Manson, R. J. Glynn and J. M. Gaziano, *JAMA*, 2008, **300**, 2123.
101. I.-M. Lee, N. R. Cook, J. M. Gaziano, D. Gordon, P. M. Ridker, J. E. Manson, C. H. Hennekens and J. E. Buring, *JAMA*, 2005, **294**, 56.
102. U. Tinggi, *Environ. Health Prev. Med.*, 2008, **13**, 102–108.
103. H. Tapiero, D. Townsend and K. Tew, *Biomed. Pharmacother.*, 2003, **57**, 134–144.
104. H. Traulsen, H. Steinbrenner, D. P. Buchczyk, L.-O. Klotz and H. Sies, *Free Radical Res.*, 2004, **38**, 123–128.
105. R. Winkler, S. Griebenow and W. Wonisch, *Cell Biochem. Funct.*, 2000, **18**, 143–146.
106. P. P. A. Smyth, *BioFactors*, 2003, **19**, 121–130.

107. C. Nimalaratne, N. Bandara and J. Wu, *Food Chem.*, 2015, **188**, 467–472.
108. C. Chen, Y.-J. Chi, M.-Y. Zhao and L. Lv, *Amino Acids*, 2012, **43**, 457–466.
109. A. Dávalos, M. Miguel, B. Bartolomé and R. López-Fandiño, *J. Food Prot.*, 2004, **67**, 1939–1944.
110. S. Sakanaka, Y. Tachibana, N. Ishihara and L. Raj Juneja, *Food Chem.*, 2004, **86**, 99–103.
111. P.-J. Park, W.-K. Jung, K.-S. Nam, F. Shahidi and S.-K. Kim, *J. Am. Oil Chem. Soc.*, 2001, **78**, 651–656.
112. N. Tsuge, Y. Eikawa, Y. Nomura, M. Yamamoto and K. Sugisawa, *Nippon Nogeikagaku Kaishi.*, 1991, **65**, 1635–1641.
113. M. Manso, M. Miguel, J. Even, R. Hernandez, A. Aleixandre and R. Lopezfandino, *Food Chem.*, 2008, **109**, 361–367.
114. S. Katayama, X. Xu, M. Z. Fan and Y. Mine, *J. Agric. Food Chem.*, 2006, **54**, 773–778.
115. S. Katayama, S.-I. Ishikawa, M. Z. Fan and Y. Mine, *J. Agric. Food Chem.*, 2007, **55**, 2829–2835.
116. P. F. Surai, P. C. M. Simons, J. E. Dvorska, F. Aradas and N. H. C. Sparks, in *The Amazing Egg: Nature's Perfect Functional Food for Health Promotion*, ed. J. S. Sim and H. H. Sunwoo, University of Alberta, Edmonton, Canada, 2006, pp. 68–93.
117. P. F. Surai and V. I. Fisinin, in *Handbook of Eggs in Human Function*, ed. R. Watson and F. Meester, Wageningen Academic Pub, Wageningen, 1st edn, 2015, pp. 133–152.
118. I. Fraeye, C. Bruneel, C. Lemahieu, J. Buyse, K. Muylaert and I. Foubert, *Food Res. Int.*, 2012, **48**, 961–969.
119. C. Lemahieu, C. Bruneel, K. Muylaert, J. Buyse and I. Foubert, in *Egg Innovations and Strategies for Improvements*, ed. P. Hester, Academic Press, Elsevier, London, UK, 1st edn, 2017, pp. 383–391.
120. D. E. Breithaupt, *Trends Food Sci. Technol.*, 2007, **18**, 501–506.
121. S. Leeson, in *The Amazing Egg: Nature's Perfect Functional Food for Health Promotion*, ed. J. S. Sim and H. H. Sunwoo, Department of Agricultural, Food and Nutritional Science, University of Alberta, Edmonton, Alberta, Canada, 2006, pp. 171–179.
122. D. R. Breithaupt, in *Carotenoids*, ed. H. Pfander, Birkhäuser Basel, 2008, vol. 4, pp. 255–264.
123. K. Zaheer, *CyTA--J. Food*, 2017, **15**, 474–487.
124. P. F. Surai, A. MacPherson, B. K. Speake and N. H. C. Sparks, *Eur. J. Clin. Nutr.*, 2000, **54**, 298–305.
125. H.-Y. Chung, H. M. Rasmussen and E. J. Johnson, *J. Nutr.*, 2004, **134**, 1887–1893.
126. J. M. Serpeloni, D. Grotto, A. Z. Mercadante, M. de Lourdes Pires Bianchi and L. M. G. Antunes, *Arch. Toxicol.*, 2010, **84**, 811–822.
127. R. L. Roberts, J. Green and B. Lewis, *Clin. Dermatol.*, 2009, **27**, 195–201.
128. J. Nataraj, T. Manivasagam, A. J. Thenmozhi and M. M. Essa, *Nutr. Neurosci.*, 2016, **19**, 237–246.
129. K. Wertz, U. Siler and R. Goralczyk, *Arch. Biochem. Biophys.*, 2004, **430**, 127–134.

130. J. B. Olson, N. E. Ward and E. A. Koutsos, *Poult. Sci.*, 2008, **87**, 2573–2580.
131. F. Akdemir, C. Orhan, N. Sahin, K. Sahin and A. Hayirli, *Br. Poult. Sci.*, 2012, **53**, 675–680.
132. G. W. Burton and M. G. Traber, *Annu. Rev. Nutr.*, 1990, **10**, 357–382.
133. S. Péter, U. Moser, S. Pilz, M. Eggersdorfer and P. Weber, *Int. J. Vitam. Nutr. Res.*, 2013, **83**, 129–136.
134. T. A. B. Sanders and A. Hinds, *Br. J. Nutr.*, 2007, **68**, 163.
135. E. E. Valk and G. Hornstra, *Int. J. Vitam. Nutr. Res.*, 2000, **70**, 31–42.
136. J. D. House, K. Braun, D. Ballance, C. O'Connor and W. Guenter, *Poult. Sci.*, 2002, **81**, 1332–1337.
137. J. D. House, C. O'Connor and W. Guenter, *J. Agric. Food Chem.*, 2003, **51**, 4461–4467.
138. B. M. Rezk, G. R. M. Haenen, W. J. van der Vijgh and A. Bast, *FEBS Lett.*, 2003, **555**, 601–605.
139. C. Antoniades, C. Shirodaria, N. Warrick, S. Cai, J. de Bono, J. Lee, P. Leeson, S. Neubauer, C. Ratnatunga, R. Pillai, H. Refsum and K. M. Channon, *Circulation*, 2006, **114**, 1193–1201.
140. M. C. Verhaar, R. M. F. Wever, J. J. P. Kastelein, T. van Dam, H. A. Koomans and T. J. Rabelink, *Circulation*, 1998, **97**, 237–241.
141. Z. Dobrzanski, H. Gorecka, G. Strzelbicka, J. Szczypel and T. Trziszka, *Electron. J. Polish Agric. Univ. Ser. Anim. Husb.*, 2001, **4**, available at http://www.ejpau.media.pl/volume4/issue2/animal/art-01.html (accessed April 2019).
142. W. Kalt, *J. Food Sci.*, 2005, **70**, R11–R19.
143. J. Shi and M. Le Maguer, *Crit. Rev. Food Sci. Nutr.*, 2000, **40**, 1–42.
144. V. Dewanto, X. Wu, K. K. Adom and R. H. Liu, *J. Agric. Food Chem.*, 2002, **50**, 3010–3014.
145. V. Dewanto, X. Wu and R. H. Liu, *J. Agric. Food Chem.*, 2002, **50**, 4959–4964.
146. S. Adefegha and G. Oboh, *Afr. J. Biotechnol.*, 2013, **10**, 632–639.
147. N. Turkmen, F. Sari and Y. S. Velioglu, *Food Chem.*, 2005, **93**, 713–718.
148. K. Ravichandran, N. M. M. T. Saw, A. A. A. Mohdaly, A. M. M. Gabr, A. Kastell, H. Riedel, Z. Cai, D. Knorr and I. Smetanska, *Food Res. Int.*, 2013, **50**, 670–675.
149. A. Ismail, Z. M. Marjan and C. W. Foong, *Food Chem.*, 2004, **87**, 581–586.
150. F. Natella, F. Belelli, A. RambertiI and C. Scaccini, *J. Food Biochem.*, 2010, 796–810.
151. D. Zhang and Y. Hamauzu, *Food Chem.*, 2004, **88**, 503–509.
152. H. Jing, M. Yap, P. Y. Y. Wong and D. D. Kitts, *Food Bioprocess Technol.*, 2009, **4**, 1489–1496.
153. Z. Tu, Y. Hu, H. Wang, X. Huang, S. Xia and P. Niu, *J. Food Sci. Technol.*, 2015, **52**, 1453–1461.
154. K. J. Albright, D. T. Gordon and O. J. Cotterill, *J. Food Sci.*, 1984, **49**, 78–81.
155. C. Nimalaratne and J. Wu, *Nutrients*, 2015, **7**, 8274–8293.
156. A. Schieber and R. Carle, *Pigm. Food*, 2005, **16**, 416–422.
157. C. Nimalaratne, P. Savard, S. F. Gauthier, A. Schieber and J. Wu, *J. Agric. Food Chem.*, 2015, **63**, 2956–2962.

158. M. Wenzel, I. Seuss-Baum and E. Schlich, *J. Agric. Food Chem.*, 2010, **58**, 1726–1731.
159. V. C. Barbosa, A. Gaspar, L. F. L. Calixto and T. S. P. Agostinho, *Rev. Bras. Zootec.*, 2011, **40**, 1540–1544.
160. J. Galobart, A. C. Barroeta, M. D. Baucells, L. Cortinas and F. Guardiola, *Poult. Sci.*, 2001, **80**, 1496–1505.
161. M. F. Caboni, E. Boselli, M. C. Messia, V. Velazco, A. Fratianni, G. Panfili and E. Marconi, *Food Chem.*, 2005, **92**, 293–303.
162. C. Nimalaratne, A. Schieber and J. Wu, *Food Chem.*, 2016, **194**, 111–116.
163. S. Lin, Y. Jin, M. Liu, Y. Yang, M. Zhang, Y. Guo, G. Jones, J. Liu and Y. Yin, *Food Chem.*, 2013, **139**, 300–306.
164. M. K. Remanan and J. Wu, *Food Funct.*, 2014, **5**, 1464–1474.
165. A. B. Stefanović, J. R. Jovanović, S. Ž. Grbavčić, N. Ž. Šekuljica, V. B. Manojlović, B. M. Bugarski and Z. D. Knežević-Jugović, *Eur. Food Res. Technol.*, 2014, **239**, 979–993.
166. I. Van der Plancken, A. Van Loey and M. E. Hendrickx, *Innovative Food Sci. Emerging Technol.*, 2005, **6**, 11–20.
167. N. Mateo Anson, R. Havenaar, A. Bast and G. R. M. M. Haenen, *J. Cereal Sci.*, 2010, **51**, 110–114.
168. C.-J. Chiang, H. Kadouh and K. Zhou, *LWT--Food Sci. Technol.*, 2013, **51**, 417–422.
169. D. Tagliazucchi, E. Verzelloni, D. Bertolini and A. Conte, *Food Chem.*, 2010, **120**, 599–606.
170. M. J. Rodríguez-Roque, M. A. Rojas-Graü, P. Elez-Martínez and O. Martín-Belloso, *Food Chem.*, 2013, **136**, 206–212.
171. I.-J. Jensen, H. Abrahamsen, H. K. Maehre and E. O. Elvevoll, *J. Agric. Food Chem.*, 2009, **57**, 10928–10932.
172. L. You, M. Zhao, J. M. Regenstein and J. Ren, *Food Chem.*, 2010, **120**, 810–816.
173. S. Rao, J. Sun, Y. Liu, H. Zeng, Y. Su and Y. Yang, *Food Chem.*, 2012, **135**, 1245–1252.
174. A. Bougatef, N. Nedjar-Arroume, L. Manni, R. Ravallec, A. Barkia, D. Guillochon and M. Nasri, *Food Chem.*, 2010, **118**, 559–565.
175. J. O. Onuh, A. T. Girgih, R. E. Aluko and M. Aliani, *Food Chem.*, 2014, **150**, 366–373.
176. J. Bouayed, L. Hoffmann and T. Bohn, *Food Chem.*, 2011, **128**, 14–21.
177. A. L. K. Faller, E. Fialho and R. H. Liu, *J. Agric. Food Chem.*, 2012, **60**, 4826–4832.
178. D. Young, F. Nau, M. Pasco and Y. Mine, *J. Agric. Food Chem.*, 2011, **59**, 9207–9218.
179. J. Wang, W. Liao, C. Nimalaratne, S. Chakrabarti and J. Wu, *NPJ Sci. Food*, 2018, **2**, 7.

CHAPTER 10

Modulation of Inflammation by Egg Components

C. J. ANDERSEN*[a] AND A. R. VAN DYKE[b]

[a]Fairfield University, Department of Biology, 1073 North Benson Road, Fairfield, CT 06824, USA; [b]Fairfield University, Department of Chemistry and Biochemistry, 1073 North Benson Road, Fairfield, CT 06824, USA
*E-mail: candersen@fairfield.edu

10.1 Introduction

Inflammation is an essential pathway in healthy immune responses, while also contributing to the pathophysiology underlying numerous chronic diseases.[1–3] In response to pathogens or tissue injury, cells of the innate and adaptive immune system coordinate sophisticated inflammatory responses involving the activation of immune cells, production of inflammatory mediators (*e.g.* cytokines, chemokines, eicosanoids), and eradication of the tissue insult.[4] While generation of these pro-inflammatory mediators is essential, resolution of inflammation is necessary to ensure tissue healing and a return to homeostasis.[5] Impairments in mounting the initial pro-inflammatory responses are linked to impaired immunity to pathogenic infection and stimuli, whereas failure to resolve inflammation is associated with acute inflammatory (*e.g.* sepsis) and autoimmune disorders.[6–8] Obesity-induced metabolic stress additionally perpetuates a chronic state of low-grade, systemic inflammation stemming from adipose tissue dysfunction, leading to

Food Chemistry, Function and Analysis No.14
Eggs as Functional Foods and Nutraceuticals for Human Health
Edited by Jianping Wu

Published by the Royal Society of Chemistry, www.rsc.org

increased risk of developing chronic diseases, such as cardiovascular disease, type 2 diabetes mellitus (T2DM), non-alcoholic fatty liver disease (NAFLD), and cancer.[2,9–11] Thus, it is essential that inflammatory pathways are regulated in a way that optimizes immune responses while mitigating the risk of developing chronic diseases.

Eggs contain a wide variety of bioactive compounds that can impact inflammatory pathways that are integral to human health and disease risk.[12] Egg-derived compounds include lipid species (*e.g.* phospholipids, sphingolipids, cholesterol, fatty acids), proteins and peptides, carotenoids (*e.g.* lutein and zeaxanthin), and vitamins and minerals.[12,13] Many of these food components are highly bioavailable, particularly when consumed within the whole food matrix of eggs.[14,15] Further, when evaluated in studies using isolated or purified forms, many of these compounds exert pro- and/or anti-inflammatory effects in various cell-, animal-, and human-based models.[16–19] Results from these studies suggest that certain compounds may serve as direct ligands for nuclear receptors involved in inflammatory pathway regulation or may exhibit indirect effects on inflammation by modulating pathways of lipid metabolism and oxidative stress.[20–25] The diverse mechanisms of these bioactive components may help to elucidate the differential effects of egg fraction intake (*i.e.* whole eggs *vs.* egg whites), dose (*i.e.* number of eggs per day), and human health status on inflammation observed across studies,[12] which are highlighted in the following sections.

10.2 Effects of Egg Intake in Human Populations

Given the essentiality of immune regulation in human health and disease, it is important to understand how egg consumption impacts inflammation within distinct dietary patterns and populations.[4,12] Evaluation of these parameters is particularly timely given the revised recommendations put forth by the American Heart Association/American College of Cardiology in 2013 and the Dietary Guidelines for Americans 2015–2020, which no longer limit daily intake of dietary cholesterol.[26,27] A recent study evaluating data from the 2001–2012 National Health and Nutrition Examination Surveys additionally found that while the proportion of U.S. adults who consume eggs has remained consistent (21–22%), *per capita* egg consumption has increased by 11%, particularly among women.[28] Further, research has demonstrated benefits to egg intake beyond inflammation, including promotion of satiety and weight maintenance, and protection against age-related macular degeneration and sarcopenia.[29–31] Egg consumers have additionally been shown to have greater overall nutrient intake and dietary quality.[32] With these findings, individuals may seek to incorporate eggs into their diets to obtain a range of health benefits. Interestingly, the effect of egg intake on inflammation appears to range from pro- to anti-inflammatory, depending on the number and fraction of eggs consumed (*i.e.* yolk *vs.* white), the health status of the population, and whether individuals are undergoing weight loss.[22,29,33–36] These findings suggest that recommendations to consume egg as a means to address inflammation may be more complex and population-specific.[12] The following sections review findings from epidemiological and intervention studies that contribute to our understanding of the relationship between egg intake and inflammation.

10.2.1 Epidemiological Studies

While a number of studies have evaluated the relationship between egg intake and risk for cardiovascular disease, fewer have examined the impact of egg intake on inflammatory markers.[37,38] In 1032 men from the Kuopio Ischaemic Heart Disease Risk Factor Study, C-reactive protein (CRP) levels did not significantly differ between men consuming different amounts of either egg or dietary cholesterol.[39] Conversely, high-sensitivity CRP levels were associated with intake of eggs and egg products in 956 young women from the International Collaboration Study for the Construction of Asian Cohort of the Korean Genome and Epidemiology Study cohort.[40] However, it is suggested, albeit unclear, that this association was lost in multiple regression analysis after controlling for age, BMI, exercise, intake of energy, alcohol, and dietary supplements.[40] Using population databases, egg intake has further been associated with decreased or neutral risk of diseases/conditions where inflammation is a common characteristic, including metabolic syndrome and cardiovascular disease.[37,38,41,42] However, conflicting results have been reported on the association between egg consumption and risk for heart failure, T2DM, and cancer.[37,38,43–49] Thus, more research is required to elucidate the effects of egg intake on inflammation at the large-scale population level, and whether these effects contribute to chronic disease development.

10.2.2 Dietary Intervention Trials

In addition to epidemiological evidence, numerous intervention trials have revealed differential effects of egg intake on markers of inflammation, depending on the dose and fraction of the egg consumed, in addition to the health and weight status of the population.[12] The following sections outline how these parameters impact the effects of egg intake on inflammation across populations. Together, these findings support the need for additional research to understand the mechanisms underlying population-specific effects.

10.2.2.1 Effects of Egg Intake on Postprandial Inflammation

A number of studies (Table 10.1) have evaluated the effects of egg consumption on postprandial inflammation, particularly in regard to the formation of trimethylamine-*N*-oxide (TMAO) – a pro-atherosclerotic

Table 10.1 Effects of egg intake on postprandial inflammation.

Treatment	Population	Effect on inflammation	Reference
0 or 1 egg yolk	Healthy adults	No effect on plasma TMAO	51
2-egg meal	Healthy adults	Increased plasma TMAO	36
2, 4, or 6 egg yolks	Healthy adults	Increased plasma TMAO levels; peak 6–8 hours post-ingestion	51
High-fat meals that include eggs	Healthy adults (meta-analysis)	Increase postprandial interleukin 6 levels; no change in CRP, TNFα, IL-1β and IL-8	52

derivative of phosphatidylcholine metabolism generated by gut microbiota.[50] Tang *et al.* found that healthy individuals with normal, unmodified intestinal microbiota exhibited increased plasma TMAO following a two-egg meal.[36] Similarly, Miller *et al.* reported increased TMAO levels in healthy adults following intake of 2, 4, or 6 egg yolks, with the greatest increases observed at 6–8 hours post-ingestion.[51] Plasma and urine TMAO levels did not increase following consumption of 0 or 1 egg yolk, and serum high-sensitivity CRP levels were not altered by any egg treatment.[51] Studies have additionally found high-fat meals that include eggs to increase postprandial interleukin 6 levels; however, these results are inconsistent, and studies are often performed using various combinations of high-fat and high-carbohydrate foods.[52,53]

10.2.2.2 Effects of Egg Dose on Inflammation

While differences may be observed between postprandial and fasting states, the dose or number of eggs consumed may further impact the inflammatory response to egg intake (Table 10.2). In a study evaluating the effects of consuming 0 eggs per day for 2 weeks, or 1, 2, or 3 eggs per day for 4 weeks, egg intake was shown to dose-dependently increase activity of paraoxonase 1 (PON1) in healthy men and women, where consumption of 3 eggs per day resulted in the greatest PON1 activity.[54] PON1 is known to exert antioxidant activity, as well as promote high-density lipoprotein (HDL)-mediated cholesterol efflux by inducing enrichment of macrophages with lysophosphatidylcholine, thereby increasing HDL binding and ABCA1-mediated efflux.[55] Accordingly, PON1 activity may serve as a predictor of coronary heart disease risk.[56] Despite TMAO levels being shown to increase postprandially in a healthy population following a two-egg meal,[36] DiMarco *et al.* demonstrated that intake of 0, 1, 2, or 3 whole eggs per day did not affect plasma TMAO levels in healthy men and women.[57]

Table 10.2 Effects of habitual egg intake on inflammation across populations.

	Treatment	Population	Effect on inflammation	Reference
Healthy adults				
	0 eggs per day for 2 weeks; 1, 2, or 3 eggs per day for 4 weeks	Healthy adults	PON1 activity increased with intake of 3 eggs per day; no effect on TMAO	54,57
	2 eggs per day for 4 weeks	Healthy adults	No effect on plasma AST or ALT	30
	4 eggs per day for 4 weeks	Lean, insulin-sensitive individuals	Increased pro-inflammatory CRP and SAA	33
Insulin-resistant adults				
	4 eggs per day for 4 weeks	Lean or obese insulin-resistant adults	No change in CRP or SAA	33
	1 egg per day for 5 weeks	Type 2 diabetic patients	Decreased plasma AST and TNFα; no changes in CRP	35
Tuberculosis patients				
	High-cholesterol diet (800 mg day^{-1}), which included egg yolks	Inpatient subjects with active tuberculosis	Faster recovery from pulmonary tuberculosis infection	64
Modified eggs				
	Standard whole eggs (6 $week^{-1}$), n-3 fatty acid-enriched whole eggs (6 $week^{-1}$), or walnuts (28.4 g, 6 times per week)	Healthy lacto-ovo-vegetarians	No differences in serum inflammatory markers; increased DHA and ALA content of erythrocyte membranes	61
	Lutein- and zeaxanthin-enriched eggs	Healthy adults	Increased serum concentrations of lutein and zeaxanthin	62

10.2.2.3 *Daily Whole Egg Intake in Healthy* vs. *Insulin-resistant Populations*

A number of studies have evaluated the inflammatory effects of egg intake in healthy populations, as well as populations exhibiting insulin resistance (*e.g.* metabolic syndrome, T2DM; Table 10.2).[29,33–35,57,58] Interestingly, while results are variable, a greater number of studies suggest that whole egg intake increases pro-inflammatory markers in healthy populations, with a neutral or beneficial anti-inflammatory effect observed in insulin-resistant individuals.[12] In a study by Tannock *et al.*, consumption of 4 eggs per day for 4 weeks increased pro-inflammatory CRP and serum amyloid A (SAA) in lean, insulin-sensitive individuals, whereas no changes were observed in lean or obese individuals who were insulin-resistant.[33] Compared to consuming an oatmeal breakfast, type 2 diabetic patients consuming 1 egg per day for 5 weeks had significantly lower plasma aspartate aminotransferase (AST) and tumor necrosis factor α (TNFα), while no changes in CRP were observed.[35] No changes in fasting plasma glucose, insulin, glycosylated hemoglobin (HbA1c) or lipids were observed, suggesting that decreases in inflammatory markers associated with egg intake occurred independently of traditional T2DM and cardiovascular disease biomarkers.[35] Conversely, consumption of 2 eggs per day for 4 weeks did not affect plasma levels of AST or alanine aminotransferase (ALT) in healthy young adults, as compared to an oatmeal breakfast.[30] The variability in results between healthy, insulin-sensitive *vs.* insulin-resistant individuals may be attributable to differences in cholesterol absorption or gut microbiota metabolism. Lean, insulin-sensitive individuals have been shown to exhibit a greater capacity to absorb dietary cholesterol as compared to insulin-resistant individuals.[59] Further, as described previously, it has also been demonstrated that postprandial TMAO production can occur in healthy individuals following egg intake, whereas this phenomenon has not been clearly elucidated in insulin-resistant individuals.[36]

10.2.2.4 *Effects of Egg Fractions (Whole Egg* vs. *Whites) on Inflammation During Weight Loss*

While consumption of whole eggs appears to have a neutral or suppressive effect on inflammatory markers in T2DM populations during weight maintenance,[35] whole egg *vs.* egg white-based substitute intake during weight loss has been shown to differentially affect inflammatory markers in overweight and metabolic syndrome populations (Table 10.3).[29,34,58] In overweight men following a carbohydrate-restricted diet for 12 weeks, consumption of 3 whole eggs per day reduced plasma CRP and increased anti-inflammatory adiponectin, as compared to men consuming an egg substitute.[29] Conversely, men consuming the egg substitute

Table 10.3 Effects of egg fractions (whole eggs *vs.* egg whites) in inflammation during weight loss.

	Treatment	Population	Effect on inflammation	Reference
Whole eggs				
	3 whole eggs per day + carbohydrate-restricted diet for 12 weeks	Overweight men	Reduced CRP; increased adiponectin	29
	3 whole eggs per day + moderate carbohydrate-restricted diet for 12 weeks	Men and women with metabolic syndrome	Reduced plasma TNFα and SAA	22
	3 whole eggs per day + moderate carbohydrate-restricted diet for 12 weeks	Men and women with metabolic syndrome	No change in LPS-induced TNFα and IL-1β secretion from *ex vivo* PBMCs[a]	34
Egg white substitute				
	Egg white substitute + carbohydrate-restricted diet for 12 weeks	Overweight men	Reduced MCP-1	29
	Egg white substitute + moderate carbohydrate-restricted diet for 12 weeks	Men and women with metabolic syndrome	Increase in LPS-induced TNFα and IL-1β secretion from *ex vivo* PBMCs[a]	34

[a]Peripheral blood mononuclear cells.

reduced monocyte chemoattractant protein 1 (MCP-1).[29] Differences between whole eggs *vs.* egg white-based substitutes were additionally observed in a study conducted in men and women classified with metabolic syndrome.[22,34] Consumption of 3 whole eggs per day for 12 weeks while following a moderate carbohydrate-restricted diet reduced plasma TNFα and SAA, as compared to subjects consuming the egg substitute.[22] Interestingly, when subject-derived peripheral blood mononuclear cells (PBMC) isolated from baseline and week 12 were stimulated with lipopolysaccharide *ex vivo*, TNFα and interleukin 1β (IL-1β) production significantly increased over time only in the egg substitute group, whereas pro-inflammatory cytokine production did not change in the group consuming whole eggs.[34] These observations may be related to whole egg-induced changes in cellular cholesterol flux and HDL function; however, further evaluation is warranted to elucidate the extent to which whole eggs *vs.* egg whites can impact leukocyte activity.[20,34,60]

10.2.2.5 Effects of Egg Composition and Modification on Inflammation

Studies have additionally evaluated the effects of modified eggs – specifically those enriched in n-3 fatty acids or lutein (Table 10.2).[61,62] In healthy lacto-ovo-vegetarians, no differences in serum inflammatory markers were observed after consuming standard whole eggs (6 week^{-1}), n-3 fatty acid-enriched whole eggs (6 week^{-1}), or walnuts (28.4 g, 6 times per week), despite intake of n-3 fatty acid-enriched eggs and α-linolenic acid-rich walnuts leading to increases in the docosahexaenoic acid (DHA) and alpha-linolenic acid (ALA) contents of erythrocyte membranes, respectively.[61] *N*-3 fatty acid-enriched eggs have additionally been shown to reduce serum triglycerides.[63] Consumption of lutein- and zeaxanthin-enriched eggs has additionally been shown to increase serum concentrations of lutein and zeaxanthin to a greater extent than standard eggs, which may lead to greater anti-inflammatory and antioxidant effects.[58,62]

10.2.2.6 Effects of Eggs During Infection or Allergy

While many of the studies outlined in the preceding sections study egg intake within the context of cardiometabolic disease, eggs can additionally modulate immune pathways and inflammation within the context of acute infection and allergic reactions (Table 10.2). Perez-Guzman *et al.* found that patients consuming a high-cholesterol diet (800 mg day^{-1}), which included egg yolks, exhibited a faster recovery from pulmonary tuberculosis infection while receiving inpatient treatment, as opposed to patients receiving a control diet (250 mg cholesterol day^{-1}).[64] Egg components, predominantly egg white-derived proteins, additionally induce allergic reaction in affected/sensitive individuals. IgE-mediated reactions are the most common forms of allergic response, leading to immune activation, inflammatory protein production, and symptoms ranging from gastrointestinal distress and atopic dermatitis to anaphylaxis.[65,66] While egg allergy typically presents within the first year of life, the extent to which individuals can develop inflammatory allergies and sensitivities to egg components in adulthood remains to be more clearly elucidated, although it is currently thought to be rare.[65,67]

10.3 Bioactive Egg Components

As outlined in the previous sections, it is clear that intake of whole eggs or egg white-based substitutes differentially impact markers of inflammation in human populations, and that effects may be dependent upon health and weight status, as well as the dose and duration of egg consumption.[12] While it is important to understand the effects of consuming egg components in their whole food form, evaluating the mechanisms by which individual components regulate pro- and anti-inflammatory pathways may help to explain that variability in these results, as well as inform the development and understanding of dietary supplements, food-derived pharmaceuticals/

therapeutics, and food technology practices.[12,16,68] The following sections highlight the individual classes of egg components and present the mechanisms by which they can exert pro- and/or anti-inflammatory activity.

10.3.1 Lipids

Eggs serve as relatively rich sources of dietary lipids, which are predominantly contained within the yolk.[69] Egg lipid species include glycerophospholipids, sphingolipids, sterols, triacylglycerols, and fatty acids (which are the primary components of complex glycerophospholipids and sphingolipids).[16,69] Chicken egg lipid composition and distribution can reflect the dietary composition of chicken feed and lipid classes can have varying degrees of bioavailability when provided as a whole food or in isolated forms.[20,70–72] The following sections describe mechanisms by which egg lipids can modulate inflammation in cell-, animal-, and human-based models.

10.3.1.1 Glycerophospholipids

Eggs are one of the richest sources of dietary phospholipids, with the majority contained within the yolk fraction.[20,69] Phosphatidylcholine represents the major class of glycerophospholipids (~72%), followed by phosphatidylethanolamine, lysophosphatidylcholine, and phosphatidylinositol (~20%, 3%, and 2%, respectively).[20] Studies have shown that glycerophospholipids provided by eggs are highly bioavailable, and readily incorporate into serum lipoproteins – primarily HDL.[14] Egg intake has also been shown to modulate the phospholipid content of subject-derived HDL, specifically enriching phosphatidylethanolamine fractions.[20] Beyond provision of glycerophospholipids, eggs serve as an important source of dietary choline, derived from egg phosphatidylcholine, which is essential for acetylcholine production, neurological function, fetal growth and development, lipid metabolism, and muscle health.[73,74] A recent study demonstrated that individuals across different life stages who consumed eggs were most likely to meet dietary recommendations for choline intake, which could not be made up for by intake of other protein-rich foods containing choline.[75]

In addition to providing exogenous choline and regulating lipid metabolism, egg-derived glycerophospholipids are known to exert anti-inflammatory activity when provided in isolated, or purified forms. Phosphatidylcholine supplementation (2.6 g choline day^{-1}) for 2 weeks reduced plasma total homocysteine in healthy men, while also reducing homocysteine levels following methionine loading.[76] Greater choline intake has also been associated with lower concentrations of CRP and TNFα in men and women in the cross-sectional ATTICA Study.[77] Phosphatidylcholine has additionally been shown to reduce gastrointestinal inflammation in Caco-2 cells and ulcerative colitis patients.[19,78,79] Anti-inflammatory effects of phosphatidylcholine supplementation have additionally been observed in animal models of neuroinflammation, as well as acute and rheumatoid arthritis.[80–82]

Phospholipids may be able to regulate inflammation by serving as direct ligands to nuclear receptors involved in inflammatory signaling. Phospholipids and their derivatives have been shown to directly bind and activate nuclear receptors in the NR5A subfamily, including steroidogenic factor 1 (SF-1) and liver receptor homolog 1 (LRH-1), as well as peroxisome proliferator-activated receptor α (PPARα).[23,24,83,84] Given the high degree of bioavailability, egg-derived glycerophospholipids may drive inflammatory responses to egg *via* these molecular mediators.

While contributing to the regulation of embryonic development, adipose-derived adiponectin production, bile acid synthesis, and reverse cholesterol transport, LRH-1 has additionally been implicated in suppression of pro-inflammatory acute-phase responses in the liver.[85] This appears to be associated with interference with C/EBP binding to DNA, thereby preventing activation of downstream pro-inflammatory pathways.[85] Certain phosphatidylcholine species, including dilauroyl phosphatidylcholine (DLPC) and diundecanoyl phosphatidylcholine (DUPC), have been shown to serve as direct LRH-1 ligands and agonists.[86] Supplementation with DLPC additionally improved measures of glucose metabolism and hepatic lipogenesis in mouse models of insulin resistance. DLPC-induced LRH-1 activation has further been shown to promote PIk3 signaling and ATF2 transcriptional pathways, which are involved in resolution of inflammatory endoplasmic reticulum stress.[87] Species of phosphatidylethanolamine – the second most abundant glycerophospholipid class in eggs – have additionally been shown to bind human LRH-1.[12,88]

An additional phosphatidylcholine species, specifically 1-palmitoyl-2-oleoyl-*sn*-glycerol-3-phosphocholine (16 : 0/18 : 1-GPC), has been shown to serve as a PPARα ligand.[84] In line with its well-established hypotriglyceridemic effects, PPARα is known to suppress arterial and hepatic inflammatory pathways associated with the development of atherosclerosis and NAFLD.[89,90] Non-esterified fatty acid components of glycerophospholipids and sphingolipids further serve as direct ligands to PPAR family receptors, as described in the following.

In addition to binding LRH-1 and PPARα, phosphatidylcholine can also directly bind SF-1.[91] SF-1 is involved in regulation of reproductive and adrenal development, and has been implicated in pathogenesis of reproductive disorders and inflammation (*e.g.* endometriosis) and cancer.[92] Interestingly, Li *et al.* identified that phosphatidylethanolamine could also serve as a direct ligand and activator of SF-1, but that these effects were dependent upon the presence of C12–18 fatty acid side chains, whereas longer fatty acid side chains induced inhibition of SF-1.[83] This may be significant, as the major fatty acid classes present in eggs are oleic (18 : 1) and palmitic (16 : 0) acid.[69] Phosphatidylinositol species, although present in relatively lower amounts in eggs, have additionally been shown to activate human SF-1 and LRH-1.[24,91,93]

Overall, research suggests that glycerophospholipids possess protective, anti-inflammatory properties in various models. As described, the most notable exception is the potential formation of gut microbiota-mediated, phosphatidylcholine-derived TMAO, which has been shown to be pro-inflammatory and pro-atherogenic.[36,74] Despite the large degree of variability in studies evaluating both inflammation and TMAO production following egg intake, it is likely that these highly bioavailable, bioactive glycerophospholipid components contribute to egg-induced regulation of inflammation in humans.[12,51,57,74]

10.3.1.2 Sphingolipids

In addition to glycerophospholipid species, eggs – particularly yolk fractions – are rich sources of sphingolipids.[16,69] The predominant species of egg sphingolipids include sphingomyelin (SM) and ganglioside, while the majority of egg sphingomyelin is composed of sphingosine backbones and palmitate tails.[16,94] Complex sphingolipid species, such as sphingomyelin, are thought to require digestion by alkaline sphingomyelinase to phosphorylcholine and ceramide prior to absorption, whereas glycosphingolipids and sphingoid bases (*i.e.* sphingosine) can be absorbed intact.[16] Interestingly, in a study conducted in men and women with metabolic syndrome, consumption of 3 whole eggs per day for 12 weeks led to the enrichment of HDL with sphingomyelin species that were present in the whole egg products, which were not present in subject HDL prior to the intervention.[20] These findings further support the notion that whole egg consumption modulates HDL lipid composition – perhaps through direct incorporation into HDL particles – and may represent a mechanism by which dietary lipids can directly modulate HDL particle functions.[20,34,60]

While endogenous cellular sphingolipid species and derivatives generated through cellular metabolism often induce pro-inflammatory signaling, various dietary/exogenous sphingolipids have been found to exhibit pro- and anti-inflammatory properties.[16] Variability in these results may be attributable to the use of different experimental models and treatment doses, where high doses of sphingolipids have been shown to induce inflammation, whereas lower levels are anti-inflammatory.[25,95] In C57BL/6J mice fed a high-fat, high-cholesterol diet for 10 weeks, the addition of 0.1% (w/w) egg sphingomyelin resulted in lower body weight, serum lipids and glucose, hepatic steatosis, and skeletal muscle triacylglycerols as compared to the control group.[96] Further, egg sphingomyelin supplementation additionally reduced markers of adipose tissue inflammation, as evidenced by a reduction in macrophage-mediated crown-like structures, and a reduction in mRNA expression of the macrophage markers CD68, CD11c, and F4/80, as well as reduced mRNA expression of the pro-inflammatory chemokine CCL2 and cytokine TNFα.[96] mRNA expression of anti-inflammatory and insulin-sensitizing adiponectin were found to be increased, whereas serum concentrations of CCL2 were also found to be reduced. Interestingly, egg sphingomyelin was found to be more effective at mitigating the hyperlipidemic and pro-inflammatory effects of high-fat and high-cholesterol feeding than milk-derived SM.[96] The authors postulate that these differences may in part be owing to variation in bioactivity, specifically related to the capacity of egg *vs.* milk SM to form hydrophobic interactions with other lipids (including ones that interfere with cholesterol absorption), intestinal hydrolysis, and ceramide formation, although further research is needed to elucidate mechanisms beyond the level of lipid absorption.[70,96–98]

One possible mechanism could be that SM alters gut microbiota composition or affects bacterial translocation and lipopolysaccharide (LPS) entry into the systemic bloodstream.[16] However, in a 4 week study evaluating the effects of egg (0.25% w/w) *vs.* milk-derived SM (0.25% w/w) during high-fat feeding, serum LPS was not affected by egg SM intake, whereas milk SM lowered serum LPS and altered gut microbiota composition.[99] In this study, egg SM was also found to increase hepatic and serum lipids – including serum SM – suggesting that this higher dose of egg SM may lead to differential effects on pathways of lipid metabolism and inflammation.[99] Dietary milk-derived SM has also been shown to mitigate inflammation in DSS-induced mouse models of colitis, whereas high doses (4 mg day^{-1}) of egg-derived SM by oral gavage worsened apoptosis and inflammation in DSS-induced and IL-10−/− mice.[95]

As outlined, egg sphingolipids may affect inflammatory mechanisms by a variety of pathways – both directly and indirectly. In addition to interfering with and reducing cholesterol absorption, dietary sphingolipids act as direct ligands for nuclear receptors involved in inflammatory signaling.[70,97,98,100] Similar to a number of glycerophospholipid species described earlier, sphingosine is a known SF-1 ligand, whereas various sphingolipids can impact factors related to gene expression, including DNA synthesis, chromatin assembly, RNA stability, and histone acetylation.[100] Sphingomyelin and sphingosine-1-phosphate serve as ligands for the anti-inflammatory, insulin-sensitizing PPARγ.[25,95] While few studies have analyzed the effects of purified egg sphingolipids on markers of inflammation in humans, findings suggest that milk-derived sphingolipids may promote postprandial anti-inflammatory responses (increased IL-10, decreased sICAM) in overweight adults fed a meal high in saturated fat, whereas minimal effects on inflammation were observed in obese adults.[101] Additional research is required to determine the contributions of sphingolipids to the pro- and anti-inflammatory effects of egg intake observed across populations.

10.3.1.3 Fatty Acids

In addition to the complex lipids highlighted previously, egg yolks are rich sources of fatty acids. Eggs predominantly contain monounsaturated fatty acids (~46%), followed by saturated fatty acids (~35%), and polyunsaturated fatty acids (~18%).[69,102] Oleic acid (18 : 1) is the most prevalent (~43%) monounsaturated fatty acid, whereas predominant saturated fatty acids include palmitic (26%) and stearic (9%) acid, and polyunsaturated fatty acids include n-6 linoleic acid (15.5%) and arachidonic acid (2%).[102] Studies have shown that the dietary composition of the hen's feed can alter the fatty acid composition of the yolk, in addition to the total relative weights of egg yolks and whites.[102] As described earlier, consumption of n-3-enriched eggs has been shown to increase the DHA content of erythrocyte membranes and lower serum triglycerides, suggesting that egg-derived fatty acids are bioavailable and bioactive.[61,63]

Fatty acids are known to affect inflammatory pathways through a variety of mechanisms. At the cellular level, fatty acids can modulate inflammatory responses by altering cell membrane fluidity, serving as precursors to eicosanoids, and acting as ligands for the PPAR family of nuclear receptors, which are involved in mediating inflammatory signaling.[103–106] DHA, an n-3 polyunsaturated fatty acid (PUFA), has been shown to alter localization and composition of lipid rafts in CD4+ T cells isolated from murine spleens, resulting in a reduction of inflammatory activation and signaling.[107,108] Although there were no changes in inflammatory markers following n-3 PUFA-enriched egg consumption and DHA enrichment of erythrocytes, these findings may have important implications for modified eggs and immune function.[61] It has further been suggested that phosphatidylethanolamine containing oleic acid may result in the formation of smaller, less stable lipid rafts, as compared to phospholipids containing PUFAs, although further research is required to determine the impact of immune inflammation.[109,110] In general, multiple human, animal, and cell studies have demonstrated anti-inflammatory, pro-inflammatory, and hyperlipidemic effects of oleic acid-rich diets.[111,112]

Certain saturated fatty acids, particularly lauric acid (12 : 0), have also been shown to directly activate toll-like receptor 4 (TLR4) and TLR2, inducing pro-inflammatory signaling.[113,114] Palmitic acid can further induce myocardial inflammation by directly binding and activating MD2 – a TLR4 accessory protein.[115] Stearic acid has additionally been shown to induce inflammatory responses in macrophages independent of TLRs, causing endoplasmic reticulum stress, shifts to M1 pro-inflammatory macrophage phenotypes, and apoptosis.[116] Recent findings also suggest that the amount and type of fat intake may alter gut microbiota populations and composition, in addition to affecting postprandial bacterial translocation of gut microbiota-derived LPS.[112] However, many of these findings have been demonstrated in animal models, and it is currently unclear whether similar effects hold true in humans. Together, the fatty acids that are predominant in eggs impact a wide variety of pro- and anti-inflammatory pathways. Given that the fatty acid composition can be altered by the chicken feed, it is possible that variations in lipid composition may contribute to discrepancies in pro- and anti-inflammatory responses to egg consumption.[71,72]

10.3.1.4 Sterols

In addition to containing a diverse range of complex lipid species, eggs are relatively rich dietary sources of cholesterol. With the majority of the cholesterol contained within the yolk fraction, one large egg typically contains approximately 186 mg of cholesterol.[13] Numerous cell- and animal-based studies have demonstrated pro-inflammatory, pro-atherogenic, and cytotoxic effects of elevated cholesterol concentrations; however, these findings have not been replicated in humans to a significant extent.[34,117] National guidelines now reflect this observation, as both the Dietary Guidelines for Americans and the American Heart Association no longer include limitations on dietary cholesterol in their guidelines owing to a lack of evidence that it increases LDL-cholesterol and risk of cardiovascular disease.[26,27] As described earlier, the bioavailability of egg-derived cholesterol is known to be diminished by glycerophospholipids and sphingolipids, and the efficiency of absorption appears to be further suppressed in insulin-resistant individuals.[59,70,97,98]

In the event of cholesterol absorption, cholesterol can promote inflammation *via* NOD-, LRR- and pyrin domain-containing 3 (NLRLP3) inflammasome activation, as well as by increasing cholesterol loading in cell membranes, leading to greater lipid raft formation and inflammatory signaling potential.[118–121] Interestingly, in men and women with metabolic syndrome who consumed 3 eggs per day while following a moderate-carbohydrate-restricted diet, there was a trend toward decreased PBMC cholesterol content between baseline and week 12, which was not observed in subjects consuming the equivalent amount of an egg white-based substitute.[34] Changes in PBMC cholesterol content over the course of the intervention additionally correlated with changes in PBMC lipid raft content. These observations may be attributable to changes in HDL composition and increased cholesterol efflux capacity in the whole egg group.[20,34] While these parameters were evaluated in the presence of weight loss, further research is required to determine the extent to which egg-derived cholesterol is bioavailable and can mediate inflammatory responses.

10.3.2 Proteins and Peptides

Advances in mass spectrometry and proteomics are starting to map the functional protein network within egg yolks and whites.[122] Many of these proteins – and the peptides liberated from them by proteases – possess antioxidant properties. They may act by quenching reactive oxygen species, scavenging free radicals, chelating prooxidative transition metals, or reducing hydroperoxides.[123] The following sections discuss inflammation-modulating proteins and peptides, respectively (Table 10.4).

10.3.2.1 Proteins

Ovotransferrin (OVT) is an iron-binding glycoprotein, comprising nearly 12% of egg white proteins.[124] Given orally, OVT reduced histological scores and suppressed the production of TNFα, IL-6, IL-1β, and IFN-γ in a murine model of inflammatory bowel disease (IBD).[125] These cytokines are important for the onset, amplification, and perpetuation of intestinal inflammation. Patients with IBD frequently suffer from increased and irregular

Table 10.4 Effects of egg proteins and peptides on inflammation.

Treatment	Model	Effect	Reference
Protein			
Ovotransferrin	IBD-induced mice	Decreased production of TNFα, IL-6, IL-1β, and IFN-γ	125
Antisecretory factor	IBD-induced mice	Decreased production of IL-1, IL-2, and leukotriene B_4 as well as less colonic damage	129
	IBD in humans	Lower erythrocyte sedimentation rate and C-reactive protein markers; improved intestinal mucosa	130–132
Peptide			
Aminopeptidase digest of egg white peptides	IBD-induced piglets	Decreased expression of TNFα, IL-6, IL-8, IL-1β, and IFN-γ	133
YAEERYPIL	*In vitro* assay	Antioxidant and ACE inhibitor	135,136
IRW	Spontaneously hypertensive rats	Lowered angiotensin II, reactive oxygen species, and peroxynitrite	137
	HUVEC[a]	Blocked TNFα-induced increases in ICAM-1, VCAM-1, MCP-1, and superoxide ions; blocked nuclear translocation of p65 and p50	138,139
IQW[b]	HUVEC[a]	Blocked nuclear translocation of p50	139
RADHPF	*In vitro* assay	Bradykinin B_1 inhibitor	141
RPLKPW[b]	*In vitro* assay	Bradykinin B_1 inhibitor	142
Tryptic digest of phosvitin phosphopeptides	HT-29 cells	Inhibited expression of IL-8, MCP-1, and IL-12	144
	LPS-stimulated macrophages	Lowered level of iNOS	145
Pepsin-digested livetins	LPS-stimulated macrophages	Lowered level of iNOS; decrease in TNFα, IL-1β, and IL-6	147
Alcalase-digested livetins	LPS-stimulated macrophages	Lowered expression of cyclooxygenase-2 and prostaglandin-E2; decrease in TNFα, IL-1β, and IL-6	147

[a]Human umbilical vein endothelial cells.
[b]Synthetic peptide.

bowel movements.[126] Antisecretory factor (AF) is a protein of interest for IBD researchers as it inhibits intestinal hypersecretion and possesses anti-inflammatory properties.[127] Eggs yolks are especially rich in AF.[128] Mice treated with 2,4,6-trinitrobenzenesulfonic acid (to model IBD) and then given an AF-rich egg yolk diet exhibited lower levels of IL-2, IL-1, and leukotriene B_4, as well as less colonic damage than those receiving a placebo.[129] In humans with IBD, AF-rich egg supplementation has improved symptoms associated with the disease,[130,131] reduced the histological severity of mucosal biopsies, and lowered inflammatory blood markers (*e.g.* erythrocyte sedimentation rate, CRP).[132] While not a panacea for IBD, further research is merited to fully appreciate egg-derived proteins as modulators of inflammation.

10.3.2.2 Peptides

Disrupting a protein's tertiary structure often leads to a net gain in antioxidant capacity as more amino acids become solvent-exposed.[123] Consequently, egg proteins are frequently hydrolyzed to peptides and then assayed for bioactivity. For example, a cocktail of peptide fragments (<10 kDa) obtained by an aminopeptidase digest of egg white proteins was found to reduce the expression of pro-inflammatory cytokines – TNFα, IL-6, IL-8, IL-1β, and IFN-γ – in a porcine model of IBD.[133] While a desirable functional outcome, the identity of the active peptide(s) must be assigned in order to elucidate its mechanism of action. The exceptional resolution afforded by high-performance liquid chromatography paired with tandem mass spectrometry (HPLC-MS/MS) is a popular technique for deconvoluting these complex mixtures and identifying specific peptide constituents.

Angiotensin I-converting enzyme (ACE) is a critical mediator of blood pressure, oxidative stress, and inflammation.[134] Egg white proteins hydrolyzed with pepsin exhibited high radical scavenging activity.[135] HPLC-MS/MS analysis identified peptide YAEERYPIL, a fragment of ovalbumin, as the strongest antioxidant and an ACE inhibitor.[136] Structure–activity relationship studies revealed that tyrosine contributes significantly to the peptide's activity and both tyrosines are necessary for maximal effect. In a separate study, Wu *et al.* identified the tripeptide IRW from a digest of egg white ovotransferrin as an ACE inhibitor.[137] In a murine model of hypertension, IRW treatment lowered oxidative stress, as evidenced by lower levels of angiotensin II, reactive oxygen species, and peroxynitrite. It was subsequently found that IRW blocks TNFα-induced increases in ICAM-1, VCAM-1, MCP-1, and superoxide ions.[138] The arginine is critical for selectivity as the tripeptide IQW only blocked increases in ICAM-1 and superoxide. These results may be explained by the peptides' differing abilities to act upon initiators of the NF-kB signaling pathway; IRW blocked nuclear translocation of both p50 and p65 whereas IQW blocked only p50.[139] Eggs offer a rich pool of proteins and peptides for the discovery of ACE and other enzyme inhibitors.[140]

Synthetic chemistry is a powerful tool for elucidating a peptide's mechanism as well as optimizing its function. For example, ovokinin(2–7) is a hexapeptide (RADHPF) obtained from a peptic digest of ovalbumin that inhibits bradykinin B_1.[141] Through systematic sequence optimization, the synthetic hexapeptide RPLKPW was obtained with 100-fold greater anti-hypertensive activity than the original RADHPF.[142]

Phosvitin constitutes ~11% of egg yolk protein and over half of its amino acids are phosphorylated serines, making it one of the most phosphorylated proteins in nature.[143] These phosphates endow the protein with a high metal binding capacity, making it a potentially strong antioxidant. Phosvitin phosphopeptides (PPPs), ranging in size from 1 to 3 kDa, have been prepared by partial dephosphorylation followed by a tryptic digest.[144] PPPs inhibited the expression of pro-inflammatory cytokines (*e.g.* IL-8, MCP-1, IL-12) in HT-29 cells and inducible nitric oxide synthase (iNOS) in lipopolysaccharide (LPS)-stimulated macrophage cells. PPPs may constitute a unique class of nutraceuticals with anti-inflammatory properties.[145]

By changing proteases, one can obtain unique peptide products from the same starting protein. The immune-modulating similarities and differences of these peptides, however, remains an area of active investigation. Livetins α, β, αvδ γ make up ~9% of egg yolk proteins, with γ-livetin (*i.e.* immunoglobulin Y) being the most abundant.[146] Livetins were digested separately with either pepsin or alcalase to approximately 10 kDa and then evaluated in LPS-stimulated macrophages.[147] Interestingly, both sets of peptides lowered levels of TNFα, IL-1β, and IL-6 in response to LPS stimulation. However, pepsin-derived peptides were more effective at reducing iNOS expression, while only alcalase-derived peptides could inhibit the expression of cyclooxygenase-2 and prostaglandin-E2.

10.3.3 Carotenoids

Egg yolks serve as one of the most bioavailable sources of the carotenoids lutein and zeaxanthin.[15,58,62,148] Whole egg consumption increases enrichment of plasma with lutein and zeaxanthin, particularly HDL fractions.[58] Consumption of lutein- and zeaxanthin-enriched eggs has additionally been shown to increase serum concentrations of lutein and zeaxanthin to a greater extent than standard eggs.[62] Numerous studies have demonstrated antioxidant and anti-inflammatory properties of lutein, including its capacity to scavenge free radicals, reduce oxidative stress, and promote the stability and integrity of DNA and chromosomes.[17,18,149–152] While it is most noted for its capacity to protect against the development of age-related macular degeneration, lutein has also been shown to reduce atherosclerosis, fatty liver, asthma, and LPS-induced septic lethality in animal models.[17,18,153–155] Lutein supplementation in guinea pigs fed a high-cholesterol diet has additionally been shown to reduce TNFα and IL-1β levels in the eye and liver,[18,68] in addition to lower hepatic NF-kB p65 DNA binding.[17] Lutein supplementation of egg yolk has additionally been shown to improve markers of retinal integrity and lipid peroxidation.[156] In LPS-challenged animals, lutein has been shown to increase mRNA expression of anti-inflammatory IL-10 in the spleen,[153] while lowering serum levels of TNFα and IL-6.[157] Lutein additionally reduced LPS-induced production of TNFα, IL-1β, and IL-6 in *ex vivo* PBMCs isolated from coronary artery disease patients.[158] However, no changes in CRP, VCAM1, or ICAM1 were observed in healthy subjects consuming lutein and zeaxanthin supplements for 8 weeks.[159] Given the high degree of bioavailability of lutein and zeaxanthin from eggs, these compounds likely contribute to the antioxidant and anti-inflammatory effects of egg intake.

10.4 Summary and Conclusions

As outlined throughout this chapter, eggs possess a variety of bioactive components that can affect pro- and anti-inflammatory pathways. Understanding the effects of egg intake across different populations, the properties of individual bioactive components, as well as the biological and molecular mechanisms mediated by these components is becoming increasingly important to inform dietary recommendations and human health practices. Further research is warranted to elucidate the effects of egg intake on markers of inflammation in different human populations of health and disease, in addition to the contributions of each bioactive egg component to the regulation of inflammation.

References

1. R. Medzhitov, *Nature*, 2008, **454**, 428–435.
2. P. Libby, Y. Okamoto, V. Z. Rocha and E. Folco, *Circ. J.*, 2010, **74**, 213–220.
3. M. Arrese, D. Cabrera, A. M. Kalergis and A. E. Feldstein, *Dig. Dis. Sci.*, 2016, **61**, 1294–1303.
4. R. Medzhitov, *Nature*, 2007, **449**, 819–826.
5. A. Ortega-Gomez, M. Perretti and O. Soehnlein, *EMBO Mol. Med.*, 2013, **5**, 661–674.
6. T. S. Rodriguez-Reyna and D. Alarcon-Segovia, *Autoimmun. Rev.*, 2006, **5**, 86–88.
7. V. Pop-Began, V. Paunescu, V. Grigorean, D. Pop-Began and C. Popescu, *J. Med. Life*, 2014, **7 Spec No. 2**, 38–41.
8. S. R. Permar, D. E. Griffin and N. L. Letvin, *Clin. Vaccine Immunol.*, 2006, **13**, 437–443.
9. N. Kloting and M. Bluher, *Rev. Endocr. Metab. Disord.*, 2014, **15**, 277–287.
10. C. E. Ndumele, K. Nasir, R. D. Conceicao, J. A. Carvalho, R. S. Blumenthal and R. D. Santos, *Arterioscler., Thromb., Vasc. Biol.*, 2011, **31**, 1927–1932.
11. G. De Pergola and F. Silvestris, *J. Obes.*, 2013, **2013**, 291546.
12. C. J. Andersen, *Nutrients*, 2015, **7**, 7889–7913.
13. U.S. Department of Agriculture, Agricultural Research Service and Nutrent Data Laboratory, *USDA National Nutrient Database for Standard Reference 1*, April 2018.

14. O. Zierenberg and S. M. Grundy, *J. Lipid Res.*, 1982, **23**, 1136–1142.
15. H. Y. Chung, H. M. Rasmussen and E. J. Johnson, *J. Nutr.*, 2004, **134**, 1887–1893.
16. G. H. Norris and C. N. Blesso, *Nutrients*, 2017, **9**(11), 1180.
17. J. E. Kim, R. M. Clark, Y. Park, J. Lee and M. L. Fernandez, *Nutr. Res. Pract.*, 2012, **6**, 113–119.
18. J. E. Kim, J. O. Leite, R. DeOgburn, J. A. Smyth, R. M. Clark and M. L. Fernandez, *J. Nutr.*, 2011, **141**, 1458–1463.
19. I. Treede, A. Braun, P. Jeliaskova, T. Giese, J. Fullekrug, G. Griffiths, W. Stremmel and R. Ehehalt, *BMC Gastroenterol.*, 2009, **9**, 53.
20. C. J. Andersen, C. N. Blesso, J. Lee, J. Barona, D. Shah, M. J. Thomas and M. L. Fernandez, *Lipids*, 2013, **48**, 557–567.
21. C. J. Andersen, J. Y. Lee, C. N. Blesso, T. P. Carr and M. L. Fernandez, *Nutrients*, 2014, **6**, 2650–2667.
22. C. N. Blesso, C. J. Andersen, J. Barona, B. Volk, J. S. Volek and M. L. Fernandez, *J. Clin. Lipidol.*, 2013, **7**(5), 463–471.
23. P. M. Musille, J. A. Kohn and E. A. Ortlund, *FEBS Lett.*, 2013, **587**, 1238–1246.
24. I. N. Krylova, E. P. Sablin, J. Moore, R. X. Xu, G. M. Waitt, J. A. MacKay, D. Juzumiene, J. M. Bynum, K. Madauss, V. Montana, L. Lebedeva, M. Suzawa, J. D. Williams, S. P. Williams, R. K. Guy, J. W. Thornton, R. J. Fletterick, T. M. Willson and H. A. Ingraham, *Cell*, 2005, **120**, 343–355.
25. K. A. Parham, J. R. Zebol, K. L. Tooley, W. Y. Sun, L. M. Moldenhauer, M. P. Cockshell, B. L. Gliddon, P. A. Moretti, G. Tigyi, S. M. Pitson and C. S. Bonder, *FASEB J.*, 2015, **29**, 3638–3653.
26. U.S. Department of Health and Human Services and U.S. Department of Agriculture, *2015–2018 Dietary Guidelines for Americans*, 8th edn, December 2015.
27. R. H. Eckel, J. M. Jakicic, J. D. Ard, J. M. de Jesus, N. Houston Miller, V. S. Hubbard, I. M. Lee, A. H. Lichtenstein, C. M. Loria, B. E. Millen, C. A. Nonas, F. M. Sacks, S. C. Smith Jr, L. P. Svetkey, T. A. Wadden and S. Z. Yanovski, *J. Am. Coll. Cardiol.*, 2014, **63**, 2960–2984.
28. Z. Conrad, L. K. Johnson, J. N. Roemmich, W. Juan and L. Jahns, *Nutrients*, 2017, **9**(4), 333.
29. J. C. Ratliff, G. Mutungi, M. J. Puglisi, J. S. Volek and M. L. Fernandez, *Nutr. Metab.*, 2008, **5**, 6.
30. A. Missimer, D. M. DiMarco, C. J. Andersen, A. G. Murillo, M. Vergara-Jimenez and M. L. Fernandez, *Nutrients*, 2017, **9**(2), 89.
31. A. Smith and J. Gray, *Br. J. Community Nurs.*, 2016, **21**, 305–309.
32. S. Vega-Lopez, G. A. Pignotti, M. Todd and C. Keller, *Nutrients*, 2015, 7, 8402–8412.
33. L. R. Tannock, K. D. O'Brien, R. H. Knopp, B. Retzlaff, B. Fish, M. H. Wener, S. E. Kahn and A. Chait, *Circulation*, 2005, **111**, 3058–3062.
34. C. J. Andersen, J. Y. Lee, C. N. Blesso, T. P. Carr and M. L. Fernandez, *Nutrients*, 2014, **6**, 2650–2667.
35. M. N. Ballesteros, F. Valenzuela, A. E. Robles, E. Artalejo, D. Aguilar, C. J. Andersen, H. Valdez and M. L. Fernandez, *Nutrients*, 2015, **7**, 3449–3463.

36. W. H. Tang, Z. Wang, B. S. Levison, R. A. Koeth, E. B. Britt, X. Fu, Y. Wu and S. L. Hazen, *N. Engl. J. Med.*, 2013, **368**, 1575–1584.
37. Y. Rong, L. Chen, T. Zhu, Y. Song, M. Yu, Z. Shan, A. Sands, F. B. Hu and L. Liu, *BMJ*, 2013, **346**, e8539.
38. J. Diez-Espino, F. J. Basterra-Gortari, J. Salas-Salvado, P. Buil-Cosiales, D. Corella, H. Schroder, R. Estruch, E. Ros, E. Gomez-Gracia, F. Aros, M. Fiol, J. Lapetra, L. Serra-Majem, X. Pinto, N. Babio, L. Quiles, M. Fito, A. Marti, E. Toledo and P. Investigators, *Clin. Nutr.*, 2017, **36**, 1015–1021.
39. J. K. Virtanen, J. Mursu, H. E. Virtanen, M. Fogelholm, J. T. Salonen, T. T. Koskinen, S. Voutilainen and T. P. Tuomainen, *Am. J. Clin. Nutr.*, 2016, **103**, 895–901.
40. A. Ko, H. Kim, C. J. Han, J. M. Kim, H. W. Chung and N. Chang, *Nutr. Res. Pract.*, 2014, **8**, 445–452.
41. H. W. Woo, B. Y. Choi and M. K. Kim, *PLoS One*, 2016, **11**, e0147729.
42. S. Shin, H. W. Lee, C. E. Kim, J. Lim, J. K. Lee, S. A. Lee and D. Kang, *Nutrients*, 2017, **9**(7), 687.
43. L. Djousse, J. M. Gaziano, J. E. Buring and I. M. Lee, *Diabetes Care*, 2009, **32**, 295–300.
44. L. Djousse, A. Kamineni, T. L. Nelson, M. Carnethon, D. Mozaffarian, D. Siscovick and K. J. Mukamal, *Am. J. Clin. Nutr.*, 2010, **92**, 422–427.
45. O. Khawaja, H. Singh, F. Luni, A. Kabour, S. S. Ali, M. Taleb, H. Ahmed, J. M. Gaziano and L. Djousse, *Front. Nutr.*, 2017, **4**, 10.
46. N. Keum, D. H. Lee, N. Marchand, H. Oh, H. Liu, D. Aune, D. C. Greenwood and E. L. Giovannucci, *Br. J. Nutr.*, 2015, **114**, 1099–1107.
47. S. T. Zeng, L. Guo, S. K. Liu, D. H. Wang, J. Xi, P. Huang, D. T. Liu, J. F. Gao, J. Feng and L. Zhang, *Clin. Nutr.*, 2015, **34**, 635–641.
48. D. Fang, F. Tan, C. Wang, X. Zhu and L. Xie, *Exp. Ther. Med.*, 2012, **4**, 906–912.
49. A. L. Frazier, C. T. Ryan, H. Rockett, W. C. Willett and G. A. Colditz, *Breast Cancer Res.*, 2003, **5**, R59–R64.
50. E. Ierardi, C. Sorrentino, M. Principi, F. Giorgio, G. Losurdo and A. Di Leo, *Hepatobiliary Surg. Nutr.*, 2015, **4**, 289–292.
51. C. A. Miller, K. D. Corbin, K. A. da Costa, S. Zhang, X. Zhao, J. A. Galanko, T. Blevins, B. J. Bennett, A. O'Connor and S. H. Zeisel, *Am. J. Clin. Nutr.*, 2014, **100**, 778–786.
52. S. R. Emerson, S. P. Kurti, C. A. Harms, M. D. Haub, T. Melgarejo, C. Logan and S. K. Rosenkranz, *Adv. Nutr.*, 2017, **8**, 213–225.
53. C. S. Teeman, S. P. Kurti, B. J. Cull, S. R. Emerson, M. D. Haub and S. K. Rosenkranz, *Nutr. Metab.*, 2016, **13**, 80.
54. D. M. DiMarco, G. H. Norris, C. L. Millar, C. N. Blesso and M. L. Fernandez, *J. Nutr.*, 2017, **147**, 323–329.
55. M. Rosenblat, J. Vaya, D. Shih and M. Aviram, *Atherosclerosis*, 2005, **179**, 69–77.
56. Y. Zhao, Y. Ma, Y. Fang, L. Liu, S. Wu, D. Fu and X. Wang, *Mol. Genet. Metab.*, 2012, **105**, 141–148.

57. D. M. DiMarco, A. Missimer, A. G. Murillo, B. S. Lemos, O. V. Malysheva, M. A. Caudill, C. N. Blesso and M. L. Fernandez, *Lipids*, 2017, **52**, 255–263.
58. C. N. Blesso, C. J. Andersen, B. W. Bolling and M. L. Fernandez, *Food Funct.*, 2013, **4**, 213–221.
59. P. Paramsothy, R. H. Knopp, S. E. Kahn, B. M. Retzlaff, B. Fish, L. Ma and R. E. Ostlund Jr, *Am. J. Clin. Nutr.*, 2011, **94**, 1182–1188.
60. C. J. Andersen and M. L. Fernandez, *Food Funct.*, 2013, **4**(9), 1304.
61. B. Burns-Whitmore, E. Haddad, J. Sabate and S. Rajaram, *Nutr. J.*, 2014, **13**, 29.
62. E. R. Kelly, J. Plat, G. R. Haenen, A. Kijlstra and T. T. Berendschot, *PLoS One*, 2014, **9**, e92659.
63. P. Bovet, D. Faeh, G. Madeleine, B. Viswanathan and F. Paccaud, *Nutr., Metab. Cardiovasc. Dis.*, 2007, **17**, 280–287.
64. C. Perez-Guzman, M. H. Vargas, F. Quinonez, N. Bazavilvazo and A. Aguilar, *Chest*, 2005, **127**, 643–651.
65. J. C. Caubet and J. Wang, *Pediatr. Clin. North Am.*, 2011, **58**, 427–443, xi.
66. P. Dhanapala, C. De Silva, T. Doran and C. Suphioglu, *Mol. Immunol.*, 2015, **66**, 375–383.
67. M. Unsel, A. Z. Sin, O. Ardeniz, N. Erdem, R. Ersoy, O. Gulbahar, N. Mete and A. Kokuludag, *J. Invest. Allergol. Clin. Immunol.*, 2007, **17**, 55–58.
68. A. G. Murillo, D. Aguilar, G. H. Norris, D. M. DiMarco, A. Missimer, S. Hu, J. A. Smyth, S. Gannon, C. N. Blesso, Y. Luo and M. L. Fernandez, *J. Nutr.*, 2016, **146**, 1961–1969.
69. J. Weihrauch and Y.-S. Son, *J. Am. Oil Chem. Soc.*, 1983, **60**, 1971–1978.
70. S. K. Noh and S. I. Koo, *J. Nutr.*, 2004, **134**, 2611–2616.
71. A. C. Beynen, *NJAS-Wagen. J. Life Sci.*, 2004, **52**, 3–10.
72. M. Schreiner, H. W. Hulan, E. Razzazi-Fazeli, J. Bohm and C. Iben, *Poult. Sci.*, 2004, **83**, 462–473.
73. S. H. Zeisel and K. A. da Costa, *Nutr. Rev.*, 2009, **67**, 615–623.
74. C. N. Blesso, *Nutrients*, 2015, **7**, 2731–2747.
75. T. C. Wallace and V. L. Fulgoni, *Nutrients*, 2017, **9**(8), 839.
76. M. R. Olthof and P. Verhoef, *Curr. Drug Metab.*, 2005, **6**, 15–22.
77. P. Detopoulou, D. B. Panagiotakos, S. Antonopoulou, C. Pitsavos and C. Stefanadis, *Am. J. Clin. Nutr.*, 2008, **87**, 424–430.
78. W. Stremmel, R. Ehehalt, F. Autschbach and M. Karner, *Ann. Intern. Med.*, 2007, **147**, 603–610.
79. W. Stremmel, U. Merle, A. Zahn, F. Autschbach, U. Hinz and R. Ehehalt, *Gut*, 2005, **54**, 966–971.
80. T. Tokes, G. Eros, A. Bebes, P. Hartmann, S. Varszegi, G. Varga, J. Kaszaki, K. Gulya, M. Ghyczy and M. Boros, *Shock*, 2011, **36**, 458–465.
81. G. Eros, S. Ibrahim, N. Siebert, M. Boros and B. Vollmar, *Arthritis Res. Ther.*, 2009, **11**, R43.
82. P. Hartmann, A. Szabo, G. Eros, D. Gurabi, G. Horvath, I. Nemeth, M. Ghyczy and M. Boros, *Eur. J. Pharmacol.*, 2009, **622**, 58–64.

83. Y. Li, M. Choi, G. Cavey, J. Daugherty, K. Suino, A. Kovach, N. C. Bingham, S. A. Kliewer and H. E. Xu, *Mol. Cell*, 2005, **17**, 491–502.
84. M. V. Chakravarthy, I. J. Lodhi, L. Yin, R. R. Malapaka, H. E. Xu, J. Turk and C. F. Semenkovich, *Cell*, 2009, **138**, 476–488.
85. N. Venteclef, J. C. Smith, B. Goodwin and P. Delerive, *Mol. Cell. Biol.*, 2006, **26**, 6799–6807.
86. J. M. Lee, Y. K. Lee, J. L. Mamrosh, S. A. Busby, P. R. Griffin, M. C. Pathak, E. A. Ortlund and D. D. Moore, *Nature*, 2011, **474**, 506–510.
87. J. L. Mamrosh, J. M. Lee, M. Wagner, P. J. Stambrook, R. J. Whitby, R. N. Sifers, S. P. Wu, M. J. Tsai, F. J. Demayo and D. D. Moore, *eLife*, 2014, **3**, e01694.
88. E. A. Ortlund, Y. Lee, I. H. Solomon, J. M. Hager, R. Safi, Y. Choi, Z. Guan, A. Tripathy, C. R. Raetz, D. P. McDonnell, D. D. Moore and M. R. Redinbo, *Nat. Struct. Mol. Biol.*, 2005, **12**, 357–363.
89. A. Zambon, P. Gervois, P. Pauletto, J. C. Fruchart and B. Staels, *Arterioscler., Thromb., Vasc. Biol.*, 2006, **26**, 977–986.
90. M. Pawlak, P. Lefebvre and B. Staels, *J. Hepatol.*, 2015, **62**, 720–733.
91. E. P. Sablin, R. D. Blind, I. N. Krylova, J. G. Ingraham, F. Cai, J. D. Williams, R. J. Fletterick and H. A. Ingraham, *Mol. Endocrinol.*, 2009, **23**, 25–34.
92. B. Ferraz-de-Souza, L. Lin and J. C. Achermann, *Mol. Cell. Endocrinol.*, 2011, **336**, 198–205.
93. R. D. Blind, E. P. Sablin, K. M. Kuchenbecker, H. J. Chiu, A. M. Deacon, D. Das, R. J. Fletterick and H. A. Ingraham, *Proc. Natl. Acad. Sci. U. S. A.*, 2014, **111**, 15054–15059.
94. W. C. Byrdwell and R. H. Perry, *J. Chromatogr. A*, 2007, **1146**, 164–185.
95. J. C. Mazzei, H. Zhou, B. P. Brayfield, R. Hontecillas, J. Bassaganya-Riera and E. M. Schmelz, *J. Nutr. Biochem.*, 2011, **22**, 1160–1171.
96. G. H. Norris, C. M. Porter, C. Jiang, C. L. Millar and C. N. Blesso, *J. Nutr. Biochem.*, 2017, **40**, 36–43.
97. Y. Jiang, S. K. Noh and S. I. Koo, *J. Nutr.*, 2001, **131**, 2358–2363.
98. S. I. Koo and S. K. Noh, *J. Nutr.*, 2001, **131**, 717–722.
99. G. H. Norris, C. Jiang, J. Ryan, C. M. Porter and C. N. Blesso, *J. Nutr. Biochem.*, 2016, **30**, 93–101.
100. N. C. Lucki, D. Li and M. B. Sewer, *Mol. Cell. Endocrinol.*, 2012, **348**, 165–175.
101. T. S. Rogers, E. Demmer, N. Rivera, E. R. Gertz, J. B. German, J. T. Smilowitz, A. M. Zivkovic and M. D. Van Loan, *Nutr. Metab.*, 2017, **14**, 36.
102. G. Cherian, T. B. Holsonbake and M. P. Goeger, *Poult. Sci.*, 2002, **81**, 30–33.
103. T. Varga, Z. Czimmerer and L. Nagy, *Biochim. Biophys. Acta*, 2011, **1812**, 1007–1022.
104. P. C. Calder, *Nutrients*, 2010, **2**, 355–374.
105. S. M. Kim, N. Neuendorff, R. S. Chapkin and D. J. Earnest, *EBioMedicine*, 2016, **7**, 100–111.

106. R. S. Chapkin, W. Kim, J. R. Lupton and D. N. McMurray, *Prostaglandins, Leukotrienes Essent. Fatty Acids*, 2009, **81**, 187–191.
107. W. Kim, Y. Y. Fan, R. Barhoumi, R. Smith, D. N. McMurray and R. S. Chapkin, *J. Immunol.*, 2008, **181**, 6236–6243.
108. T. Y. Hou, D. N. McMurray and R. S. Chapkin, *Eur. J. Pharmacol.*, 2016, **785**, 2–9.
109. S. R. Shaikh, M. R. Brzustowicz, N. Gustafson, W. Stillwell and S. R. Wassall, *Biochemistry*, 2002, **41**, 10593–10602.
110. S. R. Shaikh, A. C. Dumaual, A. Castillo, D. LoCascio, R. A. Siddiqui, W. Stillwell and S. R. Wassall, *Biophys. J.*, 2004, **87**, 1752–1766.
111. C. Carrillo, M. Cavia Mdel and S. Alonso-Torre, *Nutr. Hosp.*, 2012, **27**, 978–990.
112. K. L. Fritsche, *Adv. Nutr.*, 2015, **6**, 293S–301S.
113. J. Y. Lee, L. Zhao, H. S. Youn, A. R. Weatherill, R. Tapping, L. Feng, W. H. Lee, K. A. Fitzgerald and D. H. Hwang, *J. Biol. Chem.*, 2004, **279**, 16971–16979.
114. J. Y. Lee, K. H. Sohn, S. H. Rhee and D. Hwang, *J. Biol. Chem.*, 2001, **276**, 16683–16689.
115. Y. Wang, Y. Qian, Q. Fang, P. Zhong, W. Li, L. Wang, W. Fu, Y. Zhang, Z. Xu, X. Li and G. Liang, *Nat. Commun.*, 2017, **8**, 13997.
116. E. K. Anderson, A. A. Hill and A. H. Hasty, *Arterioscler., Thromb., Vasc. Biol.*, 2012, **32**, 1687–1695.
117. C. N. Blesso and M. L. Fernandez, *Nutrients*, 2018, **10**(4), 426.
118. P. Duewell, H. Kono, K. J. Rayner, C. M. Sirois, G. Vladimer, F. G. Bauernfeind, G. S. Abela, L. Franchi, G. Nunez, M. Schnurr, T. Espevik, E. Lien, K. A. Fitzgerald, K. L. Rock, K. J. Moore, S. D. Wright, V. Hornung and E. Latz, *Nature*, 2010, **464**, 1357–1361.
119. F. J. Sheedy, A. Grebe, K. J. Rayner, P. Kalantari, B. Ramkhelawon, S. B. Carpenter, C. E. Becker, H. N. Ediriweera, A. E. Mullick, D. T. Golenbock, L. M. Stuart, E. Latz, K. A. Fitzgerald and K. J. Moore, *Nat. Immunol.*, 2013, **14**, 812–820.
120. A. J. Armstrong, A. K. Gebre, J. S. Parks and C. C. Hedrick, *J. Immunol.*, 2010, **184**, 173–183.
121. P. Yaqoob, *Annu. Rev. Nutr.*, 2009, **29**, 257–282.
122. A. D'Alessandro, P. G. Righetti, E. Fasoli and L. Zolla, *J. Proteomics*, 2010, **73**, 1028–1042.
123. R. J. Elias, S. S. Kellerby and E. A. Decker, *Crit. Rev. Food Sci. Nutr.*, 2008, **48**, 430–441.
124. J. Kovacs-Nolan, M. Phillips and Y. Mine, *J. Agric. Food Chem.*, 2005, **53**, 8421–8431.
125. Y. Kobayashi, P. Rupa, J. Kovacs-Nolan, P. V. Turner, T. Matsui and Y. Mine, *J. Agric. Food Chem.*, 2015, **63**, 1532–1539.
126. B. Khor, A. Gardet and R. J. Xavier, *Nature*, 2011, **474**, 307–317.
127. S. Lange, E. Jennische, E. Johansson and I. Lonnroth, *Cell Tissue Res.*, 1999, **296**, 607–617.

128. S. Lange, I. Lonnroth and K. Martinsson, *Br. Poult. Sci.*, 1994, **35**, 615–620.
129. J. Mane, V. Loren, E. Pedrosa, I. Ojanguren, E. Domenech, M. A. Gassull and E. Cabre, *Br. J. Nutr.*, 2011, **106**, 1522–1528.
130. A. Laurenius, B. Wangberg, S. Lange, E. Jennische, B. K. Lundgren and I. Bosaeus, *Clin. Nutr.*, 2003, **22**, 549–552.
131. A. Eriksson, M. Shafazand, E. Jennische, I. Lonnroth and S. Lange, *Inflammatory Bowel Dis.*, 2003, **9**, 398–400.
132. A. Eriksson, M. Shafazand, E. Jennische and S. Lange, *Scand. J. Gastroenterol.*, 2003, **38**, 1045–1049.
133. M. Lee, J. Kovacs-Nolan, T. Archbold, M. Z. Fan, L. R. Juneja, T. Okubo and Y. Mine, *J. Funct. Foods*, 2009, **1**, 161–169.
134. M. C. Chappell, *Am. J. Physiol.: Heart Circ. Physiol.*, 2016, **310**, H137–H152.
135. A. Davalos, M. Miguel, B. Bartolome and R. Lopez-Fandino, *J. Food Prot.*, 2004, **67**, 1939–1944.
136. M. Miguel, I. Recio, J. A. Gomez-Ruiz, M. Ramos and R. Lopez-Fandino, *J. Food Prot.*, 2004, **67**, 1914–1920.
137. K. Majumder, S. Chakrabarti, J. S. Morton, S. Panahi, S. Kaufman, S. T. Davidge and J. Wu, *PLoS One*, 2013, **8**, e82829.
138. W. Huang, S. Chakrabarti, K. Majumder, Y. Jiang, S. T. Davidge and J. Wu, *J. Agric. Food Chem.*, 2010, **58**, 10840–10846.
139. K. Majumder, S. Chakrabarti, S. T. Davidge and J. Wu, *J. Agric. Food Chem.*, 2013, **61**, 2120–2129.
140. C. Grootaert, B. Matthijs, S. Voorspoels, S. Possemiers, G. Smagghe and J. Van Camp, *Food Funct.*, 2017, **8**, 3847–3855.
141. H. Fujita, H. Usui, K. Kurahashi and M. Yoshikawa, *Peptides*, 1995, **16**, 785–790.
142. Y. Yamada, N. Matoba, H. Usui, K. Onishi and M. Yoshikawa, *Biosci., Biotechnol., Biochem.*, 2002, **66**, 1213–1217.
143. C. Nimalaratne and J. Wu, *Nutrients*, 2015, **7**, 8274–8293.
144. B. Jiang and Y. Mine, *J. Agric. Food Chem.*, 2000, **48**, 990–994.
145. C. Xu, C. Yang, Y. Yin, J. Liu and Y. Mine, *J. Funct. Foods*, 2012, **4**, 718–726.
146. C. Meram, Y. Esparza, F. Temelli and J. Wu, *Food Biosci.*, 2017, **18**, 38–45.
147. C. Meram and J. Wu, *Food Res. Int.*, 2017, **100**, 449–459.
148. C. Nimalaratne, P. Savard, S. F. Gauthier, A. Schieber and J. Wu, *J. Agric. Food Chem.*, 2015, **63**, 2956–2962.
149. N. I. Krinsky, J. T. Landrum and R. A. Bone, *Annu. Rev. Nutr.*, 2003, **23**, 171–201.
150. J. M. Serpeloni, I. M. Colus, F. S. de Oliveira, A. F. Aissa, A. Z. Mercadante, M. L. Bianchi and L. M. Antunes, *Food Chem. Toxicol.*, 2014, **70C**, 205–213.
151. J. M. Serpeloni, G. R. Barcelos, J. P. Friedmann Angeli, A. Z. Mercadante, M. Lourdes Pires Bianchi and L. M. Antunes, *Toxicol. In Vitro*, 2012, **26**, 288–294.
152. J. M. Serpeloni, D. Grotto, A. Z. Mercadante, M. de Lourdes Pires Bianchi and L. M. Antunes, *Arch. Toxicol.*, 2010, **84**, 811–822.

153. R. Shanmugasundaram and R. K. Selvaraj, *Poult. Sci.*, 2011, **90**, 971–976.
154. J. Y. Song, C.-M. Lee and M. K. Lee, *J. Life Sci.*, 2012, **22**, 298–305.
155. L. S. Meriwether, B. D. Humphrey, D. G. Peterson, K. C. Klasing and E. A. Koutsos, *J. Anim. Physiol. Anim. Nutr.*, 2010, **94**, e115–e122.
156. P. Fernandez-Robredo, J. A. Rodriguez, L. M. Sadaba, S. Recalde and A. Garcia-Layana, *J. Nutr. Biochem.*, 2008, **19**, 40–48.
157. B. Nidhi, G. Sharavana, T. R. Ramaprasad and B. Vallikannan, *Food Funct.*, 2015, **6**, 450–460.
158. R. W. S. Chung, P. Leanderson, A. K. Lundberg and L. Jonasson, *Atherosclerosis*, 2017, **262**, 87–93.
159. R. Graydon, R. E. Hogg, U. Chakravarthy, I. S. Young and J. V. Woodside, *Br. J. Nutr.*, 2012, **108**, 334–342.

CHAPTER 11

Antiviral Properties of Egg Components

HUA ZHANG[a] AND YOSHINORI MINE*[b]

[a]Guelph Food Research Centre, Agriculture and Agri-Food Canada, 93 Stone Road West, Guelph, Ontario, Canada, N1G 5C9; [b]Department of Food Science, University of Guelph, Guelph, Ontario, N1G 2W1, Canada
*E-mail: ymine@uoguelph.ca

11.1 Introduction

Hen eggs, recognized as an extraordinary source of high-quality food proteins as well as other functional constituents, *e.g.* lipids, carbohydrates and micronutrients, are widely consumed worldwide. A whole hen egg commonly consists of approximately 63% albumen, 27.5% yolk and 9.5% eggshell by weight. Carbohydrates, lipids and proteins contained in eggs are commonly found in conjugated forms as glycoproteins or lipoproteins.[1] Nine essential amino acids, *i.e.* histidine, isoleucine, leucine, lysine, methionine, phenylalanine, threonine, tryptophan and valine, have been associated with the consumption of egg[2]. Consumers consider the hen egg as the most pleiotropic and affordable functional food, offering a unique balance of essential nutrients that contribute to sustained growth and health. In addition, eggs are consumable by people of all ages and life stages, and are particularly highly recommended for elderly, pregnant women

Food Chemistry, Function and Analysis No.14
Eggs as Functional Foods and Nutraceuticals for Human Health
Edited by Jianping Wu

Published by the Royal Society of Chemistry, www.rsc.org

and children who are at risk of low nutrient intake or have high nutrient demands for growth.[3] Despite reports that consumption of eggs might be linked to increased risks of high cholesterol and cardiovascular diseases, hen eggs remain an undeniable source of essential nutrients and molecular entities presenting health-promoting biological functions, such as antioxidant, anticancer, anti-hypertensive, antimicrobial and immunomodulatory properties.[4]

A mounting body of scientific evidence supports the observation that egg bioactive compounds exert preventive and therapeutic effects on chronic disease and infectious disease.[5–9] For instance, intake of *n*-3 polyunsaturated fatty acid-enriched eggs was shown to reduce plasma triglyceride levels, leading to reduced risks of cardiovascular disease,[10] while egg yolk lipids were incorporated into infant formula to enrich the long-chain polyunsaturated fatty acid content.[11] Egg phospholipids and sphingolipids feature as dietary compositions for digestion in the lumen, impacting gut barrier functions, cholesterol absorption and intestinal inflammation.[12] Egg-derived micronutrients, such as vitamin E, selenium and carotenoids, *e.g.* lutein, zeaxanthin and xanthophylls, contribute to the characteristic pigment of egg yolk and act as natural antioxidants through cleavage of free radicals arising from cellular metabolism. This results in the prevention of oxidative stress and suppression of increasing incidence of chronic diseases and metabolic disorders.[13–15] Taken all together, a myriad of bioactive components derived from egg proteins have been documented and exert significant health-promoting effects.

A variety of naturally occurring egg protein fractions, mainly including ovalbumin, ovotransferrin, ovomucin, ovomucoid and lysozyme present in the egg white, as well as phosvitin and lipoprotein present in the egg yolk, have been characterized with their respective and diverse biological functions. Emerging evidence has shown that these egg proteins possess antibacterial, antihypertension, antioxidant, immunomodulatory and antiadhesive properties.[16–18] Meanwhile, peptides released from egg proteins upon acidic or enzymatic hydrolysis occurring during food processing or gastrointestinal digestion have also been documented for their novel therapeutic potential. Bioactivities have been attributed to proteins as a full entity, *e.g.* ovalbumin, lysozyme and ovotransferrin, or as released peptides *e.g.*, ovomucoid peptides. Owing to their immunoregulatory potency, researchers are currently investigating their potential use in the replacement or optimisation of conventional immunomodulatory therapies.[19] These bioactive egg proteins and peptides have been shown to exhibit immunomodulatory activity by enhancing antibody production or restoring immune responsiveness, representative of their antiviral properties. Interestingly, even though the antiviral activity of egg-derived bioactive peptides has been demonstrated against a variety of viruses *in vitro*, the exact nature of their antiviral effects and the underlying mechanisms remain to be elucidated.

11.2 Antiviral Activities of Egg White Proteins

Eggs are equipped with physically and biologically functional defense systems to protect the embryo against invasion and multiplication of microorganisms. The egg white (or albumen) presents a high water and protein content and contributes about 60% of the total egg weight.[18] The primary protein constituent found in the egg white is ovalbumin, followed by ovotransferrin and ovomucoid. Other proteins are ovomucin, lysozyme, avidin, cystatin, ovoinhibitor and ovostatin. The functional protein components, which are particularly involved in immune defense properties against viral or microbial invasion, are summarized in Table 11.1.[18,20]

11.2.1 Ovomucin

Ovomucin is a glycoprotein responsible for the viscosity of the egg albumen and contributes to maintaining the structural integrity of egg white in a gel form. It was also found that both the carbohydrate and peptide moieties of a glycoprotein have binding potency to viruses.[21] Ovomucin consists of α- and β-subunits linked by disulfide bonds. As an important egg-derived glycoprotein, ovomucin has been documented for its strong hemagglutination inhibitory activity against different types of viruses invading into cells, leading to it possessing strong antiviral actions. Tsuge *et al.* have demonstrated that ovomucin and its peptides exert antiviral activity against Newcastle disease virus, bovine rotavirus and human influenza virus reliant on the structural feature of its subunits.[22–24]

11.2.2 Ovotransferrin

Another antivirus glycoprotein identified in egg albumen is ovotransferrin, representing about 12% of total egg white proteins by weight. Being a disulfide-linked homodimer, ovotransferrin acts as a superoxide dismutase (SOD)-like antioxidant to reduce oxidative stress reliant on an effective scavenging domain located in its N-terminal lobe.[25] Owing to its well-known iron binding and transporting properties, the primary physiological function of ovotransferrin is to promote growth, as well as protect the host from microbial infections by chelating available iron to prevent microbial growth, and is therefore involved in the defense mechanism

Table 11.1 Antiviral activity of egg white proteins.

Protein	Target viruses	Reference
Ovomucin	Bovine rotavirus Newcastle disease virus	22–24
Ovotransferrin	Marek's disease virus	27,29,30
Lysozyme	Norovirus Hepatitis A HIV-1	41–43

in eggs.[26] In addition, increased expression and release of ovotransferrin were observed in chicken embryo fibroblasts infected with Marek's disease virus (MDV), referred to as an avian herpes virus, suggesting that ovotransferrin has antiviral potency.[27] Ovotransferrin was reported to be more effective than human or bovine lactoferrins in inhibiting MDV infection.[28] Two main peptic fragments of ovotransferrin were reported to be the main potential contributors to its anti-herpes virus activity.[29] The peptide fragments, *i.e.* DQKDEYELL (hOTrf219–227) and KDLLFK (hOTrf269–301) and C-lobe (hOTrf633–638), were subsequently found to be capable of inhibiting MDV infection in chicken embryo fibroblasts; however, they exhibited lower inhibitory efficiency compared with the intact protein, indicating that the native conformation of the protein is an important determinant of its antiviral sensing ability.[30] In addition, a significant increase in the release of ovotransferrin was observed in a virally re-infected lymphoblastoid cell *in vitro* model in a dose-dependent manner.[27] Finally, ovotransferrin has also been identified as a major acute phase protein in chickens, and the release of ovotransferrin was shown to modulate macrophage and heterophil cell activity in response to inflammation and infections.[31,32] Taken together, these finding suggests that ovotransferrin plays a key role in avian defense mechanisms through regulation of innate immune responses.

11.2.3 Lysozyme

Lysozyme is a single polypeptide consisting of 129 amino acids cross-linked by four disulfide bridges, and is recognized as a food preservative and an essential constituent of cosmetics and medical products.[33] Owing to its high lysozyme content, hen egg white is the primary commercial source of lysozyme. Lysozyme is a well-known natural antimicrobial agent capable of preventing bacteria-induced food spoilage and food-borne disease. Similarly, we previously identified lysozyme-derived bioactive peptides with antimicrobial activity.[34] Furthermore, lysozyme was also associated with strong immunomodulatory activities, leading to therapeutic applications in various disease treatments, *e.g.* chronic sinusitis, chronic bronchitis and furunculosis, *via* hampering disease progression or reducing disease severity.[35–37] It was also reported that lysozyme is capable of promoting antibody production in hybridomas and lymphocytes cultures, leading to a restored immune response in immune-depressed patients undergoing anticancer treatments.[38] More notably, lysozyme has been documented for its antiviral actions. Several viral skin infections, including herpes simplex and chicken pox, were shown to be effectively prevented and controlled through the direct action of lysozyme.[36] Dimerized lysozyme was found to protect rainbow trout against viral diseases and treat virus-induced immune suppression through restoring their cellular and humoral defense mechanisms.[39] Dextran-conjugated lysozymes have also been reported for their inhibitory properties in the growth of viral hemorrhagic septicemia virus *in vitro*.[40] Heat-denatured lysozyme was demonstrated to effectively inactivate norovirus, resulting in reduced incidence of infection and transmission of norovirus.[41] The same authors also discovered that heat-denatured lysozyme inactivated hepatitis A virus on berry fruit.[42] The results of their studies suggest that lysozyme can be an effective disinfectant owing to its antiviral potency. Additionally, egg white lysozyme exerts effects on human immunodeficiency type 1 virus (HIV-1). Recent scientific evidence rising from an *in silico* study verified that lysozyme from egg white can block HIV-1 binding with host cell CD4.[43] All in all, these findings suggest that egg white lysozyme has strong antiviral properties, making it a promising alternative strategy for the treatment of HIV-1 infection but also as a disinfecting agent to prevent environmental transmission of viruses.

11.2.4 Cystatin and Ovoglobulin

Cystatin and ovoglobulin are two more egg white proteins that have been investigated for their antiviral properties. Cystatin is a small protein with a molecular weight of 13.3 kDa that is capable of inhibiting cysteine active site in proteases. Human cystatin found in tears and saliva has been shown to inhibit adenoviral infection,[44] suggesting that human cystatin is part of the host defense system protecting against pathogenic viral and bacterial infections.[45] Chicken cystatin was documented to reduce virus loads by altering the intracellular proteolytic process of poliovirus proteins.[46] A variety of globulin fractions are also found in the egg white, including macroglobulin, ovoglobulins (G1, G2 and G3) and ovoinhibitors. Both ovoglobulin G1 and ovoinhibitors were identified as lysozyme, indicating that they may also have antiviral potency. Ovomacroglobulin is the second largest egg glycoprotein and has a hemagglutination inhibitory activity similar to that of ovomucin.[47]

Taken altogether, many egg white proteins exhibit antiviral properties. Ovomucin inhibits viral hemagglutination, ovotransferrin acts as an acute phase protein stimulating innate immune responses against viral infection, egg white lysozyme may block the binding of HIV-1 with CD4-positive host cells, and finally, cystatin and ovoglobulin also present antiviral activity. While these proteins exist in the egg albumen, they have also been detected in embryonic blood, where they may play a role in the prevention of viral infection. In addition to their identified antimicrobial functions, egg white proteins may also exert synergistic effects on the host defense against microbial invasion.

11.3 Antiviral Properties of Egg Yolk Components

Egg yolk consists of proteins and lipids, and egg yolk proteins mainly exist in the form of lipoproteins, in both the granule and plasma fractions. High-density lipoproteins (HDL), *e.g.* α- and β-lipovitellins and phosvitin, and

Table 11.2 Antiviral activity of egg yolk proteins.

Protein	Target viruses	Reference
IgY	*Intestinal viruses* Bovine rotavirus Human rotavirus (Simian rotavirus SA 11) Porcine epidemic diarrhoea virus Transmissible gastroenteritis virus Infectious bursal disease virus Poliomyelitis virus type 2 Coxsackie B2 Norovirus *Influenza virus* H5N1 H1N1 Influenza B virus SARS	26,55,56,58–65, 72–74,76
IgY	*Influenza virus* H5N1 H1N1 Influenza B virus SARS	77–83
Sialic acids	Simian rotavirus SA 11	91

low-density lipoproteins (LDL) are the main constituents of granules.[20] LDL are primarily present in the plasma as water-soluble fractions containing livetins, which are lipid-free globular proteins, such as immunoglobulin Y.[48] Egg yolk also contains carbohydrates, most of which are oligosaccharides bound with proteins, minerals and pigments.[48] Egg yolk is an economic source of specific immunoglobulins (IgY) that have noticeable activity in preventing bacterial and viral infections, as summarized in Table 11.2. Encounters with viruses contribute to the development of a mature and functional immune system, hence contributing to the embryo defense system and ensuring healthy embryonic growth.

11.3.1 Egg Yolk Immunoglobulin (IgY)

Egg yolk immunoglobulins (Ig) Y have a similar function to mammal antibody IgG, are transferred from the hen to the egg and play a key role in establishing avian acquired immunity.[49] One application of egg yolk IgY has been passive immunization of immunocompromised patients as an alternative to traditional antibiotic treatment.[50] Passive immunity refers to the transfer of antigen-specific antibodies produced by an immunized subject to a susceptible individual with the aim of providing fast and effective protection against a given infection.[51] Passive immunization-based approaches have recently drawn researchers' attention with the aim of addressing antimicrobial- and drug-resistant microorganisms. Conventional vaccines are unable to evoke an immune response in patients presenting impaired immunity. The use of IgY has found applications in both human and veterinary medicine owing to the fact that (1) egg yolk represents an economical source of IgY production, (2) egg yolk allows for the large-scale production of IgY, (3) the phylogenetic distance between chickens and mammals is significant enough to make mammalian proteins very distinctive targets for IgY, and finally (4) IgY does not interact with mammalian Fc receptors to trigger an inflammatory response.[49,50,52,53] Emerging evidence from both *in vitro* and *in vivo* studies supports that egg yolk IgY is capable of inhibitory effects on both gastrointestinal microbial and viral infections and evokes disease symptoms.[34]

For more than two decades, egg yolk IgY antibodies have been massively produced and used to protect domesticated animals, *e.g.* pigs, poultry and calves, against diarrheic intestinal pathogens, such as bovine and human rotaviruses, bovine coronavirus, enterotoxigenic *Escherichia coli* (ETEC) and *Salmonella* spp.[54] Dietary supplementation with egg yolk IgY has been reported to prevent diarrhoea in newborn calves *via* modulation of immune responses against bovine rotavirus infections, and therefore represents a promising therapeutic intervention against group A rotavirus in calves.[55–58] Administration of egg yolk or colostrum antibodies was later found to protect neonatal calves against bovine coronavirus-caused diarrhoea.[59] Moreover, hen IgY was demonstrated to present immunoprophylactic effects against porcine epidemic diarrhoea virus and transmissible gastroenteritis virus in piglets, leading to increased survival rates.[60–62] Passively immunizing chickens with egg IgY was shown to prevent infectious bursal disease virus diseases.[63–65] Administration of egg yolk IgY has also been documented for its protective effects against intestinal viral infections and associated disease symptoms in mouse models of human and cattle infectious agents, *e.g.* human rotavirus, bovine rotavirus and enterovirus type 71, further emphasizing the clinical potential of IgY passive immunotherapy.[66–71] IgY antibodies also showed protective effects against human rotavirus (RV)-induced diarrhoea in the neonatal gnotobiotic piglet disease model.[72]

In earlier studies, egg yolk IgY antibodies were used in passive immunization studies against different intestinal viruses, including simian rotavirus SA 11, poliomyelitis type 2 and Coxsackie B2 viruses.[73] Egg yolk IgY prepared from hyperimmunized chickens was used as a dietary supplement in children to treat RV-induced diarrhoea and effectively relieved disease symptoms.[74] Both RV and norovirus (NoV) are leading causes of acute gastroenteritis that widely affect people worldwide. P--VP8-based IgY formulations were developed, comprising both RV and NoV antigens, presenting binding affinity to histo-blood group antigen (HBGA) receptor and neutralizing RV replication in Madin-Darby canine kidney (MDCK) cells.[75] The same authors reported that the NoV-specific IgY formulation could effectively block NoV antigens from binding with the HBGA receptor.[76] Evidence from recent *in vitro* and *in vivo* studies supports the oral administration of IgY as a promising strategy for prevention of rotavirus infection in low birth weight infants.[77,78] In addition to its protective effect on virus-induced gastroenteritis, egg yolk IgY also showed preventive effects on flu virus infections. Influenza A virus is a highly virulent pathogen and causes acute and fatal pulmonary diseases in humans. H5N1, an avian influenza A virus, may be transmitted from avian species to humans. IgY antibodies isolated from immunized ostrich eggs were reported to present strong neutralization activity against H5N1 virus infection in embryonated chicks.[79] Outbreak of the pandemic swine influenza A (H1N1) spread rapidly around the globe and became a significant health problem in 2009. Both H5N1- and H1N1-specific IgY antibodies were prepared from egg yolk and successfully used for the prevention of these two types of viral infection.[80] H1N1-specific IgY antibodies were subsequently found to protect infected mice by reducing viral titers while maintaining the physiological function and structure of the lungs.[81] Egg yolk IgY antibodies were demonstrated to not only protect against influenza A virus infection but also against influenza B virus (IBV) infection. IBV-specific IgY antibodies were shown to suppress influenza infection in MDCK cell culture systems and protected mice against IBV-induced lung infections.[82] Severe acute respiratory syndrome (SARS) is a viral disease characterized by acute fibrinous pneumonia with a high fatality rate. SARS coronavirus-specific IgY antibodies were isolated from immunized hen eggs and showed high stability and strong antiviral activity.[83] Altogether, these findings suggest that egg yolk IgY is a cost-effective, safe and convenient alternative therapeutic approach for the control of influenza outbreaks. Significant progress was made in the design and production of a broad variety of IgY, with future promising applications in the treatment of various types of viral diseases.[84] All in all, continuing research into IgY technology that meets the requirement of large-scale production, together with optimisation of immunization protocols, *e.g.* discovery of novel adjuvants, to increase antibody yield will lead to even broader applications of IgY immunotherapy for the benefits of both humans and animals.

11.3.2 Egg Yolk Sialic Acid and Oligosaccharides

Sialic acids include *N*-acetylneuraminic acids, as well as 30 kinds of derivatives composed of glycoproteins, glycolipids and oligosaccharides, and are widely presented in mammalian tissues as well as in bacteria.[85] Hen eggs are recognized as an excellent source of sialic acid and its oligosaccharide derivatives, and higher yields of sialic acids are found in egg yolk.[86,87] The inhibitory activity of egg white ovomucin on the virus-mediated hemagglutination of erythrocytes is primarily owing to its sialic acid content. Recent evidence suggests that egg yolk-derived sialic acid glycoproteins might interact with rotaviruses, leading to inhibition of viral replication, suggesting the utility of sialic acid derivatives in the treatment of viral gastroenteritis.[88,89] The sialylglycopeptides purified from protease-digested egg yolk have been documented for their antirotaviral potency.[90] Furthermore, a synthetic sialylphospholipid (SPL) showed strong inhibitory effects on both simian (SA-11) and human (MO) strains of rotaviruses.[91]

Interestingly, egg yolk-derived oligosaccharides may also possess antiviral activity. Nevertheless, antigenic hemagglutinin and neuraminidase proteins are expressed on the influenza A viral envelope surface. Antigenic hemagglutinin can bind with glycan receptors on the surface of host cells to induce endocytosis of the virus. These studies provide important knowledge towards in-depth understanding of the mechanisms underlying human and avian influenza virus pathogenesis and adaptation.

11.4 Conclusion

Eggs are a well-known source of functional foods containing numerous bioactive constituents with notable therapeutic effects, going beyond the provision of essential nutrients. Nowadays, hen eggs are one of the most explored sources of bioactive proteins or peptides. Recent advances in analytical techniques with improved sensitivity and efficiency along with the development of novel quantitative structure–biological activity models will benefit research into the mechanisms underlying the health-promoting effects of hen egg-derived bioactives.

Egg content can be manipulated through various methods, either as a dietary supplement or *via* immunization, for example, and is moving closer towards the development of alternative therapeutic approaches. Of the various biological activities identified in the hen egg, we highlighted the antiviral properties of egg protein and its derived peptides or oligosaccharides. In the last two decades, extensive studies have been conducted to identify or develop effective antiviral components in both egg white and yolk, seeking their possible antagonist effect on the binding of viruses to cells. Numerous egg-derived bioactive components, such as ovomucin, ovotransferrin, lysozyme, cystatin, IgY and sialic acid derivatives, have been reported for their effective antiviral activities, particularly gastroenteric and influenza viruses. Hen eggs represent a unique and extraordinary natural source for the large-scale production of bioactive components on the basis of low cost, convenience and safety, and are much less invasive than production in mammals. Continuous identification of new and existing biological functions of hen egg bioactives adds to the value of eggs as well as improving the general condition of public health and securing their role in the therapy and prevention of infectious disease.

References

1. T. Okubo, S. Akachi, and H. Hatta, in *Hen Eggs: Basic and Applied Science*, ed. T. Yamamoto, L. R. Juneja, H. Hatta and M. Kim, CRC Press, Boca Raton, FL, 1st edn, 1997, ch. 1, pp. 1–12.
2. P. Lunven, C. L. C. De St Marcq, E. Carnovale and A. Fratoni, *Br. J. Nutr.*, 1973, **30**, 189–194.
3. S. Natoli, T. Markovic, D. Lim, M. Noakes and K. Kostner, *Nutr. Diet.*, 2007, **64**, 105–111.
4. E. Abeyrathne, H. Lee and D. Ahn, *Poult. Sci.*, 2013, **92**, 3292–3299.
5. N. Sparks, *World's Poult. Sci. J.*, 2006, **62**, 308–315.
6. I. Fraeye, C. Bruneel, C. Lemahieu, J. Buyse, K. Muylaert and I. Foubert, *Food Res. Int.*, 2012, **48**, 961–969.
7. C. Bunchasak and S. Kachana, *Trop. Anim. Health Prod.*, 2009, **41**, 1583.
8. G. Cherian, in *Complementary and Alternative Therapies and the Aging Population*, ed. R. R. Watson, Elsevier, San Diego, CA, USA, 1st edn, 2009, ch. 16, pp. 333–346.
9. C. Nimalaratne and J. Wu, *Nutrients*, 2015, **7**, 8274–8293.
10. N. M. Lewis, S. Seburg and N. Flanagan, *Poult. Sci.*, 2000, **79**, 971–974.
11. D. R. Hoffman, R. C. Theuer, Y. S. Castañeda, D. H. Wheaton, R. G. Bosworth, A. R. O'Connor, S. E. Morale, L. E. Wiedemann and E. E. Birch, *J. Nutr.*, 2004, **134**, 2307–2313.
12. D. Rui-Dong, *J. Dig. Dis.*, 2011, **12**, 60–70.
13. J. D. Ribaya-Mercado and J. B. Blumberg, *J. Am. Coll. Nutr.*, 2004, **23**, 567S–587S.
14. V. I. Fisinin, T. T. Papazyan and P. F. Surai, *Crit. Rev. Biotechnol.*, 2009, **29**, 18–28.
15. I. Seuss-baum, in *Bioactive Egg Compounds*, Springer, 2007, pp. 117–144.
16. K. Watanabe, Y. Tsuge, M. Shimoyamada, N. Ogama and T. Ebina, *J. Agric. Food Chem.*, 1998, **46**, 3033–3038.
17. D. A. Omana, J. Wang and J. Wu, *Trends Food Sci. Technol.*, 2010, **21**, 455–463.
18. J. Kovacs-Nolan, M. Phillips and Y. Mine, *J. Agric. Food Chem.*, 2005, **53**, 8421–8431.
19. Y. Mine and J. Kovacs-Nolan, *World's Poult. Sci. J.*, 2006, **62**, 87–96.
20. H. Sugino, T. Nitoda and L. Juneja, in *Hen Eggs, Basic and Applied Science*, ed. T. Yamamoto, L. R. Juneja, H. Hatta and M. Kim, CRC Press, Boca Raton, FL, 1st edn, 1997, ch. 2, pp. 13–25.
21. Y. Kawasaki, H. Isoda, H. Shinmoto, M. Tanimoto, S. Dosako, T. Idota and I. Nakajima, *Biosci., Biotechnol., Biochem.*, 1993, **57**, 1214–1215.
22. Y. Tsuge, M. Shimoyamada and K. Watanabe, *Biosci., Biotechnol., Biochem.*, 1996, **60**, 1505–1506.
23. Y. Tsuge, M. Shimoyamada and K. Watanabe, *J. Agric. Food Chem.*, 1997, **45**, 2393–2398.
24. K. Watanabe, Y. Tsuge and M. Shimoyamada, *J. Agric. Food Chem.*, 1998, **46**, 4501–4506.

25. H. R. Ibrahim, M. I. Hoq and T. Aoki, *Int. J. Biol. Macromol.*, 2007, **41**, 631–640.
26. F. B. Abdallah and J. M. E. H. Chahine, *Eur. J. Biochem.*, 1999, **263**, 912–920.
27. F. Giansanti, M. F. Giardi, M. T. Massucci, D. Botti and G. Antonini, *Biochem. Cell Biol.*, 2007, **85**, 150–155.
28. F. Giansanti, P. Rossi, M. T. Massucci, D. Botti, G. Antonini, P. Valenti and L. Seganti, *Biochem. Cell Biol.*, 2002, **80**, 125–130.
29. R. Siciliano, B. Rega, M. Marchetti, L. Seganti, G. Antonini and P. Valenti, *Biochem. Biophys. Res. Commun.*, 1999, **264**, 19–23.
30. F. Giansanti, M. T. Massucci, M. F. Giardi, F. Nozza, E. Pulsinelli, C. Nicolini, D. Botti and G. Antonini, *Biochem. Biophys. Res. Commun.*, 2005, **331**, 69–73.
31. H. Xie, G. R. Huff, W. E. Huff, J. M. Balog and N. C. Rath, *Dev. Comp. Immunol.*, 2002, **26**, 805–815.
32. H. Xie, G. R. Huff, W. E. Huff, J. M. Balog, P. Holt and N. C. Rath, *Poult. Sci.*, 2002, **81**, 112–120.
33. Z. Yu, Y. Yin, W. Zhao, F. Chen and J. Liu, *J. Sci. Food Agric.*, 2014, **94**, 2839–2845.
34. Y. Mine, F. Ma and S. Lauriau, *J. Agric. Food Chem.*, 2004, **52**, 1088–1094.
35. A. Siwicki, P. Klein, M. Morand, W. Kiczka and M. Studnicka, *Vet. Immunol. Immunopathol.*, 1998, **61**, 369–378.
36. G. Sava, *EXS*, 1996, **75**, 433–449.
37. K. Asakura, T. Kojima, H. Shirasaki and A. Kataura, *Auris, Nasus, Larynx*, 1990, **17**, 33–38.
38. T. Sugahara, F. Murakami, Y. Yamada and T. Sasaki, *Biochim. Biophys. Acta, Gen. Subj.*, 2000, **1475**, 27–34.
39. A. Siwicki, M. Morand, P. Klein and W. Kiczka, *J. Appl. Ichthyol.*, 1998, **14**, 229–232.
40. J. Lee, I. Kim, S. Yeo, D. Kim and M. Kim, *Prev. Nutr. Food Sci.*, 2018, **23**, 60.
41. H. Takahashi, M. Nakazawa, C. Ohshima, M. Sato, T. Tsuchiya, A. Takeuchi, M. Kunou, T. Kuda and B. Kimura, *Sci. Rep.*, 2015, **5**, 11819.
42. M. Takahashi, Y. Okakura, H. Takahashi, M. Imamura, A. Takeuchi, H. Shidara, T. Kuda and B. Kimura, *Int. J. Food Microbiol.*, 2018, **266**, 104–108.
43. M. Behbahani, M. Nosrati and H. Mohabatkar, *Appl. Biochem. Biotechnol.*, 2018, **185**(3), 786–798.
44. A. Ruzindana-Umunyana and J. M. Weber, *Antiviral Res.*, 2001, **51**, 203–214.
45. E. Saitoh, K. Minaguchi and O. Ishibashi, *Arch. Biochem. Biophys.*, 1998, **352**, 199–206.
46. B. D. Korant, J. Brzin and V. Turk, *Biochem. Biophys. Res. Commun.*, 1985, **127**, 1072–1076.
47. A. M. Abdou, M. Kim and K. Sato, in *Bioactive Food Peptides in Health and Disease*, ed. B. Hernández-Ledesma and C. Hsie, InTech, 2013, ch. 5, pp. 115–144.

48. E. C. Li-Chan, W. D. Powrie and S. Nakai, in *Egg Science and Technology*, ed. W. Stadelman, D. Newkrik and L. Newby, CRC Press, New York, 4th edn, 1995, ch. 6, vol. 4, pp. 105–175.
49. D. Carlander, J. Stålberg and A. Larsson, *Upsala J. Med. Sci.*, 1999, **104**, 179–189.
50. D. Carlander, H. Kollberg, P.-E. Wejåker and A. Larsson, *Immunol. Res.*, 2000, **21**, 1–6.
51. J. Kovacs-Nolan and Y. Mine, *Annu. Rev. Food Sci. Technol.*, 2012, **3**, 163–182.
52. J. Sharma, *Adv. Anim. Vet. Sci.*, 1999, **41**, 481–494.
53. J. Kovacs-Nolan and Y. Mine, *Food Biotechnol.*, 2004, **18**, 39–62.
54. T. Diraviyam, B. Zhao, Y. Wang, R. Schade, A. Michael and X. Zhang, *PLoS One*, 2014, **9**, e97716.
55. C. Vega, M. Bok, P. Chacana, L. Saif, F. Fernandez and V. Parreño, *Vet. Immunol. Immunopathol.*, 2011, **142**, 156–169.
56. C. Vega, M. Bok, L. Saif, F. Fernandez and V. Parreño, *Res. Vet. Sci.*, 2015, **103**, 1–10.
57. M. Kuroki, M. Ohta, Y. Ikemori, F. Icatlo, C. Kobayashi, H. Yokoyama and Y. Kodama, *Arch. Virol.*, 1997, **142**, 843–851.
58. H. Kim, B. Lee, S. Han and Y. Jung, *Acta Virol.*, 2017, **61**, 143–149.
59. Y. Ikemori, M. Ohta, K. Umeda, F. C. Icatlo Jr, M. Kuroki, H. Yokoyama and Y. Kodama, *Vet. Microbiol.*, 1997, **58**, 105–111.
60. C.-h. Kweon, B.-j. Kwon, S.-r. Woo, J.-m. Kim, G.-h. Woo, D.-h. Son, W. Hur and Y.-s. Lee, *J. Vet. Med. Sci.*, 2001, **62**, 961–964.
61. W. Song, F. Xu, J. Wang, B. Yang, P. Lai and Y. Meng, *Acta Agric. Scand.*, 2003, **18**, 114–115.
62. Y. Zuo, J. Fan, H. Fan, T. Li and X. Zhang, *Front. Agric. China*, 2009, **3**, 104–108.
63. A. Farooq, M. Rabbani, K. Muhammad, Z. Akram, A. Ahad, Z. Fatima, T. Kamal and Z. Anwar, *Afr. J. Microbiol. Res.*, 2012, **6**, 2993–2998.
64. M. W. Malik, N. Ayub and I. Z. Qureshi, *J. Vet. Med. Sci.*, 2006, **7**, 43–46.
65. K. Muhammad, F. Rabbi, I. Hussain, A. Riaz, K. Saeed and T. Hussain, *Int. J. Agric. Biol.*, 2001, **3**, 413–415.
66. H. Hatta, K. Tsuda, S. Akachi, M. Kim, T. Yamamoto and T. Ebina, *Biosci., Biotechnol., Biochem.*, 1993, **57**, 1077–1081.
67. M. Kuroki, Y. Ikemori, H. Yokoyama, R. C. Peralta, F. C. Icatlo Jr and Y. Kodama, *Vet. Microbiol.*, 1993, **37**, 135–146.
68. T. Ebina, K. Tsukada, K. Umezu, M. Nose, K. Tsuda, H. Hatta, M. Kim and T. Yamamoto, *Microbiol. Immunol.*, 1990, **34**, 617–629.
69. S. A. Sarker, N. Pant, L. R. Juneja and L. Hammarström, *J. Health Popul. Nutr.*, 2007, **25**, 465.
70. J.-F. Liou, C.-W. Chang, J.-j. Tailiu, C.-K. Yu, H.-Y. Lei, L.-R. Chen and C. Tai, *Vaccine*, 2010, **28**, 8189–8196.
71. M. Buragohain, G. S. Dhale, G. R. Ghalsasi and S. D. Chitambar, *World J. Vaccines*, 2012, **2**, 73.

72. C. G. Vega, M. Bok, A. N. Vlasova, K. S. Chattha, F. M. Fernández, A. Wigdorovitz, V. G. Parreño and L. J. Saif, *PLoS One*, 2012, **7**, e42788.
73. G. Shirman, N. Graevskaia, I. Lavrova, V. Ginevskaia and L. Baeva, *Vopr. Virusol.*, 1988, **33**, 725–729.
74. S. A. Sarker, T. H. Casswall, L. R. Juneja, E. Hoq, I. Hossain, G. J. Fuchs and L. Hammarström, *J. Pediatr. Gastroenterol. Nutr.*, 2001, **32**, 19–25.
75. Y.-C. Dai, X.-F. Zhang, M. Tan, P. Huang, W. Lei, H. Fang, W. Zhong and X. Jiang, *Antiviral Res.*, 2013, **97**, 293–300.
76. Y.-C. Dai, Y.-Y. Wang, X.-F. Zhang, M. Tan, M. Xia, X.-B. Wu, X. Jiang and J. Nie, *J. Virol. Methods*, 2012, **186**, 126–131.
77. P. Mohan and K. Haque, *Cochrane Database Syst. Rev.*, 2003, CD003740.
78. M. Pammi and K. N. Haque, *Cochrane Database Syst. Rev.*, 2011, **10**, CD004205.
79. K. Adachi, E. Handharyani, D. K. Sari, K. Takama, K. Fukuda, I. Endo, R. Yamamoto, M. Sawa, M. Tanaka and I. Konishi, *Mol. Med. Rep.*, 2008, **1**, 203–209.
80. H. H. Nguyen, T. M. Tumpey, H.-J. Park, Y.-H. Byun, L. D. Tran, V. D. Nguyen, P. E. Kilgore, C. Czerkinsky, J. M. Katz and B. L. Seong, *PLoS One*, 2010, **5**, e10152.
81. Y.-e. Yang, J. Wen, S. Zhao, K. Zhang and Y. Zhou, *J. Virol. Methods*, 2014, **206**, 19–26.
82. J. Wen, S. Zhao, D. He, Y. Yang, Y. Li and S. Zhu, *Antiviral Res.*, 2012, **93**, 154–159.
83. C.-Y. Fu, H. Huang, X.-M. Wang, Y.-G. Liu, Z.-G. Wang, S.-J. Cui, H.-L. Gao, Z. Li, J.-P. Li and X.-G. Kong, *J. Virol. Methods*, 2006, **133**, 112–115.
84. P. T. Witkowski, D. R. Bourquain, O. Hohn, R. Schade and A. Nitsche, *J. Immunol. Methods*, 2009, **341**, 146–153.
85. A. Rosenberg and C. Schengrund, in *Biological Roles of Sialic Acid*, ed. A. Rosenberg, Springer Science & Business Media, New York, 2013, ch. 10, pp. 295–359.
86. L. R. Juneja, M. Koketsu, K. Nishimoto, M. Kim, T. Yamamoto and T. Itoh, *Carbohydr. Res.*, 1991, **214**, 179–186.
87. T. Okubo, S. Akachi and H. Hatta, in *Hen Eggs, Basic and Applied Science*, ed. T. Yamamoto, L. R. Juneja, H. Hatta and M. Kim, CRC Press: Boca Raton, FL, 1997, ch. 1, pp. 1–12.
88. R. H. Yolken, R. Willoughby, S.-B. Wee, R. Miskuff and S. Vonderfecht, *J. Clin. Invest.*, 1987, **79**, 148–154.
89. P. Isa, C. F. Arias and S. López, *Glycoconjugate J.*, 2006, **23**, 27–37.
90. M. Koketsu, A. Seko, L. R. Juneja, M. Kim, N. Kashimura and T. Yamamoto, *Carbohydr. Chem.*, 1995, **14**, 833–841.
91. M. Koketsu, T. Nitoda, H. Sugino, L. R. Juneja, M. Kim, T. Yamamoto, N. Abe, T. Kajimoto and C.-H. Wong, *J. Med. Chem.*, 1997, **40**, 3332–3335.

CHAPTER 12

Innate Antimicrobial Proteins and Peptides of Avian Egg

HISHAM R. IBRAHIM*

Department of Biochemistry and Biotechnology, Faculty of Agriculture, Kagoshima University, 1-21-24 Korimoto, Kagoshima 890-0065, Japan
*E-mail: hishamri@chem.agri.kagoshima-u.ac.jp, k2504042@kadai.jp

12.1 Introduction

Egg is a complex physiological fluid with multifunctional roles that facilitate the successful growth of the developing embryo by stimulating cellular growth and the establishment of a defense system against invading microorganisms.[1] It is an intricate mixture of bioactive proteins, lipids and carbohydrates that is unique to egg that supports the defensive role as well as providing nutrients with high bioavailability and in sufficient quantities to the rapidly growing embryo. Additionally, the functions of these bioactive factors in egg extend beyond the support of the embryo by providing nutritional benefits to humans when consumed.[2,3] Hen eggs contain complex mixtures of proteins and peptides that impart numerous benefits of defense against infections.[4] In this chapter, the role of egg proteins and peptides in defense against microbial infection is summarized, with discussion of existing data and suggestions made for future research to delineate the biology of egg and to increase its potential in the pharmaceutical and nutraceutical industries.

Food Chemistry, Function and Analysis No.14
Eggs as Functional Foods and Nutraceuticals for Human Health
Edited by Jianping Wu

Published by the Royal Society of Chemistry, www.rsc.org

12.2 Antimicrobial Defense Proteins of Egg Albumen

Beneath the shell and shell membrane, egg albumen constitutes the first defense line against microbial invasion, and is called the chemical defense line of egg.[1,5] The egg albumen provides the embryo not only with nutrients but also with different biological functions.[6] About 90% of the egg albumen is water and the rest of its mass is mostly proteins.[7] The egg albumen consists mainly of proteins having a complex structural and functional properties, which have been thought to play important biological roles during the early stages of embryonic development. There are over 40 different proteins in egg albumen and many of them are yet to be characterized.[8] Most of the proteins in the egg albumen have biological functions and appear to possess structures homologous to proteins with known functions in other species.[9] One of the major functions of these proteins is the protection of the egg from microbial attack, mainly by means of nutrient deprivation, bacteriolytic action and a physical barrier of high viscosity.[9] Proteins and peptides providing important antimicrobial effects in egg albumen are summarized in Table 12.1. In this chapter, selected proteins and peptides, with a particular focus on egg albumen, will be described owing to their distinguished defensive biological roles against microbial infection.

12.2.1 Ovotransferrin

Ovotransferrin (OTf) is a major egg albumin protein, accounting for 12% of total albumin proteins. Structurally it belongs to a family of iron-binding proteins called transferrins.[10,11] The protein is folded into two lobes, the N-terminal lobe (N-lobe) and the C-terminal lobe (C-lobe), whereas each lobe is made up of two domains, namely the alpha- and beta-domains. An atom of iron is loaded in each lobe between the two domains (Figure 12.1).[12,13] The antimicrobial activity of ovotransferrin has been attributed to its ability to deprive iron needed for microbial growth.[14–18] However, scientific evidence has shown that ovotransferrin can kill bacteria regardless of its iron-chelating property and that it contains a unique antibacterial peptide, called OTAP-92.[10,19] The antibacterial peptide OTAP-92 is released from protein by acid hydrolysis, which specifically cleaves the protein at the C-terminus of aspartic acid residues.[19] OTAP-92 is composed of 92 amino acid residues within the 109–200 sequence located at the lip of the iron-binding cleft of the N-lobe (Figure 12.1, boxed). As shown in Figure 12.2A, the structure of OTAP-92 consists of three helices, in between which is a two-stranded beta-sheet held together by three disulfide bridges, SS-1, SS-2 and SS-3, between residues Cys160–Cys174, Cys171–Cys182 and Cys115–Cys197, respectively.[11,20] The two disulfide bridges (Cys160–Cys174 and Cys171–Cys182) form a bilobal structure called a disulfide kringle, making it resemble

Table 12.1 Major proteins and peptides involved in the antimicrobial defense system of egg albumen.

Protein	% Total proteins	Antimicrobial action	Reference
Ovotransferrin	12	Deprives iron needed by microorganisms	14–18
		Antimicrobial peptide (OTAP-92) causes damage to bacterial membranes	10, 19, 21
		Self-cleaved peptides specifically kill colon and breast cancers	26
Lysozyme	3.5	Bacteriolytic action (muramidase activity)	5, 27, 28
		Partially unfolded, damage bacterial membranes	29, 30
		Fatty acylated, lethal to gram-negative bacteria	32, 34
		Helical antimicrobial peptide at the upper lip of the active site, potent bactericidal *via* membrane pore formation	35
		Helical antimicrobial peptide motifs of alpha-domain; - Bactericidal through dissipation of bacterial respiration and membrane damage - Anti-inflammatory through antagonizing TLR4 and LPS neutralization	36, 37, 40
Ovoflavoprotein	0.8	Deprives riboflavin needed by microorganisms	34–47
Avidin	0.05	Deprives biotin needed by microorganisms	48–51
Ovomucoid	11	Inhibits serine proteases of microorganisms	56, 57
Ovoinhibitor	1.5	Inhibits serine proteases of bacterial and fungal origin	52, 58
Cystatin	0.05	Inhibits thiol proteases of microorganisms	52
Ovomacroglobulin	0.5	Inhibits metalloproteinases	52

the structure of insect defensins[19,21] (Figure 12.2B). Insect defensins are cysteine-rich antimicrobial peptides that are active against Gram-positive and Gram-negative bacteria. The cysteine-rich insect defensins kill bacteria by forming a pore or ion channel in the cytoplasmic membrane. The peptide OTAP-92 exhibits strong antimicrobial activity against the Gram-positive *Staphylococcus aureus* and Gram-negative *Escherichia coli* strains. Interestingly, OTAP-92 shows the ability to damage the outer membrane

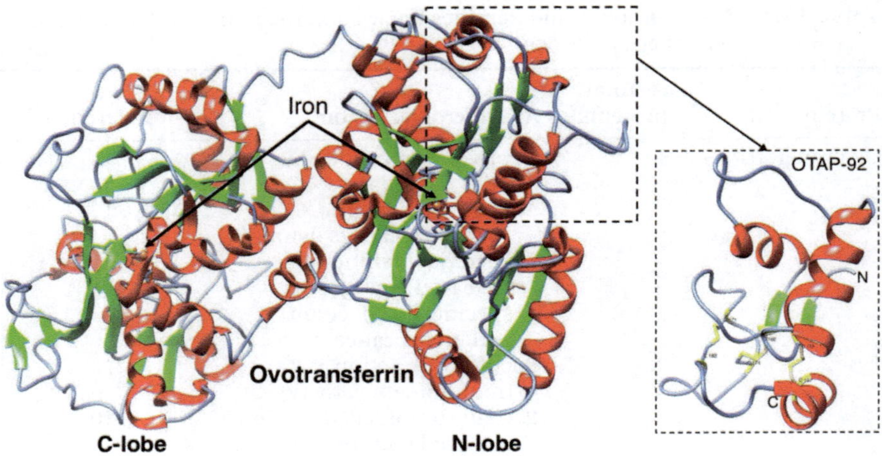

Figure 12.1 Ribbon structure of ovotransferrin showing the N-lobe and C-lobe and illustrating the location of the antimicrobial peptide (OTAP-92). The OTAP-92 peptide is displayed in the box (dashed line) at the iron-binding cleft of the N-lobe and is magnified for clarity in the right panel.

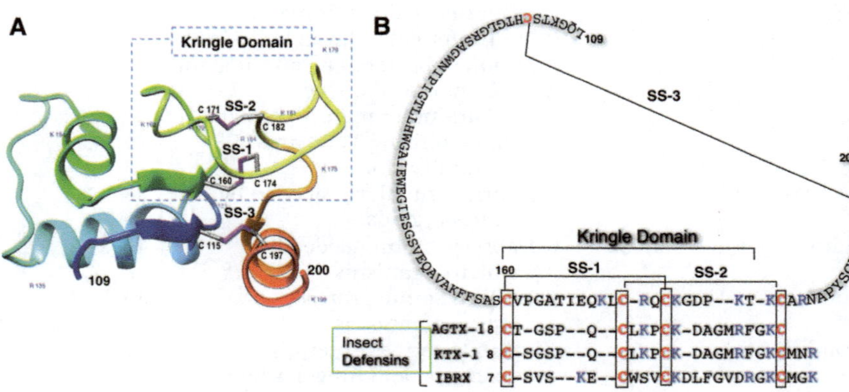

Figure 12.2 Ribbon structure and amino acid sequence of OTAP-92. (A) The fold of OTAP-92 showing the three disulfide bonds holding its rigid structure that projects the disulfide kringle domain to the exterior of the molecule. (B) The amino acid sequence of OTAP-92 showing the disulfide bridges of the kringle domain and the homology with three cysteine-rich insect defensins, scorpion agitoxin 1 (AGTX-1), kaliotoxin 1 (KTX-1) from *Androctonus mauretanicus* and iberiotoxin (IBTX) from *Mesobuthus tamulus*.

and the inner membrane of Gram-negative bacteria, where the formation of a multimeric pore into the inner membrane results in a lethal event.[21] Sequence comparison between OTAP-92 and the three cysteine-rich insect defensins (Figure 12.2B) indicates that the kringle domain of OTAP-92 constitutes the membrane insertion region.

12.2.1.1 Other Health Benefits of OTf and Its Peptides

Interestingly, OTf undergoes redox-mediated transformations leading to self-cleavage at the distinct cysteines holding the two disulfide kringle domains,[22] thus it was converted into an superoxide dismutase (SOD) mimic protein with high specificity for superoxide anions.[23] Therefore, it can be envisioned that the cysteine residues in the kringle domain of OTAP-92 may function as redox-responsive during exposure to the membrane potential of the invading bacteria. OTf can also be viewed as a multifunctional protein that is activated in response to the cellular redox environment. This is supported by the fact that OTf is selectively cleaved by chicken macrophages;[24,25] thus, the released OTAP-92 peptide may provide the first line of defense against invading bacteria until the immune system launches a full attack. The redox-dependent self-cleavage of OTf also occurred upon reduction with thioredoxin primarily at four distinct sites flanking the two disulfide kringles, leading to the liberation of the two kringle domains, including OTAP-92 (Figure 12.2B) in the N-lobe.[22] Amazingly, the self-cleavage of OTf was found to be a key process to generate kringle-containing peptides with anticancer activity specific to human colon and breast cancer cells, without effect on normal cells.[26] These findings provide new information on the multiple biofunctions of OTf and its kringle-containing peptide and offer a fascinating opportunity for the potential use of the reduced OTf or kringle peptides in therapy for the treatment of microbial infections, oxidative stress-associated diseases and cancers. The surprise occasioned by the novel discovery of these biofunctions of OTf and its peptides thus seems likely to be joined by additional surprises as the role of these peptides in other diseases is explored.

12.2.2 Lysozyme

Lysozyme (LZ) is not only present in egg albumen, but also in the shell as well as in the shell membrane and the vitelline membranes. It accounts for 3.5% of the total protein in egg albumin. Lysozyme belongs to a class of bacteriolytic enzymes that hydrolyse the beta-linkage between *N*-acetylmuramic acid and *N*-acetylglucosamine in the bacterial cell walls, where it is termed muramidase.[5] Gram-positive bacteria with less cross-linked and surface-exposed peptidoglycan are readily lysed and killed by lysozyme. However, many Gram-positive pathogens possess highly cross-linked peptidoglycan and thus show resistance to the action of lysozyme. Gram-negative bacteria are generally less susceptible to the action of lysozyme owing to their hydrophobic outer membrane lying over the peptidoglycan layer. The antimicrobial action of lysozyme has been proved to be independent of its enzymatic activity.[5,27,28] Use of recombinant DNA technology to create a catalytically inactive mutant lysozyme (D52S) provided concrete evidence that the antimicrobial action of lysozyme depends largely on structure phase change.[29–31] Interestingly, the susceptibility of Gram-negative bacteria to lysozyme was greatly enhanced by modification of two lysine residues with fatty acid chains or genetically inserted hydrophobic peptides at its C-terminus.[32–34] A helix-loop-helix peptide was found at the upper lip of the active site of lysozyme that exerts potent antimicrobial activity against Gram-negative as well as Gram-positive bacteria *via* membrane disruption.[35] Recent studies have revealed that the crystal structure of lysozyme contains a number of potent antimicrobial helical peptide motifs in the N-terminal region, which can be released by the neonate gastric pepsin or cathepsin D, aspartic proteases.[36] The peptides are a single helix (H1 or H2), two helices connected by a short loop (HLH), or the H2 extended with two beta-strands (H2–S12) or three beta-strands (H2–S13) at its C- terminal end (Figure 12.3). The peptides are highly cationic and the helices are amphiphilic in nature, which contributes to their ability to disrupt the membrane of Gram-negative bacteria and inhibit the respiration of Gram-positive bacteria.[37]

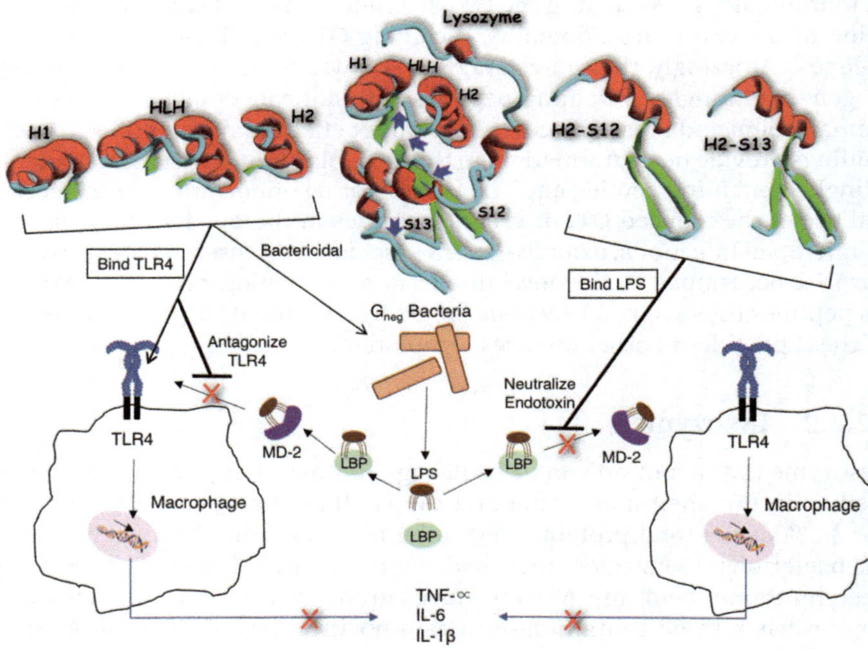

Figure 12.3 Outline of the major events in bacterial killing and anti-inflammatory actions of the five helical peptide motifs released from lysozyme by neonate pepsin (bold arrows). Three peptides, H1, H2 and HLH, attack the respiratory system of Gram-negative bacteria (G_{neg} bacteria) while antagonizing the toll-like receptor 4 (TLR4) of macrophages, thus suppressing the production of proinflammatory cytokines, *i.e.* TNF-α, IL-6 and IL-1β. The other two peptides, helix-sheet motifs H2–S12 and H2–S13, are able to bind the lipopolysaccharides (LPS) released from G_{neg} bacteria, thus neutralizing its inflammatory effect (right). LBP, LPS-binding protein; MD-2, myeloid differentiation factor 2, which forms a heterodimer with TLR4 that recognizes LPS molecules.

Lysozyme is secreted by activated immune cells and is also present in serum, saliva, breast milk and tears.[5] Upon microbial infection, activated macrophages release lysozyme into inflammatory fluids, where it acts in synergy with the cathelicidin and defensin antimicrobial peptides.[38,39] Helical peptide motifs generated by digestion of lysozyme with neonate gastric pepsin have demonstrated anti-inflammatory effects on macrophages activated by endotoxin or interferon-gamma.[40] Interestingly, three helical peptides, namely H1, H2 and HLH, were found to be capable of downregulating endotoxin-induced inflammation through antagonistic action to toll-like receptor 4 (TLR4) and the other two peptides are helix-sheet motifs, namely H2–S12 and H2–S13, that are able to neutralize the lipopolysaccharide endotoxin (Figure 12.3). While inflammation is essential for resistance to microbial infections and wound healing, excessive and uncontrolled inflammatory changes often lead to chronic diseases. The recently discovered helical peptides of lysozyme thus are not only promising for controlling infections but also suggest potential benefits in managing inflammation and associated diseases.

12.2.3 Vitamin-binding Proteins

Nutrients in eggs are transferred from the hen to the egg by vitamin-binding proteins for thiamin, riboflavin, biotin, cobalamin, retinol and cholecalciferol.[41] Because they are usually not saturated with respect to their ligand, these binding proteins are able to scavenge nutrients and thereby are thought to protect the embryo from infection by microbes that require the loaded vitamins. In this section, two vitamin-binding proteins will be described owing to their important biological activities, which seem related to the defensive role.

12.2.3.1 Riboflavin-binding Protein

Riboflavin-binding protein (RBP) is glycophosphoprotein present in both egg albumen and yolk with a molecular mass of approximately 32 000 Da and an isoelectric point of 4.0.[42] It is also referred to as ovoflavoprotein. 1 mole of RBP binds 1 mole of riboflavin (vitamin B_2). The protein is suggested to act as a carrier and store of riboflavin for the developing embryo.[41] An increase of RBP was reported during the first 9 days of egg incubation, suggesting that more riboflavin needs to be held by RBP, which may reflect the possibility that it serves as a scavenger of riboflavin and thus protects embryos against bacterial attack.[41,43,44] In egg albumen, a remarkable amount of bound riboflavin is present, suggesting both nutritional and antimicrobial functions for the RBP. However, although no systematic study has been reported on the direct antimicrobial activity of RBP, riboflavin was found to be effective in ameliorating both bacterial infection and toxin-induced septic shock in mice.[45] Interestingly, riboflavin deficiency significantly impairs the immune response of macrophages, respiratory burst and phagocytosis, and an abundance of riboflavin decreases the proinflammatory activation of macrophages.[46,47]

12.2.3.2 Avidin

Avidin is a biotin-binding glycoprotein in avian egg albumen that makes up approximately 0.05% of the total protein (Table 12.1). It is a tetrameric protein with a combined molecular mass of approximately 67 000 Da, composed of four identical subunits (128 residues each) with an isoelectric point of 10.0. Each subunit binds the vitamin biotin with a strong noncovalent bond. Because of the extraordinarily high affinity of avidin for biotin, it has been suggested that avidin, as a biotin scavenger, is a defense protein for chicken and egg against biotin-requiring microbes.[48] In particular, the biotin needed for the embryo is carried into the yolk by another protein.[49] In chicken oviducts, avidin is induced in inflammation by macrophages and after bacterial and viral infection,[50] suggesting that it may act as an antimicrobial protein in the inflammation reaction caused by infections.[51] Arguably, the high basicity of avidin (*p*I 10.0) shows that its effects on infection-induced anti-inflammatory are not only based on biotin binding because basic proteins are involved in the modulation of the inflammasome and also exert antimicrobial activity.[51] This is further supported by the finding that avidin has the ability to bind, *in vitro*, to different Gram-negative bacteria and some Gram-positive ones.[48] The porin protein of the outer membrane of *E. coli* was found to be an avidin receptor and is most likely on all Gram-negative bacteria.[51] The antimicrobial activity of avidin could be attributed to its ability to bind the cell wall of the susceptible bacteria. Future research on the antimicrobial action could reveal the defense role and mechanism of avidin and explore its potential as an antimicrobial agent.

12.3 Protease Inhibitors

Hen egg albumen is a rich source of biologically active protease inhibitors, such as ovomucoid, ovoinhibitor, cystatin and ovomacroglobulin, which are capable of inhibiting the activity of most classes of proteases.[52] Ovomucoid, a serine protease inhibitor, is the main inhibitor in hen egg albumen and the other protease inhibitors are present in smaller amounts.[53] Protease inhibitors are needed to control proteolysis during early embryogenesis, where they are passed from the albumen to the embryo during incubation.[54,55] In egg, the function of ovomucoid is to inhibit trypsin and serine proteases produced by micro-organisms[56,57].

Egg albumen contains another inhibitor of serine protease named ovoinhibitor, which is also present in egg yolk. Ovoinhibitor is able to inhibit trypsin, chymotrypsin and elastase and was found to be capable of inhibiting bacterial proteinase K and fungal proteinase from *Aspergillus* spp.[52] It was shown to exhibit antimicrobial activity against *Bacillus* spp.[58] Although there is scarce research on the antimicrobial activities of ovoinhibitor and ovomucoid, a few studies suggest that ovoinhibitor and ovomucoid play important roles in egg's antimicrobial defenses.

For the other mechanistic classes of proteases, cystatin in egg albumen is an inhibitor of cysteine proteases, including papain, ficin and cathepsins, and is present in albumen at a low concentration of 80 μg mL^{-1}.[52] Alpha 2-macroglobulin in egg albumin inhibits metalloproteinases, collagenase and thermolysin. On the assumption that the protease inhibitors in egg are antimicrobial, natural selection has favored variability in the protease inhibitors, possibly as a response to repeated microbial infections. Despite the extensive research done on the multiple protease inhibitors of egg, their contributions as defense proteins against microbial infection remain to be explored.

12.4 Conclusion and Perspectives

Egg albumen has obvious health benefits as a source of functional defense proteins that work synergistically in prevention of the pathogenesis of several diseases. This chapter focused on egg albumen, although egg yolk also contains multiple proteins homologous to those in the albumen, but the high lipid content of egg yolk and their low solubility make exploration of biological functions difficult. From a number of studies on egg albumen, it is evident that lysozyme and ovotransferrin are the key defense molecules of avian egg with the prospect that their peptides could show therapeutic potential against a number of chronic diseases. Lysozyme is a potent antimicrobial protein and its antimicrobial action is enhanced upon partial unfolding by heating, particularly with industrial applications that require thermal treatment. Peptides derived from lysozyme have been shown to have antimicrobial and anti-inflammatory activities, and have potential for use in pharmaceutical and nutraceutical applications. Ovotransferrin is an antimicrobial protein and its peptide (OTAP-92) could effectively disrupt the membranes of bacteria. Ovotransferrin also undergoes thiol-linked self-cleavage upon reduction and produces peptides, including OTAP-92, with potent anticancer effects against colon and breast cancers. Therefore, ovotransferrin and its peptides can be excellent sources of anti-infective and anticancer supplements for human health. Ovomucoid and ovoinhibitor are capable of inhibiting bacterial and fungal proteases and show antimicrobial activities, which may provide opportunity for their application in the control of biofilm formation. The health benefits of the proteins of egg albumen and their peptides are thus recognized, but much more interesting proteins or peptides may actually be responsible for various other activities. One challenging area for future research should concern exploration of the complex antimicrobial mixtures of proteins in egg albumen and multidisciplinary clinical studies involving these multifunctional proteins, which will be highly rewarding, so egg albumen remains an interesting subject for protein research.

References

1. S. Réhault-Godbert, V. Hervé-Grépinet, J. Gautron, C. Cabau, Y. Nys and M. Hincke, *Improving the Safety and Quality of Eggs and Egg Products*, Woodhead Publishing, 2011, pp. 183–208.
2. J. Kovacs-Nolan, M. Phillips and Y. Mine, *J. Agric. Food Chem.*, 2005, **53**, 8421–8431.
3. T. B. Zou, T. P. He, H. B. Li, H. W. Tang and E. Q. Xia, *Molecules*, 2016, **21**, 72.
4. M. Alabdeh, V. Lechevalier, F. Nau, M. Gautier, M. F. Cochet, F. Gonnet, S. Jan and F. Baron, *J. Food Prot.*, 2011, **74**, 24–31.
5. E. A. Charter and G. Lagarde, in *Encyclopedia of Food Microbiology*, ed. M. L. Tortorello, Academic Press, Oxford, 2nd edn, 2014, pp. 936–940.
6. Q. Xu, D. Buckley, C. Guan and H.-C. Guo, *Cell*, 1999, **98**, 651–661.
7. E. Li-Chan and S. Nakai, *Crit. Rev. Poult. Biol.*, 1989, **2**, 21–58.
8. D. V. Vadehra, K. R. Nath and R. Forsythe, *CRC Crit. Rev. Food Technol.*, 1973, **4**, 193–309.
9. L. Stevens, *Sci. Prog.*, 1996, **79**, 65–87.
10. H. R. Ibrahim, in *Natural Food Antimicrobial Systems*, ed. A. S. Naidu, CRC Press Inc., FL, 2000, pp. 211–226.
11. J. Mazurier, M. H. Metz-Boutigue, J. Jolles, G. Spik, J. Montreuil and P. Jolles, *Experientia*, 1983, **39**, 135–141.
12. W. M. Keung and P. Azari, *J. Biol. Chem.*, 1982, **257**, 1184–1188.
13. J. Williams, K. Moreton, G. D'Andrea and A. Oratore, *Biochem. Int.*, 1992, **28**, 155–160.
14. P. Valenti, C. Antonin, P. Von Hunolstein, N. O. Visca and E. Antonin, *Int. J. Tissue React.*, 1983, **1**, 97–101.
15. P. Valenti, G. Antonini, C. Von-Hunolstein, P. Visca, N. Orsi and E. Antonini, *Int. J. Tissue React.*, 1983, **5**, 97–105.
16. P. Valenti, G. Antonini, C. Von-Hunolstein, P. Visca, N. Orsi and E. Antonini, *J. Appl. Bacteriol.*, 1984, **56**, 53–61.
17. P. Valenti, P. Visca, G. Antonini and N. Orsi, *Mycopathologia*, 1985, **89**, 169–175.
18. T. Ganz, *Int. J. Hematol.*, 2018, **107**, 7–15.
19. H. R. Ibrahim, E. Iwamori, Y. Sugimoto and T. Aoki, *Biochim. Biophys. Acta*, 1998, **1401**, 289–303.
20. J. Williams, K. Moreton and A. D. Goodearl, *Biochem. J.*, 1985, **228**, 661–665.
21. H. R. Ibrahim, Y. Sugimoto and T. Aoki, *Biochim. Biophys. Acta*, 2000, **1523**, 196–205.
22. H. R. Ibrahim, T. Haraguchi and T. Aoki, *Biochim. Biophys. Acta*, 2006, **1760**, 347–355.
23. H. R. Ibrahim, M. I. Hoq and T. Aoki, *Int. J. Biol. Macromol.*, 2007, **41**, 631–640.
24. H. Xie, G. R. Huff, W. E. Huff, J. M. Balog and N. C. Rath, *Dev. Comp. Immunol.*, 2002, **26**, 805–815.

25. H. Xie, L. Newberry, F. D. Clark, W. E. Huff, G. R. Huff, J. M. Balog and N. C. Rath, *Avian Dis.*, 2002, **46**, 122–131.
26. H. R. Ibrahim and T. Kiyono, *J. Agric. Food Chem.*, 2009, **57**, 11383–11390.
27. H. R. Ibrahim, S. Higashiguchi, Y. Sugimoto and T. Aoki, *J. Agric. Food Chem.*, 1997, **45**, 89–94.
28. H. R. Ibrahim, *Food / Nahrung*, 1998, **42**, 187–193.
29. H. R. Ibrahim, T. Matsuzaki and T. Aoki, *FEBS Lett.*, 2001, **506**, 27–32.
30. H. R. Ibrahim, S. Higashiguchi, M. Koketsu, L. R. Juneja, M. Kim, T. Yamamoto, Y. Sugimoto and T. Aoki, *J. Agric. Food Chem.*, 1996, **44**, 3799–3806.
31. H. R. Ibrahim, S. Higashiguchi, L. R. Juneja, M. Kim and T. Yamamoto, *J. Agric. Food Chem.*, 1996, **44**, 1416–1423.
32. H. R. Ibrahim, T. Aoki and A. Pellegrini, *Curr. Pharm. Des.*, 2002, **8**, 671–693.
33. H. R. Ibrahim, A. Kato and K. Kobayashi, *J. Agric. Food Chem.*, 1991, **39**, 2077–2082.
34. H. R. Ibrahim, M. Yamada, K. Kobayashi and A. Kato, *Biosci., Biotechnol., Biochem.*, 1992, **56**, 1361–1363.
35. H. R. Ibrahim, U. Thomas and A. Pellegrini, *J. Biol. Chem.*, 2001, **276**, 43767–43774.
36. H. R. Ibrahim, D. Inazaki, A. Abdou, T. Aoki and M. Kim, *Biochim. Biophys. Acta*, 2005, **1726**, 102–114.
37. H. R. Ibrahim, K. Imazato and H. Ono, *J. Agric. Food Chem.*, 2011, **59**, 10336–10345.
38. S. Reitamo, J. J. Reitamo, P. Sipponen and M. Klockars, *Acta Pathol. Microbiol. Scand., Sect. A*, 1979, **87**, 451–456.
39. N. E. Hansen, H. Karle, A. Jensen and E. Bock, *Acta Neurol. Scand.*, 1977, **55**, 418–424.
40. H. R. Ibrahim, K. Hamasaki and T. Miyata, *Eur. J. Pharm. Sci.*, 2017, **107**, 240–248.
41. H. B. White 3rd, *J. Exp. Zool. Suppl.*, 1987, **1**, 53–63.
42. M. Nishikimi and Y. Kyogoku, *J. Biochem.*, 1973, **73**, 1233–1242.
43. R. Huopalahti, R. Lopez-Fandino, M. Anton and R. Schade, in *Bioactive Egg Compounds*, ed. R. Huopalahti, L. F. Rosina, M. Anton and R. Schade, Springer-Verlag, Berlin, Heidelberg, 2007, pp. 69–74.
44. H. B. White and J. A. H. Merrill, *Annu. Rev. Nutr.*, 1988, **8**, 279–299.
45. T. Toyosawa, M. Suzuki, K. Kodama and S. Araki, *Eur. J. Pharmacol.*, 2004, **25**, 273–280.
46. A. I. Mazur-Bialy, B. Buchala and B. Plytycz, *Br. J. Nutr.*, 2013, **110**, 509–514.
47. A. I. Mazur-Bialy, E. Pochec and B. Plytycz, *J. Physiol. Pharmacol.*, 2015, **66**, 793–802.
48. T. A. Kunnas, M. J. Wallen and M. S. Kulomaa, *Biochim. Biophys. Acta*, 1993, **1216**, 441–445.
49. H. B. White, *Ann. N. Y. Acad. Sci.*, 1985, **447**, 202–211.

50. B. Zerega, L. Camardella, S. Cermelli, R. Sala, R. Cancedda and F. Descalzi Cancedda, *J. Cell Sci.*, 2001, **114**, 1473–1482.
51. H. A. Elo and J. Korpela, *Comp. Biochem. Physiol., Part B: Comp. Biochem.*, 1984, **78**, 15–20.
52. I. Saxena and S. Tayyab, *Cell. Mol. Life Sci.*, 1997, **53**, 13–23.
53. I. Kato, J. Schrode, W. J. Kohr and M. Laskowski Jr, *Biochemistry*, 1987, **26**, 193–201.
54. J. E. T. Moran, *Poult. Sci.*, 2007, **86**, 1043–1049.
55. K. J. Bainter and G. Fehér, *Dev. Biol.*, 1974, **36**, 272–278.
56. I. Saxena and S. Tayyab, *Cell. Mol. Life Sci.*, 1997, **53**, 13–23.
57. R. M. Broadway, *J. Insect Physiol.*, 1997, **43**, 855–874.
58. M. Bourin, J. Gautron, M. Berges, S. Attucci, G. Le Blay, V. Labas, Y. Nys and S. Rehault-Godbert, *J. Agric. Food Chem.*, 2011, **59**, 12368–12374.

CHAPTER 13

Bioactive Egg Proteins

EMERSON NOLASCO, SNIGDHA GUHA AND KAUSTAV MAJUMDER*

University of Nebraska-Lincoln, Department of Food Science and Technology, 1901 N 21 St, Lincoln, NE, 68588-6205, USA
*E-mail: kaustav.majumder@unl.edu

13.1 Introduction

The nutritional excellence of the hen egg is profoundly related to its reproductive task. As a life-giving medium, the egg must contain the necessary nutrients to conceive well-developed embryos. The egg macronutrients are distributed in the eggshell (9.5%), egg white (63%), and egg yolk (27.5%), with protein contents of 6.4%, 9.7–11%, and 15.7–16%, respectively.[1,2] Carbohydrates, vitamins, and minerals are also present in the egg in minor amounts.[1,3] Besides its nutritional function, egg proteins also protect against exterior threats, such as microorganisms and viruses.

Proteins play a crucial role in the egg's biological activities, and they are present in the all three main compartments of the egg: egg white, egg yolk, and eggshell membrane. The major eggshell membrane proteins are collagens (types I, V, and X), cysteine-rich proteins, and glycoproteins.[4] Apart from these major proteins, eggshell also has different kinds of proteins. However, the identification, purification, and characterization of all the proteins

Food Chemistry, Function and Analysis No.14
Eggs as Functional Foods and Nutraceuticals for Human Health
Edited by Jianping Wu

Published by the Royal Society of Chemistry, www.rsc.org

present in eggshell has been delayed owing to their low solubility.[5,6] Egg white is characterized by a high protein diversity, containing over 100 different proteins, with ovalbumin, ovotransferrin, ovomucoid, ovomucin, and lysozyme as the main ones.

Moreover, low-density lipoprotein, high-density lipoprotein, livetins, phosvitin, and biotin-binding proteins are the major proteins present in egg yolk.[1] Most of these proteins account for at least one biological activity, as shown in Figure 13.1. In addition to the biological activity of these native proteins, enzymatic hydrolysis, food processing, and gastrointestinal digestion can also produce small peptides. Generally, these peptides are inactive in their parent protein sequences but can exert health-beneficial biological activities after successful liberation. These proteins are regarded as bioactive proteins owing to their biological activities above and beyond their known nutritional values.

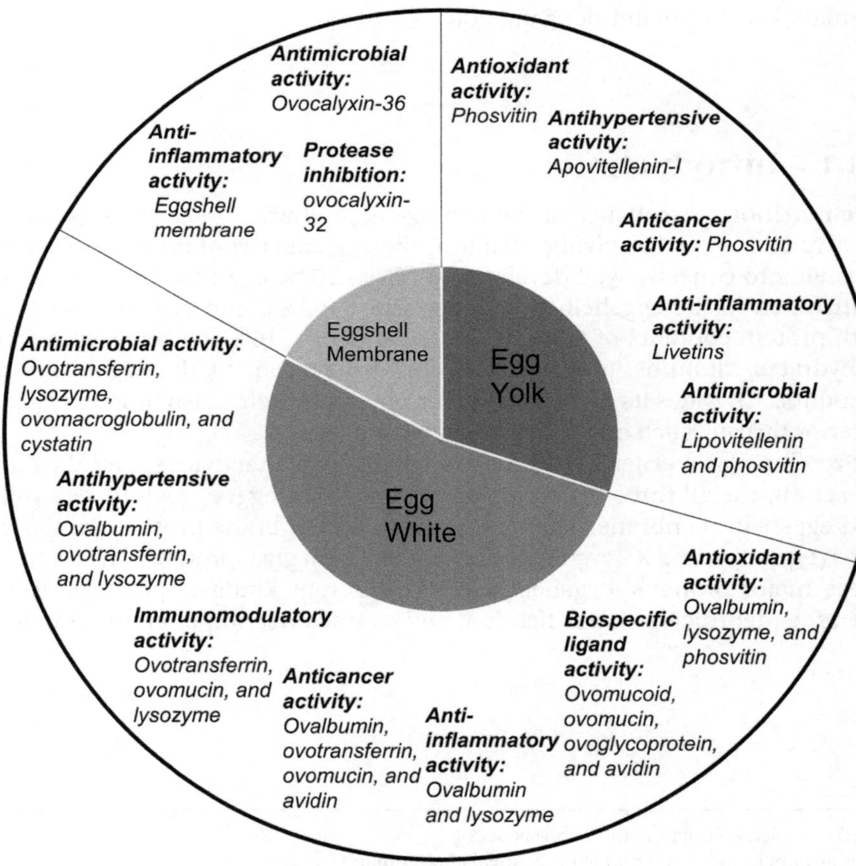

Figure 13.1 Biological activities of different egg proteins.

For instance, eggshell membrane proteins have been shown to have antimicrobial, anti-inflammatory, nerve regeneration, and tissue regeneration activity, as well as ameliorating hepatic fibrogenesis.[7–11]

Next, yolk acts as a source of antibodies, energy, and minerals for the hen's embryo, as well as proteins with antioxidant, tumor cell proliferation inhibition, antimicrobial, osteoporosis prevention, anti-inflammatory, and antihypertensive activity.[12–16] Finally, the most researched biologically active egg proteins are present in the egg white, and quite some research has been done in past decades on its bioactive proteins and peptides. Along with the most well-known antibacterial properties, egg proteins and peptides also exhibit antihypertensive, immunomodulatory, protease inhibitory, antiviral, and anticancer effects, as detailed by Kovacs-Nolan *et al.* in 2005.[1]

Besides the beneficial nutritional effects that the bioactive proteins and peptides may confer, *in vivo* bioavailability must be taken into consideration. Food proteins are most commonly ingested with food matrices, which are hydrolyzed in the gastrointestinal tract for amino acid absorption into the bloodstream. Therefore, protein-derived peptide or amino acid uptake does not depend solely on the environment but also on the affinity of the intestinal cells for the co-existing food molecules. Recent studies clarify that the absorption depends on the peptide chain length, intestinal peptide degradation, and amino acid affinity for the carrier-mediated transport route.[17] Additionally, co-existing compounds may downregulate carrier-mediated transport routes.[18] Hence, novel biological effects must be confirmed through *in vivo* studies to verify its applicability. Additionally, egg bioactive proteins can also be used as a nutritional supplement, topical ointments, or beauty products. It is evident that egg proteins have a diverse range of biological activities and thus the purpose of this chapter is to provide a brief description of the different biological activities and known mechanisms of action of the proteins present in the three separate compartments of an egg.

13.2 Beneficial Bioactivities of Major Egg Proteins

13.2.1 Egg Proteins with Antimicrobial Activity

Major proteins in all three components of egg possess antimicrobial properties, and the main reason behind this activity is to protect the embryo from possible invasion of pathogenic microorganisms. Hen egg white protects the yolk and embryo from bacterial penetration beyond the eggshell membrane. It is composed mainly of water (88%), protein (11%), and trace carbohydrates as well as minerals. Besides the harsh physicochemical properties, such as alkaline pH and high viscosity, proteins represent the main active molecules preventing bacterial proliferation.[19] The major activity has been reported by the most abundant proteins, such as ovalbumin, ovotransferrin, and lysozyme. Recently, minor proteins like gallin and avidin have also been shown to inhibit microbial growth.[19] The following sub-sections briefly describe different egg proteins that have exhibited antimicrobial activity.

13.2.1.1 Eggshell Proteins

The eggshell is the outmost layer of an egg, mainly composed of calcium carbonate ($CaCO_3$, 94%), calcium phosphate (1%), organic matter (4%), and magnesium carbonate (1%).[20] Other main components of the eggshell are a cuticle layer (10 μm thick) and three layers of the eggshell membrane (outer, inner, and limiting membrane).[21] The eggshell membrane (ESM) is composed of inner (20 μm thick) and outer (50 μm thick) membranes with a structure resembling entangled threads of randomly knitted nets.[21–23] The limiting membrane located in the innermost portion of the eggshell membrane surrounds the egg white. The primary purpose of these spider web-like nets is to trap invading microorganisms and prevent them from reaching the embryo. The ESM network is mainly composed of 70% organic compounds, 10% inorganic compounds, and 20% water. Among the organic compounds, 80% are proteins, followed by 2.3% lipids, and 3.4% carbohydrates.[22] Approximately 10% of the total protein content of ESM is collagen (types I, V, and X), and 70–75% is other proteins and glycoproteins containing lysine-derived crosslinks.[21] A total of 62 different types of proteins have been identified in ESM,[24] which makes ESM a competent biomaterial that could be a significant source of bioactive proteins with food, cosmetic, and biomedical applications. Here, different bioactivities of ESM-derived proteins are highlighted. The ESM is the first defense line against microbial invasion of the egg. The proteins from ESM have demonstrated antibacterial activity against *Pseudomonas aeruginosa*, *Bacillus cereus*, *Staphylococcus aureus*, *Escherichia coli*, and *Salmonella enteritidis*.[25] Along with the ESM protein, eggshell cuticle-derived proteins have also demonstrated antibacterial activity against *P. aeruginosa*, *Bacillus subtilis*, and *S. aureus*.[26,27] Thus, the antibacterial activities of the eggshell-derived proteins are well-known; however, the identification of the specific proteins responsible for particular antibacterial activities remains to be delineated entirely.

The five primary eggshell membrane proteins are ovocleidin-116 (OC-116), ovocleidin-17 (OC-17), ovocalyxin-36 (OCX-36), ovocalyxin-32 (OCX-32), and ovocalyxin-25 (OCX-25). Among them, OCX-36 and recombinant OCX-32 exhibit antimicrobial activity.[28,29] OCX-36 is primarily localized to the inner part of the calcified eggshell, and the protein sequence is nearly 20–25% identical to the lipopolysaccharide-binding proteins (LBP), bactericidal permeability-increasing proteins (BPI), and palate, lung, and nasal epithelium clone (Plunc) family proteins.[30] OCX-36 showed antimicrobial activity against Gram-positive *S. aureus* and significantly inhibited the bacterial growth. OCX-36 expresses both bactericidal and bacteriostatic effects against *S. aureus*, and the bacteriostatic effect of OCX-36 against *S. aureus* is dose- and time-dependent.[31] However, OCX-36 treatment did not show any effect on Gram-positive (*Listeria monocytogenes*, *Enterococcus faecalis*) and Gram-negative (*P. aeruginosa*, *E. coli*, and *Salmonella typhimurium*) bacterial strains.[31] OCX-36 showed high binding affinity with lipoteichoic acid (LTA), indicating its interaction with bacterial cell wall LTA and inhibition of *S. aureus* growth. Additionally, OCX-36 also showed significant binding with lipopolysaccharide (LPS) of *E. coli* O111 : B4, suggesting the pattern recognition function of OCX-36 as the first mechanism of action for its antibacterial effect. On the other hand, recombinant OCX-32 also inhibited the growth of *Bacillus subtilis* through alteration of the bacterial metabolism by inhibition of carboxypeptidase, an arginine-cleaving enzyme.[32] Moreover, the growth of *P. aeruginosa* has also been shown to be inhibited by the outer eggshell membrane proteins.[26] Additional proteins present in the eggshell membrane, such as β-defensin-9, -10, and -11, regarded as gallinacins, also showed antimicrobial properties.[33] For instance, recombinant gallin, corresponding to the β-defensin peptide family, inhibited *E. coli* bacterial growth through membrane pore formation.[34] Finally, GAL11, a β-defensin protein, showed antimicrobial activity against *Salmonella enteritidis* (Gram-negative) and *L. monocytogenes* (Gram-positive).[4]

13.2.1.2 Egg White Proteins

Apart from eggshell membrane proteins, several proteins from egg white also exhibit antimicrobial properties. The following sub-sections highlight the antimicrobial properties of the major egg white proteins.

13.2.1.2.1 Lysozyme. Lysozyme is present in several animals as, for example, G-, I-, and C-type lysozymes, with the latter one being the most common. Egg white lysozyme consists of 129 amino acids and is a 14.4 kDa protein with an isoelectric point (pI) of 10.7. Lysozyme present in the egg is unique as it is highly soluble and stable as compared to lysozyme present in other foods. Lysozyme is defined as a muramidase enzyme, owing to its ability to cleave the β-(1,4)-glycosidic bond between *N*-acetylmuramic acid and *N*-acetylglucosamine in the peptidoglycan bacterial cell wall.[35] Without the barrier mechanism of the cell wall, the bacterial cell swells up and is not able to survive. Owing to this characteristic, it has been stated that lysozyme is more effective against Gram-positive bacteria than Gram-negative bacteria. The presence of an extra outer membrane layer provides additional protection for Gram-negative bacteria.[57] On the other hand, lysozyme offsets this characteristic and has shown antimicrobial activity against Gram-negative bacteria through membrane conformational changes and by disturbing the normal electrostatic interactions between the components of the bacterial cell wall.[143] Therefore, lysozyme is no less effective against Gram-negative bacteria.

Additionally, lysozyme has shown two other antimicrobial mechanisms besides muramic acid cleaving. As previously mentioned, the second mechanism consists of bacterial membrane dysfunction. It occurs when a lysozyme domain binds to the cell membrane based on its cationic and hydrophobic interaction with lipids. This leads to a micelle formation, like lysozyme aggregates, which disrupts the bacterial membrane and increases its permeability.[36,37] The third mechanism involves bacterial genome disintegration, altering the transcription and replication process owing to nucleic acid binding.[38]

As a protection mechanism, bacteria have developed cell membrane glycosylation.[39] Furthermore, previous studies have reported three lysozyme inhibitors, MliC/PliC, PliI/PliG, and Ivy-1. Among these inhibitors, Ivy-1 generally forms a rigid loop, with a moiety containing the amino acids CKPHDC in its sequence, occupying lysozyme's active site and inhibiting the enzyme through a lock and key mechanism.[40] The main role of the highly conserved CKPHDC moiety in the inhibition of lysozyme was validated experimentally through directed mutagenesis. The aspartic residue in the CKPHDC moiety showed a repulsive effect against lysozyme owing to lysozyme's acidic residues in its active site. Alternatively, MliC/PliC blocks lysozyme's active site through a lock mechanism of two conserved regions.[41]

Finally, chemical or physiological modifications of lysozyme have increased its versatility. Proteins such as niacin and lactoferrin as well as organic acids help to complement Gram-negative bacteria growth inhibition through cell membrane weakening.[42,43] Furthermore, coupling lysozyme with hydrophobic peptides enhances the cell membrane penetration capability and can be effectively used to inhibit the growth of Gram-negative bacteria, such as *E. coli*.[44] Similarly, the enhanced antimicrobial activity of lysozyme has also been reported after conjugating lysozyme with polysaccharide.[45] Conjugation of lysozyme with perillaldehyde significantly reduced the growth of both Gram-positive (*S. aureus*) and Gram-negative (*E. coli*) bacteria.[46]

13.2.1.2.2 Ovotransferrin. Among egg white proteins, ovotransferrin is the second most abundant protein. Its physicochemical characteristics have been determined as a 76 kDa monomeric glycoprotein with 686 amino acid residues[47] and a pI of 5.6–6.2.[48] The chemical basis of ovotransferrin's antimicrobial properties correlates with its iron-binding capacity. The growth of microorganisms depends on their uptake of nutrients such as iron from the environment. Therefore, an iron deficiency produced by ovotransferrin can downregulate the microorganism's growth.[49] Owing to this basic mechanism, ovotransferrin-mediated reduction of microbial growth is observed in several viruses, fungi, yeast, Gram-positive bacteria, and Gram-negative bacteria.[50,51] However, ovotransferrin is most effective in preventing the growth of Gram-negative spoilage organisms in egg white.[50,51] Furthermore, induced iron deficiency is not the only antimicrobial mechanism that has been observed in ovotransferrin. A bactericidal effect was observed against

Bacillus cereus, affecting the bacterial membrane's electrochemical potential; which consequently induced membrane dysfunction.[52] Finally, ovotransferrin can form bonds with complementary cations such as sodium bicarbonate and zinc, resulting in improved antimicrobial activity against *E. coli* and *L. monocytogenes*; ovotransferrin with citric acid has shown a synergistic antimicrobial effect on *L. monocytogenes*.[53]

13.2.1.2.3 Ovomucin. Ovomucin is a glycoprotein found in egg white. It accounts for 1.5–3.5% of the total protein in egg white.[54] Besides contributing to egg white's physical characteristics, such as viscosity, ovomucin hydrolysate has been shown to have antiviral and antimicrobial properties. Pronase hydrolysis of β-ovomucin resulted in peptide fractions composed of *O*-glycoproteins with binding affinity for Newcastle Disease Virus (NDV). This interaction occurs through clustered sialic moieties. Sialic acid plays important roles in ovomucin glycopeptides and it has been attributed to influencing the antimicrobial activity against *E. coli* O157:H7. Additionally, polypeptide chains without carbohydrates have been shown to bind anti-ovomucin antibodies.[55] Finally, ovomucin binding mechanisms such as lectin-like interactions and *E. coli* fimbriae binding with sialic acid have neem shown to inhibit *E. coli* O157:H7 hemagglutination activity.[56] However, care must be taken when applying ovomucin for this purpose as heat-treated ovomucin at pH > 6.0 degrades its sialic acid group in the β-subunit while cleaving its inter- and intra-subunit disulfide bonds in the α- and β-subunits.[57]

13.2.1.2.4 Ovalbumin. Ovalbumin is the most abundant protein in egg white, making up 54% of the total egg white proteins.[1,2] It is 45 kDa in size with 386 amino acids residues[47] and a pI of 4.5.[58] Beside the functional properties of the native protein, ovalbumin, specific ovalbumin-derived peptides have shown antimicrobial activity when liberated after enzymatic digestion or fermentation. Previous studies have reported eight different antimicrobial peptides that inhibit the growth of *B. subtilis* and *Candida albicans*. The peptides responsible for the antimicrobial activity obtained from tryptic digestion were SALAM (residues 36–40), SALAMVY (residues 36–42) YPILPEYLQ (residues 111–119), ELINSW (residues 143–148), and NVLQPSS (residues 159–165). Chymotrypsin digestion produced the peptides AEERYPILPEYL (residues 127–138), GIIRN (residues 155–159), and TSSNVMEER (residues 268–276). The observation suggests that ovalbumin may support its host's immune-defense through the antimicrobial properties.[59] The ovalbumin family contains three major proteins with very high similarity in their amino acid sequences; those are ovalbumin, ovalbumin-X (OVAX), and ovalbumin-Y (OVAY). Among them, OVAX exhibits antimicrobial activities against *Listeria monocytogenes* and *Salmonella enterica* sv. Brief details of the antimicrobial activity of OVAX are presented in the minor protein section under ovalbumin-related protein (Section 13.3.7).

13.2.1.3 Egg Yolk Proteins

Egg yolk is composed of molecules that have specific antimicrobial activities to ensure the hen embryo's protection. It acts as the third and final defense line for the embryo. Egg yolk immunoglobulins transfer by passive diffusion through the ovarian follicular membranes and inhibit further microbial contamination.[60] The egg yolk protein phosvitin complements this bioactivity by relying on its serine phosphorylated structure to disrupt microbial cell membranes. Finally, yolk proteins exhibit varied antimicrobial mechanisms of action, which maximizes the embryo's development opportunity. These highlighted properties are considered alternatives to low-efficacy medication and interesting positive results could be seen for resistant bacteria. These effects are contributed by phosvitin, lipovitellin, and lipovitellenin proteins, which constitute 13.4%, 40%, and 37.3%, respectively, of egg yolk proteins.[61]

13.2.1.3.1 Lipovitellin and Lipovitellenin Fraction (High-density and Low-density Lipoproteins). Granules account for 22% of egg yolk composition and 50% of yolk protein.[62,63] Moreover, α- and β-lipovitellins constitute 70% of granule proteins, representing high-density lipoproteins, while 12% of granule proteins are low-density lipoproteins.[61,64] Plasma protein is composed of 85% low-density lipoproteins and 15% livetins.[63,64] Lipoprotein lipid-mediated antimicrobial effects were reported against *Streptococcus* mutants *in vitro*.[65] Additionally, as a result of the high-density lipoprotein protein–lipid complex, previous studies showed an anti-adhesive effect against *Salmonella* spp. and *E. coli* O157:H7.[66] Therefore, egg yolk constitutes a versatile medium capable of countering bacterial invasion with several mechanisms.

13.2.1.3.2 Phosvitin. Phosvitin, well-known for its structure, is derived from vitellogenin I and II. α- and β-phosvitin contain 344 and 223 amino acid residues[67] with molecular weights of 160 and 190 kDa, respectively, and a pI of 4.0. Its amino acids correspond to 50% phosphorylated serine, which confers its mineral-binding ability.[68] This protein configuration enables phosvitin to entrap the iron needed for microbial proliferation and growth,[69] thus exerting antimicrobial properties. For example, antimicrobial activity against *E. coli* and *S. aureus* has been reported under thermal stress at 50 °C, weakening the microbial cell outer membrane through iron and calcium destabilization.[70,71]

13.2.2 Egg Proteins with Antioxidant Activity

Reactive oxygen species (ROS) are oxygen-derived molecules inducing free radical generation in an organism. Similarly, reactive nitrogen species (RNS) are formed through reaction of nitric oxide with oxygen.[72,73] Oxidative stress generated by ROS ends in DNA, RNA, and protein damage. This effect is related to an increased risk for cardiovascular diseases, cancer, autism, and aging.[74–77] Additionally, lipid oxidation in food also leads to food spoilage. Thus, the reduction of the oxidation process can be an effective strategy for improving health and maintaining shelf-life of any food. The main purpose of antioxidants is to slow down the oxidation reactions, through hydrogen donation or lowering the damage of oxidation products by radical scavenging. For this reason, a few recent studies have searched for novel antioxidant peptides with reduced secondary effects through unique chemical and molecular analyses.[72]

13.2.2.1 Egg White Proteins

Ovalbumin has been shown to effectively reduce the oxidation of lipids through glycosylation with the polysaccharide galactomannan. Glycosylation exposed ovalbumin's sulfhydryl groups, therefore enhancing its antioxidant activity by electron donation.[78] Second, ovotransferrin has iron-binding capacity and exhibits its antioxidant property due to its unique molecular structure. Studies proposed that its antioxidant activity could be attributed to its capacity of modulating the cellular redox environment, derived from its N-terminal lobe, which has shown superoxide dismutase activity capable of metal binding.[79] On the other hand, several antioxidant peptides have been identified through mass spectrometry, such as WNIP and GWNI from the N-lobe and C-lobe of ovotransferrin when hydrolyzed by thermolysin.[80] Knowing this amino acid composition helps to foresee a peptide's antioxidant activity since the amino acid composition and peptide molecular weight play a key role in this biological activity. Likewise, the presence of aromatic amino acids and low-molecular-weight peptides has been generally reported to contribute to higher antioxidant activities owing to its higher electron donor capacity. Incidentally, quantification of ovotransferrin's antioxidant capacity has been differentiated between the parent protein and its hydrolysates. While peptides hydrolyzed by thermolysin and pepsin showed 1.69 μmol Trolox equivalent mg^{-1}, natural ovotransferrin achieved 0.2 μmol Trolox equivalent mg^{-1}, both through oxygen radical absorbance capacity (ORAC) assay.[81]

After demonstrating ovotransferrin's antioxidant activity through *in vitro* studies, research extension to a cellular level was necessary. Two of the ovotransferrin-derived peptides, IRW and IQW, exhibited antioxidant activity on human umbilical cord cells (HUVEC). It is important to emphasize that the specific capacities correspond to the specific amino acid contents and structures of these peptides, since the di-peptide configurations of these corresponding tripeptides, did not exert the same antioxidant effect.[82]

Lastly, hen egg white lysozyme has shown antioxidant activity based on its 18 amino acid domain, which binds agents as advanced glycation end-products that generate ROS. The research, based on a mice study, concluded that lysozyme protection against acute and chronic injury mechanisms involves suppression of ROS generation and oxidant stress response genes such as $p66^{Shc}$ and c-Jun.[83]

13.2.2.2 Egg Yolk Proteins

The iron-binding characteristic of phosvitin confers its antioxidant properties. Owing to its metal chelating ability, it can reduce metal-catalyzed lipid oxidation,[84] avoiding peroxide formation. Phosvitin exhibits a higher antioxidant activity for iron-catalyzed phospholipid oxidations up to a 30 : 1 Fe^{2+} to phosvitin molar ratio. Additionally, it was shown that pasteurization temperatures did not reduce phosvitin antioxidant activity, not being so when autoclaved.[85] Phosvitin has been proven to be more effective than ferritin and transferrin for inhibiting hydroxyl formation. This is owing to phosvitin's role in accelerating Fe(II) autoxidation, thus decreasing its availability for participation in the hydroxyl radical generation. As a result, it was shown that phosvitin had a protective effect on DNA against oxidative damage induced by Fe(II) or H_2O_2.[86]

Additionally, phosvitin has been glycosylated with galactomannan polysaccharide to increase its emulsifying activity while obtaining a better antioxidant capacity at different temperatures.[87] This technique enhances its functional properties in food products while maintaining its biological activity. On the other hand, phosvitin peptides hydrolyzed by alcalase enzyme yield two antioxidant peptides with 10 and 15 amino acid residues, containing leucine in their N-terminal as a common denominator. The 15 amino acid residue sequence, LELHKLRSSHWFSRR, showed antioxidant power in the thiobarbituric acid (TBA) assay that was 61% higher than that for α-tocopherol. Therefore, it is regarded that peptides containing histidine may benefit from its radical reducing ability owing to its imidazole ring.[88] After early studies proved phosvitin's antioxidant activity, research focus shifted to its biological activity at a cellular level. Katayama *et al.* observed that phosphorylated phosphopeptides (PPP) induced upregulation of glutathione biosynthesis-associated enzymes such as glutathione reductase and glutathione *S*-transferase, which are regarded as natural radical scavengers. This study laid the groundwork for the phosphopeptides' effect on tissue epithelial cells.[89] As a result, PPP showed successful antioxidant activity after digestion by up-regulating specific antioxidant genes associated with ROS metabolism. This contributed to lower intestinal oxidative stress and promoted gut health by reducing the risk of inflammation associated with ROS.[90]

13.2.3 Egg Proteins with Anti-inflammatory Activity

13.2.3.1 Eggshell Membrane Proteins

Studies have been done on the anti-inflammatory activity of the natural eggshell membrane, prepared through an aqueous extract (NEM-AQ) and *in vitro* digestions (NEM-IVD). NEM-AQ application on peripheral blood mononuclear cells (PBMC) showed lower levels of interleukin-6 (IL-6), IL-10, IFN-c, and tumor necrosis factor-α (TNF-α) when exposed to phytohemagglutinin (PHA), while in the presence of pokeweed mitogen (PWM), it only reduced IL-10 and IL-6 and decreased TNF-α cytokine levels at high dosage. On the other hand, NEM-IVD just reduced TNF-α production induced by PWM at low dosage.[91] Additionally, alcalase- and protease *S*-hydrolyzed eggshell membrane showed *in vitro* inhibition of pro-inflammatory cytokine IL-8 secretion. These studies on anti-inflammatory activities propose ESM as a potential treatment for inflammatory bowel disease.[8] The complementary research assessed the inflammatory arthritis risk reduction through key mediator regulation. As a result, eggshell membrane proteins indicated the reduction of interleukin (IL)-1β (39–44%) and TNF-α (19–32%) pro-inflammatory cytokines as well as monocyte chemotactic protein 1 (MCP-1) (67.3%), macrophage inflammatory protein 1 alpha (MIP-1α) and MIP-1β (88.4%).[92] In a randomized, double-blinded, placebo-controlled trial, supplementation with 500 mg of ESM-derived protein per day significantly reduce both joint pain and stiffness.[93] In another study, intervention using ESM hydrolysates (ESMH) showed anti-inflammatory, anti-wrinkle, and moisture protection activity.[94] The high-molecular-weight fraction (>10 kDa) of ESMH inhibits interferon-gamma (IFN-γ)-induced inflammatory responses.

13.2.3.2 Egg White Proteins

Ovalbumin's potential as an anti-inflammatory protein was observed through *in vitro* TNF-α modulation. This bioactivity is obtained when the protein is modified by methylglyoxal, inducing TNF-α at levels higher than bovine serum albumin (BSA) or RNaseA.[95] Egg white protein ovotransferrin-derived peptides (IRW and IQW) decreased the expression of inflammatory adhesion molecules such as intercellular adhesion molecule 1 (ICAM-1) and vascular cell adhesion molecule 1 (VCAM-1) on vascular tissues.[96] Finally, an immunomodulatory-antihypertensive system connection was fathomed when the IRW anti-inflammatory response by Ang-II downregulation was modulated by the NF-κB pathway, leading to reduced inflammation in vascular smooth muscle cells (VSMC).[97] Hence, this broadens the biological activity and scope of ovotransferrin-derived peptides beyond one specific pathway, showing an interdependence in the human immune and blood pressure systems.

Ovomucin's first anti-inflammatory studies suggested that the O-linked carbohydrate chains exert macrophage stimulating activity, and its structure is an important factor in reducing inflammation in tumor cell line J774.[98] Subsequently, ovomucin desalted peptides, with a molecular weight of < 30 kDa, showed anti-inflammatory activity in human dermal fibroblasts. The anti-inflammatory activity of the ovomucin-derived peptides was identified by TNF-α inhibition mediated through the NF-κB pathway. Furthermore, TNF-α inhibition mediated by ovomucin hydrolysates inhibited ICAM-1 expression in dermal fibroblasts. The importance of peptide composition and molecular weight is highlighted by the low inhibition of > 30 kDa peptides, which were generally lost during desalting.[99]

Lastly, previous studies have indicated that lysozyme inhibits the hemolytic activity of serum complement, at different doses, when tested within the levels present in normal and inflamed breast milk samples.[100] Afterward, studies induced colitis through porcine dextran sodium sulfate (DSS) supplementation and showed that lysozyme significantly reduced the local expression of pro-inflammatory cytokines such as TNF-R, IL-6, IFN-γ, IL-8, and IL-17. On the other hand, it increased the response of anti-inflammatory compounds such as IL-4 and TGF-β. This last mediator along with Foxp3 indicated a role in gut homeostasis restoration by T-cell activation, a regulator of the mucosal immune system.[101]

13.2.3.3 Egg Yolk Proteins

Recent studies have elucidated egg yolk livetins and their peptides' anti-inflammatory properties in LPS-induced RAW 264.7 macrophages. Its pepsin hydrolysates were shown to inhibit nitric oxide (NO) (22.7–39.2%), inducible nitric oxide synthase (iNOS) (58.6–62%), TNF-α (36.9–43.2%), IL-1β (26.1–50.9%), IL-6 (60.4–69.0%), and IL-10. While alcalase hydrolysates inhibited NO, prostaglandin-E2 (PGE2) (30.3%), cyclooxygenase-2 (COX-2) (55.7%), TNF-α, IL-1β, and IL-6. Furthermore, phagocytosis enhancing capacity was observed, supporting its immunomodulatory capacity.[102] Similarly, PPP downregulated pro-inflammatory markers in Caco-2 and HT-29 cells. In this study, inhibition of TNF-α induced IL-8 occurred when cells were treated with a PPP concentration of 1 mg mL^{-1}. Additionally, MCP-1 and IL-12 were inhibited in TNF-α- and LPS-stimulated HT-29 cells while LPS-stimulated macrophages in RAW 264.7 cells presented reduced expression of TNF-α, IL-1b, IL-6, and iNOS.[103]

13.2.4 Egg Proteins with Antihypertensive Activity

Hypertension is a critical risk factor associated with cardiovascular diseases (CVDs). The renin-angiotensin-aldosterone system (RAAS) pathway is one of the major signaling pathways that regulate blood pressure in the human body. The pathway maintains vascular tonicity while regulating extracellular fluid volume and arterial pressure through enzymes and receptors. Renin, secreted in the kidney by juxtaglomerular cells, hydrolyzes angiotensinogen present in the liver, producing angiotensin I (Ang-I). Ang-I is then further cleaved by angiotensin-converting enzyme (ACE) in the lungs, yielding angiotensin II (Ang-II). Upregulation of Ang-II promotes smooth muscle constriction and aldosterone secretion.[104] Finally, secreted aldosterone increases sodium reabsorption through proximal kidney tubules while potassium is lost.[105] This increases water retention, contributing to increased blood pressure. Most of the research has focused on controlling the RAAS pathway as the main factor to control hypertension. Egg proteins have shown an antihypertensive effect primarily by inhibiting the action of the ACE enzyme and modulating the RAAS pathway. Apart from ACE inhibition, egg protein-derived peptides also reduce vascular inflammation, which indirectly helps in maintaining blood pressure. The following subsections briefly describe the different egg proteins that exhibit antihypertensive effects.

13.2.4.1 Egg White Proteins

Egg white has been extensively studied for its antihypertensive and ACE inhibitory proteins. Mostly short egg white protein-derived peptides rather than the whole protein have exhibited antihypertensive activity. Ovalbumin protein and peptides have been observed to inhibit the action of ACE, therefore reducing Ang-II expression and subsequently reducing blood pressure. Ovokinin peptide (FRADHPFL) corresponding to the 358–365 amino acid residues and ovokinin (2–7) peptide (RADHPF) corresponding to the 359–365 amino acid residues of ovalbumin were isolated through peptic and chymotrypsin digestion. They regulated systolic blood pressure in a dose-dependent manner in spontaneously hypertensive rats (SHR).[106] Its antihypertensive activity is related to nitric oxide-mediated vasorelaxation and bradykinin B_2 vascular receptors, as reported in SHR model studies.[107,108] Further studies changed the ovokinin (2–7) antihypertensive activity mechanism after modifications of the C-terminal amino acids arginine and aspartic acid at positions two and three with proline and phenylalanine, respectively. The peptide (Pro^2-Phe^3)-ovokinin (2–7) with the sequence RPFHPF showed a minimum effective dose of 0.3 mg kg^{-1}, equivalent to one-thirtieth of that of ovokinin (2–7).[109,110] Additionally, enzymatic hydrolysis yielded antihypertensive peptides from crude egg white with the amino acid sequences of RADHPFL and YAEEAYPIL[111] containing ACE inhibitory activity IC_{50} values of 6.2 and 4.7 μM, respectively. Cooking methods have been shown to influence the protein activity as studies have shown a reduction in blood pressure with the administration of hydrolyzed fried whole egg, egg white, and defatted egg yolk in an 18 day period SHR model. The result showed a decrease from 170 mm Hg to 154 mm Hg at the end of the trial. Furthermore, nitric oxide-dependent vasorelaxation was achieved with a reduction of angiotensin II levels in plasma.[112]

Finally, previous studies have also elucidated the mechanisms involved in the action of antihypertensive peptides.[113] Some pathways involve the reduction of endothelial inflammation, oxidative stress, vasorelaxation, and Ang-II circulation.[96] For instance, intervention with ovotransferrin-derived peptides presented a reduction of angiotensin II proliferation and smooth cell inflammation[97] and reduced vascular inflammation and nitrotyrosine expression in SHR.[114] Furthermore, another peptide from egg white, RVPSL, was shown to reduce the mRNA level of molecules involved in the renin angiotensin system (RAS), such as renin, ACE, AT1R, and AT2R.[115] Finally, lysozyme peptides hydrolyzed with pepsin showed a strong antihypertensive activity with an IC_{50} of 12.6 μg mL^{-1}. From these, 38 peptides were identified through mass spectrometry, among which some were characterized as antihypertensive peptides, such as KVF, MKR, AMK, AKF, RGY, WIR, VAW, and GIL. Interestingly peptides RGY, WIR, and VAW presented antioxidant activities as well.[116] In conclusion, hypertension regulation is extended beyond ACE inhibition, showing, in some cases, an interdependence and cross-linking in the organism's vasorelaxation mechanisms.[117]

13.2.4.2 Egg Yolk Proteins

Egg yolk hydrolyzed by crude enzymes, containing protease and lipase, lowered systolic and diastolic pressure when administered at a 500 mg kg^{-1} weight dose over a 12 week period.[118] This assessment led to further investigation of the yolk peptide mechanism of reducing blood pressure, which was thought to be *via* ACE inhibition. In addition, a hydrolyzed egg yolk preparation with *Cucurbita ficifolia* enzyme at 1000 U mg^{-1} of yolk hydrolysates also yielded ACE inhibitory peptides. One homogenous and three heterogeneous peptides with 9–18 amino acid residues, mainly containing arginine and leucine at the N-terminal region, were obtained. From these, peptide LAPSLPGKPKPD showed ACE inhibitory activity with an IC_{50} of 1.97 µmol L^{-1}.[16] Similarly, egg yolk apovitellenin-I-derived peptide sequence YIEAVNKVSPRAGQF showed ACE inhibitory properties with an IC_{50} value of 5.6 µmol L^{-1}.[119] These active peptide sequences were identified after ethanol extraction of phospholipids, and the ACE inhibitory abilities of these peptides are highly comparable to that of the synthetic ACE inhibitor captopril.[120] Its capacity to regulate blood pressure makes it a potential alternative for current treatments.

13.2.5 Egg Proteins with Anticancer Activity

Actual trends indicate cancer as one of the leading mortality causes worldwide. However, studies have shown a trend of 26% lower death rates in the last 20 years from this disease.[121] This positive trend has been possible owing to extensive research and more equalitarian treatment throughout the population of the United States. Additionally, healthy lifestyles, including the consumption of healthy foods, such as functional foods, could contribute to maintaining this trend. Therefore, promising anticancer benefits could be obtained under specific circumstances if egg consumption is included in people's diet. The following sub-sections describe several egg proteins, occasionally present in functional foods, that have shown anticancer bioactivity.

13.2.5.1 Egg White Proteins

Heat-denatured ovalbumin has shown anti-mutagenic activity against *N*-methyl-*N*′-nitro-*N*-nitroguanidine. However, it was shown that not only heat treatment confers the protein bioactivity as pepsin and pancreatin hydrolysis also exhibits anti-mutagenic proteins from both heated and unheated ovalbumin.[122] Thus, gastrointestinal digestion is as important in increasing ovalbumin's anti-mutagenic activity. The second most abundant protein in egg white, ovotransferrin, showed anticancer properties by a thiol-linked auto-cleaving mechanism when it was in reduced form. Once peptides were obtained, they induced cytotoxicity in colon cancer cells (HTC-116) by apoptosis induction in a dose-dependent manner.[123] Furthermore, ovotransferrin protein and peptides showed 90% cytotoxicity to a cervix cancer cell line at a dose of 10 mg mL^{-1} and 95% growth inhibition in a stomach cancer cell line in further studies.[50] Overall, these results support the ovotransferrin peptide's ability to control imbalanced cell proliferation in tumors.

The first studies identifying lysozyme's anticancer activity were realized in 1991 and 1995, where lysozyme was demonstrated to reduce mice lung carcinoma metastases through a proposed mechanism of spleen and macrophage activation. As a consequence, lysozyme activated the host's immune system, increasing the efficacy of current cancer treatments.[124,125]

Finally, the egg white ovomucin structure contains glycosylated glycoproteins with disulfide bonds between its α- and β-subunits. This structure has been linked to its biological activity as an anticancer protein. Previous studies investigated its anticancer activity by pronase-treated hydrolysis on induced tumors of BALB/c mice. The obtained peptides of 220 and 120 kDa decreased the tumor growth and increased the response of serum immunosuppressive protein, indicating a parallel response of the immune system. Furthermore, it was determined that sialic acid could have an important role in avoiding the regression of tumors.[126] Yokota *et al.* described the different effects of ovomucin subunits against tumors. The β-subunit yields a cytotoxic effect on sarcoma-180 (SR-180) cells in a dose-dependent manner (5 mg kg^{-1} of body weight) over a period, resulting in degenerated and necrotic tumor cells. In contrast, SR-180 cells treated with α-subunits remained unaffected.[127] The determined mechanism suggested growth inhibition of SR-180 through basic fibroblast growth factor receptor (bFGFR) and its interaction with ovomucin β-subunits.[128]

13.2.5.2 Egg Yolk Proteins

Phosvitin's previously discussed antioxidant activity has been linked to its anticancer biological activity. Studies have indicated that consumption of egg yolk hydrolysates reduces the risk of colorectal cancer in rats.[129] Besides, studies on cellular responses demonstrated that glutathione (GLH) biosynthesis enzymes were upregulated by γ-glutamylcysteine owing to the dosage of phosvitin peptides.[14,89,118] Additionally, endogenous antioxidant enzymes such as catalase and glutathione reductase were increased by phosvitin peptides, which suggests that they could be considered as anticancer peptides. Recent studies have included cervix (HeLa), breast (MCF-7), stomach (AGS), lung (A549 and SK-MES-1), liver (HepG2), and larynx (Hep-2) cancer cell lines. Such results reported phosvitin's IC_{50} on cancer cells to fall in the range of 3.93–11.82 mg mL^{-1}.[130] Finally, the protective effect of phosvitin on human leukocytes suggests that it is a promising source of anticancer agents.

13.2.6 Immunomodulatory Activity of Egg Proteins

An organism's immune system protects the organism itself from bacteria, fungi, viruses, protozoans, and cancer cells. This system is divided into two subcategories, which are innate and adaptive immunity. Innate immunity is composed of the physiological, cellular, anatomical, and anti-inflammatory components protecting against these threats. Further, innate cellular immunity relies on natural killer (NK) cells, regulating tumors and virus-infected cells as well as macrophages and neutrophils with their phagocytosis roles. Therefore, this immunity category assesses general and recurrent infections to which the organism is exposed to in daily situations. Next, adaptive immunity consists of the gained immunity against specific organisms through consequent exposure. It is a more specific type of immunity against foreign antigens. Adaptive immunity is further divided into cell-mediated immunity, secreting immunomodulatory factors such as cytokines, and antibody-mediated immunity which produces antibodies to bind pathogens' antigens, consequently killing them *via* macrophages.[131] Research has indicated that innate and adaptive immune systems are dependent on each other, achieving a defense response together against the antigen of interest, and an imbalance among the two leads to a higher probability of chronic disease development.[132] Inflammatory responses occurring owing to this imbalance have been linked to obesity, diabetes, hypertension, and cancer.[72] Hence, the correct functioning of people's immune system is of high interest to reduce the risk of chronic diseases. The following sub-sections elucidate the egg proteins that induce immunomodulatory activities.

13.2.6.1 Egg White Proteins

Ovotransferrin has shown *in vitro* immunomodulatory activity by modulating macrophage and heterophil functions in HD11 cells and blood-isolated heterophils.[133] Additionally, mouse *in vivo* studies showed that ovotransferrin protein interaction inhibited spleen lymphocyte proliferation solely, not attributable to a function of iron transport or mitogen inactivation.[134] Moreover, reports detailed that ovotransferrin enhanced the phagocytic response of mononuclear and polynuclear cells in dogs, possibly mediated by active humoral substances produced by mononuclear cells.[135] Secondly, ovomucoid's immunomodulatory activity has been linked to its binding activity to IgG and IgE antibodies. In addition, food preparation influences the magnitude of the antibody response. For example, studies reported that ovomucoid binding to human IgG antibody was reduced when it was partially denatured by heat or modified by carboxymethylation. The results suggested that anti-ovomucoid antibodies recognized conformational and sequential epitopes, such that ovomucoid was a dominant allergen for IgE antibodies of anaphylaxis patients.[136] Further studies indicated that charged and hydrophobic amino acids were important for antibody binding, contributing to the information required for molecular design and ovomucoid allergenicity reduction.[137]

Ovomucin protein has shown immunomodulatory activity by stimulating macrophage, H_2O_2, and IL-1 generation. Ovomucin peptide digest induced immunomodulatory activity at a concentration of 100 μg mL^{-1}. Moreover, the O-linked sulfated carbohydrate chains were identified as the active components responsible for this function.[98]

Finally, the immunomodulatory activity of egg lysozyme has been proven on chronic diseases. For instance, chronic bronchitis had a lower impact owing to lysozyme activity in humoral and cellular response normalization.[138] Similarly, the clinical effects of allergy in children with chronic sinusitis tended to be better when immunotherapy included lysozyme protein.[139] Further, studies reported that lysozyme stimulates immunoglobulin production in human–human hybridoma line, HB4C5 cells and human peripheral blood lymphocytes. In this case, IgM production was enhanced in transcription-suppressed HB4C5 cells treated with actinomycin D, suggesting that lysozyme accelerates the translational process to enhance immunoglobulin production.[140] In addition, post-translationally modified peptides, by nitration of tyrosine and modified tryptophan in the T-cell contact residues, enabled CD4+ T cells to recognize and bind to class II histocompatibility molecule I-Ak.[141] This effect was further studied in type A and B T-cell subsets, which were able to recognize distinct configurations in the dominant epitope of hen lysozyme presented by I-Ak. Besides, human leukocyte antigen-DM (H2-DM) was shown to act as a conformational editor, excluding type B configuration in the late endosomes.[142]

13.2.7 Protease Inhibitory Activity of Egg Proteins

Proteases are enzymes responsible for protein hydrolysis in the host organism through peptidyl bond cleavage. Consequently, the host's damaged tissue and a limited immune system response favor microbial development. For this reason, organisms develop protection systems that minimize the degradation effect of these molecules. Egg contains such protease inhibitors, whose activity exerts a reduction in the proteolytic degradation of egg proteins.[143] Egg proteins with protease inhibitory activity include ovomucoid, cystatin, ovoinhibitor, ovostatin, and serpin 10.

13.2.7.1 Eggshell Membrane Proteins

Recent studies have shown the presence of two protease inhibitor proteins in the eggshell membrane named serpin 10 and ovocalyxin-36. Serpin 10 corresponds to the serine protease inhibitor family responsible for the proteolytic activity in an organism, such as angiogenesis and embryogenesis.[4] Moreover, a protein's protease inhibitor activity is associated with antimicrobial properties by altering the microorganism's metabolism. This effect reduces the microorganism's nutrient uptake by inhibiting it to metabolize complex proteins into simple amino acids. As an example, ovocalyxin-36's antimicrobial property was associated with its carboxypeptidase inhibition, a protease necessary for microbial development.[29]

13.2.7.2 Egg White Proteins

Egg proteases are encountered mainly in the egg white. Firstly, ovomucoid has exhibited inhibitory activity against serine proteases. Research has characterized ovomucoid's structure and established the structure–function relationship between ovomucoid's domain 3 and its protease inhibition property. Additionally, substitution of ovomucoid's P1 site alanine with methionine or lysine gave an increase in chymotrypsin or trypsin inhibition.[144] Such studies have confirmed that, besides the P1 site amino acid composition, the electrostatic properties of the amino acid residues around the protease inhibitor's reactive site influence the degree to which it inhibits proteases. The amino acid arginine at the P3′ site of the chymotrypsin inhibitor was required for leucine and methionine to be recognized as a P1 site. Similarly, non-charged residues around the reactive site of the trypsin inhibitor were needed to highlight the P1 site's positive charge.[145] Furthermore, studies have reported reduced degradation by proteolytic enzymes when ovomucoid is incorporated. Intravenous ovomucoid particularly, at levels of 16 300 ATU kg^{-1} 24 h^{-1}, reduced trypsin-like activity and trypsinogen activation peptide in an experimental pancreatitis rat model, preserving the organism's pancreas.[146] For this reason, ovomucoid trypsin inhibition has been extended for drug delivery purposes. Calcitonin, a polypeptide promoting bone formation and homeostasis, has shown enhanced oral delivery through trypsin and elastase inhibition when administered along with ovomucoid.[147]

Second, ovoinhibitor is a Kazal-type serine protease that represents 1.5% of egg white proteins and is secreted in the hen oviduct after being stimulated by estrogen and progesterone.[148] It has a molecular weight of 49 kDa and a 5–10% carbohydrate content through the *N*-glycoside bond. Like ovomucoid, ovoinhibitor exhibits multiple domains with a characteristic pattern of disulfide bridges. On the other hand, ovoinhibitor differs by being able to inhibit a wide spectrum of proteinases.[149] Previous studies have determined its protease inhibitor activity against serine proteases.

The highest activity was observed for trypsin and subtilisin. In contrast, low protease inhibition was observed against chymotrypsin.[150] This characteristic plays a significant role in egg's antibacterial defense, preventing contamination while protecting the embryo development.[143] Ovoinhibitor from different egg sources, such as quail, showed inhibition of concanavalin A- and phytohemagglutinin-induced proliferative responses of mouse splenocytes and immunoglobulin production.[151] Moreover, mouse and quail T and B lymphocyte responses were modulated by inhibiting its enzymatic activity. Even though ovoinhibitor is regarded as a potential protease inhibitor, its application is jeopardized by its stability at alkaline pH.[152] Efforts to compensate for this trait include a polysaccharide conjugation through a Maillard reaction with galactomannan, obtaining improved heat stability as well as emulsifying properties.[153]

13.2.8 Biospecific Ligand Activity

13.2.8.1 Egg White Proteins

The biospecific ligand activity enhances an active ingredient or compound's interaction with an organism's cells or tissue through affinity enhancement or degradation prevention. For instance, a glycoprotein–ovomucoid polymeric hydrogel increased absorption of a protein drug in the bloodstream by acting as a biospecific ligand to the gastrointestinal wall lectins. As a secondary benefit, the drug was protected from proteolytic enzymes, preventing its degradation.[154] Additionally, ovomucoid doubled the influx of insulin within the rat jejunum; offering an alternative to enhance insulin oral delivery.[155]

Second, ovomucin protein was found to reduce *in vitro* cholesterol uptake in Caco-2 cells by reducing micellar cholesterol solubility. Similarly, *in vivo* studies reported major cholesterol and bile excretion in a rat model study, reporting lower serum cholesterol levels with lower cholesterol concentrations in the liver. The study results convey that the interaction between cholesterol mixed micelles and ovomucin was realized in the jejunal epithelia, leading to downregulation of cholesterol absorption. Moreover, ovomucin can also inhibit the reabsorption of bile acids in the ileum, thus lowering the serum cholesterol level.[156]

13.3 Bioactivities of Minor Egg Proteins

Proteins in both egg white and yolk are distributed in distinctive proportions, thus, enabling characterization of its several proteins based on quantification and percentage composition. Minor proteins are classified by their low presence in both yolk and egg white, in contrast with major proteins. The following sub-sections highlight the bioactivity of some minor proteins from egg white and egg yolk.

13.3.1 Ovoglobulin

In general, globulin type proteins are sensitive to heat denaturation and are soluble only in low concentrations of salt solution. Globulins' classification as G1, G2, and G3 is derived from their electrophoretic mobility differences. G1 has been regarded as a lysozyme based on its egg white abundance, isoelectric point, and electrophoretic mobility.[157] For this reason, ovoglobulin is a synonym of ovoglobulin G2 and G3, the primary sequences for which remain to be characterized.[157] Ovoglobulin G2 is assumed to constitute 1–4% of the egg white proteins,[1,157,158] with a molecular weight of 49 kDa and a pI of 5.5 and 5.8 for G2 and G2, respectively.[159] However, ovoglobulin G2 presents polymorphism in the chicken egg, leading to its sequencing. G2 sequencing reported G2 to be identical to transiently expressed in neural precursor (TENP) protein, with the polymorphism attributed to an amino acid substitution.[157] Its functional properties are related to its foaming capacity, which attracts interest for commercial application in industry.[158] Studies have shown that ovoglobulins aid ovalbumin and ovomucin in forming a high-viscosity foam while diminishing the liquid drainage from the matrix.[159] Furthermore, ovoglobulin represent a potential research area as its biological and food chemical functions have not been completely elucidated.[157]

13.3.2 Ovoglycoprotein

Ovoglycoprotein constitutes only 1% of egg white proteins.[1,160,161] It contains 13.6% hexose, 13.8% hexosamine, and 3% sialic acid. Hexose constitutes mannose and galactose in the ratio 2 : 1, with hexosamine constituted as glucosamine and sialic acid as *N*-acetylneuraminic acid. Its molecular weight is 24.4 kDa, with an isoelectric point of 3.9.[160] Ovoglycoprotein is used as a chiral selector owing to its excellent chiral recognition ability, in contrast with chicken ovomucoid. Therefore, its potential for drug enantiomer separation through HPLC or capillary electrophoresis has been recognized. On the other hand, its biological function is still to be elucidated.[162,163]

13.3.3 Ovoflavoproteins

Ovoflavoproteins constitute 0.8% of egg white proteins with an isoelectric point of 4.0 and a molecular weight of 32 kDa. The protein structure is arranged in two domains: the riboflavin-binding site, located at the N-terminal (residues 1–170) and a negatively charged amino acid portion with ten glutamyl residues located in the C-terminal.[164] All 18 cysteine residues in ovoflavoprotein are convoluted in nine disulfide bridges, awarding stability to the protein structure at high temperatures.[165] The riboflavin-binding domain is a 20 Å wide and 15 Å deep hydrophobic cleft containing five out of the six tryptophan residues present in the protein.

Previous studies showed that 1 mole of ovoflavoprotein binds 1 mole of riboflavin.[166,167] As a result, no free flavin was present in the egg white.[168] Additionally, modification of one of the carbohydrates in its structure, composed of fucose, mannose, galactose, *N*-acetylglucosamine, and sialic acid, resulted in a decrease of its riboflavin-binding capacity.[169,170] Finally, ovoflavoprotein has been reported to suppress sweet and bitter flavors by its interaction with sweet and bitter taste receptors present in the tongue.[171,172]

13.3.4 Ovomacroglobulin

Ovomacroglobulin, a minor protein in egg white, is a macroglobulin-like protease inhibitor with four subunits of 195 kDa linked by disulfide bonds. It has been shown to reduce the proteolytic effect of cysteine, serine, and aspartic proteases, and metalloproteases. Studies have elucidated the inhibitory effect against Gram-negative *S. marcescens*' 56K, 60K, and 73K proteases, as well as thermolysin and alkaline protease by 55 to 75% in a 20 min period. Moreover, research has determined its anti-protease activity towards trypsin, papain, subtilisin, and thermolysin under different conditions.[173] Even though early studies stated that ovomacroglobulin did not exhibit protease inhibition activity, in the presence of substrates such as Nα-Benzoyl-L-arginine 4-nitroanilide hydrochloride (BAPNA) and casein ovomacroglobulin showed anti-protease activity towards trypsin.[174] As previously mentioned, protease inhibition relates to ovomacroglobulin's antimicrobial effect, which has also been proven against Gram-positive microorganisms, such as *P. aeruginosa*.[175] Furthermore, *in vivo* studies found that ring abscess in guinea pig cornea owing to *P. aeruginosas* strain IFO 3455 was significantly inhibited when ovomacroglobulin was applied. Its protease inhibitor activity enables migration of polymorphonuclear leukocytes to the central lesion, which is otherwise prevented by *P. aeruginosas*' elastase, *Pseudomonas*' endotoxin, and endotoxin A.[176] Lastly, ovomacroglobulin's immunomodulatory activity has been shown when applied to accelerated fibroblast growth, collagen deposition, and capillary formation in granulation tissue. These results indicated that ovomacroglobulin could be a useful healing promoter for flap surgery.[177]

13.3.5 Cystatin

Hen egg cystatin protein is a type 2 cystatin within the cystatin superfamily. It has about 115 amino acids, two disulfide bonds, and no carbohydrate presence with a molecular weight of 12.7 kDa.[178] Cystatin protein is an inhibitor of lysosomal cysteine proteases, such as cathepsins, and plant proteases, such as papain, actinidin, and ficin. This function protects the organism from endogenous and exogenous cysteine proteases. Cystatin's mechanism of action involves tight equimolar complexes through hydrophobic interactions with a low dissociation constant of 20 nM–10 fM, blocking the active site of proteinases. The crystal structures of cystatin and cystatin–papain complex have three contact regions acting as binding sites to form complementary wedge-shaped edges on the inhibitor. These insert swiftly into the active site cleft of papain with minimal conformational change.[179,180] Initial studies determined the antimicrobial activity of cystatin against *P. gingivalis*, *A. lwoffii*, *E. coli*, *Oligella* sp. and *P. aeruginosa*.[181,182] Consequently, it was shown that cathepsin B cysteine protease activity was reduced by 50% at a concentration cystatin of 120 μg mL^{-1} after 2 h incubation.[182] Furthermore, cystatin has shown immunomodulatory activity using the host's response through the cytokine network. It upregulated the production of IL-6 by two human gingival fibroblast cell lines or murine splenocytes and IL-8 production by gingival fibroblasts at physiological concentrations. However, the papain-inhibitory site was not involved in the cytokine-inducing activity.[183] Moreover, cystatin protein induced synthesis of TNF-α and IL-10, stimulating the production of nitric oxide by interferon-γ-activated or mouse peritoneal macrophages.[184] Recently, studies indicated a relationship between cystatins and pathological conditions by playing a role in cancer development,[185] through inhibition of endogenous cysteine peptidase, such as cathepsin B. In cancer, the peptidase inhibitor balance is altered, leading to harmful degradation of the extracellular matrix.[186] This phenomenon has been found in malignant progression of human tongue cancer, where exogenous addition of cystatin to the patient's sera effectively reduced cathepsin B activities.[187] Furthermore, cathepsin inhibition was shown in human breast epithelial cells and gastric tissues, decreasing by 18-fold the cathepsins activity after treatment with 5 nM of purified egg cystatin in the latter.[188,189] Application of cystatin, however, may involve off-target side effects as they inhibit all cysteine peptidases nonselectively.[186]

13.3.6 Avidin

Avidin is a glycoprotein present in egg white that was first noted for the antinutritive effect given by its biotin binding.[190] Its molecular structure is a basic tetrameric glycoprotein composed of four identical subunits, each containing 128 amino acids with molecular weights of 15 and 15.8 kDa, giving a final molecular weight of 66–69 kDa.[191] Each subunit has a disulfide bond between Cys4 and Cys83. Furthermore, avidin's carbohydrate moiety consists of a single oligosaccharide chain with four or five mannose and three *N*-acetylglucosamine residues per subunit linked to Asp17 of the polypeptide chain.[180,192] The avidin–biotin interaction is a noncovalent protein–ligand interaction with a dissociation constant of 10^{-15} M^{-1}. This strong interaction has been used in systems such as bacteriophage inactivation, gene and cellular mapping, macromolecule immobilization, cell-selective absorption, and quantitative enzyme immunoassay.[193] Additionally, avidin's biotin-binding property has gained interest in food safety as a natural compound to control the microbial growth of microorganisms that rely on this essential vitamin for growth.[194] Studies have shown that *E. coli K-12, K. pneumoniae, S. marcescens, P. aeruginosa, S. aureus*, and *Staphylococcus epidermidis* were inhibited by avidin's binding ability to Gram-negative and positive bacterial cells.[195] Moreover, its heparin–sepharose binding suggests an alternative antimicrobial role by attaching to the phospholipid layer of certain microorganisms.[196]

Next, avidin's anticancer activity has been shown through tumor pre-targeting, which improved TNF's antitumor effect with systematically administered biotin–TNF conjugates by at least five-fold. This antitumor effect was related to indirect mechanisms, such as the host-mediated response.[197] Further, reported avidin-driven tumor bridging was shown to be essential for T-cell specificity and activity on murine tumors WEHI-164 fibrosarcoma and RMA lymphoma as it delayed tumor growth at the early stages.[198] Finally, avidin-biospecific ligand activity has been shown as the avidin–biotin system enables chimeric peptide coupling with a blood–brain barrier drug transport vector. This alternative allows a high-yield coupling of any biotinylated therapeutic, facilitating its delivery to the brain.[199]

13.3.7 Ovalbumin-related Protein X and Y Fragment (OVAX/OVAY)

The ovalbumin-expressing gene in egg contains three genes present in a 46 kb locus of chromosome 2, being: ovalbumin, ovalbumin-related protein Y (OVAY), and ovalbumin-related protein X (OVAX). These genes are expressed by the influenced of estrogen, but their protein concentrations in egg are distinctive. OVAX along with ovalbumin does not express protease inhibition, unlike OVAY, based on the consensus sequence for inhibitory serpins. However, OVAX interacts with heparin, a glycosaminoglycan, through an uncovered domain containing a positive charge in the outer part of the molecule. OVAY's further functions are still to be elucidated, but new studies suggest a relevant impact on embryonic development. Finally, OVAX has demonstrated antibacterial activity against *L. monocytogenes* and *S. enteritidis*.[200] Its mechanism adopts different modes of action besides the peptide's heparin interaction, which evidence suggests aids the host's defense against pathogens.

13.3.8 Ovosecretoglobin

A minor egg protein named ovosecretoglobin with a 7 kDa molecular mass has a 40–48% similar sequence to mammalian secretoglobins. It is the first non-mammalian compound of the secretoglobin/uteroglobin family. Previous studies have shown that some of these family members bind steroids. However, its function is still unknown. It has been concluded that its concentration is at least similar to those for avidin or cystatin.[201]

13.3.9 TENP

Initial studies identified a gene transiently expressed in neural precursors (tenp), whose mRNA was detected in the developing retina and brain of embryonic chicks while being absent in the heart, kidney, or liver. Additionally, tenp gene expression might be involved in an early neurogenic event after terminal mitosis, not being specific for a particular developmental stage.[202] The gene-expressed protein, TENP, was immunodetected in membrane fractions, suggesting it might be a membrane protein. Consequently, TENP protein was shown to have strong homology to bacterial permeability-increasing protein family (BPI) and VMO-1, an outer layer vitelline membrane protein. This homology suggests that TENP could participate in the antibacterial activity, which is yet to be confirmed experimentally. Its content is between 0.1–0.5% of egg proteins.[203] Recent studies had reported ovoglobulin G2 sequencing as identical to TENP, also known as BPI-fold containing family B.[157]

13.3.10 Other Minor Egg Proteins

Hep21 protein in egg white was first identified through 2D-PAGE, protein spot 71, and polymerase chain reaction (PCR) cloning. It is composed of 106 amino acids with a cysteine spacing pattern, being a member of the uPAR/CD59/Ly-6/snake neurotoxin superfamily. Hep21 is predominantly expressed in the oviduct and especially the magnum.[204] Studies elucidated significant differences among hep21 content in egg whites of vitamin-enriched, lutein-enriched, and organic eggs compared to white-shell eggs.[205] A protein similar to acyloxyacyl hydrolase has been identified in egg with 62% sequence homology to the mammalian counterpart. Its structure consists of two disulfide-bonded subunits, and the identified peptides of the chicken egg white enzyme were from these subunits. Mammalian acyloxyacyl hydrolase cleaves acyl chains from bacterial lipopolysaccharides (LPS), abolishing the effect of these toxic bacterial products. Lymphocyte antigen 86 (MD-1) is a 17 kDa extracellular protein detected in the eggshell membrane matrix while occurring in egg white at high concentration. It has been found to be involved in triggering cellular response to LPS. Furthermore, its function in the egg white is not clear as its effect takes place in a complex with protein RP105. Next, a 74 kDa protein was found in a proteomic analysis of egg whose homology relates to human and mouse M130, which suggests its involvement in the clearance of hemoglobin–haptoglobin complexes and the clearance of iron. Similarly, an egg protein homologous to protein PIT 54 was found with a 60% sequence homology. Such a protein has been found in chicken serum and eggshell matrix. Finally, a protein like oncoprotein-induced transcript 1 was identified with a 59% sequence homology to FAM3D; belonging to the cytokine-like family proteins. Intracellular proteins present in egg white include ubiquitin, histones, HMG-1, and glutathione *S*-transferase.[201]

13.4 Novel Bioactivities of Egg Proteins

13.4.1 Adipogenic Differentiating Peptides from Egg White

Adipose tissue's role in lipid and glucose metabolism has been determined by the effect of insulin on differentiation of pre-adipocytes and mature adipocytes, which secretes anti-inflammatory adipokines, through PPARγ (peroxisome proliferator associated receptor gamma). However, RAS-mediated insulin resistance promotes adipose dysfunction and lowers glucose uptake. On the other hand, angiotensin receptor blockers increase adipose tissue insulin-stimulated glucose uptake by enhanced PPARγ expression. Hydrolyzed ovalbumin and ovotransferrin yielded adipogenic differentiating peptides. It is suggested that Asp, Leu, and Lys in ovalbumin sequences WEKAFKDED, QAMPFRVTEQE, ERYPIL, and VFKGL increased pre-adipocyte PPARγ expression, leading to adequate mature adipocyte differentiation and glucose uptake.[206]

13.4.2 Calcium-binding Activity of Phosvitin

Previous studies on phosvitin have elucidated its capacity to avoid the formation of insoluble calcium complexes, an ability attributed to its phosphorylated serine in the polypeptide structure. When tryptic digested phosvitin was obtained, an increase in its calcium-binding ability was reported with 14.2 ppm Ca^{+2} per 600 mg of solubilized phosvitin. PPP's ability to weakly bind Ca^{+2} molecules enables the body to absorb it, obtaining high *in vivo* calcium absorption.[207] Recent studies on MG-63 cells have shown the effect of egg yolk-derived peptides by increasing MG-63 cell proliferation, collagen synthesis, and calcium deposition. It was observed that ERK1/2 activation by egg yolk peptides induced ELK1 phosphorylation, suggesting that ELK1 is a mediator of osteogenic gene expression upregulation in MG-63 cells.[208] Finally, egg yolk-derived peptides showed an anti-osteoporotic effect by maintaining bone mineral density for 6 months in a group of 65 perimenopausal women. It is suggested that supplementation with a 100 mg dose could enable the consumer to benefit from its anti-resorptive and anti-fracture effects on bones.[209] Therefore, its use and implementation as a nutraceutical ingredient hold potential benefits for consumers searching to reduce the risk and suffering of osteoporosis.

13.5 Egg Allergenic Proteins

Despite the high nutritional quality of egg proteins, it has been shown that egg proteins can trigger allergic reactions in infants and children. The reactions take place in the nose and throat, which could lead to anaphylaxis, and are detected by IgE-mediated symptoms. Ten egg allergens have been identified, the major ones being ovalbumin, ovomucoid, ovotransferrin, and lysozyme.[210] Additionally, yolk allergens include chicken serum albumin and YGB 42. Egg allergy is developed through raw and cooked egg consumption. However, cooking methods decrease the allergenic response of patients, even when the protein allergy is not dependent on heat and enzyme resistance. Studies indicated that continuous exposure to cooked eggs is associated with allergy tolerance through immunological changes similar to the changes observed for raw eggs.[211] The changes include an increase in IgG4 levels and a reduction in egg white-specific skin prick testing.[212]

13.5.1 Egg White Allergenic Proteins

Ovomucoid is categorized as one of the principal allergens in egg white, being a serine protease inhibitor glycoprotein. The molecular structure of ovomucoid consists of nine disulfide bonds and no free sulfhydryl groups with three tandem domains, homologous to pancreatic secretory trypsin inhibitor (Kazal-type).[58] On the other hand, ovomucoid's putative reactive site for trypsin inhibition is limited to the second domain. It has been suggested that the structure of the IgE-binding epitopes of ovomucoid, which correspond to amino acids 4–20, 46–59, and 91–104, is linear owing to its resistance to heat and proteinase activity.[212,213] Therefore, heat treatment up to 100 °C under acidic conditions does not display a relevant change in ovomucoid's physical or chemical properties.[58]

Second, ovalbumin, being the most abundant egg protein (54%) in egg white, is responsible for egg allergic reactions and hypersensitivity. It is suggested that anti-ovalbumin IgE primarily recognizes linear epitopes rather than conformational epitopes. This is owing to ovalbumin's IgE-binding capacity, which has been shown to remain unaffected by heat denaturation (95 °C), urea treatment, and carboxymethylation.[214] On the other hand, it has been shown that digestive enzymes might reduce its allergenicity. Moreover, ovalbumin belongs to the protein serpin family, characterized by protease inhibition. However, this activity is absent in ovalbumin owing to the serpin conformational change in the reactive center loop of ovalbumin.[212,215]

Third, the role of ovotransferrin's carbohydrate moiety in its allergenic activity is controversial. In addition to ovotransferrin's natural glycosylation, a relevant modification occurs between non-reducing sugars and specific protein amino acids induced by heat, giving a Maillard reaction. This reaction is suggested to introduce neoantigens and affect its allergic activity.[216,217] Therefore, it is suggested that cooking methods may induce allergic reaction hypersensitivity.[212]

Finally, lysozyme's allergic activity was shown through sera obtained from patients who reacted to egg ingestion. Lysozyme sensitization studies reported that 35% of egg-allergic patients had anti-lysozyme IgE, suggesting its inclusion in food labels as a potential allergen.[218] However, lysozyme is a weak allergen, suggested to be denatured by boiling temperatures.[219] Owing to the occurrence of lysozyme in foods and pharmaceutical products, it is an important target in egg allergy research.[212]

13.5.2 Egg Yolk Allergenic Proteins

Chicken serum albumin has been regarded as an egg yolk allergen as IgE from patients with bird-egg syndrome identifies the 70 kDa chicken serum albumin or α-livetin. Therefore, it was suggested that chicken serum albumin leads to cross-sensitization and bird-egg syndrome.[220] Initial sensitization to egg yolk proteins induces respiratory allergic symptoms. Therefore, serum albumin has been confirmed as an inhalant allergen through bronchial provocation.[212] Regarding its allergenicity, serum albumin's allergic activity was reduced by 88% after a 90 °C heat treatment for 30 min. Finally, ELISA inhibition indicated that only partial cross-reactivity between chicken albumin and conalbumin had occurred.[221]

Second, egg yolk glycoprotein 42, a vitellogenin-1 precursor, has recently been characterized as a secondary egg yolk allergen. Previous research showed that the 35 kDa protein induced an allergic reaction in 18% of the patients involved in the study. In addition, denaturation methods such as heating and reduction treatments did not affect its allergic activity. On the other hand, proteolytic digestion did diminish the IgE-binding capacity of the allergen. This new egg yolk allergen has been identified as Gal d 6.[222]

13.6 Conclusion

Protein's value has now been extended beyond its nutritional contribution. Besides providing the organism's building blocks, it has now been shown to interact with several systems in the human body and can exhibit physiological effects. Nowadays, increased demand for functional and nutraceutical foods has put egg proteins and protein-derived peptides in the spotlight. Along with egg being a dietary source of all essential amino acids, consumption of egg proteins has been proven to have beneficial effects both *in vitro* and, in some cases, *in vivo*. Some of these include antihypertensive and antimicrobial activity as the most well-known, but new biological activities continue to arise.[206] However, more often than not, a complete understanding of these effects in an organism's pathways is not achieved, even though past unknowns have been clarified. Consequently, a better application of egg compounds will be accomplished as further studies continue to enlighten current gaps in the area.

References

1. J. Kovacs-Nolan, M. Phillips and Y. Mine, *J. Agric. Food Chem.*, 2005, **53**, 8421.
2. Y. Mine, *World's Poult. Sci. J.*, 2002, **58**, 31.
3. N. E. Ward, in *Egg Innovations and Strategies for Improvements*, ed. P. Y. Hester, Academic Press, San Diego, 2017, p. 207.
4. C. M. M. Cordeiro and M. T. Hincke, *J. Proteomics*, 2016, **130**, 11.
5. J. L. Arias, M. S. Fernandez, J. E. Dennis and A. I. Caplan, *Connect. Tissue Res.*, 1991, **26**, 37.
6. V. K. Kodali, S. A. Gannon, S. Paramasivam, S. Raje, T. Polenova and C. Thorpe, *PLoS One*, 2011, **6**, 1.
7. Y. Shi, J. Kovacs-Nolan, B. Jiang, R. Tsao and Y. Mine, *J. Funct. Foods*, 2014, **11**, 571.
8. Y. Shi, P. Rupa, B. Jiang and Y. Mine, *Int. J. Mol. Sci.*, 2014, **15**, 22728.
9. H. Jia, W. Aw, K. Saito, M. Hanate, Y. Hasebe and H. Kato, *Sci. Rep.*, 2014, **4**, 1.
10. G. H. Farjah, B. Heshmatian, M. Karimipour and A. Saberi, *Iran. J. Basic Med. Sci.*, 2013, **16**, 901.
11. J. Jia, G. Liu, Z. X. Guo, J. Yu and Y. Duan, *J. Nanomater.*, 2012, **2012**, 1–7.
12. A. Zambrowicz, A. Dabrowska, L. Bobak and M. Szoltysik, *Postepy Hig. Med. Dosw.*, 2014, **68**, 1524.
13. X. Gao, N. Chen, Y. Zhang, X. Zhang and X. Bing, *Aquaculture*, 2017, **479**, 69.
14. E. Eckert, A. Zambrowicz, M. Pokora, A. Polanowski, J. Chrzanowska, M. Szoltysik, A. Dabrowska, H. Rózański and T. Trziszka, *World's Poult. Sci. J.*, 2013, **69**, 375.
15. H. Yoshii, N. Tachi, R. Ohba, O. Sakamura, H. Takeyama and T. Itani, *Comp. Biochem. Physiol., Part C: Pharmacol., Toxicol. Endocrinol.*, 2001, **128**, 27.
16. E. Eckert, A. Zambrowicz, M. Pokora, B. Setner, A. Dabrowska, M. Szołtysik, Z. Szewczuk, A. Polanowski, T. Trziszka and J. Chrzanowska, *J. Proteomics*, 2014, **110**, 107.
17. W. Shen and T. Matsui, *Food Funct.*, 2017, **8**, 4306.
18. J. Takeda, H. Y. Park, Y. Kunitake, K. Yoshiura and T. Matsui, *Food Chem.*, 2013, **138**, 2140.
19. F. Baron, F. Nau, C. Guérin-Dubiard, S. Bonnassie, M. Gautier, S. C. Andrews and S. Jan, *Food Microbiol.*, 2016, **53**, 82.
20. E. M. Rivera, M. Araiza, W. Brostow, V. M. Castaño, J. R. Díaz-Estrada, R. Hernández and J. R. Rodríguez, *Mater. Lett.*, 1999, **41**, 128.
21. M. Baláž, in *Acta Biomaterialia*, Elsevier, 2014, vol. 10, p. 3827.
22. K. Park, J. Yoo and Y. Shin, *Korean J. Food Sci. Anim.*, 2012, **32**, 308.
23. J. Wu, in *Food Processing: Principles and Applications*, ed. S. Clark, S. Jung and B. Lamsal, John Wiley & Sons, Ltd., Hoboken, New Jersey, 2nd edn, 2014, p. 383.

24. K. Kaweewong, W. Garnjanagoonchorn, W. Jirapakkul and S. Roytrakul, *Protein J.*, 2013, **32**, 297.
25. Y. Mine, C. Oberle and Z. Kassaify, *J. Agric. Food Chem.*, 2003, **51**, 249.
26. O. Wellman-Labadie, J. Picman and M. T. Hincke, *Br. Poult. Sci.*, 2008, **49**, 133.
27. O. Wellman-Labadie, J. Picman and M. T. Hincke, *Comp. Biochem. Physiol., Part B: Biochem. Mol. Biol.*, 2008, **149**, 640.
28. J. E. Presslitz and V. A. Ray, *Antimicrob. Agents Chemother.*, 1975, **7**, 578.
29. J. Xing, O. Wellman-Labadie, J. Gautron and M. T. Hincke, *Comp. Biochem. Physiol., Part B: Biochem. Mol. Biol.*, 2007, **147**, 172.
30. M. T. Hincke, J. Gautron, K. Mann, M. Panhéleux, M. D. McKee, M. Bain, S. E. Solomon and Y. Nys, *Connect. Tissue Res.*, 2003, **44**, 16.
31. C. M. M. Cordeiro, H. Esmaili, G. Ansah and M. T. Hincke, *PLoS One*, 2014, **8**, e84112.
32. J. Xing, O. Wellman-Labadie, J. Gautron and M. T. Hincke, *Comp. Biochem. Physiol., Part B: Biochem. Mol. Biol.*, 2007, **147**, 172.
33. M. Rose-Martel, S. Smiley and M. T. Hincke, *J. Proteomics*, 2015, **116**, 81.
34. D. Gong, P. W. Wilson, M. M. Bain, K. McDade, J. Kalina, V. Hervé-Grépinet, Y. Nys and I. C. Dunn, *BMC Immunol.*, 2010, **11**, 1.
35. L. Callewaert and C. Michiels, *J. Biosci.*, 2010, **35**, 127.
36. H. R. Ibrahim, T. Matsuzaki and T. Aoki, *FEBS Lett.*, 2001, **506**, 27.
37. T. Silvetti, S. Morandi, M. Hintersteiner and M. Brasca, in *Egg Innovations and Strategies for Improvements*, Elsevier, 2017, p. 233.
38. L. K. Steinrauf, D. Shiuan, W. J. Yang and M. Y. Chiang, *Biochem. Biophys. Res. Commun.*, 1999, **266**, 366.
39. K. M. Davis and J. N. Weiser, *Infect. Immun.*, 2011, **79**, 562.
40. C. Abergel, V. Monchois, D. Byrne, S. Chenivesse, F. Lembo, J.-C. Lazzaroni and J.-M. Claverie, *Proc. Natl. Acad. Sci.*, 2007, **104**, 6394.
41. S. Yum, M. J. Kim, Y. Xu, X. L. Jin, H. Y. Yoo, J. W. Park, J. H. Gong, K. M. Choe, B. L. Lee and N. C. Ha, *Biochem. Biophys. Res. Commun.*, 2009, **378**, 244.
42. J. Losso, S. Nakai and E. Charter, in *Natural Food Antimicrobial Systems*, ed. A. Naidu, CRC Press, New York, 2000, p. 185.
43. F. Baron and S. Rehault, in *Bioactive Egg Compounds*, ed. R. Huopalahti, R. Lopez-Fandiño, M. Anton and R. Schade, Springer International Publishing, Berlin, 2007, p. 191.
44. H. R. Ibrahim, M. Yamada, K. Matsushita, K. Kobayashi and A. Kato, *J. Biol. Chem.*, 1994, **269**, 5059.
45. Z. Alahdad, R. Ramezani, M. Aminlari and M. Majzoobi, *J. Agric. Food Chem.*, 2009, **57**, 6449.
46. H. R. Ibrahim, H. Hatta, M. Fujiki, M. Kim and T. Yamamoto, *J. Agric. Food Chem.*, 1994, **42**, 1813.
47. W. J. Stadelman and O. J. Cotterhill, *Egg Science and Technology*, AVI Publishing Company Inc., Westport, CT, 4th edn, 2001.
48. E. Holen and S. Elsayed, *Int. Arch. Allergy Immunol.*, 1990, **91**, 136.

49. R. Finkelstein, C. Sciortino and M. McIntosh, *Rev. Infect. Dis.*, 1983, **5**, S759.
50. S. H. Moon, J. H. Lee, Y. J. Lee, K. H. Chang, J. Y. Paik, D. U. Ahn and H. D. Paik, *Poult. Sci.*, 2013, **92**, 424.
51. P. Valenti, V. Paolo, G. Antonini and N. Orsi, *Mycopathologia*, 1985, **89**, 169.
52. F. Baron, S. Jan, F. Gonnet, M. Pasco, J. Jardin, B. Giudici, M. Gautier, C. Guérin-Dubiard and F. Nau, *J. Food Prot.*, 2014, **77**, 955.
53. K. Y. Ko, A. F. Mendonca and D. U. Ahn, *Poult. Sci.*, 2008, **87**, 2660–2670.
54. S. D. Robinson and J. B. Monsey, *Biochem. J.*, 1971, **121**, 537.
55. Y. Tsuge, M. Shimoyamada and K. Watanabe, *J. Agric. Food Chem.*, 1997, **45**, 2393.
56. K. Kobayashi, M. Hattori, Y. Hara-Kudo, T. Okubo, S. Yamamoto, T. Takita and Y. Sugita-Konishi, *J. Agric. Food Chem.*, 2004, **52**, 5740.
57. Y. Tsuge, M. Shimoyamada and K. Watanabe, *J. Agric. Food Chem.*, 1997, **45**, 4629.
58. A. M. Abdou, M. Kim and K. Sato, in *Bioactive Food Peptides in Health and Disease*, ed. B. Hernández-Ledesma and C.-C. Hsieh, InTech, Rijeka, 2013, p. 115.
59. A. Pellegrini, A. J. Hülsmeier, P. Hunziker and U. Thomas, *Biochim. Biophys. Acta, Gen. Subj.*, 2004, **1672**, 76.
60. K. Kitaguchi, K. Osada, F. Horio and A. Murai, *Vet. Immunol. Immunopathol.*, 2008, **121**, 290.
61. J. Kovacs-Nolan and Y. Mine, *Avian Poult. Biol. Rev.*, 2004, **15**, 25.
62. M. Anton and G. Gandemer, *J. Food Sci.*, 1997, **62**, 484.
63. M. Anton, *J. Sci. Food Agric.*, 2013, **93**, 2871.
64. R. W. Burley and W. H. Cook, *Can. J. Biochem. Physiol.*, 1961, **39**, 1295.
65. D. Brady, S. Gaines, L. Fenelon, J. McPartlin and C. O'Farrelly, *J. Food Sci.*, 2002, **67**, 3096.
66. Z. G. Kassaify, E. W. Y. Li and Y. Mine, *J. Agric. Food Chem.*, 2005, **53**, 4607.
67. D. Czernick, J. Liu, D. Serge and E. Salih, *J. Proteomics*, 2013, **83**, 76.
68. R. C. Clark, *Int. J. Biochem.*, 1985, **17**, 983.
69. S. T. Ong, J. Z. Shan Ho, B. Ho and J. L. Ding, *Immunobiology*, 2006, **211**, 295.
70. M. A. Sattar Khan, S. Nakamura, M. Ogawa, E. Akita, H. Azakami and A. Kato, *J. Agric. Food Chem.*, 2000, **48**, 1503.
71. J. Ma, H. Wang, Y. Wang and S. Zhang, *Mol. Immunol.*, 2013, **53**, 355.
72. W. Liao, F. Jahandideh, H. Fan, M. Son and J. Wu, in *Advances in Food and Nutrition Research*, ed. M. Eskin, Academic Press, 83rd edn, 2018, p. 1.
73. J.-M. Lü, P. H. Lin, Q. Yao and C. Chen, *J. Cell. Mol. Med.*, 2010, **14**, 840.
74. G. I. Giles and C. Jacob, *Biol. Chem.*, 2002, **383**, 375.
75. R. H. Liu and J. H. Hotchkiss, *Mutat. Res., Genet. Toxicol.*, 1995, **339**, 73.
76. D. A. Geier, *Neurochem. Res.*, 2009, **34**, 386.

77. B. N. Ames, M. K. Shigenaga and L. S. Gold, *Environ. Health Perspect.*, 1993, **101**, 35.
78. S. Nakamura and A. Kato, *Food/Nahrung*, 2000, **44**, 201.
79. J. Wu and A. Acero-Lopez, *Food Res. Int.*, 2012, **46**, 480.
80. S. Shen, B. Chahal, K. Majumder, S.-J. You and J. Wu, *J. Agric. Food Chem.*, 2011, **58**, 7664.
81. J. Kim, S. H. Moon, D. U. Ahn, H. D. Paik and E. Park, *Poult. Sci.*, 2012, **91**, 2747.
82. K. Majumder, S. Chakrabarti, S. T. Davidge and J. Wu, *J. Agric. Food Chem.*, 2013, **61**, 2120.
83. H. Liu, F. Zheng, B. Cao, B. Ren, L. Zhu, G. Striker and H. Vlassara, *Am. J. Physiol.: Endocrinol. Metab.*, 2006, **290**, E824.
84. J. Hegenauer, P. Saltman and G. Nace, *Biochemistry1*, 1979, **18**, 3865–3879.
85. C. L. Lu and R. C. Baker, *Poult. Sci.*, 1986, **65**, 2065.
86. S.-I. Ishikawa, Y. Yano, K. Arihara and M. Itoh, *Biosci., Biotechnol., Biochem.*, 2004, **68**, 1324.
87. S. Nakamura, M. Ogawa, S. Nakai, A. Kato and D. D. Kitts, *J. Agric. Food Chem.*, 1998, **46**, 3958.
88. P. J. Park, W. K. Jung, K. S. Nam, F. Shahidi and S. K. Kim, *J. Am. Oil Chem. Soc.*, 2001, **78**, 651.
89. S. Katayama, S. I. Ishikawa, M. Z. Fan and Y. Mine, *J. Agric. Food Chem.*, 2007, **55**, 2829.
90. D. Young, F. Nau, M. Pasco and Y. Mine, *J. Agric. Food Chem.*, 2011, **59**, 9207.
91. K. F. Benson, K. J. Ruff and G. S. Jensen, *J. Med. Food*, 2012, **15**, 360–368.
92. K. J. Ruff and D. P. Devore, *Mod. Res. Inflammation*, 2014, **3**, 19.
93. K. J. Ruff, D. P. DeVore, M. D. Leu and M. Robinson, *Clin. Interventions Aging*, 2009, **4**, 235.
94. J. Yoo, K. Park, Y. Yoo, J. Kim, H. Yang and Y. Shin, *Korean J. Food Sci. Anim.*, 2014, **34**, 26.
95. X. Fan, R. Subramaniam, M. Weiss and V. Monnier, *Arch. Biochem. Biophys.*, 2003, **409**, 274.
96. K. Majumder, S. Chakrabarti, J. S. Morton, S. Panahi, S. Kaufman, S. T. Davidge and J. Wu, *PLoS One*, 2013, **8**, e82829.
97. W. Liao, S. Chakrabarti, S. T. Davidge and J. Wu, *J. Agric. Food Chem.*, 2016, **64**, 7342.
98. H. Tanizaki, H. Tanaka, H. Iwata and A. Kato, *Biosci., Biotechnol., Biochem.*, 1997, **61**, 1883.
99. X. Sun, S. Chakrabarti, J. Fang, Y. Yin and J. Wu, *Nutr. Res.*, 2016, **36**, 648.
100. M. O. Ogundele, *Mediators Inflammation*, 1998, **7**, 363.
101. M. Lee, J. Kovacs-Nolan, C. Yang, T. Archbold, M. Z. Fan and Y. Mine, *J. Agric. Food Chem.*, 2009, **57**, 2233.
102. C. Meram and J. Wu, *Food Res. Int.*, 2017, **100**, 449.
103. C. Xu, C. Yang, Y. Yin, J. Liu and Y. Mine, *J. Funct. Foods*, 2012, **4**, 718.

104. J. Yatabe, M. Yoneda, M. S. Yatabe, T. Watanabe, R. A. Felder, P. A. Jose and H. Sanada, *Endocrinology*, 2011, **152**, 1582.
105. A. Chiolero, J. Nussberger, G. Brunner and M. Burnier, *Hypertension*, 2000, **36**, 631.
106. H. Fujita, H. Usui, K. Kurahashi and M. Yoshikawa, *Peptides*, 1995, **16**, 785.
107. N. Matoba, H. Usui, H. Fujita and M. Yoshikawa, *FEBS Lett.*, 1999, **452**, 181.
108. P. Scruggs, C. M. Filipeanu, J. Yang, J. K. Chang and N. J. Dun, *Regul. Pept.*, 2004, **120**, 85.
109. N. Matoba, Y. Yamada, H. Usui, R. Nakagiri and M. Yoshikawa, *Biosci., Biotechnol., Biochem.*, 2001, **65**, 736.
110. Y. Yamada, N. Matoba, H. Usui, K. Onishi and M. Yoshikawa, *Biosci., Biotechnol., Biochem.*, 2002, **66**, 1213.
111. M. Miguel, I. Recio, J. A. Gomez-Ruiz, M. Ramos and R. Lopez-Fandino, *J. Food Prot.*, 2004, **67**, 1914.
112. F. Jahandideh, K. Majumder, S. Chakrabarti, J. S. Morton, S. Panahi, S. Kaufman, S. T. Davidge and J. Wu, *PLoS One*, 2014, **9**, 1.
113. K. Majumder and J. Wu, *Int. J. Mol. Sci.*, 2014, **16**, 256.
114. K. Majumder, S. Chakrabarti, J. S. Morton, S. Panahi, S. Kaufman, S. T. Davidge and J. Wu, *J. Funct. Foods*, 2015, **13**, 50.
115. Z. Yu, Y. Yin, W. Zhao, F. Chen and J. Liu, *J. Agric. Food Chem.*, 2014, **62**, 912.
116. S. Rao, J. Sun, Y. Liu, H. Zeng, Y. Su and Y. Yang, *Food Chem.*, 2012, **135**, 1245.
117. J. Wu, W. Liao and C. C. Udenigwe, *Trends Food Sci. Technol.*, 2017, **69**, 214.
118. S. Katayama, X. Xu, M. Z. Fan and Y. Mine, *J. Agric. Food Chem.*, 2006, **54**, 773.
119. A. Zambrowicz, M. Pokora, B. Setner, A. Dąbrowska, M. Szołtysik, K. Babij, Z. Szewczuk, T. Trziszka, G. Lubec and J. Chrzanowska, *Amino Acids*, 2015, **47**, 369.
120. M. Yousr and N. Howell, *Int. J. Mol. Sci.*, 2015, **16**, 29161.
121. R. L. Siegel, K. D. Miller and A. Jemal, *Ca-Cancer J. Clin.*, 2018, **68**, 7.
122. E. H. Vis, A. F. Plinck, G. M. Alink and M. A. J. S. Van Boekel, *J. Agric. Food Chem.*, 1998, **46**, 3713.
123. H. R. Ibrahim and T. Kiyono, *J. Agric. Food Chem.*, 2009, **57**, 11383–11390.
124. G. Sava, V. Ceschia, S. Pacor and G. Zabucchi, *Anticancer Res.*, 1991, **11**, 1109.
125. G. Sava, S. Pacor, G. Dasic and A. Bergamo, *Anticancer Res.*, 1995, **15**, 1883.
126. K. Watanabe, Y. Tsuge, M. Shimoyamada, N. Ogama and T. Ebina, *J. Agric. Food Chem.*, 1998, **46**, 3033.
127. T. Yokota, H. Ohishi and K. Watanabe, *Food Sci. Technol. Res.*, 1999, **5**, 273.

128. T. Yokota, H. Tani, H. Ohishi, T. Oguro and K. Watanabe, *Food Sci. Technol. Res.*, 2000, **6**, 275.
129. D. P. Belobrajdic, G. H. McIntosh and J. A. Owens, *Cancer Lett.*, 2003, **198**, 43.
130. S. H. Moon, J. H. Lee, M. Lee, E. Park, D. U. Ahn and H. D. Paik, *Poult. Sci.*, 2014, **93**, 2103.
131. M. Chalamaiah, W. Yu and J. Wu, *Food Chem.*, 2018, **245**, 205.
132. G. S. Hotamisligil, *Nature*, 2006, **444**, 860.
133. H. Xie, G. R. Huff, W. E. Huff, J. M. Balog and N. C. Rath, *Dev. Comp. Immunol.*, 2002, **26**, 805.
134. H. Otani and M. Odashima, *Food Agric. Immunol.*, 1997, **9**, 193.
135. Y. Hirota, M. P. Yang, S. Araki, K. Yoshihara, S. Furusawa, M. Yasuda, A. Mohamed, Y. Matsumoto and T. Onodera, *J. Vet. Med. Sci.*, 1995, **57**, 825.
136. Y. Mine and J. W. Zhang, *J. Agric. Food Chem.*, 2002, **50**, 2679.
137. Y. Mine and J. Wei Zhang, *Biochem. Biophys. Res. Commun.*, 2002, **292**, 1070.
138. G. Sava, *EXS*, 1996, **75**, 433.
139. K. Asakura, T. Kojima, H. Shirasaki and A. Kataura, *Auris, Nasus, Larynx*, 1990, **17**, 33.
140. T. Sugahara, F. Murakami, Y. Yamada and T. Sasaki, *Biochim. Biophys. Acta, Gen. Subj.*, 2000, **1475**, 27.
141. J. Herzog, Y. Maekawa, T. P. Cirrito, B. S. Illian and E. R. Unanue, *Proc. Natl. Acad. Sci.*, 2005, **102**, 7928.
142. S. B. Lovitch and E. R. Unanue, *Immunol. Rev.*, 2005, **207**, 293.
143. M. Bourin, J. Gautron, M. Berges, S. Attucci, G. Le Blay, V. Labas, Y. Nys and S. Rehault-Godbert, *J. Agric. Food Chem.*, 2011, **59**, 12368.
144. K. Shuichi, F. Noriko, I. Atsuko, K. Izumi and M. Kin-ichiro, *Gene*, 1994, **143**, 239.
145. S. Kojima, N. Takagi, T. Minagawa, N. Fushimi and K.-I. Miura, *Protein Eng.*, 1999, **12**, 857.
146. T. A. Valueva, N. L. Matveev, V. V. Mosolov and V. A. Penin, *Agents Actions Suppl.*, 1992, **38**(Pt 2), 203.
147. R. Shah and M. A. Khan, *J. Pharm. Sci.*, 2003, **93**, 392.
148. I. Saxena and S. Tayyab, *Cell. Mol. Life Sci.*, 1997, **53**, 13.
149. M. Laskowski and I. Kato, *Annu. Rev. Biochem.*, 1980, **49**, 593.
150. Y. Sugimoto, T. Kusakabe, S. Nagaoka, T. Nirasawa, K. Tatsuguchi, M. Fujii, T. Aoki and K. Koga, *Biochim. Biophys. Acta, Protein Struct. Mol. Enzymol.*, 1996, **1295**, 96.
151. M. Odashima, F. Takano and H. Otani, *Anim. Sci. J.*, 2000, **71**, 92.
152. R. Nakamura and T. Matsuda, *J. Agric. Food Chem.*, 1984, **32**, 483.
153. S. Begum, A. Saito, X. Xu and A. Kato, *Biosci., Biotechnol., Biochem.*, 2003, **67**, 1897.
154. N. A. Plate, I. L. Valuev, G. A. Sytov and L. I. Valuev, *Biomaterials*, 2002, **23**, 1673.
155. V. Agarwal, S. Nazzal, I. K. Reddy and M. A. Khan, *J. Pharm. Pharmacol.*, 2001, **53**, 1131.

156. S. Nagaoka, M. Masaoka, Q. Zhang, M. Hasegawa and K. Watanabe, *Lipids*, 2002, **37**, 267.
157. K. Kinoshita, T. Shimogiri, H. R. Ibrahim, M. Tsudzuki, Y. Maeda and Y. Matsuda, *PLoS One*, 2016, **11**, e0159571.
158. H. H. Sunwoo and N. Gujral, in *Handbook of Food Chemistry*, ed. P. Cheung, Springer, Heidelberg, Berlin, 2014, p. 1.
159. C. A. Alleoni, *Sci. Agric.*, 2006, **63**, 291–298.
160. B. Ketterer, *Biochem. J.*, 1965, **96**, 372.
161. C. Chang, T. Lahti, T. Tanaka and M. T. Nickerson, *J. Sci. Food Agric.*, 2018, **98**, 5547–5558.
162. J. Haginaka, C. Seyama and N. Kanasugi, *Anal. Chem.*, 1995, **67**, 2539.
163. J. Haginaka and N. Kanasugi, *J. Chromatogr. A*, 1997, **782**, 281.
164. M. S. Miller, M. T. Mas and H. B. White, *Biochemistry*, 1984, **23**, 569.
165. Y. Hamazume, T. Mega and T. Ikenaka, *J. Biochem.*, 1987, **101**, 217.
166. G. Blankenhorn, *Eur. J. Biochem.*, 1978, **82**, 155.
167. H. L. Monaco, *EMBO J.*, 1997, **16**, 1475.
168. E. Fee, B. Rhodes and N. Bennett, *J. Biol. Chem.*, 1959, **234**, 2054.
169. T. Croguennec, C. Guérin-Dubiard and F. Nau, in *Bioactive Egg Compounds*, Springer, Berlin, Heidelberg, 2007, vol. 200, p. 69.
170. M. S. Miller, E. G. Buss and C. O. Clagett, *Biochim. Biophys. Acta, Gen. Subj.*, 1981, **677**, 225.
171. K. Maehashi, M. Matano, A. Kondo, Y. Yamamoto and S. Udaka, *Chem. Senses*, 2007, **32**, 183.
172. K. Maehashi, M. Matano, M. Nonaka, S. Udaka and Y. Yamamoto, *Chem. Senses*, 2008, **33**, 57.
173. A. Molla, Y. Matsumura, T. Yamamoto, R. Okamura and H. Maeda, *Infect. Immun.*, 1987, **55**, 2509.
174. H. Nagase, E. D. Harris, J. F. Woessner, K. Brew and H. Nagaset, *J. Biol. Chem.*, 1983, **258**, 7481.
175. S. Miyagawa, N. Nishino, R. Kamata, R. Okamura and H. Maeda, *Microb. Pathog.*, 1991, **11**, 137.
176. Y. Ijiri, T. Yamamoto, R. Kamata, H. Aoki, K. Matsumoto, R. Okamura and T. Kambara, *Graefe's Arch. Clin. Exp. Ophthalmol.*, 1993, **231**, 521.
177. Y. Ofuji, T. Suzuki, H. Yoshie, K. Hara and M. Adachi, *Periodontal Clin. Invest.*, 1992, **14**, 13.
178. A. J. Barrett, *Biomed. Biochim. Acta*, 1986, **45**, 1363.
179. M. T. Stubbs, B. Laber, W. Bode, R. Huber, R. Jerala, B. Lenarcic and V. Turk, *EMBO J.*, 1990, **9**, 1939.
180. Y. Mine and I. D'Silva, in *Egg Bioscience and Biotechnology*, ed. Y. Mine, John Wiley & Sons, Inc., Hoboken, New Jersey, 2008, p. 141.
181. M. Blankenvoorde, W. van't Hof, E. Walgreen-Weterings, T. van Steenbergen, H. Brand, E. Veerman and A. Nieuw Amerongen, *Biol. Chem.*, 1998, **379**, 1371.
182. E. Wesierska, Y. Saleh, T. Trziszka, W. Kopec, M. Siewinski and K. Korzekwa, *World J. Microbiol. Biotechnol.*, 2005, **21**, 59.

183. T. Kato, T. Imatani, T. Miura, K. Minaguchi, E. Saitoh and K. Okuda, *Biol. Chem.*, 2000, **381**, 1143.
184. L. Verdot, G. Lalmanach, V. Vercruysse, J. Hoebeke, F. Gauthier and B. Vray, *Eur. J. Biochem.*, 2001, **266**, 1111.
185. A. Shamsi and B. Bano, *Int. J. Biol. Macromol.*, 2017, **102**, 674.
186. J. Kos, A. Mitrovic and B. Mirkovic, *Future Med. Chem.*, 2014, **6**, 1355.
187. Y. Saleh, J. Wnukiewicz and T. Trziszka, *J. Cancer Mol.*, 2006, **2**, 67.
188. A. Premzl, V. Puizdar, V. Zavašnik-Bergant, N. Kopitar-Jerala, T. T. Lah, N. Katunuma, B. F. Sloane, V. Turk and J. Kos, *Biol. Chem.*, 2001, **382**, 853.
189. S. Yousif, S. Maciej, K. Wojciech, Z. Piotr, G. Marian and R. Jacek, *J. Exp. Ther. Oncol.*, 2003, **3**, 319.
190. W. C. Kett, R. I. Osmond, L. Moe, S. E. Skett, B. F. Kinnear and D. R. Coombe, *Biochim. Biophys. Acta, Gen. Subj.*, 2003, **1620**, 225.
191. J. Korpela, *Med. Biol.*, 1984, **62**, 5.
192. R. C. Bruch, R. C. Bruch and H. B. White, *Biochemistry*, 1982, **21**, 5334.
193. J. L. Guesdon, T. Ternynck and S. Avrameas, *J. Histochem. Cytochem.*, 1979, **27**, 1131.
194. N. M. Green, *Adv. Protein Chem.*, 1975, **29**, 85.
195. J. Korpela, E. M. Salonen, P. Kuusela, M. Sarvas and A. Vaheri, *FEMS Microbiol. Lett.*, 1984, **22**, 3.
196. N. Guyot, V. Labas, G. Harichaux, M. Chessé, J. C. Poirier, Y. Nys and S. Réhault-Godbert, *Sci. Rep.*, 2016, **6**, 1.
197. A. Gasparri, M. Moro, F. Curnis, A. Sacchi, S. Pagano, F. Veglia, G. Casorati, A. G. Siccardi, P. Dellabona and A. Corti, *Cancer Res.*, 1999, **59**, 2917–2923.
198. M. Guttinger, F. Guidi, M. Chinol, E. Reali, F. Veglia, G. Viale, G. Paganelli, A. Corti and A. G. Siccardi, *Cancer Res.*, 2000, **60**, 4211–4215.
199. U. Bickel, T. Yoshikawa and W. M. Pardridge, *Adv. Drug Delivery Rev.*, 2001, **46**, 247.
200. S. Réhault-Godbert, V. Labas, E. Helloin, V. Hervé-Grépinet, C. Slugocki, M. Berges, M. C. Bourin, A. Brionne, J. C. Poirier, J. Gautron, F. Coste and Y. Nys, *J. Biol. Chem.*, 2013, **288**, 17285.
201. K. Mann, *Proteomics*, 2007, **7**, 3558.
202. R. T. Yan and S. Z. Wang, *J. Neurobiol.*, 1998, **34**, 319.
203. C. Guérin-Dubiard, M. Pasco, D. Mollé, C. Désert, T. Croguennec and F. Nau, *J. Agric. Food Chem.*, 2006, **54**, 3901.
204. F. Nau, C. Guérin-Dubiard, C. Désert, J. Gautron, S. Bouton, J. Gribonval and S. Lagarrigue, *Poult. Sci.*, 2003, **82**, 242.
205. J. Wang, Y. Liang, D. A. Omana, N. N. V. Kav and J. Wu, *J. Agric. Food Chem.*, 2012, **60**, 272.
206. F. Jahandideh, P. Liu and J. Wu, *Food Chem.*, 2018, **259**, 25.
207. B. Jiang and Y. Mine, *Biosci., Biotechnol., Biochem.*, 2001, **65**, 1187.
208. H. K. Kim, M. G. Kim and K. H. Leem, *Molecules*, 2014, **19**, 12909.
209. A. M. Abdou, K. Watabe, T. Yamane, T. Isono, Y. Okamura, S. Kawahito, K. Takeshima, K. Masuda and M. Kim, *Food Sci. Nutr.*, 2014, **2**, 193.

210. Y. Zhu, S. K. Vanga, J. Wang and V. Raghavan, *Trends Food Sci. Technol.*, 2018, **78**, 188.
211. H. Lemon-Mulé, H. A. Sampson, S. H. Sicherer, W. G. Shreffler, S. Noone and A. Nowak-Wegrzyn, *J. Allergy Clin. Immunol.*, 2008, **122**, 977.
212. P. Dhanapala, C. De Silva, T. Doran and C. Suphioglu, *Mol. Immunol.*, 2015, **66**, 375.
213. H. Matsuo, T. Yokooji and T. Taogoshi, *Allergol. Int.*, 2015, **64**, 332.
214. Y. Mine and J. W. Zhang, *J. Agric. Food Chem.*, 2002, **50**, 2679.
215. J. A. Huntington and P. E. Stein, *J. Chromatogr. B: Biomed. Sci. Appl.*, 2001, **756**, 189.
216. P. J. Davis, C. M. Smales and D. C. James, *Allergy Eur. J. Allergy Clin. Immunol. Suppl.*, 2001, **56**, 56.
217. P. Tong, J. Gao, H. Chen, X. Li, Y. Zhang, S. Jian, H. Wichers, Z. Wu, A. Yang and F. Liu, *Food Chem.*, 2012, **131**, 603.
218. S. Frémont, G. Kanny, J. P. Nicolas and D. A. Moneret-Vautrin, *Allergy Eur. J. Allergy Clin. Immunol.*, 1997, **52**, 224.
219. D. R. Hoffman, *J. Allergy Clin. Immunol.*, 1983, **71**, 481.
220. Z. Szépfalusi, C. Ebner, R. Pandjaitan, F. Orlicek, O. Scheiner, G. Boltz-Nitulescu, D. Kraft and H. Ebner, *J. Allergy Clin. Immunol.*, 1994, **93**, 932.
221. S. Quirce, F. Marañón, A. Umpiérrez, M. De Las Heras, E. Fernández-Caldas and J. Sastre, *Allergy Eur. J. Allergy Clin. Immunol.*, 2001, **56**, 754.
222. A. Amo, R. Rodríguez-Pérez, J. Blanco, J. Villota, S. Juste, I. Moneo and M. L. Caballero, *J. Agric. Food Chem.*, 2010, **58**, 7453.

CHAPTER 14

Bioactive Minor Egg Components

J. GAUTRON*, N. GUYOT, A. BRIONNE AND S. RÉHAULT-GODBERT

INRA, BOA, Université de Tours, 37380 Nouzilly, France
*E-mail: joel.gautron@inra.fr

14.1 Introduction

A limited number of egg white proteins (less than 10) represent more than 85% of the whole amount of egg proteins. Until 2006, only 40 to 50 proteins, representing the most abundant, were identified in egg. This number has dramatically increased in the last decade, thanks to the results of functional genomic studies, which have dramatically transformed biology and biotechnology, including egg science. The recent development of high-throughput methods used in combination with the newly available chicken genome sequence[1] and bioinformatics tools to predict functions has generated new insights for the characterization of about 1000 egg components.[2,3] This large number of proteins constitutes a small quantity in the egg and they are designated as minor egg proteins. These proteins are involved in the protection and development of the chicken embryo and participate in the nutritive values of this basic food ingredient. Furthermore, the egg compartments

Food Chemistry, Function and Analysis No.14
Eggs as Functional Foods and Nutraceuticals for Human Health
Edited by Jianping Wu

Published by the Royal Society of Chemistry, www.rsc.org

contain molecules with a broad range of biological activities with potential interest for several areas, including pharmaceutical, cosmetic, food and materials industries.[4–7]

In this chapter, we will review how high-throughput and data mining technologies were used to identify and to integrate the huge amount of proteins within the whole egg and in each individual compartment. We will then report on the functionality of the numerous newly identified minor proteins, constituting a small amount in egg, but about 95% of the total number of egg proteins. In particular, we will describe how the identification of shell matrix proteins is important for shell quality improvement or biomimetic interpretation for material sciences. We will also highlight the egg as a major source of bioactive molecules including antimicrobial, immunomodulating, antioxidant and anticancer activities.

14.2 Integrative Analysis of Egg Proteomes

Since the beginning of this century, chicken (*Gallus gallus*) gene transcripts have been characterized. Sequencing of cDNAs yielded short nucleotide sequences (200–500 bp), known as expressed sequence tags (ESTs), representing a comprehensive catalogue of global or tissue-specific mRNA sequences expressed in the chicken. The combination of joint international projects allowed the characterization of 600 434 ESTs (http://www.ncbi.nlm.nih.gov/dbEST/dbEST_summary.html). These sequences were assembled to yield a genome-wide non-redundant catalogue of mRNAs (UniGene; http://www.ncbi.nlm.nih.gov/UniGene/UGOrg.cgi?TAXID=9031). The publication of the chicken genome sequence was another major advance in identifying and characterizing chicken genes and proteins.[1] With the development of next-generation sequencing technologies (NGS), several tens of millions of chicken transcript fragments are now available (NCBI Sequence Read Archive, http://www.ncbi.nlm.nih.gov/sra/?term=chicken). In March 2018, the International Chicken Genome Consortium released the Gallus_gallus-6a assembly of the chicken genome (https://www.ncbi.nlm.nih.gov/genome/annotation_euk/Gallus_gallus/104/). It consists of 34 chromosomes, and predicted 24 012 genes and 49 661 transcripts. The existence of genes and their corresponding proteins in a database is fundamental for the use of high-throughput technologies (proteomics and transcriptomics) to identify proteins in the various milieus composing the egg. Indeed, these sequences in databases are required in proteomics studies to ascribe experimental mass spectra to existing proteins.

These recent advances make possible the investigation of the egg proteome, or egg compartment sub-proteomes, using mass spectrometry-based high-throughput methods, as shown for the organic matrix of the chicken calcified eggshell layer, the egg white, the egg yolk and the vitelline membrane.

The first major proteomic analysis of egg came in 2006, with the eggshell proteome. Mann *et al.*[8] identified the acid-soluble eggshell organic matrix and completed this approach with a phosphoproteome of the soluble eggshell proteins.[9] Both studies identified 528 different proteins as constituents of the soluble eggshell matrix. The insoluble fraction of the eggshell matrix was also investigated.[10–13] Rose-Martel *et al.*[14] performed a proteomic analysis of the outermost layer of the shell (cuticle), suspected to play a major role in preventing microbial penetration. A more recent proteomic survey allowed the identification of novel components[15,16] and the quantification of about 300 eggshell proteins at the key steps of shell calcification.[17] Finally, a recent proteomic survey on shell membranes characterized about 300 eggshell membrane proteins.[18]

Guerin-Dubiard *et al.*[19] firstly explored the egg white proteome, but the largest number of proteins identified in the egg white came from the studies of Mann and Righetti's laboratories.[20–22] Mann analyzed egg white proteins using LC-MS/MS and MS^3 of peptide mixtures prepared by in-solution cleavage of egg white proteins, which allowed the identification of 78 proteins, 54 of which were identified in egg white for the first time.[21] D'Ambrosio *et al.*[20] explored the chicken egg white proteome using combinatorial peptide ligand libraries. This method enabled the identification of 70 additional egg white proteins. By using a novel dual pressure linear ion trap instrument, the LTQ Orbitrap Velos, which increased sensitivity, Mann and Mann[22] identified 44 additional proteins. Additionally, the egg white composition was explored in different egg varieties[23] and under various storage temperatures.[24]

The chicken egg yolk is separated from the white by the proteinaceous extracellular vitelline membrane. 137 proteins were identified in the chicken egg vitelline membrane proteome.[25] Only 13 were previously known to be components of the vitelline membrane. Most of the identified components were already identified in eggshell, yolk and egg white, questioning those that are specifically constitutive of the membranes. Additionally, Mann described supplementary sequences, which improved the number of identified proteins.[25]

The egg-yolk proteome was investigated using 1D electrophoresis and LC-MS/MS; Mann and Mann[26] identified 119 egg-yolk proteins, 86 of which were not previously identified in this egg compartment. The chicken egg-yolk cytoplasmic proteome was also investigated using combinatorial peptide ligand libraries,[27] as previously reported for egg white.[20] This approach enabled the identification of 255 new yolk proteins with 54 in common with the previously determined yolk proteome.[26]

The proteomic studies allowed the identification of hundreds of egg proteins, with some of them being present in the various egg compartments. One gap in this methodology is the presence of redundancy between proteins because the proteomic studies used identifiers originated from different databases. Mann described proteins using IPI (International Protein Index database, http://www.ebi.ac.uk/IPI), which is now closed and was a merged database of ENSEMBL and GeneBank, with numerous changes to protein identifiers between 2006 (first eggshell proteomic study) and 2011 (database closing date). The other egg proteomic studies reported the proteins using identifiers originated from

GeneBank (http://www.ncbi.nlm.nih.gov/genbank/), ENSEMBL (http://www.ensembl.org) or UniProt (Universal Protein Resource, http://www.uniprot.org/). Altogether, egg proteomic studies described thousands of different protein identifiers. However, one unique protein often possesses various identifiers. To fix this problem, we have loaded the entire protein sequences originated from these different identifiers, which were aligned using a BLAST algorithm to eliminate all redundancies.

A total of 1261 non-redundant protein sequences (gene products) were finally determined using the egg proteomic studies. The different proteins were classified in the different compartments of the egg (Figure 14.1). Egg yolk, vitelline membranes and egg white constituted at least of 230, 144 and 273 different proteins, respectively. Finally, the eggshell is the compartment with the lowest amount of proteins, but it exhibits the largest variety of proteins as 904 were reported in this single compartment.

Figure 14.1 gives a representation of the specific, common and shared proteins. The egg proteins only specific to one compartment represent 82.6% (1042) of the total number, with 143 proteins specific to the yolk, 41 only found in the vitelline membranes, 149 unique proteins of the white and 709 proteins only observed in the eggshell. Surprisingly, the number of shared proteins between two or more egg compartments is limited to 219 proteins, representing less than 20% of the total number of egg proteins. Only 13 proteins are common to all egg compartments. They are riboflavin-binding protein, ovotransferrin, apolipoprotein B, glutathione peroxidase 3, immunoglobulin lambda-like polypeptide 1, vitellogenin 1, keratin 6A and 7, hemopexin, transmembrane protease serine 9, ovalbumin, ovalbumin-related X and glyceraldehyde-3-phosphate dehydrogenase. The other 206 are found within two or three egg compartments.

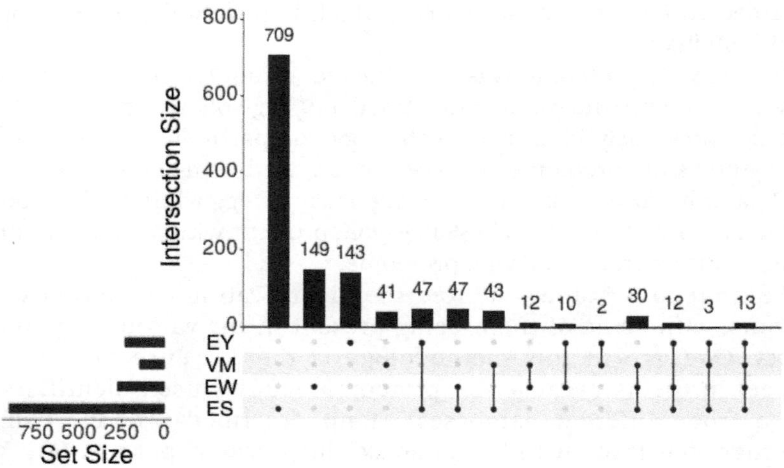

Figure 14.1 Number of proteins in the egg yolk (EY), vitelline membrane (VM), egg white (EW) and eggshell (ES). Line connectors represent the proteins shared between egg compartments.

14.3 Functional Activities of Minor Egg Proteins

14.3.1 Biomineralization of Egg

The main function of the eggshell is to protect the embryo from external aggression during its development. Consequently, the eggshell as a physical barrier must have remarkable mechanical properties. It has to be solid but also easy breakable from inside to allow hatching. Mineralized eggshell deposition occurs in the distal part of the oviduct and this process has been widely described.[28–30] Calcification is initiated in the red isthmus/uterus region (5 hours post ovulation) by deposition of spherulitic microcrystals of calcite (calcium carbonate polymorph of the chicken eggshell) on specific sites (mammillary knobs) on the surface of shell membranes. Metastable amorphous calcium carbonate (ACC) is present as an early and transient precursor phase, which rapidly evolves to supply ions to form the calcite in the shell.[31] Calcite crystals then develop into columnar crystal units with their faster growth direction (*c*-axis) nearly perpendicular to the surface developing a preferential orientation of crystals. We described four major events in the shell formation:[31] (1) Metastable ACC is first deposited and accumulated over the entire eggshell membrane, then (2) there is a rapid evolution and redistribution of ACC on specific nucleation sites (mammillary knobs) on eggshell membranes to form calcite aggregates. (3) Calcite aggregates are then enlarged into larger calcite crystals to form the mammillary layer, followed by (4) the development of columns of crystals with a preferred orientation perpendicular to the surface to form the shell's compact palisade layer. This linear deposition of mineral continues until the process is inhibited (22 hours post ovulation), and the organic cuticle is deposited on the surface of the calcified shell (22–24 hours post ovulation). Finally, the egg is laid about 24 hours after the ovulation of the yolk. Shell therefore results from the assembly of aggregated ACC particles in calcite crystals to allow a very fast controlled process during the various steps of shell calcification. These distinct phases are associated with the formation of different layers in the shell: the inner mammillary cones, the palisade layer and the cuticle.

The shell constitutes about 10% of the egg content, representing 5 to 6 g per egg. The shell is mainly composed of 95% calcium carbonate in calcitic form. Only 3.5% (175 mg) constitutes the organic shell matrix made of proteoglycans and proteins. Consequently, the 900 proteins identified in the shell represent less than 150 mg in the complete egg. In comparison, the 273 egg white proteins represent a 20–30 times greater amount. Although these shell proteins are at very low concentrations, they play a key role during the shell calcification events. Matrix proteins stabilize the ACC mineral form of calcium carbonate and select the calcite polymorph into which it is converted. Organic matrix proteins also specifically adsorb on crystal faces to control the growth and morphology of calcite, which determines the orientation of crystals in the shell.[17,29–32] The matrix–mineral interactions result in a complex ultrastructure of the eggshell, which determines its mechanical properties. A number of experimental observations support the role of the eggshell matrix proteins in the fabric of the eggshell and its resulting mechanical properties. The first is relevant to the nature of the chicken eggshell matrix in its content of specific components (ovocleidins and ovocalyxins), which are synthesized and expressed only in tissues where eggshell calcification takes place, namely, the uterus and red isthmus. Putative functions related to the mineralization process were predicted for matrix proteins using bioinformatics. They were classified into various groups (proteins associated with shell mineralization, proteins involved in the regulation of proteins driving the mineralization, antimicrobial proteins and other functions).[17] Changes in the organic composition of the uterine fluid and in the shell during the fabrication of the eggshell allowed determination of proteins potentially associated with the shell fabric. Each phase of shell mineralization is associated with a specific electrophoretic profile in the uterine fluid, suggesting specific roles for the organic contents during the calcification process.[33] Marie *et al.*[17] used quantitative proteomics on 200 shell matrix proteins and determined patterns of abundance at the different key steps of shell formation. This study highlights 21 matrix proteins suspected to have predominant roles in the control of the different stages of shell calcification.

The role of shell matrix proteins was also evidenced by laboratory experiments. Investigations have demonstrated that eggshell organic fractions exhibit calcium binding properties owing to proteins[34–36] or keratan and dermatan sulfate proteoglycans.[37] Similarly, in the uterine fluid, protein bands corresponding to ovalbumin, ovotransferrin and the 36 kDa band during the active phase of calcification, display affinity for calcium.[33] This last band was further characterized as corresponding to clusterin[38] and ovocalyxin-36.[39] Calcite crystals grown *in vitro* with soluble eggshell protein extracts and uterine fluid delay the precipitation of calcium carbonate in a dose-dependent manner.[33,37,40,41] The uterine fluid dramatically affected the precipitation kinetics, the size and the morphology of crystals grown *in vitro*.[41–44] Similar results were observed in the presence of purified lysozyme, ovotransferrin and ovocleidin-17, which showed large modifications of the calcite morphology.[44–47] Metadynamics simulations reveal that ovocleidin-17 induces the formation of calcite crystals from amorphous calcium carbonate nanoparticles.[48–50] The strong stabilization of the amorphous calcium carbonate emulsion is attributed to ovalbumin complexes acting as nucleation centers for the amorphous phase because of their enrichment by Ca^{2+} ions.[51,52] Additionally, the dermatan sulfate glycosaminoglycan chain containing ovocleidin-116 as the protein core, ovoglycan, is polyanionic and acidic with high calcium affinity and is likely to modulate crystal growth during palisade formation.[53]

The involvement of eggshell matrix proteins was also reinforced by *in vivo* relationships between matrix proteins and eggshell quality parameters. If the eggshell matrix participates in establishing the morphology of calcite crystals, it would affect the texture (crystal size and orientation) of the eggshell and influence its mechanical properties. This hypothesis was confirmed by quantifying components of matrix proteins in parallel with variations in eggshell mechanical properties.[54,55] Both studies showed variation of the abundance of matrix proteins (ovalbumin, ovotransferrin, and ovocleidin-116 and-17) related to shell mechanical properties and the size and orientation of crystals. These observations suggest that changes in organic matrix protein levels affect eggshell crystal size and provide mechanisms for improving the shell solidity. A complementary avenue to establish the role of matrix proteins in the variability of the eggshell physical and mechanical properties has been taken using genetic and genomic approaches.[56] These were aimed at determining the association between alleles of some eggshell matrix proteins (ovocleidins and ovocalyxins, osteopontin and ovalbumin) and measurements of eggshell solidity. This study revealed a number of significant associations between genotype (the marker) and phenotype (the trait, *e.g.*, acoustic resonance data, quasi-static compression test data and the thickness of specific components of the shell).[56] When expressed as allele substitution/standard deviation of the trait, the effect of a coding region polymorphism in ovocalyxin-32 was over 12% for breaking strength and 17% for deformation. Ovocalyxin-32 polymorphism also affects the size and the crystal orientation of the mineralized structure.[57] Takahashi *et al.*[58,59] identified the ovocalyxine-32 gene in the quantitative trait locus (QTL) region associated with shell quality in divergent lines. The effect of a coding region polymorphism in ovocleidin-116 was 17% for shell stiffness and polymorphism in the promoter of this gene accounted for around 10% of the thickness of the mammillary layer and its proportion in the shell.[56] Recently, a genome-wide association study (GWAS) associated different egg quality parameters with QTL in egg layers containing many proteins identified in the shell.[60]

The huge number of proteins identified in the shell will allow genomic improvement and will give insights for material sciences. Genes coding matrix proteins will be used as biological markers for genomic selection to reinforce eggshell breaking strength. The corresponding transcripts will be associated with published and private single nucleotide polymorphisms and mapped in QTLs related to shell quality. They will constitute candidate genes to gain precision for genomic selection to reinforce shell mechanical properties. Industrial ceramics are made at high temperature and pressure. Material science explores the biomineralization to investigate how living organisms build their shells under physiological conditions. Among various biominerals, the chicken shell is the most widely documented. Information on shell matrix proteins and how they contribute to the mechanical properties gives a chance to establish a list of natural organic compounds of added value usable in the fabrication of calcium carbonate materials/ceramics.

14.3.2 Antimicrobial Proteins

Besides the major antimicrobial proteins (lysozyme and ovotransferrin), many minor egg proteins also exhibit antimicrobial properties and contribute to the efficiency and complexity of egg defenses. These minor compounds can be classified in different groups according to their structural or functional properties.

14.3.2.1 Protease Inhibitors

The egg contains large amounts of active protease inhibitors (antiproteases). Among the most representative egg antiproteases are ovomucoid, ovoinhibitor, ovostatin and cystatin. They are ubiquitously distributed within all egg compartments but more specifically concentrated in egg white. They target proteases with more or less enzymatic specificity. Proteases are proteolytic enzymes catalyzing the cleavage/degradation of peptidic chains and are involved in many biological processes in eukaryotes and prokaryotes. Some bacteria are able to produce extracellular proteases involved in their survival, growth or invasive capacity and which play critical roles in host–pathogen interactions. Therefore, the neutralization of these virulent factors by antiproteases may lead to the inhibition of bacteria. Although the physiological function of egg antiproteases has not been well established to date, it is likely that they could potentially inhibit protease-secreting bacteria and/or have a direct bactericidal activity.

Ovomucoid is a 28 kDa protein that is highly glycosylated and possesses nine disulfide bonds. This glycoprotein contains three functional homologous Kazal-like inhibitory domains and exhibits antitrypsin and antichymotrypsin activities. The antibacterial role of ovomucoid and its participation in the protection of the egg against bacterial contamination have not been clearly demonstrated. However, some bacterial proteases, like subtilisins and *Streptomyces griseus* proteases A and B, are inhibited by turkey ovomucoid.[61]

Ovoinhibitor is a 48 kDa glycoprotein possessing seven Kazal-like inhibitory domains and 21 disulfide bonds. Ovoinhibitor can inhibit several serine proteases, such as trypsin, chymotrypsin and elastase, as well as subtilisin, a serine protease produced by *Bacillus* spp. Antibacterial activities have been reported *in vitro* against *Bacillus thuringiensis*.[62]

Ovostatin (or ovomacroglobulin) is a large homotetrameric protein belonging to the alpha-2-macroglobulin family, consisting of four disulfide-linked subunits (4 × 165 kDa). Ovostatin is known to bind and inhibit various proteases from different classes (serine-, cysteinyl-, metallo- and aspartyl-proteases) but with better efficiency towards metalloproteases (collagenase, thermolysin and stromelysin). Because of its ability to inhibit proteases produced by several virulent bacteria inducing corneal tissue damage (*Serratia marcescens, Pseudomonas aeruginosa*),[63] ovostatin can be considered as an antimicrobial.

Cystatin is a non-glycosylated protein (12.7 kDa, pI 5.1) containing two disulfide bonds and targeting mostly cysteine proteases, including ficin, papain, and cathepsins B, H and L. Cystatin exhibits antibacterial activity by preventing the growth of group A *Streptococcus*,[64] *Salmonella* Typhimurium[65] and *Porphyromonas gingivalis*.[66] Bactericidal activity has been observed for cystatin at low dose against *Acinetobacter lwoffii*, *E. coli*, *Oligella* spp. and *Pseudomonas aeruginosa*.[67] Cystatin is active not only against bacteria but also against viruses and fungi. Antiviral activities have been demonstrated *in vitro* and *in vivo*. In human cultured cells infected with poliovirus, the addition of chicken cystatin can alter the intracellular proteolytic processing of poliovirus proteins and reduce the production of viruses.[68] Another study demonstrated that chicken cystatin was able to protect mice infected by human rotavirus.[69] The antiviral effect of cystatin observed in these studies is likely to be mediated by the inhibition of proteases involved in viral replication. Cystatin exhibits antifungal activities against azole-sensitive *Candida albicans* isolates, as well as *Candida parapsilosis* and *Candida tropicalis*. *Candida glabrata* is also inhibited but it seems to be comparatively more resistant to the action of cystatin. The inhibition of azole-sensitive *Candida albicans* isolates is achieved with minimal inhibitory concentration values comparable to those obtained with fluconazole and histatin 5.[70] Cystatin may also be antiparasitic as it is a potent inhibitor of cysteine proteases expressed by *Trypanosoma cruzi*, a parasite responsible for trypanosomiasis.[71,72]

14.3.2.2 Vitamin-binding Proteins

Among the main egg vitamin-binding proteins are avidin and riboflavin-binding protein, which are present within all egg compartments. Their physiological function is likely related to the supply of the egg and the developing embryo with vitamins: biotin and riboflavin, respectively. However, it is hypothesized that they could also be indirectly involved in antimicrobial defenses by inhibiting microorganisms' growth that requires these vitamins.

Avidin is a cationic homotetrameric glycoprotein (68.3 kDa, pI 10) exhibiting a very high affinity for biotin (vitamin B8/H). The dissociation constant is around 10^{-15} M,[73] which is one of the strongest non-covalent interactions found in nature. This protein can potentially inhibit the growth of biotin-requiring microorganisms.[74] Interestingly, avidin is able to bind to various Gram-negative and Gram-positive bacteria, including *E. coli*, *Klebsiella pneumonia*, *Serratia marcescens*, *Pseudomonas aeruginosa*, *Staphylococcus aureus* and *Staphylococcus epidermis*.[75]

Riboflavin-binding protein (RfBP) is a phosphoglycoprotein of ~32 kDa with a pI of about 4. The apoprotein has a high affinity for riboflavin (vitamin B2) with a dissociation constant of 1.3×10^{-9} M.[76] RfBP has a critical role in embryonic development.[77] Present in the egg white of many avian species, the concentrations and the proportion of the apoform of RfBP can vary over a ten-fold range, which may reflect the possibility that RfBP in egg white possesses antimicrobial functions.[77]

14.3.2.3 Defensins

Defensins are cysteine-rich cationic peptides of about 2–6 kDa that are involved in the host innate defense. They are found in many living species, including vertebrates, invertebrates and plants. These antimicrobial peptides contain six conserved cysteines involved in three disulfide bonds, making them extremely compact and stable. Most of these molecules possess a broad-spectrum activity directed against Gram-positive and Gram-negative bacteria, but also against fungi and viruses. The antibacterial effect of defensins mainly results from direct interaction with the bacterial cell wall and disruption of the structure of cell membranes. Mammalian defensins are categorized into three families – alpha, beta and theta – according to the position and pairing of conserved cysteine residues; however, in birds, only beta-defensins have been identified. They are organized into two groups: the avian beta-defensins (AvBDs) and the ovodefensins (OvoDs). Proteomic studies conducted on chicken egg compartments revealed the presence of several defensins, including AvBD11 (vitelline membrane, egg white and eggshell), AvBD10 (eggshell), AvBD9 (yolk), and the ovodefensins gallin/OvoDA1 (egg white, vitelline membrane) and OvoDB1 (egg white).

AvBD11 (previously named vitelline membrane outer layer protein 2 or VMO-2) is a long size beta-defensin (9.2 kDa) composed of two beta-defensin motifs. Consequently, it contains 12 cysteines involved in six disulfide bonds. Such a structure is quite unique since no double defensins have been found in mammals to date. In chicken egg, AvBD11 is present within all compartments with the exception of yolk, but it is noteworthy that the vitelline membrane is likely the egg part where AvBD11 is the most abundant. Indeed, it is one of the major proteins of the outer layer of the vitelline membrane, together with ovomucin, lysozyme and VMO-1.[78] This antimicrobial polypeptide is active against *Salmonella* serovars Enteritidis and Typhimurium, *E. coli*, *Listeria monocytogenes* and *Staphylococcus aureus*.[79] AvBD11 is able to bind to heparin, a negatively charged glycosaminoglycan, which is used to purify this defensin from egg vitelline membrane by affinity chromatography. In turn, heparin can also inhibit the antibacterial activity of AvBD11, which suggests that the heparin-binding site on the protein may be involved in the mechanism of action.[80] AvBD10 (gallinacin-8) and AvBD9 (gallinacin-6) were identified in eggshell (matrix and membrane)[8,18] and egg-yolk plasma,[26] respectively. The physiological roles and antibacterial activities of these two defensins need to be further investigated.

Gallin or OvoDA1 (4.7 kDa) is an ovodefensin, a sub-family of beta-defensins initially found in the egg white from different avian species (chicken, turkey, swan and duck).[81] This cationic antimicrobial peptide is detected not only in chicken egg white but also in the vitelline membrane and eggshell membrane. In the egg white, this ovodefensin is gradually altered during egg storage,[82] which may affect its antimicrobial potential. Gallin/OvoDA1 is active against pathogenic and non-pathogenic *E. coli* strains, but not against *Salmonella* serovars Enteritidis and Typhimurium.[81,83,84] Avian pathogenic *E. coli* (APEC) seems, however, to be more resistant. Of note, a discrepancy regarding the susceptibility/resistance of *S. aureus* to gallin/OvoDA1 could be observed depending on the technique used to assess antibacterial activities (gelose or liquid phase).[81,84] Although the antibacterial spectrum of gallin/OvoDA1 needs to be further defined, it seems however that its antibacterial activity is limited compared to that of AvBD11. The three-dimensional structure of synthetic gallin contains a β-defensin fold but with significant variations, which might be related to its antibacterial specificity or other yet unknown functions.[84]

Recently, another ovodefensin, OvoDB1, has been identified in chicken egg white.[85] OvoDB1 is able to inhibit *E. coli* DH5α but with lower efficiency than OvoDA1, and faint/no activity was observed with APEC, *Salmonella* and *S. aureus*.[81]

14.3.2.4 Proteins of the LBP-BPI-Plunc Family

The LBP (LPS-binding protein)/BPI (bactericidal permeability increasing protein)/PLUNC (palate, lung and nasal epithelium clone protein) family consists of proteins involved in host defense against bacteria. Members of this family are able to bind bacterial lipopolysaccharide (LPS), a surface component of Gram-negative bacteria, and mediate alterations of the outer membrane and damage to the inner membrane of bacteria. These events lead to the inhibition of bacterial growth.[86] The chicken egg contains several members of this family, including OCX-36 and TENP (transiently expressed in neural precursor).

OCX-36 (Ovocalyxin-36) is a 36 kDa protein present in the eggshell and vitelline membrane,[25,39] and exhibits growth inhibitory activity against *Staphylococcus aureus* ATCC 6538.[87] OCX-36 was shown to possess lipopolysaccharide and lipoteichoic binding activities. Interestingly, a significant difference in *S. aureus* lipoteichoic acid binding activity was observed for two natural forms of OCX-36, Pro-71 and Ser-71, with a higher binding activity detected for Pro-71.[87]

TENP or ovoglobulin G2 is a protein of about 49 kDa. By analogy with other members of this family, TENP is assumed to be antibacterial but further investigations on this protein need to be performed to characterize and confirm chicken TENP's predicted function. TENP isolated from emu egg white, however, exhibits antibacterial activities against the Gram-positive bacteria *Micrococcus luteus* and *B. subtilis*, but not against the Gram-negative bacteria *E. coli* and *Salmonella* Typhimurium.[88]

14.3.2.5 Heparin-binding Proteins

A number of proteins present at low abundance in the egg are able to interact with heparin and possess antibacterial properties. Owing to its structure and negative charges, heparin can be seen as a compound with similarities to the negatively charged molecules present at the surface of bacteria. A previous study carried out on peptides with affinity for heparin demonstrated that these peptides have antibacterial properties.[89] This observation stimulated the development of a strategy based on heparin-affinity chromatography aiming at identifying novel antimicrobial egg molecules. The approach conducted on egg white allowed the identification of 20 proteins, including known antimicrobials and new potential candidates.[80] Five proteins contained in the egg white heparin fraction were isolated and characterized: AvBD11 (see Section 14.3.2.3 Defensins), ovalbumin-related protein X, beta-microseminoprotein-like, pleiotrophin and vitelline membrane outer layer protein 1. Antibacterial activities were confirmed *in vitro* for all these candidates and, interestingly, the heparin-binding site(s) of these molecules are likely to be involved, at least in part, in the antibacterial mechanism.

Ovalbumin-related protein X (OVAX) is a glycosylated heparin-binding protein of about 45–50 kDa, present in all egg compartments. It belongs to the ov-serpin family, which includes the major egg white protein ovalbumin. The ov-serpins are structurally related to serpins, a class of serine protein inhibitors, but functionally they are devoid of any antiprotease activities. In egg white, OVAX is estimated to be 100 times less concentrated than ovalbumin. Although OVAX and ovalbumin share high sequence identity, OVAX seems to be antimicrobial, as demonstrated for two foodborne disease pathogens, *Listeria monocytogenes* and *Salmonella* Enteritidis, whereas ovalbumin has no antibacterial activity.[90] Its activity may depend on the ability of OVAX, but not ovalbumin, to bind to the anionic surfaces/molecules (*e.g.*, heparin) since heparin (negatively charged glycosaminoglycan) can inhibit the anti-*Salmonella* properties of OVAX, presumably by blocking the heparin-binding site and therefore competing with bacteria at the antibacterial site of OVAX. A cluster of positively charged amino acid residues present at the surface of OVAX is thought to interact with heparin and participate in the antibacterial mechanism.[90] Interestingly, it has been shown that an alkaline treatment of OVAX can alter the presumed heparin-binding site,[91] suggesting that egg storage and the progressive pH increase observed in egg white may alter the antibacterial activities of OVAX.

VMO-1 (vitelline membrane outer layer protein 1) is a cationic protein of about 18 kDa containing four disulfide bonds and exhibiting antibacterial activities against *Listeria monocytogenes* but not against *Salmonella enterica* Enteritidis.[80] However, it is likely that this protein possesses other physiological roles in the egg, especially within the vitelline membrane where VMO-1 is abundant.[25] The tridimensional structure of VMO-1 is organized into a singular structural motif called a beta-prism, also found in domain II of the insecticidal delta-endotoxin (a pore-forming toxin produced by *Bacillus thuringiensis*) and in the plant jacalin-like lectin domain.[92,93] Beta-prism motifs are thought to interact with carbohydrates. The heparin-binding property of VMO-1 is partly involved in the anti-*Listeria* activity of VMO-1 but other mechanisms might act complementarily to this carbohydrate-binding property to destroy or inhibit bacteria.

Pleiotrophin (15.2 kDa, five disulfide bonds) is a cationic growth factor known for its high affinity for heparin. This protein is found in the egg white,[20] vitelline membrane[80] and eggshell.[8] The pleiotrophin sequence is extremely conserved across different species, with a sequence identity of more than 90% between chicken and mammalian sequences.[94] The human homolog is antibacterial against Gram-positive and Gram-negative bacterial strains and exerts its antibacterial action *via* a membrane disruption mechanism.[95] Antibacterial activities have also been reported for the chicken form, against *Listeria monocytogenes* and *Salmonella enterica* Enteritidis.[80]

Beta-microseminoprotein-like (gi:513191195/LOC101750704) is a small-size cationic cysteine-rich protein (9.9 kDa) recently identified in the egg white by heparin affinity. This protein also exhibits antibacterial activities against *Listeria monocytogenes* and *Salmonella enterica*.[80] Human beta-microseminoprotein possesses a potent fungicidal activity against *Candida albicans* whereas no antibacterial activity was observed against *E. coli*, *S. agalactiae*, *S. pyogenes*, *S. aureus* and *E. faecalis*.[96]

14.3.2.6 Other Antimicrobial Proteins

Ovomucin is a sulfated and heavily glycosylated protein belonging to the family of mucins, a group of proteins found in the numerous secretions of epithelial tissues and involved in the gel-like properties of secretions in which they are present. This large protein is composed of two subunits: an alpha subunit (MUC5B) low in carbohydrates and a carbohydrate-rich beta subunit (MUC6). The gel structure of egg white is attributed to the presence of ovomucin and more particularly to the complex it forms with lysozyme. The egg white's viscosity inhibits the migration of bacteria towards the yolk. Ovomucin also exhibits antibacterial and antiviral properties. The protein demonstrated inhibitory activity against colonization of *Helicobacter pylori* (a bacterium associated with peptic ulcer disease) in the stomach.[97] This effect might result from direct binding to *H. pylori* urease. In addition, hemagglutination inhibition activity was reported for ovomucin against bovine rotavirus and hen Newcastle Disease Virus.[98] While both subunits were active against the rotavirus, hemagglutination inhibition activity against Newcastle Disease Virus only requires the beta subunit moiety.

Ovocleidin-17 (OC-17) is a 17 kDa eggshell-specific protein. It belongs to the C-type lectin superfamily, a group of calcium-dependent carbohydrate-binding proteins with functions associated with cell–cell adhesion, immune response to pathogens and apoptosis. Purified OC-17 was shown to be bactericidal against Gram-positive bacteria *B. subtilis* and *S. aureus*, and exhibited enhanced activity in the presence of calcium.[99]

Histones are positively charged proteins that are able to bind to DNA. They are usually located in the eukaryotic cell nuclei nucleus, where they play critical roles in DNA compaction and chromatin regulation. However, these molecules can also be detected in the cytoplasm and in extracellular fluids. There is compelling evidence showing that extracellular histones may exert functions related to host defense and inflammatory responses. A number of studies have demonstrated the antibacterial potential of these proteins. Several histones have been identified in egg, including H1 and H2A. These two chicken histones, isolated from the hen's reproductive system, were shown to inhibit Gram-negative and Gram-positive bacteria.[100]

14.3.3 Other Activities

Many varied activities have been suggested for major proteins like ovalbumin, ovotransferrin and lysozyme. In contrast, besides antimicrobial activities, there is only limited (but promising) data illustrating the bioactive potential of egg components of lower abundance (Figure 14.2). Considering the numerous proteins and peptides, including bird-specific proteins, that have no associated functions in gene ontology databases but that are all assumed to support embryonic development, it is believed that the egg proteins still bear myriad biological surprises that deserve higher considerations.

14.3.3.1 Egg Proteins and Cancer

Cancer is associated with abnormal growth/proliferation of cells and their potential to invade or spread to other parts of the body (invasive activities). The following sub-sections present an overview of the various applications of egg proteins in cancer: (1) proteins with anti-cancerous potential (either anti-proliferative or anti-invasive), (2) proteins exhibiting specific physicochemical properties that may be useful for targeted therapy, and finally, (3) how immunoglobulins Y that are secreted into the egg yolk can also constitute a relevant approach for cancer diagnosis.

14.3.3.1.1 Anti-cancerous Activity. There is increasing evidence that food-derived proteins and peptides can be beneficial for preventing and curing cancer diseases.[101] Several studies have confirmed the tumor-inhibitory activity of lysozyme using experimental tumors, activity which essentially relies on immunopotentiation.[102] Here we will focus on emerging data on other less known egg-derived proteins such as the protease inhibitors cystatin and Kazal-like inhibitors (ovoinhibitor and ovomucoid), and phosvitin.

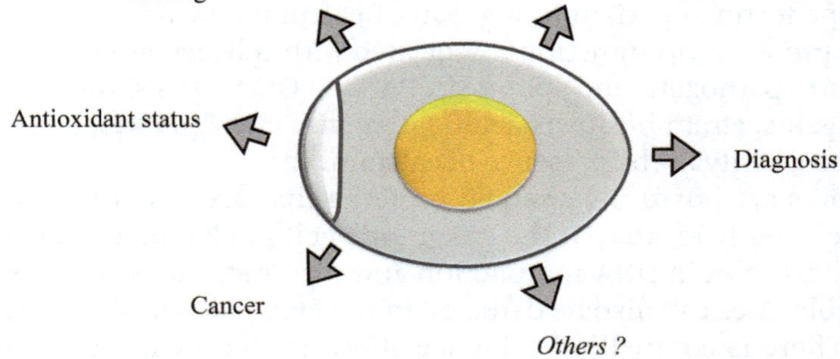

Figure 14.2 Potential therapeutic uses of minor egg proteins besides the treatment of infectious diseases. This scheme summarizes some potential applications for low abundance proteins that include avidin, glutathione peroxidases, immunoglobulin Y, OCX-36, ovomacroglobulin/ovostatin, ovomucin, ovomucoid, phosvitin and pleiotrophin.

Cancer progression is usually associated with proteolytic activities (cathepsins, serine proteases and metalloproteases) that degrade extracellular matrix proteins allowing for the proliferation and dissemination of cancerous cells. There are now compelling data that certain protease inhibitors, essentially extracted from plants, have strong anticarcinogenic activity.[103] Interestingly, egg white is characterized by several abundant protease inhibitors,[104] whose biological roles are still unclear. At least one of them, cystatin, a cysteine protease inhibitor, has revealed some anticancer properties.

Cystatins or cystatin-like proteins are present in mammals, birds, fish, insects, plants and some protozoa and regulate numerous physiological processes by inhibiting cysteine proteases (cathepsin L and B) that have a pivotal role in extracellular matrix degradation and tissue remodeling and whose activity is upregulated in metastatic progression.[105] Cystatins, either native or modified, have been proposed as anti-metastatic or cytotoxic molecules in many published studies.[106–114] In addition, ovomucoid and ovoinhibitor, which contain three and seven Kazal domains, respectively, might also have promising effects considering the antitumor activity reported for serine protease inhibitor Kazal-type 6.[115] Conversely, some Kazal inhibitors might also act as growth factors and are associated with the aggressiveness of some tumors.[116] It would be very interesting to assess such activities for both egg-specific inhibitors, which are omnipresent in egg white, whose expressions are indeed under hormonal control and which therefore may have a major role during embryonic development to drive yolk sac development/progression onto the vitelline membrane matrix.

More recently, phosvitin has revealed some cytotoxic activity against various cancer cell lines while having protective effects against the oxidative stress-induced DNA damage in leucocytes.[117]

Further studies will be needed to better appreciate the potential of all these egg molecules for cancer therapy and it might also be relevant to evaluate the synergistic activity of several of these egg candidates (or partly purified fractions) on cancer cell progression.

14.3.3.1.2 Egg Proteins in Targeting Cancer Cells. Another interesting feature of some of these egg proteins is their high affinity for some vitamins or other molecules, suggesting that they could constitute some promising carriers to deliver drugs and bioactive compounds to the tumor site and for the development of targeted therapy. The goal of such an approach is to increase the concentration of the drug in the vicinity of the cancerous cells without affecting healthy cells and while limiting side-effects. The egg archetype for such use is probably egg white avidin, *via* its very high affinity for biotin[118] and its ability to bind lectins, which are highly expressed at the surface of tumor cells.[119] A very recent article reported that ovomucin might also be a potential candidate as a mucoadhesive carrier to efficiently encapsulate and deliver drugs in various mucosal tissues.[120] Another approach is to inject peptide or protein biomarkers for cancer cells into hens, which will further produce specific antibodies (immunoglobulin Y) that will be transferred into the yolk, which thereby serves as a noninvasive source of bioactive antibodies. This approach using chicken IgY has shown promising results in killing breast cancer cells.[121,122]

14.3.3.1.3 Egg Proteins and Diagnosis of Cancer. In parallel, the immunoglobulin Y strategy to produce antibodies against cancerous biomarkers has been extensively used to develop tools (ELISA/immunohistochemistry) that contribute to the diagnosis/prognosis of the disease.[123–130]

14.3.3.2 Egg Proteins and Tissue Remodeling/Wound Healing

Although cell proliferation and migration play a major role in pathological processes including cancer, they also have a major role in wound healing and tissue remodeling. Many proteins constituting the vitelline membrane, which supports the growth of the embryo and that of the vascularized yolk sac, are assumed to promote/regulate embryonic cell proliferation/migration onto the vitelline membrane and embryonic development. Such activities have been described for some proteins, such as ovomacroglobulin, ovomucin and pleiotrophin, which are components of the vitelline membrane and the egg white, as well as egg-yolk phosvitin, which may also act in interaction with the embryo.

Ovomacroglobulin is a broad-spectrum protease inhibitor that belongs the superfamily of alpha2-macroglobulins. Alpha-2-macroglobulins also act as carrier proteins for cytokines and growth factors. The exact role of ovomacroglobulin in eggs is not clear but some studies on mouse embryonic and primary human skin fibroblasts have shown that ovomacroglobulin was triggering cell migration by enhancing cell adhesion to the extracellular matrix, reducing inter-cellular aggregation and strengthening the cytoskeleton.[131] Ovomucin, a glycoprotein composed of alpha-ovomucin/MUC5B and beta-ovomucin/MUC6 is responsible for the gel-like structure of egg white and has also been identified in the vitelline membrane. Mucins participate in lubrication of mucous-type epithelia and modulate the cell and substratum adhesion. An ovomucin-like protein was demonstrated to be expressed by chicken primordial germ cells during early embryonic development. Ovomucin was suggested to favor migration of primordial germ cells by facilitating their aggregation and by preventing their adhesion to fibroblasts until primordial germ cells reach the gonadal ridges.[132] Better knowledge of the biological activities of these candidates on cell migration and invasion in interaction with the chicken embryo and at various stages of development may help to identify egg proteins involved in organogenesis and morphogenesis that could further constitute interesting candidates for wound healing and tissue regeneration. In this respect, various publications have also highlighted the potential role of phosvitin and pleiotrophin in bone organogenesis.

Phosvitin is an egg-yolk protein naturally generated after limited proteolysis of vitellogenins. It has unique properties suspected to be critical during egg embryo development as it stimulates differentiation of osteoblasts, collagen synthesis, hydroxyproline formation and biomineralization, similarly to ascorbate (vitamin C), which is the only vitamin that is actually absent in egg[133,134]. In mammals, pleiotrophin is a secreted heparin-binding peptide expressed in mesodermal and neuroectodermal cells during development, but rarely in mature cartilage. However, it may be re-expressed in chondrocytes to participate in cartilage repair in the early stages of osteoarthritis.[135–137] Pleiotrophin has been identified in egg white, the vitelline membrane and in the eggshell and is highly conserved between species. To conclude, both phosvitin and chicken pleiotrophin may have interesting applications in tissue engineering and regenerative medicine.

14.3.3.3 Bioactive Proteins and Inflammation

Inflammation is a natural biological response to infections, damaged cells or irritants to maintain homeostasis, initiate repair and eliminate aggressors. Inflammation is a complex process that involves immune cells, blood vessels and molecular mediators. Chicken eggs contain several different pro- and anti-inflammatory components, such as egg phospholipids, cholesterol, the carotenoids lutein and zeaxanthin, and bioactive proteins, mainly ovalbumin and ovotransferrin or derived peptides.[138] In addition to these major proteins, recent studies have reported that the livetin fraction of yolk (and its resulting hydrolysates) may have anti-inflammatory activity by enhancing the phagocytic activity of macrophages[139] and that eggshell membrane extract also had a positive impact by reducing the secretion of pro-inflammatory molecules while stimulating those of anti-inflammatory cytokines.[140] The identity of the proteins that are responsible for such activities is still not known, but some publications have described similar effects for some proteins that were identified in the eggshell (ovocalyxin-36) or the egg white/vitelline membranes (pleiotrophin). Ovocalyxin-36 is an eggshell-specific protein initially described as an antimicrobial molecule that exhibits immunostimulatory activities after stimulation with lipopolysaccharide and that inhibits the production of pro-inflammatory cytokines *in vivo*.[141] Pleiotrophin is a universal multifunctional heparin-binding protein that possesses cytokine properties, among many other activities. Chicken pleiotrophin purified from egg white has recently been described as an antimicrobial protein, but it might also have interesting immunomodulatory activities in promoting lymphocyte survival and chemotaxis, like its human homolog with which it shares 93% sequence identity.[142,143]

14.3.3.4 Antioxidant Activities

Most organisms possess many cellular and molecular mechanisms to overcome environmental stresses, which trigger the accumulation of toxic oxygen radicals, which are associated with numerous functional dysregulations. In normal situations, potent antioxidant molecules, including dietary polyphenols and vitamins, but also multiple endogenous enzymes, limit the toxic effects of these radicals. Chicken egg contains many antioxidant compounds that encompass vitamins, carotenoids, minerals and trace elements but also major proteins, such as ovotransferrin or egg-yolk phosvitin.[144–146] There are also increasing data related to the antioxidant capacity of hydrolytic peptides[147–150] but the antioxidant potential of minor proteins has not yet been investigated. However, proteomic approaches revealed the presence of some enzymes catalyzing the reduction of peroxides in egg white and yolk: glutathione peroxidase 3, P22352, egg white; similar to glutathione peroxidase, NP_001156704, egg yolk.[20,21,25,27]

14.3.3.5 Unexplored Potential of Enzyme Inhibitors

Egg contains several enzymes inhibitors, such as antiproteases and a lipase inhibitor of high abundance, that are bird/oviparous specific and that are distributed between the egg white and egg-yolk compartments. The fact that they accumulate in the egg suggests that they have an important role during embryonic development. For most of these molecules, the biological function is not known, likely owing to the fact that the targeted proteases have not yet been identified. Antiproteases are involved in many biological processes by regulating proteolytic/degrading activities that can have adverse effects when uncontrolled. It is quite intriguing to realize that egg is a major source of protease inhibitors with still unknown functions. In many invertebrates, Kazal-type proteinase inhibitors (a family encompassing egg white ovomucoid and ovoinhibitor) are described as defensive molecules since they alter the digestion of predators by inhibiting their digestive enzymes.[151] These mechanisms of defense are also widely encountered in plants that contain potent protease inhibitors and there is compelling evidence that they may have powerful chemopreventive applications.[103,152,153] Whether such egg inhibitors have similar physiological activities would be interesting to investigate and the increasing data published on plant antiproteases suggest that egg antiproteases may have similar positive effects on egg eaters/predators, including humans, especially when eating raw eggs. The broad-spectrum potent inhibitory activities of these molecules may have some interest for treating pathological situations associated with protease overactivity. Similarly, in the search for innovative molecules to treat obesity, there is increasing consideration of developing lipase inhibitors to counteract the excessive accumulation of fat observed in patients.[154,155] To our knowledge, there are no available studies that have investigated the potential of egg-yolk lipase inhibitor (apovitellin) in inhibiting human lipases. Apovitellenin is indeed a very potent molecule, whose physiological function is to prevent the loss of lipids from chicken very-low-density lipoproteins during their transport from the liver to the growing yolk follicles.[156]

14.4 Conclusions

Chicken egg contains many abundant molecules likely to bear original functions. Many of these proteins would be of great interest for non-food uses in human health (antimicrobials, anticancer or diagnosis molecules) and material sciences (proteins involved in biomineralization as biomimetics for ceramics). Nevertheless, a better appreciation of the functional activities of egg proteins will need further studies to consider their intimate functions that are assumed to be related to embryonic development. So far, the biological activity of egg components has been investigated using proteins or peptides that were purified from freshly unfertilized laid eggs. However, there is some evidence that these molecules may undergo some changes during incubation/embryonic development, which occurs at higher temperature (37.8 °C), that are likely to activate some latent activities. Additionally, usually, the bioactivities of eggs are screened based on the presence of domains or homologies with annotated molecules. Knowing that several egg proteins are bird-specific and do not have annotated functions in databases, the list of egg bioactive molecules is likely to be underestimated. The key is probably to analyze the kinetics of the assimilation/use of these various molecules by the embryo and to develop some specific models allowing for the depletion of one or the other candidate[157,158] to explore its impact on embryonic development. A better connection between egg protein biochemists and fundamental development biologists would be helpful to decipher the potential of egg proteins. Moreover, some differences exist in egg protein abundance or composition, and in protein sequences between avian species, which have adapted their egg contents during evolution to face various environmental challenges.[85,88,159] Thus, we believe that avian egg proteins still harbor many secrets and hidden bioactivities that may be of high value for human health.

References

1. International Chicken Genome sequencing Consortium, *Nature*, 2004, **432**, 695–716.
2. J. Gautron, F. Nau, K. Mann, C. Guerin-Dubiard, S. Rehault, M. T. Hincke and Y. Nys, *World's Poult. Sci. J.*, 2007, **63**, 82–90.
3. J. Gautron, S. Réhault-Godbert and Y. Nys, in *Improving the Safety and Quality of Eggs and Egg products*, ed. Y. Nys, M. Bain and F. Van Immerseel, Egg Chemistry, Production and Consumption, Woodhead Publishing limited, Cambridge, 2011, vol. 1, pp. 133–150.
4. M. Anton, F. Nau and Y. Nys, *World's Poult. Sci. J.*, 2006, **62**, 429–438.
5. Y. Mine and J. Kovacs-Nolan, *World's Poult. Sci. J.*, 2006, **62**, 87–95.
6. S. Rehault, M. Anton, F. Nau, J. Gautron and Y. Nys, *INRA Prod. Anim.*, 2007, **20**, 337–347.

7. S. Réhault-Godbert, V. Hervé, J. Gautron, C. Cabau and Y. Nys, in *Improving the Safety and Quality of Eggs and Egg products*, ed. Y. Nys, M. Bain and F. Van Immerseel, Egg Chemistry, Production and Consumption, Woodhead Publishing Ltd, Cambridge, 2011, vol. 1, pp. 183–208.
8. K. Mann, B. Macek and J. V. Olsen, *Proteomics*, 2006, **6**, 3801–3810.
9. K. Mann, J. V. Olsen, B. Macek, F. Gnad and M. Mann, *Proteomics*, 2007, **7**, 106–115.
10. I. Miksik, J. Charvatova, A. Eckhardt and Z. Deyl, *Electrophoresis*, 2003, **24**, 843–852.
11. I. Miksik, A. Eckhardt, P. Sedlakova and K. Mikulikova, *Connect. Tissue Res.*, 2007, **48**, 1–8.
12. I. Mikšík, P. Ergang and J. Pácha, *Anal. Bioanal. Chem.*, 2014, **406**, 7633–7640.
13. I. Mikšik, P. Sedláková, K. Lacinová, S. Pataridis and A. Eckhardt, *Anal. Bioanal. Chem.*, 2010, **397**(1), 205–214.
14. M. Rose-Martel, J. Du and M. T. Hincke, *J. Proteomics*, 2012, **75**, 2697–2706.
15. T. A. E. Ahmed, H. P. Suso and M. T. Hincke, *J. Proteomics*, 2017, **155**, 49–62.
16. C. J. Sun, G. Y. Xu and N. Yang, *Proteomics*, 2013, **13**, 3523–3536.
17. P. Marie, V. Labas, A. Brionne, G. Harichaux, C. Hennequet-Antier, A. B. Rodriguez-Navarro, Y. Nys and J. Gautron, *J. Proteomics*, 2015, **126**, 140–154.
18. S. Makkar, R. Liyanage, L. Kannan, B. Packialakshmi, J. O. Lay Jr. and N. C. Rath, *J. Agric. Food Chem.*, 2015, **63**, 9888–9898.
19. C. Guerin-Dubiard, M. Pasco, D. Molle, C. Desert, T. Croguennec and F. Nau, *J. Agric. Food Chem.*, 2006, **54**, 3901–3910.
20. C. D'Ambrosio, S. Arena, A. Scaloni, L. Guerrier, E. Boschetti, M. E. Mendieta, A. Citterio and P. G. Righetti, *J. Proteome Res.*, 2008, **7**, 3461–3474.
21. K. Mann, *Proteomics*, 2007, **7**, 3558–3568.
22. K. Mann and M. Mann, *Prot. Sci.*, 2011, **9**, 6.
23. J. P. Wang, Y. Liang, D. A. Omana, N. N. V. Kav and J. P. Wu, *J. Agric. Food Chem.*, 2012, **60**, 272–282.
24. N. Qiu, M. Ma, L. Zhao, W. Liu, Y. Li and Y. Mine, *J. Agric. Food Chem.*, 2012, **60**, 7746–7753.
25. K. Mann, *Proteomics*, 2008, **8**, 2322–2332.
26. K. Mann and M. Mann, *Proteomics*, 2008, **8**, 178–191.
27. A. Farinazzo, U. Restuccia, A. Bachi, L. Guerrier, F. Fortis, E. Boschetti, E. Rasoli, A. Citterio and P. G. Righetti, *J. Chromatogr. A*, 2009, **1216**, 1241–1252.
28. M. T. Hincke, Y. Nys and J. Gautron, *J. Poult. Sci.*, 2010, **47**, 208–219.
29. M. T. Hincke, Y. Nys, J. Gautron, K. Mann, A. B. Rodriguez-Navarro and M. D. McKee, *Front. Biosci.*, 2012, **17**, 1266–1280.
30. Y. Nys, J. Gautron, J. M. Garcia-Ruiz and M. T. Hincke, *C. R. Palevol*, 2004, **3**, 549–562.
31. A. B. Rodríguez-Navarro, P. Marie, Y. Nys, M. T. Hincke and J. Gautron, *J. Struct. Biol.*, 2015, **190**, 291–303.

32. J. Gautron and Y. Nys, in *Bioactive Egg Compounds*, ed. R. Huopalahti, R. Lopez-Fandino, M. Anton and R. Schade, Springer-Verlag, Germany, 2007, pp. 109–115.
33. J. Gautron, M. T. Hincke and Y. Nys, *Connect. Tissue Res.*, 1997, **36**, 195–210.
34. G. Abatangelo, D. Dagagordini, I. Castellani and R. Cortivo, *Calcif. Tissue Res.*, 1978, **26**, 247–252.
35. R. Cortivo, I. Castellani, M. Martelli, G. Michelotto and G. Abatangelo, *J. Chromatogr.*, 1982, **237**, 127–135.
36. M. T. Hincke, A. M. Bernard, E. R. Lee, C. P. Tsang and R. Narbaitz, *Br. Poult. Sci.*, 1992, **33**, 505–516.
37. J. L. Arias, D. A. Carrino, M. S. Fernandez, J. P. Rodriguez, J. E. Dennis and A. I. Caplan, *Arch. Biochem. Biophys.*, 1992, **298**, 293–302.
38. K. Mann, J. Gautron, Y. Nys, M. D. McKee, T. Bajari, W. J. Schneider and M. T. Hincke, *Matrix Biol.*, 2003, **22**, 397–407.
39. J. Gautron, E. Murayama, A. Vignal, M. Morisson, M. D. McKee, S. Rehault, V. Labas, M. Belghazi, M. L. Vidal, Y. Nys and M. T. Hincke, *J. Biol. Chem.*, 2007, **282**, 5273–5286.
40. J. L. Arias, D. J. Fink, S. Q. Xiao, A. H. Heuer and A. I. Caplan, *Int. Rev. Cytol.*, 1993, **145**, 217–250.
41. J. Gautron, M. Bain, S. Solomon and Y. Nys, *Br. Poult. Sci.*, 1996, **37**, 853–866.
42. J. M. Dominguez-Vera, J. Gautron, J. M. Garcia-Ruiz and Y. Nys, *Poult. Sci.*, 2000, **79**, 901–907.
43. A. Hernandez-Hernandez, J. Gomez-Morales, A. B. Rodriguez-Navarro, J. Gautron, Y. Nys and J. M. Garcia-Ruiz, *Cryst. Growth Des.*, 2008, **8**, 4330–43339.
44. C. Jimenez-Lopez, A. Rodriguez-Navarro, J. M. Dominguez-Vera and J. M. Garcia-Ruiz, *Geochim. Cosmochim. Acta*, 2003, **67**, 1667–1676.
45. J. Gautron, M. T. Hincke, M. Panhéleux, J. M. Garcia-Ruiz, T. Boldicke and Y. Nys, *Connect. Tissue Res.*, 2001, **42**(4), 255–267.
46. M. T. Hincke, J. Gautron, M. Panheleux, J. M. Garcia-Ruiz, M. D. McKee and Y. Nys, *Matrix Biol.*, 2000, **19**, 443–453.
47. J. P. Reyes-Grajeda, A. Moreno and A. Romero, *J. Biol. Chem.*, 2004, **279**, 40876–40881.
48. C. L. Freeman, J. H. Harding, D. Quigley and P. M. Rodger, *J. Phys. Chem.*, 2011, **115**(16), 8175–8183.
49. C. L. Freeman, J. H. Harding, D. Quigley and P. M. Rodger, *Phys. Chem. Chem. Phys.*, 2012, **14**(20), 7287.
50. C. L. Freeman, J. H. Harding, D. Quigley and P. M. Rodger, *Phys. Chem. Chem. Phys.*, 2015, **17**(26), 17494–17500.
51. V. Pipich, M. Balz, S. E. Wolf, W. Tremel and D. Schwahn, *J. Am. Chem. Soc.*, 2008, **130**(21), 6879–6892.
52. S. E. Wolf, J. Leiterer, V. Pipich, R. Barrea, F. Emmerling and W. Tremel, *J. Am. Chem. Soc.*, 2011, **133**(32), 12642–12649.
53. M. S. Fernandez, A. Moya, L. Lopez and J. L. Arias, *Matrix Biol.*, 2001, **19**, 793–803.

54. A. M. Ahmed, A. B. Rodriguez-Navarro, M. L. Vidal, J. Gautron, J. M. Garcia-Ruiz and Y. Nys, *Br. Poult. Sci.*, 2005, **46**, 268–279.
55. M. Panheleux, Y. Nys, J. Williams, J. Gautron, T. Boldicke and M. T. Hincke, *Poult. Sci.*, 2000, **79**, 580–588.
56. I. C. Dunn, N. Joseph, M. Bain, A. Edmond, P. W. Wilson, P. Milona, Y. Nys, J. Gautron, M. Schmutz, R. Preisinger and D. Waddington, *Anim. Genet.*, 2009, **40**, 110–114.
57. I. C. Dunn, A. B. Rodriguez-Navarro, K. McDade, M. Schmutz, R. Preisinger, D. Waddington, P. W. Wilson and M. M. Bain, *Anim. Genet.*, 2012, **43**, 410–418.
58. H. Takahashi, O. Sasaki, K. Nirasawa and T. Furukawa, *Anim. Genet.*, 2010, **41**(5), 541–544.
59. H. Takahashi, D. Yang, O. Sasaki, T. Furukawa and K. Nirasawa, *Anim. Genet.*, 2009, **40**, 779–782.
60. H. Rome, A. Varenne, F. Herault, H. Chapuis, C. Alleno, P. Dehais, A. Vignal, T. Burlot and P. Le Roy, *Genet., Sel., Evol.*, 2015, **47**, 11.
61. W. Ardelt and M. Laskowski Jr, *Biochemistry*, 1985, **24**, 5313–5320.
62. M. Bourin, J. Gautron, M. Berges, S. Attucci, G. Le Blay, V. Labas, Y. Nys and S. Rehault-Godbert, *J. Agric. Food Chem.*, 2011, **59**, 12368–12374.
63. A. Molla, Y. Matsumura, T. Yamamoto, R. Okamura and H. Maeda, *Infect. Immun.*, 1987, **55**, 2509–2517.
64. L. Bjorck, *Mol. Microbiol.*, 1990, **4**, 1439–1442.
65. S. Nakai, in *Egg Nutrition and Biotechnology*, ed. J. S. Sim, S. Nakai and W. Guenter, CAB International, Wallingford, UK, 2000, pp. 205–217.
66. M. F. Blankenvoorde, Y. M. Henskens, W. van't Hof, E. C. Veerman and A. V. Nieuw Amerongen, *Biol. Chem. Hoppe-Seyler*, 1996, **377**, 847–850.
67. E. Wesierska, Y. Saleh, T. Trziszka, W. Kopec, M. Siewinski and K. Korzekwa, *World J. Microbiol. Biotechnol.*, 2005, **21**, 59–64.
68. B. D. Korant, J. Brzin and V. Turk, *Biochem. Biophys. Res. Commun.*, 1985, **127**, 1072–1076.
69. T. Ebina and K. Tsukada, *Microbiol. Immunol.*, 1991, **35**, 583–588.
70. A. Kolaczkowska, M. Kolaczkowski, A. Sokolowska, H. Miecznikowska, A. Kubiak, K. Rolka and A. Polanowski, *Mycoses*, 2010, **53**, 314–320.
71. A. P. C. A. Lima, F. C. G. dos Reis, C. Serveau, G. Lalmanach, L. Juliano, R. Ménard, T. Vernet, D. Y. Thomas, A. C. Storer and J. Scharfstein, *Mol. Biochem. Parasitol.*, 2001, **114**, 41–52.
72. C. Serveau, G. Lalmanach, M. A. Juliano, J. Scharfstein, L. Juliano and F. Gauthier, *Biochem. J.*, 1996, **313**, 951–956.
73. N. M. Green, *Biochem. J.*, 1963, **89**, 585–591.
74. R. G. Board and R. Fuller, *Biol. Rev.*, 1974, **49**, 15–49.
75. J. Korpela, E.-M. Salonen, P. Kuusela, M. Sarvas and A. Vaheri, *FEMS Microbiol. Lett.*, 1984, **22**, 3–10.
76. J. Becvar and G. Palmer, *J. Biol. Chem.*, 1982, **257**, 5607–5617.
77. H. B. White 3rd and A. H. Merrill Jr, *Annu. Rev. Nutr.*, 1988, **8**, 279–299.
78. S. Kido, A. Morimoto, F. Kim and Y. K. Doi, *Biochem. J.*, 1992, **286**, 17–22.

79. V. Herve-Grepinet, S. Rehault-Godbert, V. Labas, T. Magallon, C. Derache, M. Lavergne, J. Gautron, A. C. Lalmanach and Y. Nys, *Antimicrob. Agents Chemother.*, 2010, **54**, 4401–4409.
80. N. Guyot, V. Labas, G. Harichaux, M. Chesse, J. C. Poirier, Y. Nys and S. Rehault-Godbert, *Sci. Rep.*, 2016, **6**, 27974.
81. N. Whenham, T. C. Lu, M. B. Maidin, P. W. Wilson, M. M. Bain, M. L. Stevenson, M. P. Stevens, M. R. Bedford and I. C. Dunn, *Biol. Reprod.*, 2015, **92**, 154.
82. M. Y. Liu, W. L. Yu, F. Z. Ren and J. P. Wu, *Food Chem.*, 2018, **263**, 135–141.
83. D. Gong, P. W. Wilson, M. M. Bain, K. McDade, J. Kalina, V. Herve-Grepinet, Y. Nys and I. C. Dunn, *BMC Immunol.*, 2010, **11**, 12.
84. V. Herve, H. Meudal, V. Labas, S. Rehault-Godbert, J. Gautron, M. Berges, N. Guyot, A. F. Delmas, Y. Nys and C. Landon, *J. Biol. Chem.*, 2014, **289**, 7211–7220.
85. C. Sun, J. Liu, W. Li, G. Xu and N. Yang, *Proteomics*, 2017, **17**, 1770137.
86. P. Elsbach and J. Weiss, *Curr. Opin. Immunol.*, 1998, **10**, 45–49.
87. C. M. M. Cordeiro, H. Esmaili, G. Ansah and M. T. Hincke, *PLoS One*, 2013, **8**(12), e84112.
88. K. Maehashi, M. Ueda, M. Matano, J. Takeuchi, M. Uchino, Y. Kashiwagi and T. Watanabe, *J. Agric. Food Chem.*, 2014, **62**, 5156–5162.
89. E. Andersson, V. Rydengard, A. Sonesson, M. Morgelin, L. Bjorck and A. Schmidtchen, *Eur. J. Biochem.*, 2004, **271**, 1219–1226.
90. S. Rehault-Godbert, V. Labas, E. Helloin, V. Herve-Grepinet, C. Slugocki, M. Berges, M.-C. Bourin, A. Brionne, J.-C. Poirier, J. Gautron, F. Coste and Y. Nys, *J. Biol. Chem.*, 2013, **288**, 17285–17295.
91. T. Akazawa, M. Ogawa, S. Hayakawa, M. Hirata and T. Niwa, *Poult. Sci.*, 2018, **97**, 1730–1737.
92. R. Sankaranarayanan, K. Sekar, R. Banerjee, V. Sharma, A. Surolia and M. Vijayan, *Nat. Struct. Biol.*, 1996, **3**, 596–603.
93. T. Shimizu and K. Morikawa, *Trends Biochem. Sci.*, 1996, **21**, 3–6.
94. H. Rauvala, H. J. Huttunen, C. Fages, M. Kaksonen, T. Kinnunen, S. Imai, E. Raulo and I. Kilpeläinen, *Matrix Biol.*, 2000, **19**, 377–387.
95. S. L. Svensson, M. Pasupuleti, B. Walse, M. Malmsten, M. Morgelin, C. Sjogren, A. I. Olin, M. Collin, A. Schmidtchen, R. Palmer and A. Egesten, *J. Biol. Chem.*, 2010, **285**, 16105–16115.
96. A. M. Edstrom Hagerwall, V. Rydengard, P. Fernlund, M. Morgelin, M. Baumgarten, A. M. Cole, M. Malmsten, B. B. Kragelund and O. E. Sorensen, *PLoS Pathog.*, 2012, **8**, e1002625.
97. Y. Kodama and K. Nobutake, *US Pat.* US6235709 B1, 2001.
98. Y. Tsuge, M. Shimoyamada and K. Watanabe, *Biosci., Biotechnol., Biochem.*, 1996, **60**, 1505–1506.
99. O. Wellman-Labadie, R. Lakshminarayanan and M. T. Hincke, *FEBS Lett.*, 2008, **582**, 699–704.
100. U. Silphaduang, M. T. Hincke, Y. Nys and Y. Mine, *Biochem. Biophys. Res. Commun.*, 2006, **340**, 648–655.

101. B. Hernandez-Ledesma and C. C. Hsieh, *Crit. Rev. Food Sci. Nutr.*, 2017, **57**, 2358–2376.
102. G. Sava, A. Benetti, V. Ceschia and S. Pacor, *Anticancer Res.*, 1989, **9**, 583–591.
103. A. Clemente and C. Arques Mdel, *World J. Gastroenterol.*, 2014, **20**, 10305–10315.
104. I. Saxena and S. Tayyab, *Cell. Mol. Life Sci.*, 1997, **53**, 13–23.
105. M. Abrahamson, M. Alvarez-Fernandez and C. M. Nathanson, *Biochem. Soc. Symp.*, 2003, 179–199.
106. R. Colella and S. F. Casey, *Biotech. Histochem.*, 2003, **78**, 101–108.
107. J. Krol, C. Kopitz, A. Kirschenhofer, M. Schmitt, U. Magdolen, A. Kruger and V. Magdolen, *Biol. Chem.*, 2003, **384**, 1097–1102.
108. J. Krol, S. Sato, P. Rettenberger, I. Assfalg-Machleidt, M. Schmitt, V. Magdolen and U. Magdolen, *Biol. Chem.*, 2003, **384**, 1085–1096.
109. B. Muehlenweg, I. Assfalg-Machleidt, S. G. Parrado, M. Burgle, S. Creutzburg, M. Schmitt, E. A. Auerswald, W. Machleidt and V. Magdolen, *J. Biol. Chem.*, 2000, **275**, 33562–33566.
110. A. Premzl, V. Puizdar, V. Zavasnik-Bergant, N. Kopitar-Jerala, T. T. Lah, N. Katunuma, B. F. Sloane, V. Turk and J. Kos, *Biol. Chem.*, 2001, **382**, 853–857.
111. A. Premzl, V. Zavasnik-Bergant, V. Turk and J. Kos, *Exp. Cell Res.*, 2003, **283**, 206–214.
112. Y. Saleh, M. Siewinski, W. Kielan, P. Ziolkowski, M. Grybos and J. Rybka, *J. Exp. Ther. Oncol.*, 2003, **3**, 319–324.
113. M. Malicka-Blaszkiewicz, N. Filipczak, K. Golab, K. Juszczynska, T. Sebzda and J. Gburek, *Acta Biochim. Pol.*, 2014, **61**, 753–758.
114. M. Cegnar, A. Premzl, V. Zavasnik-Bergant, J. Kristl and J. Kos, *Exp. Cell Res.*, 2004, **301**, 223–231.
115. K. Ge, J. Huang, W. Wang, M. Gu, X. Dai, Y. Xu, H. Wu, G. Li, H. Lu, J. Zhong and Q. Huang, *Oncotarget*, 2017, **8**, 5965–5975.
116. K. Rasanen, O. Itkonen, H. Koistinen and U. H. Stenman, *Clin. Chem.*, 2016, **62**, 449–457.
117. S. H. Moon, J. H. Lee, M. Lee, E. Park, D. U. Ahn and H. D. Paik, *Poult. Sci.*, 2014, **93**, 2103–2107.
118. H. P. Lesch, M. U. Kaikkonen, J. T. Pikkarainen and S. Yla-Herttuala, *Expert Opin. Drug Delivery*, 2010, **7**, 551–564.
119. Z. Yao, M. Zhang, H. Sakahara, T. Saga, Y. Arano and J. Konishi, *J. Natl. Cancer Inst.*, 1998, **90**, 25–29.
120. A. Akbari and J. Wu, *Drug Delivery Transl. Res.*, 2017, **7**, 598–607.
121. S. Amirijavid, M. Entezari, A. Movafagh, M. Hashemi, A. Mosavi-Jarahi and H. Dehghani, *Asian Pac. J. Cancer Prev.*, 2016, **17**, 293–297.
122. Y. Xiao, X. Gao, O. Taratula, S. Treado, A. Urbas, R. D. Holbrook, R. E. Cavicchi, C. T. Avedisian, S. Mitra, R. Savla, P. D. Wagner, S. Srivastava and H. He, *BMC Cancer*, 2009, **9**, 351.
123. A. Lupicka-Slowik, M. Walczak, R. Grzywa, K. Bobrek, M. Lecka, S. Boivin, A. Gawel, T. Stefaniak, J. Oleksyszyn and M. Sienczyk, *Bioanalysis*, 2014, **6**, 3197–3213.

124. S. Al-Haddad, Z. Zhang, E. Leygue, L. Snell, A. Huang, Y. Niu, T. Hiller-Hitchcock, K. Hole, L. C. Murphy and P. H. Watson, *Am. J. Pathol.*, 1999, **155**, 2057–2066.
125. M. Esslimani-Sahla, A. Kramar, J. Simony-Lafontaine, M. Warner, J. A. Gustafsson and H. Rochefort, *Clin. Cancer Res.*, 2005, **11**, 3170–3174.
126. F. Noack, D. Helmecke, R. Rosenberg, S. Thorban, H. Nekarda, U. Fink, J. Lewald, M. Stich, K. Schutze, N. Harbeck, V. Magdolen, H. Graeff and M. Schmitt, *Int. J. Oncol.*, 1999, **15**, 617–623.
127. V. Sriram, C. E. Jebaraj and G. Yogeeswaran, *Indian J. Exp. Biol.*, 1999, **37**, 639–649.
128. Y. Xiao and X. Gao, *Biomarkers Med.*, 2010, **4**, 227–239.
129. Y. Xiao, X. Gao, G. Gannot, M. R. Emmert-Buck, S. Srivastava, P. D. Wagner, M. D. Amos and P. E. Barker, *Int. J. Cancer*, 2008, **122**, 2178–2186.
130. Y. Sun, Y. Yang, L. Wang, L. Lv, J. Zhu, W. Han, E. Wang, X. Guo and Y. Zhen, *Biologicals*, 2015, **43**, 165–170.
131. F. Geng, X. Huang and M. Ma, *J. Sci. Food Agric.*, 2016, **96**, 3188–3194.
132. W. Halfter, B. Schurer, H. M. Hasselhorn, B. Christ, E. Gimpel and H. H. Epperlein, *Development*, 1996, **122**, 915–923.
133. J. Liu, D. Czernick, S. C. Lin, A. Alasmari, D. Serge and E. Salih, *Dev. Biol.*, 2013, **381**, 256–275.
134. Q. Liu, C. Li, F. Geng, X. Huang and M. Ma, *J. Sci. Food Agric.*, 2017, **97**, 4532–4538.
135. R. Mentlein, *Expert Opin. Ther. Targets*, 2007, **11**, 861–867.
136. T. Pufe, M. Bartscher, W. Petersen, B. Tillmann and R. Mentlein, *Osteoarthr. Cartil.*, 2003, **11**, 260–264.
137. T. Pufe, G. Groth, M. B. Goldring, B. Tillmann and R. Mentlein, *Osteoarthr. Cartil.*, 2007, **15**, 155–162.
138. C. J. Andersen, *Nutrients*, 2015, **7**, 7889–7913.
139. C. Meram and J. Wu, *Food Res. Int.*, 2017, **100**, 449–459.
140. T. T. Vuong, S. B. Ronning, H. P. Suso, R. Schmidt, K. Prydz, M. Lundstrom, A. Moen and M. E. Pedersen, *J. Inflammation Res.*, 2017, **10**, 83–96.
141. J. Kovacs-Nolan, C. Cordeiro, D. Young, Y. Mine and M. Hincke, *Vet. Immunol. Immunopathol.*, 2014, **160**, 1–11.
142. A. Achour, J. P. M'Bika, F. Baudouin, D. Caruelle and J. Courty, *Biochimie*, 2008, **90**, 1791–1795.
143. N. Sorrelle, A. T. A. Dominguez and R. A. Brekken, *J. Leukocyte Biol.*, 2017, **102**, 277–286.
144. J. Kim, S. H. Moon, D. U. Ahn, H. D. Paik and E. Park, *Poult. Sci.*, 2012, **91**, 2747–2754.
145. C. Nimalaratne and J. Wu, *Nutrients*, 2015, **7**, 8274–8293.
146. E. Abeyrathne, X. Huang and D. U. Ahn, *Poult. Sci.*, 2018, **97**, 1462–1468.
147. C. Chen, Y. J. Chi, M. Y. Zhao and L. Lv, *Amino Acids*, 2012, **43**, 457–466.
148. S. Rao, J. Sun, Y. Liu, H. Zeng, Y. Su and Y. Yang, *Food Chem.*, 2012, **135**, 1245–1252.
149. S. Sun, H. Niu, T. Yang, Q. Lin, F. Luo and M. Ma, *J. Sci. Food Agric.*, 2014, **94**, 3195–3200.

150. M. Yousr and N. Howell, *Int. J. Mol. Sci.*, 2015, **16**, 29161–29178.
151. V. Rimphanitchayakit and A. Tassanakajon, *Dev. Comp. Immunol.*, 2010, **34**, 377–386.
152. P. J. Magee, R. Owusu-Apenten, M. J. McCann, C. I. Gill and I. R. Rowland, *Nutr. Cancer*, 2012, **64**, 741–748.
153. E. T. Johnson, C. Skory and P. F. Dowd, *J. Agric. Food Chem.*, 2014, **62**, 5458–5465.
154. R. B. Birari and K. K. Bhutani, *Drug Discovery Today*, 2007, **12**, 879–889.
155. N. A. Lunagariya, N. K. Patel, S. C. Jagtap and K. K. Bhutani, *EXCLI. J.*, 2014, **13**, 897–921.
156. W. J. Schneider, R. Carroll, D. L. Severson and J. Nimpf, *J. Lipid Res.*, 1990, **31**, 507–513.
157. T. S. Park, H. J. Lee, K. H. Kim, J. S. Kim and J. Y. Han, *Proc. Natl. Acad. Sci. U. S. A.*, 2014, **111**, 12716–12721.
158. I. Oishi, K. Yoshii, D. Miyahara, H. Kagami and T. Tagami, *Sci. Rep.*, 2016, **6**, 23980.
159. G. O. Oladipo and E. O. Ibukun, *Food Sci. Nutr.*, 2017, **5**, 334–343.

CHAPTER 15

Bioactivities and Mechanisms of Egg Protein-derived Peptides

WANG LIAO AND JIANPING WU*

Department of Agricultural, Food and Nutritional Science, 4-10 Agriculture/Forestry Centre, Edmonton, Alberta, T6G 2P5, Canada
*E-mail: jwu3@ualberta.ca

15.1 Introduction

Food protein-derived bioactive peptides are excellent ingredients for nutraceutical and functional food development. They are inactive within the parent proteins but can function as regulatory compounds to exert various physiological effects in the body, apart from their nutritional value, once they are liberated during gastrointestinal digestion or food processing.[1] Peptides from different food protein sources with various activities have been reported, mainly including antioxidant, anticancer, immunomodulatory, antimicrobial, antihypertensive and antidiabetic peptides.[2] These peptides have been implicated in the intervention or treatment of a wide range of chronic diseases;[3–6] because of their health-promoting potential, food protein-derived bioactive peptides have gained substantial interest during recent decades.

Egg is an important protein source in the human diet. One large egg contains ~6 g of protein, contributing ~11% of the daily protein intake.[7] Moreover, egg protein is high-quality and affordable, which makes it a model

Food Chemistry, Function and Analysis No.14
Eggs as Functional Foods and Nutraceuticals for Human Health
Edited by Jianping Wu

Published by the Royal Society of Chemistry, www.rsc.org

candidate for the identification of bioactive peptides. To date, research on egg protein-derived bioactive peptides has mainly focused on preparation, activity characterization and absorption. Progress in these areas has been comprehensively reviewed.[7–9]

Enzymatic digestion is the major approach to produce bioactive peptides from egg proteins. Pepsin and trypsin are two major gastrointestinal (GI) enzymes that have been applied widely to produce bioactive peptides from egg proteins.[10–13] It has also been conceived that the assistance of non-GI proteases could further improve the production of egg protein peptides.[9,14,15] Subcritical water hydrolysis is a novel technology that has been applied in recent years to generate bioactive peptides from egg proteins. Without using any organic solvents or enzymes, higher efficiency and cost-effectiveness are advantages of subcritical water hydrolysis, while non-specific cleavage of peptide bonds is the major limitation of this technique in producing bioactive peptides.[16] In addition to different types of hydrolysis, quantitative structure–activity relationships (QSAR)-aided *in silico* prediction, which is a bioinformatics-based method, has been considered to identify new bioactive peptides. This time- and cost-saving method has been successfully applied in predicting bioactive peptides from egg white ovotransferrin.[17] However, application of QSAR-aided prediction of egg protein-derived bioactive peptides should be expedited.

The activity of bioactive peptides is usually measured by chemical-based *in vitro* assays. A typical example is antioxidant assays. A number of *in vitro* assays targeting oxygen radical absorbance capacity (ORAC) have been involved in evaluating the antioxidant activity of egg protein-derived bioactive peptides.[3] Surprisingly, antioxidant peptides identified by ORAC methods did not show comparable activity in endothelial cells,[18] which indicated a lack of biological relevance of *in vitro* chemical assays. It is impractical to perform all assays *in vivo*; selection of the assay method should consider the physiological conditions associated with the *in vivo* environment. Indeed, cellular-based methods are intermediate methods to assess the bioactivity of peptides in physiologically relevant conditions and are thus encouraged for use in identification of bioactive peptides from egg proteins.[19]

Bioactive peptides need to be absorbed in the small intestine to exert physiological functions. There are at last two intestinal transport routes of egg protein-derived bioactive peptides, including through PepT1 transporter and paracellular transportation.[7] Interestingly, egg white ovotransferrin-derived tripeptides IRW, IQW and LKP could be transported by both routes.[20,21] However, we have limited understanding of the metabolic rates of egg protein-derived bioactive peptides; future research may focus on the behavior of these peptides in systemic circulation.

Research progress on egg protein-derived bioactive peptides has promoted further focus on the mechanisms of these peptides. Indeed, molecular mechanisms of food protein-derived bioactive peptides are more complicated than expected. For instance, most antihypertensive peptides were characterized by angiotensin-converting enzyme (ACE)-inhibitory assay, while *in vivo* study indicated that various signaling pathways were involved in the antihypertensive mechanisms of these peptides.[22,23] The objective of this book chapter is to visit the mechanisms of action of egg protein-derived bioactive peptides, which could help to build up a more comprehensive view on these peptides.

15.2 Antihypertensive Peptides

Hypertension, which was redefined to be above 130/80 mm Hg rather than 140/90 mm Hg for systolic/diastolic blood pressure by the American Heart Association and the American College of Cardiology in 2017, is a major predisposing factor for cardiovascular diseases.[24]

The pathophysiology of hypertension is complex. Especially for essential hypertension, which accounts for ~95% of all cases of hypertension, it could be affected by both genetic predisposition and environmental factors.[25] The renin–angiotensin system (RAS) has long been considered as the major contributor to blood pressure regulation. In the classic view of the RAS, angiotensin II (Ang II), a potent vasoconstrictor, is generated from angiotensin I (Ang I) with the aid of ACE. Angiotensin type I receptor (AT1R) and angiotensin type II receptor (AT2R) are two membrane G-protein-coupled receptors of Ang II. AT1R mediates the detrimental effects of Ang II, which mainly include increased vasoconstriction, pro-inflammation and pro-fibrosis. On the contrary, the counterbalancing effects against Ang II/AT1R axis could be exerted *via* AT2R.[26] Hence, inhibiting ACE or blocking AT1R are common strategies for the development of antihypertensive drugs.[27] However, prolonged use of antihypertensive drugs is associated with side effects[28] and thus efforts have been focused on developing safer alternatives to hypertension therapy.

ACE-inhibitory peptides were first identified from snake venom in 1971,[29] which then triggered the research in this area. Various ACE-inhibitory peptides have been identified from a wide range of food protein sources.[30,31] Egg ranks as an ideal candidate among food proteins to identify ACE-inhibitory peptides, and both egg white and egg yolk proteins are considered as sources.[32,33] Following their identifications, the blood pressure-lowering effects of some ACE-inhibitory peptides were validated in spontaneously hypertensive rats (SHRs). Surprisingly, the *in vivo* blood pressure-reducing effect was sometimes incomparable with the *in vitro* IC_{50} value (the concentration of the peptide required to inhibit 50% of ACE activity).[7] More interestingly, mechanistic study found that the antihypertensive effects of some egg protein-derived peptides were exerted through modulating expressions of key molecules within the RAS instead of solely *via* ACE inhibition (Figure 15.1). Thermoase- and pepsin-digested egg white hydrolysate was shown to reduce the blood pressure of SHRs *via* down-regulating ACE and AT1R expressions but up-regulating AT2R expression in the aorta.[34] Egg white ovotransferrin-derived RVPSL was reported to modulate expressions of ACE, AT1R and AT2R in SHRs to exert its blood pressure-reducing effect.[35] Transcriptomics study showed that the gene expression profile of the mesenteric artery of SHRs

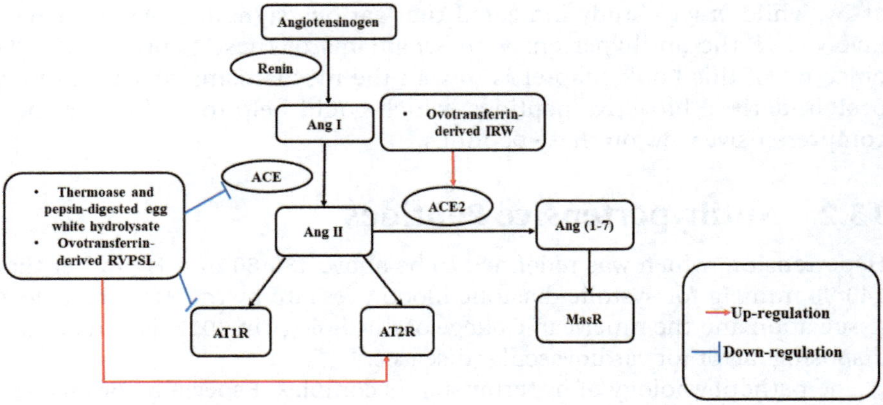

Figure 15.1 Molecular targets of egg protein-derived antihypertensive peptides in the RAS. Thermoase- and pepsin-digested egg white hydrolysate as well as egg white ovotransferrin-derived RVPSL down-regulated expressions of ACE and AT1R but up-regulated AT2R expression in SHRs. Egg white ovotransferrin-derived IRW could target the counter-regulatory arm of the RAS as it could up-regulate ACE2 in SHRs.

could be altered by oral administration of egg white ovotransferrin-derived IRW.[36] These findings shed light on the multiple roles of egg protein-derived ACE-inhibitory peptides in reducing blood pressure *via* regulating the expressions of molecules.

In 2000, the view on the RAS evolved with the identification of angiotensin-converting enzyme 2 (ACE2).[37] ACE2 is a homologue of ACE but with an opposite role in the RAS. ACE2 degrades Ang II into Ang (1–7), thus exerting counterbalancing effects against the Ang II/AT1R axis, mainly mediated *via* the Mas receptor (MasR).[26,38] The essential roles of ACE2 in regulating cardiovascular functions have been recognized. It was found that ACE2 knockout (ACE2KO) mice showed enhanced Ang II-induced hypertrophic cardiomyopathy.[39] In SHRs, increased ACE2 expression could contribute to reduced blood pressure and attenuated cardiac remodelling.[40] Therefore, ACE2 is now considered as a novel target for cardiovascular therapy.

Our previous study showed that the mRNA level of ACE2 in the mesenteric artery of SHRs could be up-regulated by oral administration of egg white ovotransferrin-derived antihypertensive peptide IRW,[36] which was the first report showing the involvement of ACE2 in the antihypertensive mechanism of egg protein-derived peptides. Our further study found that protein expression of ACE2 in the aorta of SHRs could be up-regulated by IRW (*Unpublished data*). More importantly, the blood pressure-reducing effect of IRW in SHR is dependent on the ACE2/Ang (1–7)/MasR axis (*Unpublished data*). These findings revealed the novel mechanism of an egg protein-derived antihypertensive peptide. However, whether up-regulation of ACE2 is a common feature of ACE-inhibitory peptides from egg proteins requires further investigation.

Table 15.1 Egg protein-derived antihypertensive peptides improving NO-dependent vasorelaxation.

Parent protein	Hydrolysate/peptide sequence	Reference
Egg white	Thermoase- and pepsin-digested hydrolysate	34
Whole egg	Pepsin- and pancreatin-digested hydrolysate	47
Egg white ovalbumin	RADHPF	43
Egg white	RADHPFL, RADHPF, RADHP, RAILNQ, FRADHPFL and YRGGLEPINF	44
Egg white ovotransferrin	IRW, IQW and LKP	45,46

The vascular endothelium is a single layer of cells present in the inner surface of blood vessels, which is a selective barrier to prevent the diffusion of macromolecules.[41] The vascular endothelium also participates in regulating vascular tone by secreting vasodilatory nitric oxide (NO).[42] Thus, improving endothelium-dependent vasodilation by enhanced bioavailability of NO is another major mechanism of egg protein-derived antihypertensive peptides. Egg protein-derived peptides that could improve NO-dependent vasorelaxation have been reported (Table 15.1).[34,43–47] Production of NO in vascular endothelium could be mediated by endothelial NO synthase (eNOS) through phosphatidylinositol 3-kinase-protein kinase B (PI3K-Akt) pathway.[48] However, only egg white ovotransferrin-derived IRW has been demonstrated to up-regulate eNOS expression in SHRs.[45] Molecular mechanisms of egg protein-derived peptides with the property of enhancing endothelium-dependent vasorelaxation should be further explored.

Almost all the *in vivo* mechanistic studies of egg protein-derived antihypertensive peptides was performed using male SHRs, since generally males have a higher risk of hypertension as compared with age-matched females before menopause.[49] However, to rely on a single model may restrict our insight into the mechanisms of these antihypertensive peptides. Future research is encouraged to apply different hypertensive models as well as to explore potential differentially regulatory roles of antihypertensive peptides from egg proteins in different genders.

15.3 Antidiabetic Peptides

Homeostasis of blood glucose is essential to maintain various physiological functions. A well-known complication associated with impaired glucose metabolism is type II diabetes. The prevalence of type II diabetes is in an upward trend; it is estimated that 439 million people will be affected worldwide by 2030.[50] α-amylase and intestinal brush border α-glucosidase are the two key enzymes responsible for carbohydrate digestion and releasing glucose for absorption and utilization by cells in the body. Long-chain carbohydrates are broken down by α-amylase and absorbable monosaccharides are cleaved by α-glucosidase.[51] Therefore, inhibition of α-glucosidase to reduce glucose absorption and postprandial blood glucose is a strategy for type II diabetes treatment.[52]

Food-derived α-glucosidase inhibitors have been identified from different protein sources, including egg proteins.[53,54] Two peptides with the sequences of RVPSLM and TPSPR were identified from an alcalase-digested egg white hydrolysate with IC_{50} values of 23.07 μM and 40.02 μM, respectively.[55] Another α-glucosidase-inhibitory peptide, KLPGF, was identified from alcalase-prepared albumin digestion with an IC_{50} value of 59.5 μM.[56] It is important to note that these peptides were only shown with the *in vitro* α-glucosidase-inhibitory activity; *in vivo* efficacy as well as their mechanisms of action are unknown.

Insulin, a hormone secreted by pancreatic β-cells, plays a primary role in blood glucose metabolism. After dietary intake, the insulin concentration rises from a basal level to make cells utilize glucose. Specifically, insulin secretion occurs in two phases. The first phase is after meal ingestion to suppress hepatic gluconeogenesis. In the second phase, gut-derived hormones glucose-dependent insulinotropic polypeptide (GIP) and glucagon-like peptide-1 (GLP-1) stimulate pancreatic insulin secretion, which further stimulates glucose uptake by skeletal muscle and adipose tissue.[57] However, GIP and GLP-1 are endogenous substrates of dipeptidyl peptidase IV (DPP-IV), which could be inactivated by DPP-IV rapidly.[58] Hence, DPP-IV inhibitors are another type of intervention introduced for type II diabetes. Egg protein-derived DPP-IV inhibitors have been reported. Pepsin-digested lipid-free egg yolk protein showed DPP-IV-inhibitory activity, and four peptides with the sequences of YIEAVNKVSPRAGQF, YINQMPQKSRE, YINQMPQKSREA and VTGRFAGHPAAQ were identified from this hydrolysate.[59] Egg yolk-derived RNDDLNYIQ was shown to have both DPP-IV and α-glucosidase inhibitory activities.[60] An *in vivo* study was also reported whereby oral administration of alcalase-digested egg lysozyme inhibited plasma DPP-IV in Zucker diabetic rats.[61] However, similar to α-glucosidase peptides, the molecular mechanisms of these DPP-IV-inhibitory peptides are poorly understood.

Insulin signaling has been characterized as including the insulin receptor, insulin receptor substrate (IRS), IRS-mediated phosphoinositide 3-kinases (PI3K) and mitogen-activated protein kinases (MAPK) cascades, as well as the downstream glucose transporter (GLUT).[62,63] The defect of target cells in responding to normal levels of circulating insulin, known as insulin resistance, is an essential feature of type II diabetes.[64] Recently, it was shown that egg ovotransferrin-derived IRW could improve insulin sensitivity in skeletal muscle cells *via* insulin signaling.[65] Interestingly, IRW, which was initially characterized as an ACE-inhibitory peptide, could down-regulate AT1R expression in skeletal muscle cells at the same time.[65] Indeed, a relationship between RAS blockade and improvement of insulin sensitivity has been reported. Results from several clinical studies indicated that treatment with an ACE inhibitor or AT1R blocker could contribute to a lower risk of developing type II diabetes in hypertensive patients.[66,67] Therefore, future study may focus on further elucidations of the potential insulin-sensitizing effect of egg protein-derived ACE-inhibitory peptides.

Apart from skeletal muscle cells, insulin also functions in adipose tissues. Under normal conditions, insulin improves adipocyte differentiation involving incorporating neutral lipids into these cells *via* up-regulation of peroxisome proliferator-activated receptor γ (PPAR-γ).[68,69] On the contrary, the normal effects of insulin are perturbed under pathological conditions, leading to abnormal adipogenesis.[70] Hence, compounds that can induce adipocyte differentiation may also improve insulin sensitivity and/or act as insulin memetics.[71,72] It has been documented that thermoase- and pepsin-digested egg white hydrolysate showed insulin memetic and sensitizing effects in adipocytes *via* up-regulating PPAR-γ and CCAAT/enhancer binding protein alpha (C/EBP-α), meanwhile increasing the release of adiponectin.[73] Such an *in vivo* effect has been validated in high-fat-diet-induced insulin-resistant rats. The blood glucose level in the high-fat-diet plus 4% egg white hydrolysate-fed rats was significantly lower as compared with the only high-fat-diet-fed rats.[74]

Research on egg protein-derived antidiabetic peptides has been evolved from *in vitro* screening of α-glucosidase and DPP-IV inhibitors to the insulin-sensitizing effects of potential peptides as well as the regulatory roles of these peptides in insulin signaling, advancing our knowledge on the mechanisms of egg protein-derived antidiabetic peptides.

15.4 Anticancer Peptides

Cancer, a leading cause of death worldwide, is caused by mutation of the DNA of normal cells, which can be triggered by both internal factors (hormones, immune conditions and inherited mutations) and external factors (chemicals, infectious agents and radiation). As a result, the uncontrolled proliferation of anaplastic cells could invade into surrounding tissues and metastasize to other organs, followed by setting up secondary foci of cancerous growth at distant sites.[75,76] Conventionally, chemotherapy and radiation are common treatments against cancer; these treatments, however, are associated with severe side effects as well as high cost,[77] which initiated the search for natural compounds with anticancer potential.

As a promising candidate for natural health product development, anticancer peptides have been reported from food proteins, including egg proteins.[78–81] The potential of nine ovotransferrin hydrolysates was studied in seven types of cancer cells. Although different cancer cells responded differentially towards these hydrolysates, AGS cells, a human gastric cancer cell line, generally had a higher sensitivity to ovotransferrin hydrolysate, as compared with the other cancer cells used in this study. More importantly, although ovotransferrin treatment could also reduce the viability of these cancer cells, the effect of ovotransferrin was weaker than the hydrolysates, which confirmed the necessity of hydrolysis to release peptides from ovotransferrin in reducing the viability of cancer cells.[82] Glycopeptides from egg white ovomucin were shown to inhibit the growth of tumors in a double grafted tumor system in mice.[83] However, the molecular mechanisms underlying the anticancer activity of ovotransferrin or ovomucin hydrolysate were unclear.

The cell cycle represents a series of tightly integrated events that enable cells to grow and proliferate. A standard eukaryotic cell cycle is divided into four phases. The cell is preparing for DNA synthesis in the G1 phase, followed by the S phase, when DNA duplication occurs. In the subsequent G2 phase, the cell undergoes growth and is thus prepared for cell division in the M phase. Defects in cell cycle regulation can lead to cancerous growth.[84] On the contrary, arrest of cell cycle checkpoints can activate the apoptotic cascade, which finally results in cell death. Therefore, targeting abrogation of the cell cycle and inducing cell apoptosis is a widely accepted strategy to develop anticancer agents.[78] Numerous reports on plant-derived phytochemicals show that they initiate cell cycle arrest and apoptotic cascade, which were considered as the anticancer mechanisms of these compounds.[85,86] More interestingly, lactoferricin, a milk-derived peptide, was also demonstrated with such effects,[87] which suggested the potential of bioactive peptides in regulating the cell cycle and exerting anticancer activity. However, there is little evidence showing the mechanisms of egg protein-derived peptides *via* cell cycle arrest and the apoptotic pathway. A fraction of egg white hydrolysate was reported to block the G2/M phase of a mouse lymphoma cell line and induce apoptosis.[88] However, *in vivo* evidence of such results is lacking.

Taken together, some egg protein-derived peptides with anticancer activity have been reported, but compared with phytochemicals, knowledge on the mechanisms of these anticancer peptides is in its infancy. In addition, most anticancer peptides were studied in cells; future *in vivo* study is expected to substantiate the evidence.

15.5 Immunomodulatory Peptides

The immune system in our body is a network of cells, tissues and organs acting to provide host defense against foreign organisms.[89] The immune system is composed of innate immunity and adaptive immunity. Innate immunity, which is non-specific immunity, provides the first line of defense through barriers, immune cells (macrophages, leukotrienes, dendritic cells and natural killer (NK) cells), and inflammatory constituents (cytokines, interferons, acute phase proteins, *etc.*).[89] On the contrary, adaptive immunity is highly specific to antigens. T lymphocytes (T cells) and B lymphocytes (B cells) are the most important cells in adaptive immunity. T cells are responsible for cell-mediated immunity by secreting immune regulatory factors. B cells play a role in producing antibodies, which bind to the antigens of invading pathogens and label them for destruction.[89,90]

Table 15.2 Immunomodulatory peptides from egg proteins.

Parent protein	Peptides	Cell/animal model	Mechanisms	Reference
Egg white	Aminopeptidase-digested hydrolysate with molecular weight lower than 1.3 kDa	Cultured spleen cells of egg allergy-sensitized mice	Suppression of IL-4 and interferon γ (INF- γ) production	93
Egg white	Aminopeptidase-digested hydrolysate with a molecular weight between 0.07 and 1.3 kDa	Dextran sodium sulfate-induced colitis in piglets	Downregulation of TNF-α, IL-6, IL-1β, INF- γ, IL-8 and IL-17 expression	94
Whole egg white; egg white ovalbumin; egg white lysozyme	Alcalase-digested hydrolysates	Concanavalin A-stimulated lymphocyte	Reduction of lymphocyte proliferation; suppression of IL-13, IL-10 and TNF-α production	95
Low lipid egg yolk	Pepsin-digested hydrolysates	Murine	Increase of IgA^+ cells; reduction of IL-6 production	96
Egg yolk livetins	Pepsin-, alcalase- and trypsin-digested hydrolysates with molecular weight lower than 10 kDa	Lipopolysaccharide-induced RAW 264.6 macrophages	Inhibition of TNF-α, IL-6, IL-1β and NO secretion	14

An immunomodulator is any substance that can modify the immune responses by altering any part of the immune system to strengthen the health of the immune system.[89] Food protein-derived immunomodulatory peptides were firstly characterized from human casein tryptic hydrolysate,[91] since then various immunomodulatory peptides have been reported from a wide range of food proteins, including egg proteins.[89,92] The mechanisms of egg protein-derived immunomodulatory peptides are summarized in Table 15.2.[14,93–96] These peptides were implicated in improving the immune system *via* altering innate or adaptive immunity.

Inflammation is a typical response to injury. Acute inflammation is essential for combating infection and tissue repair. In contrast, chronic and uncontrolled inflammation is associated with chronic diseases, including hypertension, atherosclerosis, diabetes, obesity and certain types of cancer.[3] Since there is a link between local inflammation and certain types of chronic disease, the bioactivity of some egg protein-derived peptides could be attributed, at least partially, to their anti-inflammatory effects.

The vascular endothelium is considered as the largest endocrine organ in the body.[41] Endothelial cells secrete both vasodilatory and vasoconstrictory agents to regulate vascular tone.[97] Endothelial dysfunction, one of the common features of cardiovascular diseases, results from endothelial inflammation.[98] Specifically, pro-inflammatory cytokines could up-regulate adhesion molecules, mainly including intercellular adhesion molecule-1 (ICAM-1) and vascular cell adhesion molecule-1 (VCAM-1), which subsequently lead to the development of atherosclerotic lesions and increased peripheral resistance.[99] It was found that egg white ovotransferrin-derived antihypertensive peptides IRW and IQW showed anti-inflammatory activities in tumor necrosis factor α (TNFα)-induced vascular endothelial cells. IRW and IQW inhibited the activation of the nuclear factor κB (NF-κB) pathway and down-regulated expressions of cell adhesion molecules.[100] The anti-inflammatory potentials of these two peptides in vascular endothelial cells have been considered to contribute to their blood pressure lowering effects *in vivo*.[45,46] Interestingly, IRW could abolish nuclear translocations of both p65 and p50 in the NF-κB pathway and down-regulate expressions of both ICAM-1 and VCAM-1. Although it differs by one amino acid residue, IQW only inhibited the nuclear translocation of p50 and down-regulated the expression of ICAM-1.[100] The differentially regulatory roles of IRW and IQW in TNFα-induced vascular endothelial cell suggested the significance of the structure and function relationships of bioactive peptides.

Apart from vascular endothelial cells, vascular smooth muscle cells (VSMCs) are another essential cellular component in the vascular wall in regulating blood vessel diameter as well as blood flow.[101] Indeed, Ang II is more than a potent vasoconstrictor as it plays multiple roles in maintaining the functional and structural integrity of the vascular walls. Over-stimulation of Ang II in VSMCs could result in inflammation, which would further facilitate vascular remodelling.[102] It was found that IRW also had an anti-inflammatory effect in Ang II-stimulated VSMCs. Similar to its effect in vascular endothelial cells, IRW restored degradation of inhibitory κBα and inhibited phosphorylation of p65 in the NF-κB pathway, which consequently down-regulated expressions of cyclooxygenase 2 (COX2) and inducible nitric oxide synthase (iNOS) in Ang II-stimulated VSMCs.[103] Taken together, the effects of IRW in mitigating vascular endothelial and smooth muscle inflammations are a part of the mechanism underlying its antihypertensive activity.

Inflammation in adipose tissue can lead to the release of harmful cytokines, which is a major factor underlying the altered metabolic state characterizing metabolic syndrome and its complications.[104] It was shown that thermoase- and pepsin-digested egg white hydrolysate could down-regulate TNFα-induced upregulation of COX2 in 3T3-F442A preadipocytes and the activator protein 1 (AP-1) pathway was involved in the action as phosphorylation of c-Jun could be reduced.[73] The above results indicated that attenuation of adipose tissue inflammation is a mechanism of thermoase- and pepsin-digested egg white hydrolysate in regulating glucose homeostasis.[73,74]

In summary, egg protein-derived immunomodulatory peptides were reported with their activities in enhancing innate or/and adaptive immunity. However, as there is a cross-talk between local inflammation and chronic diseases, attenuation of inflammation at a specific site may be a contributor to the bioactivity exerted by certain egg protein-derived peptides.

15.6 Antioxidant Peptides

Free radicals are atoms, molecules or ions with unpaired electrons. In physiological conditions, free radicals can be generated through reactions during respiration.[105] In the biological system, there are three main categories of free radicals, including reactive oxygen species (ROS), reactive nitrogen species (RNS) and reactive sulfur species (RSS).[106] Under normal conditions, free radicals generated in the body can be removed by the antioxidant defense system through enzymatic and non-enzymatic-mediated ways.[107] However, oxidative stress occurs when the endogenous defense system fails to protect the body against reactive radicals (*i.e.* excessive production of free radicals).[108] It has been widely recognized that oxidative stress in certain organs is associated with the pathogenesis of a number of chronic diseases,[109–113] which raises the need to identify antioxidant compounds to repair the impaired biological functions resulting from oxidative stress.

Antioxidants are considered as molecules that can neutralize free radicals by accepting or donating an electron to eliminate the unpaired condition of the free radical. Antioxidants may directly react with reactive radicals or remove free radicals indirectly by regulating ROS-related enzymes.[114] Since the 1990s, research on naturally derived antioxidant compounds has been substantially expanded owing to their health benefits.

Various peptides with antioxidant capacity have been identified from a wide range of food proteins, including egg proteins. Conventionally, these egg protein-antioxidant peptides (Table 15.3) were identified using *in vitro* chemical assays focusing on evaluating the ORAC of the peptide. However, such a way of characterization does not consider the complexity of the biological system or the potential of peptides in regulating ROS-related enzymes. It was not a big surprise that antioxidant peptides identified from egg white ovotransferrin based on ORAC assays actually did not show activity in vascular endothelial cells.[18] Therefore, developing a biologically relevant, efficient and cost-effective strategy to identify antioxidant peptides from egg proteins remains a challenge. On the other hand, molecular mechanisms of the already identified egg protein-derived antioxidant peptides have been rarely explored.

As accumulated oxidative stress is associated with some pathogenic changes in the body, similar to some peptides with an anti-inflammatory effect, the bioactivity of some egg protein-derived peptides is associated with the antioxidant potential at specific sites. It was reported that egg

Table 15.3 Egg protein-derived antioxidant peptides identified from *in vitro* assays.

Parent protein	Peptides identified	References
Whole egg white	DHTKE, FFGFN, MPDAHL, AEERYP, DEDTQAMP, PVDENDEG, SVDSQTAF, LPDEVSG, QPSSVDSQTAM and EERYP	117,118
Egg white lysozyme	VAWRNRCKGTD, WRNRCKGTD, AWIRGCRL, WIRGCRL and IRGCRL	119
Egg white ovomucin	LDEPDPL and NIQTDDFRT	120
Egg yolk protein	TMFPSA, WIHNENQGF, WYGPD, MPVHTDAD, KLSDW, YPSPV, IQVPL, KGLWE, YINQMPQKSRE, YIEAVNKVSPRAGQF, YINQMPQKSREA, VTGRFAGHPAAQ, ITMIAPSAF, RASDPLLSV, RNDDLNYIQ, LAPSLPGKPKPD and AGTTCLFTPLALPYDYSH	59,60

white ovotransferrin-derived antihypertensive peptide IRW could abolish TNFα-induced ROS in vascular endothelial cells, which was considered as an antihypertensive mechanism of IRW in improving endothelial dysfunction.[100] Indeed, IRW could also reduce the Ang II-stimulated ROS level in VSMCs, indicating the potential of IRW in mitigating vascular remodelling,[115] a checkpoint in hypertension development. However, the mechanisms of IRW in reducing ROS levels in vascular cells have not been elucidated. On the contrary, the mechanism of IRW in reducing oxidative stress in insulin-resistant skeletal muscle cells has been studied. It was shown that two subunits of nicotinamide adenine dinucleotide phosphate (NADPH) oxidase (p67phox and p47phox) were involved in the action of IRW, suggesting the regulatory role of this peptide in ROS-related enzymes. It was also thought to be a mechanism of IRW to modify insulin resistance in skeletal muscle cells.[65] In addition, we recently characterized three peptides from cooked egg with the sequences of DSTRQT, DVYSF and ESKPV showing activity in reducing ROS levels in VSMCs.[116] Future study will explore the potential of these peptides in treating or preventing ROS-related chronic diseases.

The blood pressure-lowering effect of thermoase- and pepsin-digested egg white hydrolysate has been validated in SHRs. Interestingly, nitrotyrosine expression in the aorta of SHRs was down-regulated by the treatment with this hydrolysate. Superoxide anion could react with peroxynitrite, a free radical under the category of RNS, which could modify tyrosine to form nitrotyrosine.[34] The down-regulation of nitrotyrosine by egg white hydrolysate in SHRs indicated that the antioxidant activity of egg protein-derived peptides may not be limited to influencing ROS, but also RNS.[34]

15.7 Conclusion

A market for functional foods has emerged during recent decades. Food protein-derived bioactive peptides are a major category of natural bioactive compounds with the potential to be developed into functional foods. As a rich source of protein, egg proteins have been used as parent proteins for identifications of various bioactive peptides, prompting the utilization of egg protein beyond its nutritional value. The bioactivities of some egg protein-derived peptides have been demonstrated in animal models and the mechanisms of actions of these peptides have been elucidated as well, which suggests the potentials of these peptides to improve human health. Further research into the activities and mechanisms of egg protein-derived peptides is suggested as follows:

1. *In vitro* chemical assay was widely used to identify egg protein-derived bioactive peptides. Owing to a lack of biological relevance, results from *in vitro* tests may not truly reflect the activity of the peptide. Thus, it is highly suggested to evaluate the bioactivity of the peptides in cellular systems or *in vivo*.
2. Although some bioactive peptides have been clinically studied,[121–126] very few egg protein-derived peptides have been moved to clinical trial. The translation from animal models to human study is central to prove the efficacy and safety of egg peptides and then to marketing these peptides as functional foods or nutraceuticals.
3. Our understanding of the molecular mechanisms of many egg protein-derived bioactive peptides is far from clear. Membrane receptors may be the first line to respond to peptide treatment, followed by triggering various intracellular signaling pathways and downstream protein expressions to exert the physiological functions of bioactive peptides. Therefore, it would be interesting to characterize membrane receptors responding to egg protein-derived bioactive peptides.
4. As discussed in this book chapter, some peptides may possess multiple activities and they are crossed-linked (Figure 15.2), in which antihypertensive peptides and antidiabetic peptides were also shown to possess antioxidant and immunomodulatory activities. Given the widely accepted roles of inflammation and oxidative stress in cancer development,[113] studying the anti-inflammatory and antioxidant effects of anticancer peptides may advance our understanding of the regulatory roles of these peptides. In addition, the RAS, which is mainly responsible for regulating blood pressure, is implicated in the pathogenesis of cancer.[127,128] As several egg protein-derived antihypertensive peptides have been demonstrated to modulate expressions of the RAS components, it would be interesting to investigate the anticancer potential of these antihypertensive peptides.

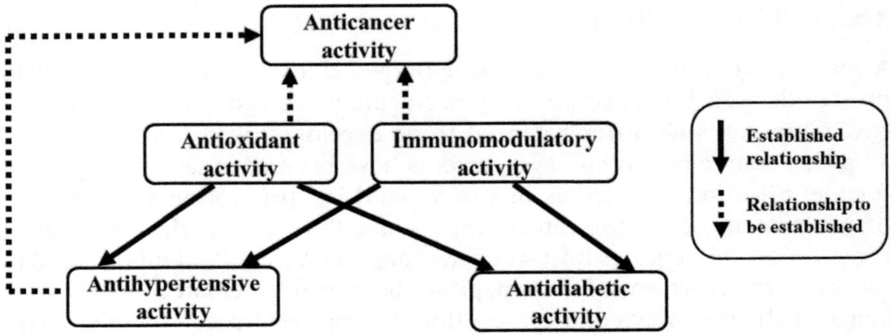

Figure 15.2 Interactions of egg protein-derived bioactive peptides. Several egg protein-derived bioactive peptides show multiple functions as some antihypertensive and antidiabetic peptides also show antioxidant and immunomodulatory effects. Given the universally accepted roles of oxidative stress and inflammation in cancer progression, it is suggested to further explore the activity of antihypertensive, antidiabetic, antioxidant and immunomodulatory peptides in relation with their anticancer potential.

5. Gut microbiota is considered to participate in the development of various diseases, including cardiovascular diseases, diabetes, obesity and cancer.[129–131] Some natural compounds have been implicated in intervening with chronic diseases *via* modulating gut dysbiosis.[132,133] As egg protein-derived peptides show a number of bioactivities, the gut microbiota may also get involved in the action of these peptides. Therefore, establishing the potential relationship between bioactivity and effects on gut microbiota is another area for future research on egg protein-derived bioactive peptides.

References

1. V. Vermeirssen, J. Van Camp and W. Verstraete, *Br. J. Nutr.*, 2004, **92**, 357–366.
2. C. C. Udenigwe and R. E. Aluko, *J. Food Sci.*, 2012, **77**, R11–R24.
3. S. Chakrabarti, F. Jahandideh and J. Wu, *BioMed Res. Int.*, 2014, 608979.
4. E. C. Li-Chan, *Curr. Opin. Food Sci.*, 2015, **1**, 28–37.
5. A. R. Madureira, T. Tavares, A. M. P. Gomes, M. E. Pintado and F. X. Malcata, *J. Dairy Sci.*, 2010, **93**, 437–455.
6. H. Korhonen and A. Pihlanto, *Int. Dairy J.*, 2006, **16**, 945–960.
7. W. Liao, F. Jahandideh, H. Fan, M. Son and J. Wu, *Adv. Food Nutr. Res.*, 2018, **85**, 1–58.
8. E. D. N. S. Abeyrathne, H. Y. Lee and D. U. Ahn, *Poult. Sci.*, 2013, **92**, 3292–3299.

9. Y. Liu, I. Oey, P. Bremer, A. Carne and P. Silcock, *Crit. Rev. Food Sci. Nutr.*, 2018, **15**, 2508–2530.
10. M. Garces-Rimon, C. Gonzalez, J. A. Uranga, V. Lopez-Miranda, R. Lopez-Fandino and M. Miguel, *PLoS One*, 2016, 0151193.
11. M. Yousr and N. Howell, *Int. J. Mol. Sci.*, 2015, **16**, 29161–29178.
12. A. Zambrowicz, M. Pokora, B. Setner, A. Dabrowska, M. Szoltysik, K. Babij and J. Chrzanowska, *Amino Acids*, 2015, **47**, 369–380.
13. C. Xu, C. Yang, Y. Yin, J. Liu and Y. Mine, *J. Funct. Foods*, 2012, **4**, 718–726.
14. C. Meram and J. Wu, *Food Res. Int.*, 2017, **100**, 449–459.
15. X. Sun, S. Chakrabarti, J. Fang, Y. Yin and J. Wu, *Nutr. Res.*, 2016, **36**, 648–657.
16. A. Shitu, S. Izhar and T. M. Tahir, *Global J. Environ. Sci. Manage.*, 2015, **1**, 255–264.
17. K. Majumder and J. Wu, *Food Res. Int.*, 2010, **43**, 1371–1378.
18. F. Jahandideh, S. Chakrabarti, S. T. Davidge and J. Wu, *J. Agric. Food Chem.*, 2016, **64**, 113–119.
19. C. López-Alarcón and A. Denicola, *Anal. Chim. Acta*, 2013, **763**, 1–10.
20. S. Bejjani and J. Wu, *J. Agric. Food Chem.*, 2013, **61**, 1487–1492.
21. Q. Xu, H. Fan, W. Yu, H. Hong and J. Wu, *J. Agric. Food Chem.*, 2017, **65**, 7406–7414.
22. K. Majumder and J. Wu, *Int. J. Mol. Sci.*, 2015, **16**, 156–183.
23. J. Wu, W. Liao and C. C. Udenigwe, *Trends Food Sci. Technol.*, 2017, **69**, 214–219.
24. P. K. Whelton, R. M. Carey, W. S. Aronow, D. E. Casey, K. J. Collins, C. Dennison Himmelfarb, S. M. DePalma, S. Gidding, K. A. Jamerson, D. W. Jones, E. J. MacLaughlin, P. Muntner, B. Ovbiagele, S. C. Smith, C. C. Spencer, R. S. Stafford, S. J. Taler, R. J. Thomas, K. A. Williams, J. D. Williamson and J. T. Wright, *J. Am. Coll. Cardiol.*, 2018, **71**, e127–e248.
25. O. A. Carretero and S. Oparil, *Circulation*, 2000, **101**, 329–335.
26. F. Fyhrquist and O. Saijonmaa, *J. Intern. Med.*, 2008, **264**, 224–236.
27. R. M. A. van de Wal, D. J. van Veldhuisen, W. H. van Gilst and A. A. Voors, *Eur. Heart J.*, 2005, **26**, 2361–2367.
28. A. Khanna, L. Lefkowitz and W. B. White, *Curr. Opin. Nephrol. Hypertens.*, 2008, **17**, 477–483.
29. M. A. Ondetti, N. J. Williams, E. Sabo, J. Pluscec, E. R. Weaver and O. Kocy, *Biochemistry*, 1971, **10**, 4033–4039.
30. D. Martínez-Maqueda, B. Miralles, I. Recio and B. Hernández-Ledesma, *Food Funct.*, 2012, **3**, 350–361.
31. A. Iwaniak, P. Minkiewicz and M. Darewicz, *Compr. Rev. Food Sci. Food Saf.*, 2014, **13**, 114–134.
32. H. Yoshii, N. Tachi, R. Ohba, O. Sakamura, H. Takeyama, T. Itani and C. Physiology, *Comp. Biochem. Toxicol. Pharmacol.*, 2001, **128**, 27–33.
33. M. Miguel, M. J. Alonso, M. Salaices, A. Aleixandre and R. López-Fandiño, *Food Chem.*, 2007, **104**, 163–168.

34. F. Jahandideh, S. Chakrabarti, K. Majumder, Q. Li, S. Panahi, J. S. Morton, S. T. Davidge and J. Wu, *J. Funct. Foods*, 2016, **27**, 667–673.
35. Z. Yu, Y. Yin, W. Zhao, F. Chen and J. Liu, *J. Agric. Food Chem.*, 2014, **62**, 912–917.
36. K. Majumder, G. Liang, Y. Chen, L. Guan, S. T. Davidge and J. Wu, *Mol. Nutr. Food Res.*, 2015, **59**, 1735–1744.
37. M. Donoghue, F. Hsieh, E. Baronas, K. Godbout, M. Gosselin, N. Stagliano, M. Donovan, B. Woolf, K. Robison, R. Jeyaseelan, R. E. Breitbart and S. Acton, *Circ. Res.*, 2000, **87**, e1–e9.
38. R. A. S. Santos, A. C. S. e. Silva, C. Maric, D. M. R. Silva, R. P. Machado, I. de Buhr, S. Heringer-Walther, S. V. B. Pinheiro, M. T. Lopes, M. Bader, E. P. Mendes, V. S. Lemos, M. J. Campagnole-Santos, H. P. Schultheiss, R. Speth and T. Walther, *Proc. Natl. Acad. Sci.*, 2003, **100**, 8258–8263.
39. M. S. Alghamri, N. M. Weir, M. P. Anstadt, K. M. Elased, S. B. Gurley and M. Morris, *J. Cardiovasc. Pharmacol. Ther.*, 2012, **18**, 138–151.
40. C. Díez-Freire, J. Vázquez, M. F. Correa de Adjounian, M. F. R. Ferrari, L. Yuan, X. Silver, R. Torres and M. K. Raizada, *Physiol. Genomics*, 2006, **27**, 12–19.
41. T. Münzel, C. Sinning, F. Post, A. Warnholtz and E. Schulz, *Ann. Med.*, 2008, **40**, 180–196.
42. J. O. Lundberg and E. Weitzberg, *Arterioscler., Thromb., Vasc. Biol.*, 2005, **25**, 915–922.
43. N. Matoba, H. Usui, H. Fujita and M. Yoshikawa, *FEBS Lett.*, 1999, **452**, 181–184.
44. A. B. Garcia-Redondo, F. R. Roque, M. Miguel, R. López-Fandiño and M. Salaices, *J. Sci. Food Agric.*, 2010, **90**, 1988–1993.
45. K. Majumder, S. Chakrabarti, J. S. Morton, S. Panahi, S. Kaufman, S. T. Davidge and J. Wu, *PLoS One*, 2013, **8**, e82829.
46. K. Majumder, S. Chakrabarti, J. S. Morton, S. Panahi, S. Kaufman, S. T. Davidge and J. Wu, *J. Funct. Foods*, 2015, **13**, 50–60.
47. F. Jahandideh, K. Majumder, S. Chakrabarti, J. S. Morton, S. Panahi, S. Kaufman and J. Wu, *PLoS One*, 2014, **9**, e115006.
48. M. P. Haynes, D. Sinha, K. S. Russell, M. Collinge, D. Fulton, M. Morales-Ruiz, W. C. Sessa and J. R. Bender, *Circ. Res.*, 2000, **87**, 677–682.
49. J. F. Reckelhoff, *Hypertension*, 2001, **37**, 1199–1208.
50. J. E. Shaw, R. A. Sicree and P. Z. Zimmet, *Diabetes Res. Clin. Pract.*, 2018, **87**, 4–14.
51. A. G. H. B. Bayer, *Eur. J. Clin. Invest.*, 2010, **24**, 3–10.
52. S. A. Ross, E. A. Gulve and M. Wang, *Chem. Rev.*, 2004, **104**, 1255–1282.
53. I. M. E. Lacroix and E. C. Y. Li-Chan, *J. Agric. Food Chem.*, 2013, **61**, 7500–7506.
54. P. Patil, S. Mandal, S. K. Tomar and S. Anand, *Eur. J. Nutr.*, 2015, **54**, 863–880.

55. Z. Yu, Y. Yin, W. Zhao, Y. Yu, B. Liu, J. Liu and F. Chen, *Food Chem.*, 2011, **129**, 1376–1382.
56. Z. Yu, Y. Yin, W. Zhao, J. Liu and F. Chen, *Food Chem.*, 2012, **135**, 2078–2085.
57. B. E. Grayson, R. J. Seeley and D. A. Sandoval, *Nat. Rev. Neurosci.*, 2013, **14**, 24–37.
58. N. Irwin and P. R. Flatt, *Curr. Opin. Pharmacol.*, 2013, **13**, 989–995.
59. A. Zambrowicz, M. Pokora, B. Setner, A. Dabrowska, M. Szoltysik, K. Babij, Z. Szewczuk, T. Trziszka, G. Lubec and J. Chrzanowska, *Amino Acids*, 2015, **47**, 369–380.
60. A. Zambrowicz, E. Eckert, M. Pokora, L. Bobak, A. Dabrowska, M. Szoltysik and J. Chrzanowska, *RSC Adv.*, 2015, **5**, 10460–10467.
61. A. Amerongen, M. J. C. Beelen, L. A. M. Wolbers, W. H. Gilst, J. H. Buikema and J. W. P. M. Nelissen, *WO Pat.* 2009128713, 2009.
62. K. D. Copps and M. F. White, *Diabetologia*, 2012, **55**, 2565–2582.
63. A. R. Saltiel and C. R. Kahn, *Nature*, 2001, **414**, 799–806.
64. F. Angelico, M. Del Ben, R. Conti, S. Francioso, K. Feole, S. Fiorello, M. G. Cavallo, B. Zalunardo, F. Lirussi, C. Alessandri and F. Violi, *J. Clin. Endocrinol. Metab.*, 2005, **90**, 1578–1582.
65. M. Son, C. B. Chan and J. Wu, *Mol. Nutr. Food Res.*, 2018, **64**, 1700602.
66. L. Hansson, L. H. Lindholm, L. Niskanen, J. Lanke, T. Hedner, A. Niklason, K. Luomanmäki, B. Dahlöf, U. de Faire, C. Mörlin, B. E. Karlberg, P. O. Wester and J. E. Björck, *Lancet*, 1999, **353**, 611–616.
67. E. J. Henriksen, *Am. J. Physiol. Integr. Comp. Physiol.*, 2007, **293**, R974–R980.
68. H. Lu, H. Wang, Y. Wen, M. Zhang and H. Lin, *World J. Gastroenterol.*, 2006, **12**, 1747–1751.
69. M. Zamboni, V. Di Francesco, U. Garbin, A. Fratta Pasini, G. Mazzali, C. Stranieri, E. Zoico, F. Fantin, O. Bosello and L. Cominacini, *Int. J. Obes.*, 2007, **31**, 1104–1109.
70. A. Smorlesi, A. Frontini, A. Giordano and S. Cinti, *Obes. Rev.*, 2012, **13**, 83–96.
71. J. E. Beh, L. T. Khoo, J. Latip, M. P. Abdullah, N. B. M. Alitheen, Z. Adam, A. Ismail and M. Hamid, *J. Ethnopharmacol.*, 2013, **150**, 339–352.
72. M. Nakano, F. Otsuka and R. Virmani, *Circulation*, 2011, **123**, 2954–2963.
73. F. Jahandideh, S. Chakrabarti, S. T. Davidge and J. Wu, *PLoS One*, 2017, **12**, e0185653.
74. F. Jahandideh, PhD thesis, University of alberta, 2017.
75. A. Zong, H. Cao and F. Wang, *Carbohydr. Polym.*, 2012, **90**, 1395–1410.
76. I. J. Fidler, *Nat. Rev. Cancer*, 2003, **3**, 453.
77. B. Hernández-Ledesma and C. C. Hsieh, *Crit. Rev. Food Sci. Nutr.*, 2017, **57**, 2358–2376.
78. S. K. Bhutia and T. K. Maiti, *Trends Biotechnol.*, 2008, **26**, 210–217.

79. S. E. Kim, K. H. Hwa, K. J. Yeon, K. Y. Im, W. H. Jong and L. H. Joo, *BioFactors*, 2008, **12**, 151–155.
80. I. C. Sheih, T. J. Fang, T. K. Wu and P. H. Lin, *J. Agric. Food Chem.*, 2010, **58**, 1202–1207.
81. G. M. Suarez-Jimenez, A. Burgos-Hernandez and J. M. Ezquerra-Brauer, *Mar. Drugs*, 2012, **10**, 963–986.
82. S. H. Moon, J. H. Lee, Y. J. Lee, K. H. Chang, J. Y. Paik, D. U. Ahn and H. D. Paik, *Poult. Sci.*, 2013, **92**, 424–434.
83. T. Yokota, H. Ohishi and K. Watanabe, *Food Sci. Technol. Res.*, 1999, **5**, 279–283.
84. V. Katrien, D. R. Van Bockstaele and Z. N. Berneman, *Cell Proliferation*, 2003, **36**, 131–149.
85. P. Fresco, F. Borges, M. P. M. Marques and C. Diniz, *Curr. Pharm. Des.*, 2010, **16**, 114–134.
86. S. M. Hadi, S. F. Asad, S. Saurabh and A. Aamir, *IUBMB Life*, 2008, **50**, 167–171.
87. J. S. Mader, A. Richardson, J. Salsman, D. Top, R. de Antueno, R. Duncan and D. W. Hoskin, *Exp. Cell Res.*, 2007, **313**, 2634–2650.
88. K. H. Kim, *Food Sci. Biotechnol.*, 2003, **12**, 224–227.
89. M. Chalamaiah, W. Yu and J. Wu, *Food Chem.*, 2018, **245**, 205–222.
90. T. J. Kindt, R. A. Goldsby, B. A. Osborne and J. Kuby, *Kuby Immunology*, W. H. Freeman, 2007.
91. P. Jolles, F. Parker, F. Floc'h, D. Migliore, P. Alliel, A. Zerial and G. H. Werner, *J. Immunopharmacol.*, 1981, **3**, 363–370.
92. H. S. Gill, F. Doull, K. J. Rutherfurd and M. L. Cross, *Br. J. Nutr.*, 2000, **84**, 111–117.
93. M. Yang, C. Yang, F. Nau, M. Pasco, L. R. Juneja, T. Okubo and Y. Mine, *J. Agric. Food Chem.*, 2009, **57**, 2241–2248.
94. M. Lee, J. Kovacs-Nolan, C. B. Yang, T. Archbold, M. Z. Fan and Y. Mine, *J. Agric. Food Chem.*, 2009, **57**, 2233–2240.
95. D. Lozano-Ojalvo, E. Molina and R. López-Fandiño, *Food Funct.*, 2016, **7**, 1048–1056.
96. R. Nelson, S. Katayama, Y. Mine, J. Duarte and C. Matar, *Food Agric. Immunol.*, 2007, **18**, 1–15.
97. P. M. Vanhoutte, *Hypertension*, 1989, **13**, 658–667.
98. G. Giannotti and U. Landmesser, *Herz Kardiovaskuläre Erkrankungen*, 2007, **32**, 568–572.
99. C. W. Smith, *Semin. Hematol.*, 1993, **30**, 45–53.
100. K. Majumder, S. Chakrabarti, S. T. Davidge and J. Wu, *J. Agric. Food Chem.*, 2013, **61**, 2120–2129.
101. A. Rudijanto, *Acta Med. Indones.*, 2007, **39**, 86–93.
102. R. M. Touyz and E. L. Schiffrin, *Pharmacol. Rev.*, 2000, **52**, 639–672.
103. W. Liao, S. Chakrabarti, S. T. Davidge and J. Wu, *J. Agric. Food Chem.*, 2016, **64**, 7342–7347.
104. C. E. M. Rodrigues, M. B. Vendramini, C. Bueno, E. Bonfá and J. F. de Carvalho, *Clin. Exp. Rheumatol.*, 2012, **30**, 871–878.

105. J. L. Evans, I. D. Goldfine, B. A. Maddux and G. M. Grodsky, *Diabetes*, 2003, **52**, 1–8.
106. J. Lu, P. Lin, Q. Yao and C. Chen, *J. Cell. Mol. Med.*, 2009, **14**, 840–860.
107. J. S. Johansen, A. K. Harris, D. J. Rychly and A. Ergul, *Cardiovasc. Diabetol.*, 2005, **4**, 5.
108. B. H. Sarmadi and A. Ismail, *Peptides*, 2010, **31**, 1949–1956.
109. U. Singh and I. Jialal, *Pathophysiology*, 2006, **13**, 129–142.
110. M. F. Hill, *Curr. Cardiol. Rev.*, 2008, **4**, 259–268.
111. W. Huang, X. Zhang and W. Chen, *Biomed. Rep.*, 2016, **4**, 519–522.
112. A. D. Romano, G. Serviddio, A. de Matthaeis, F. Bellanti and G. Vendemiale, *J. Nephrol.*, 2010, **15**, S29–S36.
113. S. Reuter, S. C. Gupta, M. M. Chaturvedi and B. B. Aggarwal, *Free Radicals Biol. Med.*, 2010, **49**, 1603–1616.
114. V. Lobo, A. Patil, A. Phatak and N. Chandra, *Pharmacogn. Rev.*, 2010, **4**, 118–126.
115. W. Liao, S. Chakrabarti, S. T. Davidge and J. Wu, *J. Agric. Food Chem.*, 2016, **64**, 7342–7347.
116. J. Wang, W. Liao, C. Nimalaratne, S. Chakrabarti and J. Wu, *NPJ. Sci. Food*, 2018, **2**, 7.
117. J. Liu, Y. Jin, S. Lin, G. S. Jones and F. Chen, *Food Chem.*, 2014, **175**, 258–266.
118. C. Nimalaratne, N. Bandara and J. Wu, *Food Chem.*, 2015, **188**, 467–472.
119. W. Carrillo, J. A. Gómez-Ruiz, B. Miralles, M. Ramos, D. Barrio and I. Recio, *Eur. Food Res. Technol.*, 2016, **242**, 1777–1785.
120. O. K. Chang, G. E. Ha, G. S. Han, K. H. Seol, H. W. Kim, S. G. Jeong, M. H. Oh, B. Y. Park and J. S. Ham, *J. Agric. Food Chem.*, 2013, **61**, 7294–7300.
121. A. F. G. Cicero, B. Gerocarni, L. Laghi and C. Borghi, *J. Hum. Hypertens.*, 2011, **25**, 425–436.
122. A. M. Turpeinen, S. Järvenpää, H. Kautiainen, R. Korpela and H. Vapaatalo, *Ann. Med.*, 2013, **45**, 51–56.
123. A. M. Turpeinen, M. Ikonen, A. S. Kivimäki, H. Kautiainen, H. Vapaatalo and R. Korpela, *Food Funct.*, 2012, **3**, 621–627.
124. T. Hirota, K. Ohki, R. Kawagishi, Y. Kajimoto, S. Mizuno, Y. Nakamura and M. Kitakaze, *Hypertens. Res.*, 2007, **30**, 489–496.
125. H. Li, N. Prairie, C. C. Udenigwe, A. P. Adebiyi, P. S. Tappia, H. M. Aukema, P. J. H. Jones and R. E. Aluko, *J. Agric. Food Chem.*, 2011, **59**, 9854–9860.
126. T. Kawasaki, E. Seki, K. Osajima, M. Yoshida, K. Asada, T. Matsui and Y. Osajima, *J. Hum. Hypertens.*, 2000, **14**, 519–523.
127. A. J. George, W. G. Thomas and R. D. Hannan, *Nat. Rev. Cancer*, 2010, **10**, 745.
128. D. Herr, M. Rodewald, H. M. Fraser, G. Hack, R. Konrad, R. Kreienberg and C. Wulff, *Gynecol. Oncol.*, 2018, **109**, 418–425.
129. W. H. W. Tang and S. L. Hazen, *J. Clin. Invest.*, 2014, **124**, 4204–4211.

130. G. Musso, R. Gambino and M. Cassader, *Diabetes Care*, 2010, **33**, 2277–2284.
131. P. Louis, G. L. Hold and H. J. Flint, *Nat. Rev. Microbiol.*, 2014, **12**, 661–672.
132. M. Van Hul, L. Geurts, H. Plovier, C. Druart, A. Everard, M. Ståhlman, M. Rhimi, K. Chira, P. L. Teissedre, N. M. Delzenne, E. Maguin, A. Guilbot, A. Brochot, P. Gérard, F. Bäckhed and P. D. Cani, *Am. J. Physiol. Metab.*, 2017, **314**, E334–E352.
133. F. Z. Marques, E. Nelson, P. Y. Chu, D. Horlock, A. Fiedler, M. Ziemann, J. K. Tan, S. Kuruppu, N. W. Rajapakse, A. El-Osta, C. R. Mackay and D. M. Kaye, *Circulation*, 2017, **135**, 964–977.

CHAPTER 16

Applications of Egg Yolk Antibody (IgY) in Diagnosis Reagents and in Prevention of Diseases

HAJIME HATTA*[a] AND YASUMI HORIMOTO[b]

[a]Department of Food and Nutrition, Kyoto Women's University, Kyoto, Japan; [b]Department of Food Science, University of Guelph, Ontario, Canada
*E-mail: jimhatta@gmail.com

16.1 Introduction

Immunoglobulin (Ig) has been used in diagnostics, therapy, and pure research. Over the last few decades, the use of Ig has received much attention in the treatment of bacterial infections owing to the increasing resistance of bacteria to antibiotics. In particular, oral administration of Ig is an attractive approach to preventing infections caused by bacteria and viruses in the mouth and gastrointestinal tract of human beings, domestic animals, and fish (for a review, please see ref. 1 and 2).

Animals produce Ig against the invasion of foreign substances such as bacteria and viruses. Ig is found in the bodily fluids of jawed vertebrates, including blood, saliva, nasal mucous, and lactation. Ig is also

Food Chemistry, Function and Analysis No.14
Eggs as Functional Foods and Nutraceuticals for Human Health
Edited by Jianping Wu

Published by the Royal Society of Chemistry, www.rsc.org

found in avian egg whites and yolks; Ig in egg yolk has been referred to as immunoglobulin Y (IgY). Traditionally, immunoassay testing has been performed with immunoglobulin G (IgG), which has been purified from the blood serum of animals such as goats and rabbits. However, in this system, blood collection is required and the amount of blood that can be collected is limited. Therefore, egg-yolk-derived IgY has received much attention as an attractive alternative to mammalian-derived IgG. Specific forms of IgY can be obtained from eggs laid by hens immunized against specific antigens. Compared to IgG preparation from animal blood, the immunized hen egg method is more cost-effective for large-scale production of antibodies.

This chapter begins with a brief discussion of the advantages of IgY compared to IgG. Then, we discuss the two main applications of IgY for human health. The first application is in diagnostics owing to IgY's binding specificity to given antigens: the use of IgY in immunological assays for clinical testing can eliminate the interference and false positives normally experienced when using mammalian IgG. In this section, we provide an overview of diagnostics and describe ABO blood typing and our work on the measurement of C-reactive protein and insulin using IgY.

The second important use of IgY is in passive immunization therapy, wherein its ability to bind to specific antigens (pathogens, venoms, *etc.*) serves to neutralize their pathogenicity. The following topics are included: neutralization of poisons, xenotransplantation, rotavirus diarrhea, dental caries, infection with gastric bacteria *Helicobacter pylori*, cystic fibrosis, aspiration pneumonia, and inflammatory bowel disease. Then recent research on the therapeutic potential of IgY for the prevention of obesity and the treatment of celiac disease is introduced. Finally, monoclonal IgY antibodies and their applications are discussed. This chapter focusses on human health; related applications of IgY in the field of disease prevention and treatment in fish and domestic animals can be found elsewhere (for a review, please see ref. 1, 3 and 4).

16.2 Advantage of IgY Compared to IgG

16.2.1 Immunoglobulin Y

Ig is a glycoprotein secreted by plasma cells that functions as an antibody in the immune system. An antibody has the ability to bind to a particular antigen, and the immune system produces the specific antibody required to neutralize an antigen. While there are five classes of Ig in mammals (IgG, IgM, IgA, IgD and IgE), birds have three classes in their blood (IgG, IgM and IgA).[5] These avian Igs are also found in hen's eggs: IgM and IgA are found in the egg white, while only IgG is found in the egg yolk. The total IgG concentration in the yolk is estimated to be between 5 and 25 mg mL^{-1}.[6] The IgG found in the serum of hens is transferred into egg yolk to provide acquired immunity to the offspring. During the development of a chicken embryo in the egg, the IgG of the egg yolk is transferred into

Table 16.1 Comparison between egg-yolk-derived IgY and mammalian blood-derived IgG.

	IgY	IgG
Molecular weight	~18 0000	~15 0000
Isoelectric point	~6.0	~7.0
Heat denaturation temperature	73.9 °C	77.0 °C
Activation of mammalian complements	Negative	Positive
Reaction with protein A or G	Negative	Positive
Reaction with rheumatoid factor	Negative	Positive
Reaction with Fc receptor	Negative	Positive

the chick's blood serum while the IgA and IgM of the egg white go into its intestinal tract. These Igs help to prevent any infection until the chick can make antibodies by itself.

16.2.2 Egg Yolk IgY *Versus* Mammalian IgG

IgG found in egg yolk is called IgY in the field of comparative immunology[1] owing to several key differences between the IgG found in animal blood and in egg yolk; they are different in terms of protein chemistry and immunochemistry (Table 16.1).[7] For example, the molecular weight of IgY (~18 kDa) is larger than that of IgG (~15 kDa). Their isoelectric points are also different (6.0 for IgY and 7.0 for IgG) and IgY is more hydrophobic than IgG. IgY also does not activate mammalian complements and Protein A produced by *Staphylococcus aureus*.

Shimizu *et al.*[8] compared egg-yolk-derived IgY with rabbit blood-derived IgG and found that IgY had less β-sheet structures in the antibody's constant region and was much less flexible in the hinge region. IgY also loses its activity under acidic conditions. The unique properties of IgY lead to different biochemical behaviors, such as an antigen-neutralizing role and structural stability. The differences between egg-yolk-derived IgY and mammalian-blood-derived IgG have been well documented elsewhere.[3,7,9]

16.2.3 Production Efficiency of Specific Antibodies

The production efficiency of IgY has received much attention. Traditionally, polyclonal IgG has been produced using mammals such as rabbits and goats. First, an antigen is injected into mammals and IgG is then purified from their blood. The obtained IgG has been used as antibodies in research and as diagnostic reagents. As one of the advantages of the use of IgY, drawing blood samples is not required during its production as it is derived from a hen egg. Moreover, cost-effective mass production is possible.[1] For example, the same amount of IgG from 30 rabbits' blood could be obtained using roughly 300 eggs, which one hen produces per year (Figure 16.1).

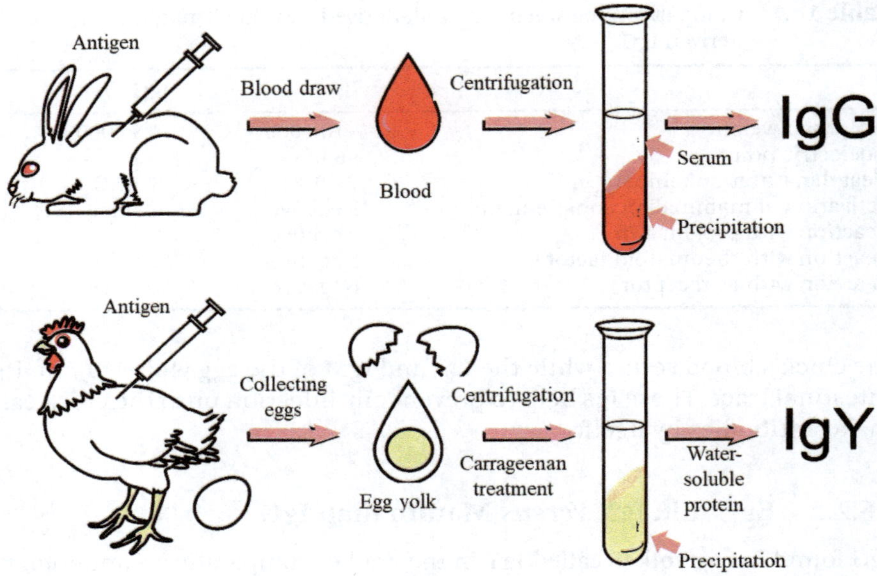

Figure 16.1 Preparation of specific polyclonal antibodies. Reproduced from ref. 19 with permission from John Wiley and Sons, Copyright 2007.

16.2.4 Suitability for Functional Food Applications

The consumer trend towards a healthy lifestyle has been increasing. IgY has broad potential for passive immunization applications *via* functional foods because it can be safely ingested. For example, an oral application of IgY has been commercialized to prevent pathogen adhesion in infections in the mouth or gastrointestinal tract.[10,11] Further examples are provided in Section 16.4.

The challenge of using IgY in functional food is the stability of IgY in the digestive system. Bioactive agents such as IgY are often protected within small capsules or particle matrices to overcome processing/storage degradation and undesirable taste/odor issues. However, mechanisms to activate the release of the encapsulated species are needed to achieve an optimal delivery rate at the target sites. While IgY is stable in the presence of trypsin and chymotrypsin, its stability is reduced under pepsin digestion.[12] Several techniques have been developed to stabilize or control the release of IgY for gastrointestinal applications.[13–15]

16.3 Development of Diagnostic Reagents Using IgY

In this section, we provide an overview of diagnostics and describe the use of IgY in the ABO blood typing test and our work on the measurement of C-reactive protein and insulin.

16.3.1 IgY as a Diagnostic Tool

Polyclonal IgY produced by immunizing chickens with an antigen can be used for the development of research and diagnostic reagents in place of IgG purified from the blood of animals such as rabbits and goats. IgY is useful in diagnostic tests that require the measurement of blood composition because IgY has no cross-reactivity with rheumatoid factors (RF), which react with IgG from mammalian species.[16] Moreover, IgY is useful in diagnostic tests for the detection of pathogens from fecal samples because IgY does not bind to protein A, which is a cell surface receptor produced by *Staphylococcal aureus*.[17] Protein A can also bind to IgG from a large number of other species. Because of its reduced reactivity with RF and protein A, IgY has fewer false positives than IgG in human diagnostic tests.

Research on the use of IgY has concentrated on several areas. For example, studies have been reported on applications of IgY that quantify both IgG and IgM in human blood samples or detect pathogenic plant and human viruses (*e.g.*, rotavirus, adenovirus, influenza virus, and papillomavirus).[1] In addition, some studies involve applications that use IgY as a diagnostic tool in the measurement of human plasma kallikrein, transferrin, IgA dimer, mucin-like glycoprotein of the milk fat globule membrane, and human thymidine kinase 1.[18] Additional studies have focused on the measurements of antigens with low molecular weight, such as prostaglandin, the active form of vitamin D, and ochratoxin.[18] There are also studies on the application of IgY against the difficult detection of antigens that have a low antigenicity among mammals, making production of an antibody difficult. For example, IgY has been suggested as a diagnostic tool to measure RNA polymerase 2, hematoside (NeuGc), human insulin, rat glutathione peroxidase, heat shock protein, parathyroid hormone, and erythropoietin receptor.[19]

More recently, Lupicka-Slowik *et al.*[20] developed a sensitive IgY-based adenosine deaminase (ADA) detection assay. The anti-ADA IgY antibodies were able to specifically recognize ADA in human cancer cell lysates. In a healthy organism, the tissue and blood concentrations of adenosine are low; however, the adenosine concentration increases significantly during inflammation, ischemia, or hypoxia. Therefore, through measuring enzyme activity, IgY-based tests can help to detect cancer in its early stages. Further examples using monoclonal IgY antibody are provided in Section 16.5.

16.3.2 ABO Blood Typing

In 1901, the ABO blood type antigen was discovered by Karl Landsteiner.[21] A blood type antigen is composed of glycoproteins and glycolipids. The ABO blood type antigens are carbohydrate chains attached to the red blood cell

Blood type O type (antigen H) Galβ1 → 3(4)GlcNAcβR
2
↑
Fuc α1

Blood type A type (antigen A) GalNAcα1 → 3Galβ1 → 3(4)GlcNAcβR
2
↑
Fuc α1

Blood type B type (antigen B) Galα1 → 3Galβ1 → 3(4)GlcNAcβR
2
↑
Fuc α1

Figure 16.2 Antigens in the ABO blood type group system.

surface. Figure 16.2 shows the blood type antigens in the ABO blood type system. Blood type A has antigen A, type B has antigen B, and type AB has both antigens A and B. Blood type O has antigen H.

Traditionally, an antibody prepared from an immunized animal has been used to determine human blood types in clinical settings. To prepare these antibodies, red blood cells with H, A, or B antigens are injected in a rabbit or a chicken, and antibodies are purified from their blood. Then, the patient's blood type is determined by mixing a drop of their blood with the anti-H, -A, and -B antibodies. Each of the blood types, A, B, and O, has an agglutination reaction to a single antibody (anti-A antibody, anti-B antibody, and anti-H antibody). The AB blood type has a reaction with both anti-A and -B antibodies.

Traditionally, the anti-H antibody has been obtained from the blood serum in immunized hens. However, the immunization process and blood collection from hens is not easy. The potential for egg-yolk-derived IgY to be used for blood type testing was investigated by Yazawa *et al.*[22] First, hens were immunized *via* the wing vein with 3 mL of 10% human type O red blood cells every 3 days over a 15 day period. Then, haemagglutination reactions of the antibodies from egg yolk and the serum were examined. Anti-H antibody appeared in the blood serum at day 10 after immunization. At day 12, the antibody also appeared in egg yolk. Agglutination increased and a high level of titer was maintained for about 1 month, after which it decreased gradually. At day 65, a final immunization was performed. Shortly thereafter, the agglutination of egg yolk antibodies increased again. The amount of anti-H antibodies from roughly 10 eggs was equal to the amount typically obtained from the blood of one immunized chicken. This study demonstrated that a specific IgY antibody for blood type testing can be obtained from egg yolks. In another study by the same group, the anti-B antibody was obtained from egg yolk.[23]

16.3.3 Immunoturbidimetric Ratio Measurement for C-reactive Protein

When inflammation or tissue damage is present in the human body, C-reactive protein (CRP) is synthesized in the liver and excreted into the blood (for a review, please see ref. 24). CRP was named for its interaction with the *Pneumococcal* C-polysaccharide. The concentration of CRP in human blood increases positively with the strength of an inflammation reaction. CRP measurement is a popular diagnostic test used by medical professionals as a marker for infection, autoimmune disease, and malignant tumors.[24]

Turbidimetric immunoassay is the most common procedure used to detect CRP using IgG.[25] The principle of this method is based on a photometric measurement of turbidity, which corresponds to the antigen–antibody reaction. Specifically, latex particles coated with the CRP antibody react with antigens, resulting in an increase in turbidity, which is then measured optically. A variety of optical turbidity detectors have been developed, including automatic analysis units for use in clinical tests.[26]

In the work of Ota *et al.*,[27] the turbidimetric method was extended to use with IgY. Generally, the CRP antibody is produced by injecting CRP into rabbits and goats and then purifying IgG from blood serum. However, because CRP measurement is so widely used, a different method with the potential to be cost-effective and mass produced is needed. A large amount of CRP antibodies could be obtained from hen eggs. The authors compared the turbidimetric immunoassay results of IgY and rabbit IgG. Sixty CRP-positive serums were analyzed. The correlation between the two methods was 0.9943, indicating the potential for the use of IgY to measure CRP using turbidimetric immunoassays (Figure 16.3).

16.3.4 Detection of Insulin

Insulin is a hormone found in the pancreas that controls the metabolism of carbohydrates and the homeostasis of blood sugar. An insulin antibody that has been labeled with a radioisotope (iodine 125) has been used to measure the concentration of insulin to diagnose diabetes, its severity, and the function of the pancreas.[28] In many modern societies, rates of diabetes and prediabetes have been increasing, leading to increased demand for an insulin-measuring reagent. Therefore, a large number of insulin antibodies are needed for use in a diagnostic tool.

The production of insulin antibody is difficult owing to its small molecular weight (6 kDa). The antibody response to compounds with a molecular weight of less than 30 000 kDa was shown to be poor in hens.[29] Insulin is a peptide hormone that is composed of chain A, which has 21 amino acids, and chain B, which has 30 amino acids. The two chains are connected by

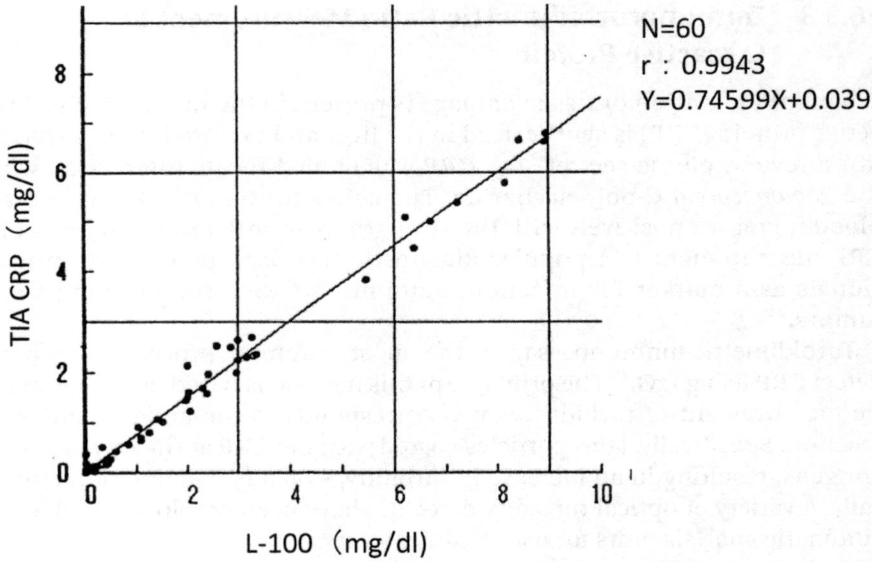

Figure 16.3 Correlation of immunoturbimetric ratio measurement for C-reactive protein.

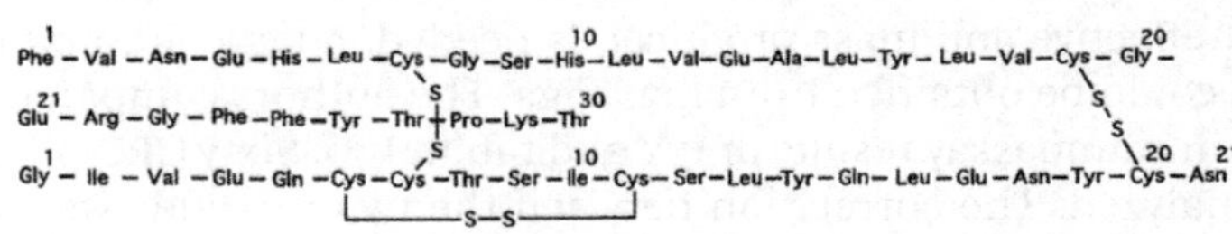

	B1	2	3	5	9	10	13	14	16	17	18	20	21	25	27	29	30	A4	8	9	10	13	14	17	18	22
Human	F	V	N	H	S	H	E	A	Y	L	V	G	E	F	T	K	T	E	T	S	I	L	Y	E	N	
Guinea pig	Y		S	R		Q	D	T		S		R	H		R	N	D	D		N		R	N	M	S	D
Mouse			K		S											M	S	D								
Rabbit																	S									
Sheep																	A		A	G	V					
Goat																	A		A	G	V					
Chicken	A	A													S		A		H	N	T					

Figure 16.4 Amino acid conservation of insulin across different animals.

two disulfide bridges. The amino acid composition is generally conserved among mammals. For instance, rabbit insulin has only one amino acid in its sequence that is different from human insulin; goat insulin has only four amino acids that vary, and mouse insulin has five. Therefore, fewer antibodies are produced when human insulin is introduced into the blood of these animals. However, insulin from marmots has 18 amino acids that differ from human insulin (Figure 16.4). Therefore, the anti-insulin antibody has been produced from the purification of marmot blood serum, but severe hypoglycemia can be induced, leading to their death.

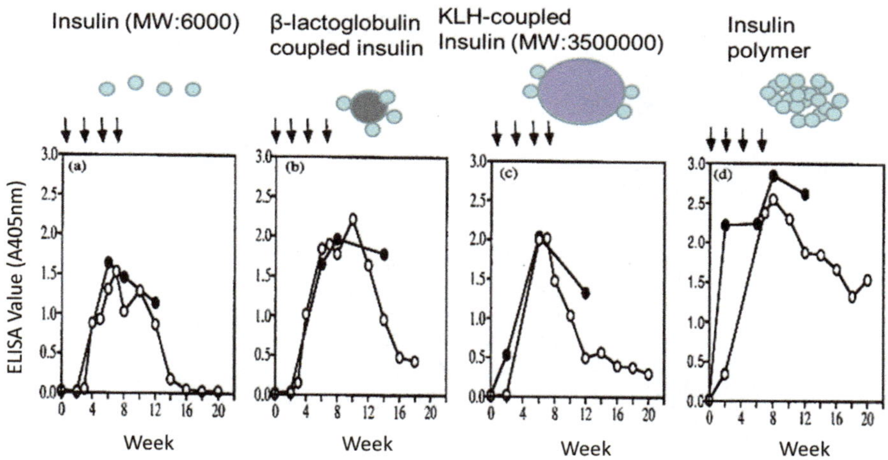

Figure 16.5 Changes of antibody responses in the serum and egg yolk from chickens immunized with insulin, insulin conjugates, and insulin polymer. Anti-insulin antibody titers were measured by ELISA using insulin (a), β-lactoglobulin-coupled insulin (b), KLH-coupled insulin (c), or insulin polymer (d) as an immunogen and expressed as ELISA value for serum (•) and egg yolk (o) at 1 : 1000 dilution. Arrows indicate weeks of injection. Insulin (N) was used as a coating antigen on the ELISA.

Based on the fact that hen insulin has seven amino acids that differ from human insulin, Lee *et al.*[30] investigated the production of an anti-insulin antibody using hens. Four different types of insulin were prepared: native insulin, insulin coupled with β-lactoglobulin, insulin coupled with Keyhole Limpet Hemocyanin, and insulin polymer. These insulin samples were administered to hens and the insulin polymer had the highest antigenicity. In addition, the antibody titer in hen egg yolk increased significantly (Figure 16.5). The results indicated that the antibody titer with the insulin polymer was several times higher than that with the monomer insulin in egg yolk. The authors also compared a sandwich enzyme-linked immunosorbent assay (ELISA) method using anti-insulin IgY with the traditional radioimmunoassay method. The correlation between the two methods was 0.96796, suggesting the potential use of IgY for enzyme immunoassay (Figure 16.6). Therefore, it appears that hens' eggs have the potential to be used to create insulin antibodies.

16.4 Prevention of Diseases Using IgY

16.4.1 Passive Immunization

Passive immunization is based on two therapeutic approaches: antiserum therapy and oral administration therapy. In anti-serum therapy, a specific antibody is injected *via* intramuscular or intravenous injection to prevent infection or to neutralize snake bites and bacterial toxins.

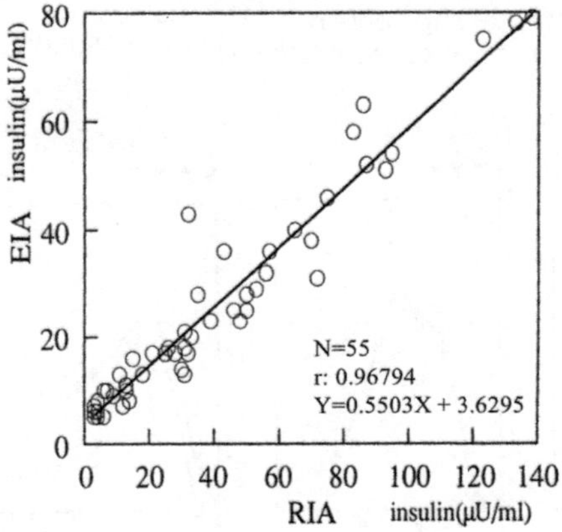

Figure 16.6 Correlation of two methods (enzyme immunoassay (EIA) and radioimmunoassay (RIA)) for human insulin measurement.

Traditionally, a horse anti-serum is used. However, egg-yolk-derived IgY has been studied as an alternative method owing to the potential to produce large quantities of IgY with a high level of purity. In oral administration therapy, a specific antibody is administered to prevent pathogen adhesion inside the mouth and gastrointestinal tract in human beings. Since IgY is produced from edible egg yolk in large-scale production, the oral administration of IgY has been studied as a possible functional food. In the following sub-sections, we discuss applications of anti-serum therapy and oral administration therapy. Then, recent research on the therapeutic potential of IgY for the prevention of obesity and the treatment of celiac disease is introduced.

16.4.2 Neutralization of Poisons

Poisonings from snakes, scorpions, spiders, and jellyfish are common around the world, resulting in a significant number of human fatalities.[31,32] Generally, a horse anti-serum is injected into patients to neutralize toxins; however, this method has high costs and side effects. For example, impurity in the horse serum can cause serum sickness, and these antibodies often cause inflammation owing to cross-reaction between horse-derived IgG and human complements.

Owing to the potential for the mass production of IgY, applications for detoxification against poisons have been studied. IgY purified from egg yolk is unable to activate the mammalian complement system.[16] Therefore, the IgY antibody is likely to be a safe detoxification antibody that can be used to replace conventional horse serum. For example, using mice as a model, Thalley *et al.*[33] reported the effective neutralization of toxins from rattlesnake and scorpion bites using IgY. In addition, Lee *et al.*[34] studied the effects of poly- and mono-clonal egg-yolk-derived IgY antibodies on *Bungarus multicinctus* snake venom, which is composed of complicated proteins. The major lethal toxins, bungarotoxins, along with other active components (*e.g.*, phospholipase A2), make the development of therapeutic agents for specific components difficult. A mixture of monoclonal IgY antibodies provided only partial protection, whereas the polyclonal IgY antibody was found to provide complete protection to the mice. Therefore, IgY antibodies show potential for use in the neutralization of poisons.

16.4.3 Xenotransplantation

Pigs have received much attention as an alternative to humans for donor organs. In particular, the pig heart is a potential source of xenotissues for humans owing to its anatomical similarity to the human heart. In addition, large-scale production would be possible as pig breeding is relatively easy. However, the main problems in pig-to-human xenotransplantation are hyper-acute rejection and rapid-onset intravascular coagulation, caused by galactose-α-1,3-galactose (αGal).[35]

The αGal epitopes are found on the cell surfaces of mammals except humans and apes. Humans have xenoreactive natural antibodies that react with αGal epitopes expressed on the surface of pig heart cells, leading to acute organ rejection.[35] Therefore, in xenotransplantation, it is important to block αGal epitopes on the cells of transplanted organs.

The use of chicken IgY antibody could be a potential strategy for preventing organ rejection because chickens do not express αGal epitopes. In addition, the chicken-derived anti-αGal IgY antibody does not activate the human complement system and does not react with Fc receptors.[36] Fryer *et al.*[37] immunized chickens with the αGal epitope antigen and prepared an anti-αGal IgY antibody. The anti-αGal IgY antibody prevented the interaction between human xenoreactive natural antibodies and the transplanted porcine tissue. Furthermore, the chicken IgY antibody blocked the complement-mediation of lysis of the porcine aortic endothelial cells by human serum. Therefore, IgY antibodies may be useful in the prevention of the rejection of xenotransplants.

16.4.4 Diarrhea Caused by Human Rotavirus

Human rotavirus (HRV) is transmitted orally and adheres on intestinal epithelial cells, resulting in vomiting and severe diarrhea. In developing countries, many infants and young children suffer or die from intestinal HRV infections every year.[38] Even in developed nations such as Japan, HRV-associated gastroenteritis outbreaks are reported.[39] Even though much effort has been made to develop vaccines, an effective solution has not been found because the infection is colonized on intestinal cells in infants who have immature immune systems.

An oral administration of the HRV antibody has been suggested to prevent the localization of HRV in the intestines. Hatta *et al.*[40] studied productivity, specificity, and resistance against heat, pH, and digestive enzymes of an anti-HRV antibody. First, chickens were immunized using HRV (Wa strain, serotype 1 and Mo strain, serotype 3). Immunized hens produced over 40 g of IgY each per year, which is equal to the amount of IgG produced by the blood serum of 30 immunized rabbits. The total production of anti-HRV IgY was 120 times (anti-Mo) more than that of rabbit-serum-derived IgG. Egg-yolk-derived IgY is relatively stable against trypsin and chymotrypsin activity, denatures at 73.9 °C, and structural denaturation occurs below pH 3.5. However, IgY loses its activity in the presence of pepsin below pH 2.0. At pH 4.4, which is similar to the pH in an infant's stomach, over 50% of the antibody activity remains. In another study by Hatta *et al.*,[12] baby mice were infected orally with HRV to induce diarrhea. The results indicated that the administration of 22.5 μg of IgY to a mouse before infection with HRV was able to prevent diarrhea. Anti-HRV IgY also prevented localized viral infection on intestinal cells immunohistochemically. In conclusion, some research supports the use of IgY in the creation of oral antibodies.

16.4.5 Dental Caries by *Streptococcus mutans*

Streptococcus mutans causes dental caries.[41] The bacteria colonize on the teeth's surface in the mouth and form insoluble polysaccharides from sucrose using glycosyltransferase (GTase). *S. mutans* produces two types of GTase: the cell-associated form, which produces water-insoluble glucan, and the cell-free form, which produces water-soluble glucan. In particular, water-insoluble glucan appears to be an essential source for adhesive polysaccharides. Owing to these adhesive polysaccharides, *S. mutants* can attach on the surface much more strongly, resulting in the formation of plaque. Inside the plaque, lactic acid is produced by lactic acid bacteria, dissolving teeth and forming caries. Therefore, IgY specific to *S. mutans* GTase could inhibit dental caries.

Otake *et al.*[42] studied the prevention of the attachment of *S. mutans* to the teeth surface. *S. mutans* MT8148 serotype c, which was subjected to formalin treatment, was immunized to chickens to produce anti-dental-caries IgY. The control IgY was prepared from unimmunized hen egg yolk. Rats were fed with anti-dental-caries IgY along with a high concentration of sugar in their feed. At day 56 after infection of *S. mutans* MT8148 serotype c, the rats were dissected and the severity of the dental caries (caries score) was measured. Compared to control rats, the caries score in rats fed with anti-caries IgY decreased significantly.

Hatta *et al.*[43] studied the effect of a mouth wash solution including anti-dental-caries IgY using 11 healthy males with a randomized double-blind crossover test. The mouth wash solution included 10% sugar solution and 1% anti-dental-caries IgY. For the control group, the mouse wash solution included 10% sugar solution and 1% IgY purified from non-immunized chicken. Saliva was collected before and after the mouth rinse test. Subjects used 10 mL of the mouth wash solution for 1 min. After 2 hours, the wash was repeated. Then, after 2 hours, saliva was collected and the ratio of *S. mutans* to total *Streptococci* bacteria was calculated. While the ratio increased in the control group, the ratio decreased using the mouth wash solution including anti-dental-caries IgY. This result suggests that anti-dental-caries IgY can suppress colonization on the surface of teeth, even in the presence of sugar.

16.4.6 Infection with the Gastric Bacteria *Helicobacter pylori*

Helicobacter pylori causes gastritis, leading to conditions such as stomach ulcer and stomach cancer. 95% of stomach cancer patients have *H. pylori*.[44] Therefore, it is important to remove *H. pylori* from the stomach to help prevention of stomach cancer.

A recent study investigated the development of a functional food to reduce the number of *H. pylori*. Because *H. pylori* urease may be mainly responsible for colonization of the bacteria on the gastric mucosa, Horie *et al.*[10] studied a novel prophylaxis for *H. pylori* using anti-*H. pylori*-urease IgY (Figure 16.7). 16 patients diagnosed as *H. pylori*-positive ate yogurt including anti-*H. pylori*-urease IgY. Before administration of the yogurt, patients were examined and

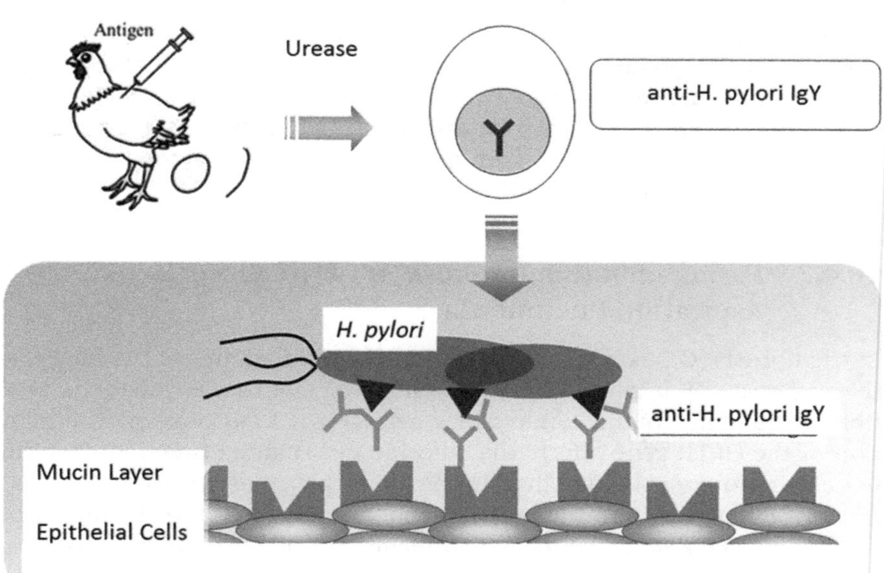

Figure 16.7 Competitive inhibition of *H. pylori* adherence by anti-*H. pylori* IgY. Reproduced from ref. 19 with permission from John Wiley and Sons, Copyright 2007.

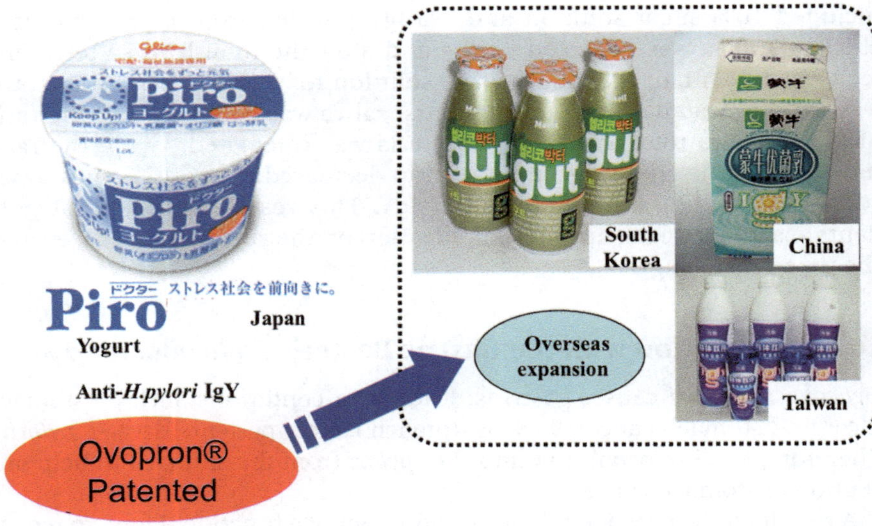

Figure 16.8 Products using anti-*H. pylori* IgY.

the number of *H. pylori* was measured using fecal samples and urea breath tests (UBT). Then, patients with a strong positive UBT value were given an anti-*H. pylori*-urease IgY yogurt. At 8 weeks after administration, the concentration of *H. pylori* in feces and the UBT value decreased significantly. At 3 months after administration, a further decrease was observed. The results suggest that IgY yogurt can be used as a functional food. Currently, yogurt including anti-*H. pylori*-urease IgY is commercialized in Japan, South Korea, and China (Figure 16.8). Work in other areas has suggested that both antibiotic treatment and the daily administration of functional food is the most effective method of treating the disorder.[45]

16.4.7 *Pseudomonas aeruginosa* in Cystic Fibrosis and Aspiration Pneumonia

Cystic fibrosis (CF) is a serious inherited disease that affects the lungs and the pancreas. CF is caused by mutations in a gene that encodes the cystic fibrosis transmembrane conductance regulator (CFTR) protein. The mutation of the CFTR gene affects the chloride ion channel function, resulting in dehydration of epithelial fluid in the lungs, pancreas, and other organs.[46] *P. aeruginosa* causes chronic lung infections in CF patients. Treating chronically colonized *P. aeruginosa* is very difficult. Antibiotics have been used as a main agent to treat lung infections in CF patients; however, there is growing concern about antibiotic resistance and antibiotic-associated toxicities (for a review, please see ref. 47).

Immunotherapy with an anti-*P. aeruginosa* antibody can be a complement to antibiotics. Several studies suggested an oral prophylactic treatment with egg yolk antibodies against *P. aeruginosa*.[48,49] Nilsson *et al.*[50] reported a decrease in the number of *P. aeruginosa* after gargling with an anti-*P. aeruginosa* IgY solution. The CF patients in their study received prophylactic IgY treatment for more than 10 years. The number of *P. aeruginosa*-positive cultures per 100 treatment months was 2.5 in the IgY group, compared with 13.7 in the control group. IgY treatment could also prevent initial *P. aeruginosa* colonization of the oropharynx; therefore, *P. aeruginosa* colonization in lower airways could be delayed. As a result, the number of antibiotic treatments would be decreased. The authors suggest that a combination of IgY and antibiotic treatment would have advantages to prevent bacterial colonization, in particular during the initial stage of CF, and could minimize the development of antibiotic resistance and its side effects.

P. aeruginosa is also an important cause of aspiration pneumonia. As a result of the aging population in many countries, the number of deaths caused by aspiration pneumonia has been increasing.[51] Aspiration pneumonia is caused mainly by bacteria and viruses, which enter the lungs along with saliva and stomach acids. Recurrent pneumonia is common, leading to antibiotic resistance. Therefore, antibiotic treatment is becoming more difficult, resulting in increasing mortality. The IgY rinses previously mentioned could be useful in preventing this disorder as well.[48]

16.4.8 Inflammatory Bowel Disease

Crohn's disease and ulcerative colitis are classified as inflammatory bowel diseases (IBD).[52] Crohn's disease is most commonly diagnosed among young people in their teens and twenties. In this disorder, the entire gastric tube from mouth to anus has chronic inflammation and ulcers. Ulcerative colitis is typically diagnosed among adolescents and adults. In this disease, inflammation occurs on the colonic mucosa. While the causes of IBD are unclear, cytokine and tumor necrosis factor (TNF-α) are implicated in its pathogenesis.[53] Anti-inflammatory drugs, immunosuppressants, and antibiotics have been used in the treatment of IBD;[54] however, the efficacy of these drugs is limited owing to factors such as side effects and immunosuppression.

Worledge *et al.*[55] reported a preventive effect of oral administration of anti-TNFα IgY on acute and chronic induced colitis in rats. Anti-TNFα IgY was more effective than standard anti-inflammatory drugs such as sulfasalazine and dexamethasone. In particular, anti-TNF IgY penetrated inflamed regions of the colon, localizing within the tissue containing TNFα. This suggests that an oral administration of anti-TNFα IgY would have fewer side effects than anti-inflammatory drugs. As a result, this treatment might be better tolerated by patients, allowing repeated use for disease recurrence or as a maintenance therapy.

16.4.9 Potential Applications

16.4.9.1 *Obesity*

Obesity is a serious problem in many modern societies, causing metabolic syndrome, which leads to serious medical issues, such as insulin resistance, hypertension, hyperlipidemia, and atherosclerosis.[56] Pancreatic lipase inhibitors are an effective approach to preventing and treating obesity.[57] Orlistat, a pancreatic lipase inhibitor, has been used in current clinical practice.[58] However, one of the challenges of using orlistat is its side effects, such as diarrhea, cholelithiasis, and cholesteric hepatitis.[58] Recently, Hirose *et al.*[59] studied the effect of egg-yolk-derived IgY on pancreatic lipase using an animal model. The authors successfully produced anti-lipase IgY by immunizing chickens with a porcine pancreatic lipase. In mice fed a high-fat diet, anti-lipase IgY showed significant inhibition of pancreatic lipase along with increased triglyceride excretion in the feces, suggesting an anti-obesity effect.

16.4.9.2 *Celiac Disease*

Celiac disease (CD) is an autoimmune enteropathy caused by ingestion of gluten. CD is found exclusively in people carrying the human leucocyte antigen DQ2 and/or DQ8.[60] The incidence of CD and other forms of gluten intolerance is growing worldwide. For people with CD, eating gluten damages the mucosa of the small intestine, resulting in malabsorption of important nutrients, such as fat, calcium, iron, and folate. Furthermore, CD can lead to associated diseases, such as osteoporosis and anemia. Currently, a gluten-free diet is the only treatment for CD and must be maintained throughout the patient's lifetime.

Gliadin, a component of wheat protein, is considered to be the most problematic component for celiac individuals because it is resistant to gastrointestinal enzymatic degradation. Undigested fractions of gliadin induce inflammation. Gujral *et al.*[61] produced specific anti-gliadin IgY and evaluated its effectiveness in inhibiting gliadin-induced intestinal complications, gliadin absorption, and the inflammatory response induced by gliadin using a CaCo-2 cell culture model. Anti-inflammatory markers, such as TNF-α and IL-1β, were measured and the results showed that gliadin absorption was inhibited, suggesting the potential usefulness of the anti-gliadin IgY. In 2012, Gujral *et al.*[15] also reported on the use of a spray-dried IgY antibody formulation using sugar protectants in a mouse model. Results suggested that mannitol-preserved IgY powder has potential as a treatment for CD patients.

16.5 Monoclonal Antibodies

Polyclonal preparations of IgY are suitable for many routine diagnostic applications; however, monoclonal antibodies are ideal antibody therapeutic agents owing to their higher specificity against antigens.

Monoclonal antibodies were first generated in mice in 1975.[62] However, their use was limited owing to side effects. To avoid an allergic-like human antimouse antibody (HAMA) response, chimeric (34% murine content) and humanized (5–10% murine content) monoclonal antibodies were developed.[63] Then, to further reduce the risk of immunogenicity, fully human antibodies containing 100% human proteins were developed. Humanized and fully human monoclonal antibodies are playing an increasingly important role in therapeutic applications.[64] For example, two-thirds of the new monoclonal antibodies approved in 2017 were fully human.[63]

Currently, most immunotests are based on murine monoclonal antibodies. However, because some antigens have low antigenicity among mammals, it is difficult to produce these monoclonal antibodies using mice and rats. Chickens can be useful for developing antigens from proteins that are highly conserved among mammals and IgY is advantageous because of the ability to economically produce these antibodies on a large scale. In this section, we provide a brief overview of monoclonal IgY antibodies and their application in diagnostics.

16.5.1 Monoclonal IgY Antibodies

For a traditional preparation of murine monoclonal antibodies, antibody-producing B cells with infinite proliferation (hybridoma) are produced by fusing antibody-producing B cells with myeloma cells. (For a review, please see ref. 65.) Once prepared, these cells are cultured for the large-scale production of homogeneous monoclonal antibodies.

The preparation of monoclonal IgY antibodies was pioneered by Matsuda's research group at Hiroshima University, Japan. This group developed a thymidine kinase-deficient chicken B cell line.[66] Briefly, thymidine kinase-deficient B cells were fused to spleen cells that were immunized by the antigen of interest. Over 10^9 lymphocytes can be harvested from the spleen of an immunized chicken. Hybridomas were then selected in the presence of a hypoxanthine-aminopterin-thymidine (HAT) medium.[66]

Recently, a single-chain antibody preparation has been investigated for use in developing therapeutic antibodies using IgY monoclonal antibodies. (For a review, please see ref. 67.) Briefly, in this procedure, the V_H and V_L genes are assembled to form full-length single-chain variable fragments (scFv) using peptide linkers. The scFv antibody, which recognizes a single antigenic epitope, has higher potential to be used as a diagnostic and therapeutic agent.

The B cell line DT40 method has been established and has gained attention. (For a review, please see ref. 68.) In this method, there is no need to immunize chickens with the antigen of interest. Culturing the DT40 cell line can create diverse libraries of antibodies, aiding the effectiveness of screening using monoclonal antibodies. The following sub-sections discuss two applications of monoclonal IgY.

16.5.2 Monoclonal IgY Antibody-based Applications

16.5.2.1 *Hanganutziu-Deicher Antigen*

Animals have a natural antibody against Hanganutziu-Deicher (HD) antigen without infections. In the late 1970s, it was discovered that the HD antigen is *N*-glycolylneuraminic acid (NeuGc) and that it is expressed on the surface of cells of a variety of cancers; therefore, anti-HD monoclonal antibody can be used to detect a variety of cancers in diagnostics.[69] In most animals, both NeuGc and *N*-acetylneuraminic acid (NeuAc) coexist. In chickens and humans, only the NeuAc is found. Therefore, the antibody against NeuGc cannot be produced in animals other than humans and chickens; anti-HD monoclonal IgY can be prepared from chickens immunized with the HD antigen. Asaoka *et al.*[70] reported the preparation of anti-NeuGc monoclonal IgY antibody for the first time.

16.5.2.2 *Bovine Spongiform Encephalopathy (BSE)*

The BSE prion has over 80% homology among mammals; therefore, it is difficult to get an effective antibody against it using mammals.[71] The successful production of a monoclonal IgY antibody against the prion protein in BSE has been reported.[72] Monoclonal antibodies against prion and scFv were prepared by cell fusion and phage display technology. The resulting IgY antibodies could recognize the prion proteins that are conserved across mammals. The authors suggested that the anti-prion monoclonal IgY antibody could be applied to detect scrapie disease in sheep and human Creutzfeldt–Jakob disease, as well as BSE in cows.

16.6 Conclusions

This chapter described the applications of yolk-derived IgY as a diagnostic tool for clinical testing and as a means to prevent and reduce infections. For these applications, a significant amount of specific antibody is necessary, and large amounts of IgY can be created quickly, easily, and in a cost-effective manner. Furthermore, chicken-derived IgY is optimal as an oral passive immunization tool.

It is generally desirable for specific antibodies to be administered orally. Since eggs are eaten in our daily lives, egg-derived IgY is an attractive approach for functional foods. Currently, food products including IgY have been commercialized to prevent dental caries and to remove *H. pylori* from the stomach. Other applications require a pharmaceutical approach. For example, research has shown potential for the use of IgY in the prevention of diarrhea caused by rotavirus in infants. For the commercialization of these applications, further demonstrations of safety and effectiveness are required.

Recently, avian IgY has received attention as an alternative to mouse monoclonal antibodies in situations where the target molecules are low in antigenicity among mammals. In the future, monoclonal IgY antibodies will be attractive for use as diagnosis and treatment agents, including for diseases for which specific antibodies were not able to be produced using mammals. Furthermore, a variety of antibody drugs will continue to be developed using a humanized monoclonal IgY antibody.

References

1. H. Hatta, M. Ozeki and K. Tsuda, Egg yolk antibody IgG and its application, in *Hen Eggs: Their Basic and Applied*, ed. T. Yamamoto, L. R. Juneja, H. Hatta and M. Kim, CRC press, New York, 1997, pp. 151–178.
2. Y. Horimoto and H. Hatta, The nutritional and physiological functions of egg yolk components, in *Achieving Sustainable Production of Egg*, ed. J. Roberts, United Kingdom:Burleigh Dodds Science Publishing, 2017.
3. R. Shade, E. G. Galzado, R. Sarmiento, P. A. Chacana, J. Porankiewica-Asplund and H. R. Terzolo, Chicken egg yok antibodies (IgY-technology): A review of progress in production and use in research and human veterinary medicine, *ATLA*, 2005, **33**, 1–26.
4. Y. Xu, X. Li, L. Jin, Y. Zhen, Y. Lu, S. Li, J. You and L. Wang, Application of chicken of terrestrial and aquatic animal diseases: A review, *Biotechnol. Adv.*, 2011, **29**, 860–868.
5. D. Parra, F. Takizawa and J. O. Sunyer, Evolution of B cell immunity, *Annu. Rev. Anim. Biosci.*, 2013, **1**, 65–97.
6. X. Li, T. Nakano, H. H. Sunwoo, B. H. Paek, H. S. Chae and J. S. Sim, Effects of egg and yolk weights on yolk antibody (IgY) production in laying chickens, *Poult. Sci.*, 1998, **77**, 266–270.
7. H. Hatta and M. Shimizu, Production of hen egg antibody and its characteristics, in *Egg Science*, ed. R. Nakamura, Asakura Publishing Co. Ltd., Tokyo, 1998, pp. 146–152, [Jpn].
8. M. Shimizu, H. Nagashima, K. Sano, K. Hashimoto, M. Ozeki, K. Tsuda and H. Hatta, Molecular stability of chicken and rabbit immunoglobulin G., *Biosci., Biotechnol., Biochem.*, 1992, **56**, 270–274.
9. W. D. da Silva and D. V. Tambourgi, IgY: A promising antibody for use in immunodiagnostic and in immunotherapy, *Vet. Immunol. Immunopathol.*, 2010, **135**, 173–180.
10. K. Horie, N. Horie, A. M. Abdou, J.-O. Yang, S.-S. Yun, H.-N. Hun, C.-K. Park, M. Kim and H. Hatta, Suppressive effect of functional drinking yogurt containing specific egg yolk immunoglobulin on *Helicobacter pylori* in humans, *J. Dairy Sci.*, 2004, **87**, 4073–4079.
11. S. Rahman, S. V. Nguyen, F. C. Icatlo Jr, K. Umeda and Y. Kodama, Oral passive IgY-based immunotherapeutic, *Hum. Vaccines Immunother.*, 2013, **9**, 1039–1048.

12. H. Hatta, K. Tsuda, S. Akachi, M. Kim, T. Yamamoto and T. Ebina, Oral passive immunization effect of anti-human rotavirus IgY and its behavior against proteolytic enzymes, *Biosci., Biotechnol., Biochem.*, 1993, **57**, 1077–1081.
13. M. Shimizu, Y. Miwa, K. Hashimoto and A. Goto, Encapsulation of chicken egg yolk immunoglobulin G (IgY) by liposomes, *Biosci., Biotechnol., Biochem.*, 1993, **57**, 1445–1449.
14. M. Shimizu, H. Nagashima, K. Hashimoto and T. Suzuki, Egg yolk antibody (IgY) stability in aqueous solution with high sugar concentrations, *J. Food Sci.*, 1994, **59**, 763–765.
15. N. Gujral, R. Lobenberg, M. Suresh and H. Sunwoo, In-vitro and in-vivo binding activity of chicken egg yolk immunoglobulin Y (IgY) against gliadin in food matrix, *J. Agric. Food Chem.*, 2012, **60**, 3166–3172.
16. A. Larsson, A. Karlsson-Parra and J. Sjoquist, Use of chicken antibodies in enzyme immunoassays to avoid interferences by rheumatoid factors, *Clin. Chem.*, 1991, **37**, 411–414.
17. G. Kronvall, U. S. Seal, S. Svensson and R. C. Williams Jr, Phylogenetic aspects of staphylococcal protein A-reactive serum globulins in birds and mammals, *Acta Pathol. Microbiol. Scand., Sect. B*, 1974, **82**, 12–18.
18. J. Kovacs-Nolan, Y. Mine and H. Hatta, Avian immunoglobulin Y and its application in human health and disease, in *Nutraceutical Proteins and Peptides in Health and Disease*, ed. Y. Mine and F. Shahidi, CRC Press, Inc., Boca Raton, FL, 2005, pp. 161–189.
19. H. Hatta, M. P. Kapoor and L. R. Juneja, Bioactive Components in Egg Yolk, in *Egg Bioscience and Biotechnology*, ed. Y. Mine, John Wiley & Sons, Inc., New Jersey, 2008, pp. 185–237.
20. A. Lupicka-Slowik, M. Psurski, R. Grzywa, K. Bobrek, P. Smok, M. Walczak, A. Gawel, T. Stefaniak, J. Oleksyszyn and M. Sienczyk, Development of adenosine deaminase-specific IgY antibodies: diagnostic and inhibitory application, *Appl. Biochem. Biotechnol.*, 2018, **184**, 1358–1374.
21. K. Landsteiner, Uber Ablutinationssersheinumben normalen menshlichen Blutes, *Wien. Klin. Wochenschr.*, 1901, **14**, 1132–1134.
22. S. Yazawa, O. Hosomi and A. Takeya, Isolation and characterization of anti-H antibody from egg yolk of immunized hens, *Immunol. Invest.*, 1991, **20**, 569–581.
23. O. Hosomi, A. Takeya and S. Yazawa, Purification and characterization of anti-B antibody from egg yolk of immunized hens, *Anim. Sci. Technol.*, 1991, **62**, 1055–1061.
24. T. W. Du Clos and C. Mold, C-reactive protein: an activator of innate immunity and a modulator of adaptive immunity, *Immunol. Res.*, 2004, **30**, 261–277.
25. C. P. Price, A. K. Trull, D. Berry and E. G. Gorman, Development and validation of a particle-enhanced turbidimetric immunoassay for C-reactive protein, *J. Immunol. Methods*, 1987, **99**, 205–211.

26. C. P. Price, J. Calvin, S. A. Walker, A. Trull, D. J. Newman and E. G. Gorman, A rapid sensitive automated light scattering immunoassay for serum C-reactive protein and the definition of a reference range in healthy blood donors, *Clin. Chem. Lab. Med.*, 1999, **37**, 109–113.
27. M. Ota, A. Maeda, H. Itagaki and H. Hatta and Y. Shitahaku, Turbidimetric immune assay of CRP using IgY, Research report of Ogata Institute for Medical and Chemical Research, 1990, pp. 9–16 [Jpn].
28. S. Blumenthal, The insulin immunoassay after 50 years: a reassessment, *Perspect. Biol. Med.*, 2009, **52**, 343–354.
29. A. Polson, M. B. von Wechmar and G. Fazakerley, Antibodies to proteins from yolk of immunized hens, *Immunol. Commun.*, 1980, **9**, 495–514.
30. K. Lee, A. Ametani, M. Shimizu, H. Hatta, T. Yamamoto and S. Kaminogawa, Production and characterization of anti-human insulin antibodies in the hen's egg, *Agric. Biol. Chem.*, 1991, **55**, 2141–2143.
31. J. P. Chippaux and M. Goyffon, Epidemiology of scorpionism: a global appraisal, *Acta Trop.*, 2008, **107**, 71–79.
32. A. Kasturiratne, A. R. Wickremasinghe, N. de Silva, N. K. Gunawardena, A. Pathmeswaran, R. Premaratna, L. Savioli, D. G. Lalloo and H. J. de Silva, The global burden snakebite: a literature analysis and modelling based on regional estimates of envenoming and deaths, *PLoS Med.*, 2008, e218.
33. B. S. Thalley and S. B. Carroll, Rattlesnake and scorpion antivenin from the egg yolks of immunized hens, *Biotechnology*, 1990, **8**, 934–937.
34. C. H. Lee, Y. C. Lee, S. J. Leu, L. T. Lin, J. R. Chiang, W. J. Hsu and Y. Y. Yang, Production and characterization of neutralizing antibodies against *Bungarus multicinctus* snake venom, *Appl. Environ. Microbiol.*, 2016, **82**, 6973–6982.
35. M. S. Sandrin and I. F. Mckenzie, Galα(1,3)Gal, the major xenoantigen(s) recognised in pigs by human natural antibodies, *Immunol. Rev.*, 1994, **141**, 169–190.
36. A. Larsson and J. Sioquist, Chicken IgY: utilizing the evolutionary difference, *Comp. Immunol. Microbiol. Infect. Dis.*, 1990, **13**, 199.
37. J. Fryer, J. Firca, J. Leventhal, B. Blondie, A. Malcolm, D. Ivancic, R. Gandhi, A. Shah, W. Pao, M. Abecassis, D. Kaufman, F. Stuart and B. Anderson, Igy antiporcine endothelial cell antibodies effectively block human antiporcine xenoantibody binding, *Xenotranspantation*, 1999, **6**, 98–109.
38. U. D. Parashar, C. J. Gibson, J. S. Bresee and R. I. Glass, Rotavirus and severe childhood diarrhea, *Emerging Infect. Dis.*, 2006, **12**, 304–306.
39. S. P. Yamamoto, A. Kaida, H. Kubo and N. Iritani, Gastroenteritis outbreaks caused by a DS-1-like G1P[8] rotavirus strain, Japan, 2012–2013, *Emerging Infect. Dis.*, 2014, **20**, 1030–1033.
40. H. Hatta, K. Tsuda, S. Akachi, M. Kim and T. Yamamoto, Productivity and some properties of egg yolk antibody (IgY) against human rotavirus compared with rabbit IgG, *Biosci., Biotechnol., Biochem.*, 1993, **57**, 450–454.

41. W. J. Loesche, J. Rowan, L. H. Straffon and P. J. Loos, Association of *Streptococcus mutans* with human dental decay, *Infect. Immun.*, 1975, **11**, 1252–1260.
42. S. Otake, Y. Nishihara, M. Makimura, H. Hatta, M. Kim, T. Yamamoto and M. Hirasawa, Protection of rats against dental caries by passive immunization with hen-egg-yolk antibody (IgY), *J. Dent. Res.*, 1991, **70**, 162–166.
43. H. Hatta, K. Tsuda, M. Ozeki, M. Kim, T. Yamamoto, S. Otake, M. Hirasawa, J. Katx, N. K. Childers and S. M. Michalek, Passive immunization against dental plaque formation in humans: effect of a mouth rinse containing egg yolk antibodies (IgY) specific to *Streptococcus mutans*, *Carries Res.*, 1997, **31**, 268–274.
44. N. Uemura, S. Okamoto, S. Yamomoto, N. Masumura, S. Yamguchi, M. Yamakido, K. Taniyama, N. Sasaki and R. J. Schlemper, *Helicobacter pylori* infection and the development of gastric cancer, *N. Engl. J. Med.*, 2001, **345**, 784–789.
45. B. S. Sheu, J. J. Wu, C. Y. Lo, H. W. Wu, J. H. Chen, Y. S. Lin and M. D. Lin, Impact of supplement with Lactobacillus- and Bifidobacterium-containing yogurt on triple therapy for *Helicobactoer pylori* eradication, *Aliment. Pharmacol. Ther.*, 2002, **16**, 1669–1675.
46. R. D. Frizzell, Functions of the cystic fibrosis transmembrane conductance regulator protein, *Am. J. Respir. Crit. Care Med.*, 1995, **151**, S54–S58.
47. V. Waters and A. Smyth, Cystic fibrosis microbiology: Advances in antimicrobial therapy, *J. Cystic Fibrosis*, 2015, **14**, 551–560.
48. D. Carlander, H. Kollberg, P. E. Wejaker and A. Larsson, Prevention of chronic *Pseudomonas aeruginosa* colonization by gargling with specific antibodies: a preliminary report, in *Egg Nutrition and Biotechnology*, ed. J. S. Sim, S. Nakai and W. Guenter, CABI Publishing, New York, 2000, pp. 371–374.
49. H. Kollberg, D. Carlander, H. Olesen, P. E. Wejaker, M. Johannesson and A. Larsson, Oral administration of specific yolk antibodies (IgY) may prevent *Pseudomonas aeruginosa* infections in patients with cystic fibrosis: a phase I feasibility study, *Pediatr. Pulmonol.*, 2003, **35**, 433–440.
50. E. Nilsson, H. Kollberg, M. Johannesson, P.-E. Wejåker, D. Carlander and A. Larsson, More than 10 years' continuous oral treatment with specific immunoglobulin Y for the prevention of *Pseudomonas aeruginosa* infections: a case report, *J. Med. Food*, 2008, **10**, 375–378.
51. M. H. Delegge, Aspiration pneumonia: Incidence, mortality, and at-risk populations, *J. Parenter. Enteral Nutr.*, 2002, **26**, S19–S25.
52. D. K. Podolosky, Inflammatory bowel disease, *N. Engl. J. Med.*, 1991, **325**, 928–937.
53. E. J. Breese, C. A. Michie, S. W. Nicholls, S. H. Murch, C. B. Williams, P. Domizio, J. A. Walker-Smith and T. T. MacDonald, Tumor necrosis factor α-producing cells in the intestinal mucosa of children with inflammatory bowel disease, *Gastroenterology*, 1994, **106**, 1455–1466.

54. D. C. Baumgart and W. J. Sandborn, Inflammatory bowel disease: clinical aspects and established and evolving therapies, *Lancet*, 2007, **369**, 1641–1657.
55. K. L. Worledge, R. Godiska, T. A. Barrett and J. A. Kink, Oral administration of avian tumor necrosis factor antibodies effectively treats experimental colitis in rats, *Dig. Dis. Sci.*, 2000, **45**, 2298–2305.
56. J. P. Despres and I. Lemieux, Abdominal obesity and metabolic syndrome, *Nature*, 2006, **444**, 881–887.
57. R. B. Birari and K. K. Bhutani, Pancreatic lipase inhibitors from natural sources: unexplored potential, *Drug Discovery Today*, 2007, **12**, 879–889.
58. A. Ballinger and S. R. Peikin, Orlistat: its current status as an anti-obesity drug, *Eur. J. Pharmacol.*, 2002, **440**, 109–117.
59. M. Hirose, T. Ando, R. Shofiqur, K. Umeda, Y. Kodama, S. V. Nguyen, T. Goto, M. Shimada and S. Nagaoka, Anti-obesity activity of hen egg anti-lipase immunoglobulin yolk, a novel pancreatic lipase inhibitor, *Nutr. Metab.*, 2013, **10**, 70–75.
60. S. Husby, S. Koletzko, I. R. Korponay-Szabo, M. L. Mearin and A. Philips, *et al.*, European society for pediatric gastroenterology, hepatology, and nutrition for the diagnosis of coeliac disease, *J. Pediatr. Gastroenterol. Nutr.*, 2012, **54**, 136–160.
61. N. Gujral, J. W. Suh and H. H. Sunwoo, Effect of anti-gliadin IgY antibody on epithelial intestinal integrity and inflammatory response induced by gliadin, *BMC Immunol.*, 2015, **16**, 41–51.
62. G. Kohler and C. Milstein, Continuous cultures of fused cells secreting antibody of predefined specificity, *Nature*, 1975, **256**, 495–497.
63. A. L. Grilo and A. Mantalaris, The increasingly human and profitable monoclonal antibody market, *Trends Biotechnol.*, 2019, **37**(1), 9–16.
64. A. K. Pavlou and M. J. Belsey, The therapeutic antibodies market to 2008, *Eur. J. Pharm. Biopharm.*, 2005, **59**, 389–396.
65. A. R. Costa, M. E. Rodrigues, M. Henriques, J. Azeredo and R. Oliveira, Guidelines to cell engineering for monoclonal antibody production, *Eur. J. Pharm. Biopharm.*, 2010, **74**, 127–138.
66. S. Nishinaka, H. Matsuda and M. Murata, Establishment of a chicken x chicken hybridoma secreting specific antibody, *Int. Arch. Allergy Immunol.*, 1989, **89**, 416–419.
67. W. Lee, A. S. Atif, S. C. Tan and C. H. Leow, Insights into the chicken IgY with emphasis on the generation and applications of chicken recombinant monoclonal antibodies, *J. Immunol. Methods*, 2017, **447**, 71–85.
68. P. Winding and M. W. Berchtold, The chicken B cell line DT40: a novel tool for gene disruption experiments, *J. Immunol. Methods*, 2000, **249**, 1–16.
69. T. Nishimaki, K. Kano and F. Milgrom, Hanganutziu-Deicher antigen and antibody in pathologic sera and tissues, *J. Immunol.*, 1979, **122**, 2314–2318.

70. H. Asaoka, S. Nishinaka, N. Wakamiya, H. Matsuda and M. Murata, Two chicken monoclonal antibodies specific for heterophil Hanganutziu-Deicher antigens, *Immunol. Lett.*, 1992, **32**, 91–96.
71. H. Matsuda, Chicken derived monoclonal antibody, *J. Grad. Sch., Bishop. Sci. Hiroshima Univ.*, 2009, **48**, 73–76.
72. K. Miyamoto, T. Shimamoto, M. Aosasa, S. Kimura, N. Nakamura, Y. Okubo, T. Yokoyama, H. Horiuchi, S. Furusawa and H. Matsuda, Development of recombinant chicken IgY from single chain fragment of variable region for diagnosis BSE, *Biologicals*, 2007, **35**, 31–34.

CHAPTER 17

Advances in the Separation of Functional Egg Proteins – Egg White Proteins

E. D. N. S. ABEYRATHNE[a], X. HUANG[b] AND D. U. AHN*[c]

[a]Department of Animal Science, Uva Wellassa University, Badulla 90000, Sri Lanka; [b]College of Food Science & Technology, Huazhong Agricultural University, Egg Processing Technology Local Joint National Engineering Research Center, National R&D Center for Egg Processing, Wuhan, Hubei 430070, China; [c]Department of Animal Science, Iowa State University, Ames, IA 50010, USA
*E-mail: duahn@iastate.edu

17.1 Introduction

Egg white consists of 88% water and 12% solids, of which >90% is protein.[1] Ovalbumin, ovotransferrin, ovomucoid, ovoglobulins (G2 and G3), ovomucin, and lysozyme are considered as the major proteins, while ovoinhibitor, ovomacroglobulin, ovoglycoprotein, ovoflavoprotein, thiamine-binding proteins, ficin/papain inhibitor (cystatin), and avidin are the minor egg white proteins (Table 17.1). These proteins have been recognized for their functional importance with foaming, antioxidant, antimicrobial, metal-binding, antibacterial, antiviral, anti-tumor, protease inhibitory, protein-binding, and angiotensin-converting enzyme (ACE)-inhibitory activities.

Food Chemistry, Function and Analysis No.14
Eggs as Functional Foods and Nutraceuticals for Human Health
Edited by Jianping Wu

Published by the Royal Society of Chemistry, www.rsc.org

Table 17.1 Composition of egg white proteins and their characteristics.[a,e]

Protein	Amount (%)[b]	PI[c]	MW (kDa)	Td[d] (°C)	Characteristics
Ovalbumin	54	4.5	45	84	Phosphoglycoprotein, metal binder
Ovotransferrin	13	6.0	77.8	61	Binds iron and other metal ions
Ovomucoid	12	6.1	28	70	Inhibits trypsin and serine proteases
G2 globulin	4	5.0	36	92.5	Foaming agent
G3 globulin	4	4.8	45	—	Foaming agent
Ovomucin	3.5	4.5–5.0	220	—	Sialoprotein. Complex with lysozyme
Lysozyme (G1 globulin)	3.4	10.7	14.3	75	Lyses bacterial cell walls
Ovoinhibitor	1.5	5.1	49	—	Inhibits serine proteases
Ovoglycoprotein	1.0	3.9	24.4	—	Sialoprotein
Ovoflavoprotein	0.8	4.0	32–36	—	Binds riboflavin
Ovomacroglobulin	0.5	4.5	650	—	Strongly antigenic, protease inhibitor
Thiamine-binding protein	0.5	—	38	—	Binds thiamine
Avidin	0.06	10	68	—	Binds biotin
Ficin/papain inhibitor	0.05	5.1	13	—	Cystatin. Inhibits cysteine proteases
Other minor proteins[b]	—	—	—	—	—

[a]Sources: Vadehra *et al.* (1973);[122] Li-Chan and Nakai (1989);[62] Stevens (1991);[124] Awade and Efstathiou (1999);[17] Stadelman and Cotterill (2001);[1] Davis and Reeves (2002);[128] Renault *et al.* (2007);[129] Gautron *et al.* (2007).[130]
[b]% of egg white protein.
[c]PI: isoelectric point.
[d]Td: denaturation temperature.
[e]Other minor proteins include lipocalins, extracellular fatty acid-binding protein, aminopeptidases, clusterin, HEP21, TENP, *etc.*

Over the past several decades, numerous methods for the separation of the functional proteins from egg white have been developed, and the functions of each egg white protein have been studied, but the separation efforts were largely limited to a single component and the methods were for laboratory scale. Separation of functional proteins from egg white can dramatically increase the value of an egg, and the modification of the separated egg white proteins can further improve the functional activities, utilization, and value of the proteins. However, the commercial use of the isolated egg white proteins is highly limited because commercial-scale separation methods for separating egg white proteins are not well established at present. Therefore, developing simple, low-cost, and scalable separation protocols for multiple proteins is essential if the isolated proteins are to be used in the food and drug industries. Moreover, the developed method should not use any harmful chemicals and should be environmentally friendly if the separation methods are to be used by industry. This chapter will cover the advances in the separation methods of the selected proteins from egg white and discuss their potential for food and non-food applications.

17.2 Separation of Egg White Proteins

17.2.1 Separation of Major Egg White Proteins

Among the major egg white proteins, ovalbumin was the first protein that was isolated using high levels of ammonium sulfate under acidic conditions.[2,3] In the 1950s, a chromatography technique was first introduced to separate ovalbumin from egg white.[4,5] Subsequently, various chromatographic methods, including anion exchange chromatography, Q Sepharose Fast Flow, Carboxymethyl (CM) Sepharose, and CM Sephadex, were tested for separating ovalbumin from egg white.[6,7] The use of the chromatographic techniques provided a high yield and purity of the isolated proteins. However, the use of these methods to separate ovalbumin was not practical and was very expensive for scale-up separation. Another approach used to separate ovalbumin from egg white was using SDS-PAGE and 2-dimensional electrophoresis,[8] but the separated protein was denatured during the separation process, the method was not economical, and it was only useful at laboratory scale. Ward and his group used foam fractionation to separate ovalbumin from egg white.[9] This method used air at a low flow rate to denature and precipitate ovalbumin from egg white, but the purity of the separated ovalbumin was low. Recently, Datta and co-workers used a low concentration of NaCl followed by ultrafiltration to separate ovalbumin.[10] However, the use of ultrafiltration to separate ovalbumin directly from egg white was difficult owing to the foaming properties of the protein as well as difficulties in controlling *trans*-membrane pressure, stirrer speed, and pH, even though the separation can be carried out in large volume. Recently, acidic ammonium sulfate was used to separate ovalbumin from egg white.[11] They removed lysozyme and ovomucin first and then precipitated ovotransferrin using acidic ammonium sulfate. The resulting supernatant was rich in ovalbumin and was then desalted and concentrated using ultrafiltration. The separated ovalbumin had a high yield owing to some impurities such as ovomucoid and ovoinhibitor contained in the ovalbumin, but its purity was still higher than 88%. The process was simple, easy, and could be scaled up.

Ovotransferrin was also first separated from egg white using high levels of ammonium sulfate at low pH conditions.[12] However, using high levels of chemicals cannot work in large-scale separation owing to the high cost of the chemicals and the need for subsequent recovery of the chemicals to reduce pollution. Later, various chromatographic methods, including CM-cellulose ion exchange, affinity chromatography,[13] Cu Sepharose 6B and diethylaminoethyl (DEAE) affinity gel,[14] Q Sepharose Fast Flow chromatography,[15–18] and an electrophoretic method,[8] were developed to separate ovotransferrin.

These techniques separated ovotransferrin in high purity and yield, but they were only good for laboratory-scale preparations. Development of a more practical, scalable separation method for ovotransferrin was started in the 2000s. Ko and Ahn developed a method to separate ovotransferrin using ethanol: they used 43% ethanol (final concentration) to precipitate all the proteins in egg white except for ovotransferrin and then used 59% ethanol (final concentration) to precipitate ovotransferrin from the ovotransferrin-containing supernatant fraction.[19] They obtained over 95% yield and >80% purity using the developed method. The method was suitable and effective for the scale-up preparation of ovotransferrin from egg white, but the ovotransferrin produced was the holo-form and needed to be converted to the apo-form if it was intended to be used as an antimicrobial agent. However, converting from holo-form to apo-form was difficult, even though this method produced high yield and purity, and could be easily scaled up. Abeyrathne *et al.* developed a method to separate ovotransferrin from chicken egg white without using organic solvents.[20] They used a two-step precipitation method using combinations of 5.0% (wt/vol) ammonium sulfate and 2.5% (wt/vol) citric acid followed by 2.0% (wt/vol) ammonium sulfate and 1.5% (wt/vol) citric acid. The method separated ovotransferrin with >85% purity and >83% yield. Although the yield of this method was not as high as that of Ko and Ahn's ethanol precipitation method, this method showed good scale-up capabilities. Furthermore, the separated ovotransferrin was in apo-form, and the method was simple and cost-effective compared with most other previously published methods.

Ovomucoid was first separated using trichloroacetic acid (TCA) and acetone,[21] and TCA and ethanol.[22] However, the use of TCA in the separation of ovomucoid limits the applications for human use. Forsythe and Foster used 50% ethanol (final concentration),[23] and others used 25% ethanol[24] (final concentration) to separate ovomucoid from egg white, but the purity of ovomucoid separated was not reported and the recovery of the protein was relatively low (around 70%). Yousif and Kan used SDS-PAGE with a linear gradient (4–20%) to separate ovomucoid from egg white,[25] but this method could not be scaled up and the protein was denatured during the separation owing to the 2-mercaptoethanol used in the protocol. A three-step chromatographic method using CM-cellulose[26] and DEAE-cellulose[27] was also used to separate ovomucoid, but this method was also not appropriate for scale-up even though it gives good purity and yield of the protein. Abeyrathne *et al.* separated ovomucoid as a part of the sequential separation method for ovotransferrin and ovomucoid, and the method is further discussed in the sequential separation part of this section.[20]

Lysozyme is commonly separated using ion exchange chromatography mainly owing to its high PI value.[28] Many different ion exchange resins were used to separate lysozyme from egg white: Strang used carboxymethylcellulose (CMC) resin to separate lysozyme from egg white, but large-scale production of lysozyme using CMC resin was not easy owing to its fine granule size, which made it difficult to have a high flow rate when used in column chromatography.[29] The fine granule size of the CM-cellulose resin also made it difficult to handle when used in batch systems. Cation exchange chromatography packed with magnetic cation exchange resin and porous glass fiber membranes coated with monophenyl trimethoxysilane (MPh),[30,31] affinity chromatography,[32–35] and gel filtration[36] were also used to separate lysozyme from egg white. However, these chromatographic methods were not suitable for the large-scale production due to the complexity of the separation, the separation efficiency, and the cost of the resins, even though they produced high-purity lysozymes with high yields. Instead of using ion exchange resins, Ghosh *et al.* used a polysulfone hollow fiber membrane (H1P30-20, MWCO 30 kDa) to separate lysozyme.[37] The method separated lysozyme with 80–90% purity but was not suitable for commercial use owing to its complexity. Recently, Abeyrathne *et al.* developed another ion exchange chromatography method to separate lysozyme.[11] They used FPC 3500 cation exchange resin under alkaline conditions. The resin used was easy to handle and suitable for both batch and column chromatography, and the method was simple and could be used for a scale-up separation of lysozyme from egg white. Using their new method, they separated lysozyme with >85% yield and >95% purity. The resin could also be easily regenerated and repeatedly reused without loss of function. Wan *et al.* used two different ultrafiltration membranes (Biomax 30 kDa and Ultracel Amicon 30 kDa) to separate lysozyme, but the method was also done only at laboratory scale and could not be scaled up owing to the equipment used.[38] The reductant β-mercaptoethanol was used at low concentrations (0.4–1.0%) to separate lysozyme.[39] In this method, eggs were pickled in saturated NaCl solution for 35 days to bring the NaCl level in egg white to 5–6%. Thus, this method took too long a time to be practical and the use of mercaptoethanol is prohibited for human foods. An affinity filtration using Cibcron blue F3GA immobilized to yeast cells was reported recently.[35] This method was tested at the bench level and produced lysozyme with >90% purity but scaling up was problematic owing to its complexity.

Ovomucin is mainly separated using isoelectric precipitation. Hiidenhovi *et al.* used isoelectric precipitation followed by gel filtration to separate ovomucin from egg white and observed three subunits (β, α1, and α2 subunits).[40] Omana and Wu used calcium chloride and potassium chloride in combination with isoelectric point precipitation and then gel filtration to purify ovomucin.[41] The use of potassium chloride produced ovomucin with high impurities while the use of $CaCl_2$ produced ovomucin with high purity. Nevertheless, this method cannot be used for scale-up production of ovomucin because of the low sample handling capacity of the gel filtration. Hiidenhovi *et al.* used dual-column gel filtration to separate ovomucin subunits and observed eight peaks during the separation, but the purity of the separated ovomucin was not reported.[42] Electrophoresis was also used to separate ovomucin from egg white,[8] but the major limitation of this method was difficulties in scale-up production and the denaturation of the protein during separation owing to 10-fold dilution of egg white.

High-speed centrifugation was another method used to separate ovomucin in several instances: Robinson and Monsey used isoelectric precipitation of ovomucin in Tris-HCl buffer and high-speed centrifugation (35 000 × *g*),[43] Guérin-Dubiard *et al.* (2005) used alkaline pH conditions and centrifugation at 24 000 × *g* for 30 minutes at 4 °C,[44] Omana and Wu used NaCl and centrifugation twice at 10 000 × *g* for 10 minutes,[45] and Omana *et al.* soaked egg overnight in 100 mM NaCl solution and then centrifuged at 15 300 × *g* for 10 minutes at 4 °C.[46] Although the method separated ovomucin with high yield, high-speed centrifugation can be impractical for the commercial-scale preparation of ovomucin owing to the equipment costs. A two-step separation with pH and NaCl treatments was used to separate ovomucin,[47] but this method produced ovomucin with a low purity. Although ovomucin was first separated in 1898, further studies were difficult owing to its insolubility and heterogeneity.[48] Ovomucin is insoluble in neutral pH conditions if a denaturing agent such as SDS, urea, or β-mercaptoethanol is not added.[42,49,51] The combination of SDS and β-mercaptoethanol dissolved ovomucin well,[42] but β-mercaptoethanol cannot be used in human foods. Guanidinium chloride (6 M) along with 0.1 M sodium acetate buffer was also used to dissolve ovomucin[43] but the use of high levels of guanidinium chloride is not practical because of the high cost and guanidine is not suitable for use in human foods. Homogenization and sonication improved the solubility of ovomucin[51] to a certain degree by either cleaving the disulfide bonds or releasing the attached carbohydrate from the main protein chain.[46] Abeyrathne *et al.* reported that ovomucin could easily be dissolved at high pH (pH 12.0) without adding any chemicals.[11]

17.2.2 Sequential Separation of Major Egg White Proteins

The separation methods for the major egg white proteins from egg white discussed above are mainly for single proteins. However, sequential separation methods for separating multiple proteins from egg white have also been developed: Vachier *et al.* separated lysozyme, ovotransferrin, and ovalbumin in sequence using ion exchange chromatography.[16] The yield of lysozyme was as low as 60%, but the yield of ovalbumin was 83%, and that for ovotransferrin was 100%. The purity of ovotransferrin was 75% whereas those of lysozyme and ovalbumin were 99% and 88%, respectively. Again, the major drawback of this method was difficulties in scaling up owing to difficulties in using the Q Sepharose Fast Flow anion exchange column. Shibusawa *et al.* separated ovotransferrin, lysozyme, and ovalbumin using counter-current columns with different flow rates but scale-up to produce large amounts of those proteins in a single sequence was not easy because the method used was complicated.[52] Shibusawa *et al.* further improved the earlier sequential separation method for lysozyme, ovotransferrin, ovalbumin, and ovomucin from egg white using counter-current chromatography with a cross-axis coil centrifuge method.[53] Tankrathok *et al.* (2009) developed a two-step sequential separation method using Q Sepharose Fast Flow anion exchange chromatography in the first step and then CM-Toyopearl 650M cation exchange chromatography in the second step to separate ovalbumin, lysozyme, ovotransferrin, and ovomucoid.[18] However, this method separated the proteins with 54, 55, 21, and 21% yields respectively. Lysozyme, ovotransferrin, ovalbumin, and ovoflavoproteins were also separated using fast flow anion exchange chromatography,[54] but scale-up was not easy owing to the cost of the ion exchange resins used. A novel approach was taken to separate lysozyme and ovotransferrin using radial flow membrane adsorption chromatography.[55] Even though over 96% purity and yield was obtained for lysozyme and over 80% was obtained for ovotransferrin, scaling up of this method has limitations owing to the viscosity of the egg white and the complex nature of the separation method. Abeyrathne and his group put together individual separation methods and developed a few sequential separation methods for multiple proteins from egg white.[11,20,56–58] They used Amberlite FPC 3500 ion exchange resin to separate lysozyme first and then used acidified ammonium sulfate to separate ovotransferrin and ovalbumin.[11]

Ovotransferrin and ovomucoid were separated in sequence using two different approaches after extracting the ovotransferrin- and ovomucoid-containing fraction from egg white.[20,57] Fe^{3+} was added to diluted egg white (2×) to stabilize ovotransferrin and all the egg white proteins, except for ovotransferrin and ovomucoid, were precipitated with 43% ethanol (final concentration). The supernatant after centrifugation was collected and treated with either high-concentration ethanol (61% final concentration) or acidic ammonium sulfate (2.5% each) to separate ovotransferrin and ovomucoid. For the ethanol precipitation method, ovotransferrin, soluble in 43% ethanol, was precipitated at 61% ethanol, while ovomucoid remained soluble. For the acidic salt precipitation method, the ethanol in the supernatant was removed and concentrated first using ultrafiltration, and then the concentrated solution was treated with a combination of 2.5% ammonium sulfate and 2.5% citric acid. After centrifugation, the precipitant was used as the ovotransferrin fraction and the supernatant as the ovomucoid fraction. Both of the protocols separated ovotransferrin and ovomucoid effectively, and the methods were simple, fast, and easy to scale-up. The yields of ovomucoid and ovotransferrin were >96% and >92%, respectively and the purities were >89% and >88%, respectively. The ELISA results confirmed that the activity of the separated ovotransferrin was >95%. A sequential separation of lysozyme, ovomucin, ovotransferrin, and ovalbumin was also developed by Abeyrathne *et al.*[11] In this method, they used ion exchange chromatography for lysozyme, isoelectric precipitation for ovomucin, and acidic ammonium sulfate for ovotransferrin and ovalbumin. They successfully applied each of the separation strategies in sequence without interrupting the separation of the subsequent proteins. This sequential separation method produced all four proteins with 83–100% yield and 82–96% purity. Moreover, the method was simple and economical, and easily scaled up. However, further refinement and improvement are needed for this method to increase the purity of some proteins, especially those of ovalbumin and ovomucin. Brand *et al.* separated ovotransferrin and lysozyme in sequence after adjusting the viscosity of ovalbumin with high-pressure homogenization and removing ovomucin.[59] This method released the lysozyme trapped in ovomucin, resulting in a higher yield than the existing methods. Recently, Brand *et al.* used another approach to isolate lysozyme and ovotransferrin from egg white using radial flow membrane adsorption chromatography.[55] The purity of the lysozyme and ovotransferrin separated was 96% and 84%, respectively, and the yield was 99% and 97%, respectively. However, this method had some limitations in scaling up even though the protocol separated the proteins with very high purity and yields.

17.2.3 Separation of Other Egg White Proteins

In addition to the major egg white proteins discussed above, there are many other important proteins present in egg white. Ovoglobulins G2 and G3 are present at relatively high levels in egg white (4% each). Feeney *et al.* purified G2 and G3 globulin from egg white using a method involving 0.1 N NaCl extraction, ammonium sulfate precipitation, and then DEAE-cellulose and CM-cellulose chromatography.[60] Huopalahti *et al.* separated G2 and G3 globulins using 2D-electrophoresis coupled with mass spectroscopy (LC-MS/MS) and ion exchange chromatography.[50] Qu *et al.* developed a zwitterionic ion chromatography method that can separate three kinds of egg white components, including ovalbumin, G2 ovoglobulin, and ovotransferrin with >95% purity in a single step.[61] However, the practicality of the methods is questionable owing to the cost of the resins. Some other minor proteins, such as ovoglycoprotein, thiamine-binding proteins, and cysteine protease, also show important biological functions, but not much information on separation methods for these proteins is available.

Flavin-binding protein (flavoprotein) is a globular monomeric phosphoglycoprotein with a molecular weight of 29.2 kDa and a high affinity to riboflavin (vitamin B2). Egg white flavoprotein constitutes approximately 0.8% of the total egg white protein.[62] Flavoprotein is one of the most acidic proteins in egg white, with an isoelectric point close to 4.0. Froehlich *et al.* successfully separated flavoprotein from laying hen liver, blood, and egg yolk using affinity chromatography.[63] Using the very low isoelectric point of flavoprotein, Rao *et al.* developed a single-step method to isolate flavoprotein from chicken egg white. Egg white was first diluted with nine volumes of 50 mM sodium phosphate buffer, pH 6.5, and the diluted egg white was applied to a DEAE-Toyopearl 650 M column.[64] After washing the column, the adsorbed flavoprotein was fractionated using a linear salt gradient. The flavoprotein separated was electrophoretically pure and the yield was about 75%. Guérin-Dubiard *et al.* separated large amounts of flavoprotein from hen egg white using displacement anion exchange chromatography on a Q Sepharose Fast

Flow column. Guérin-Dubiard *et al.* also used anion and cation chromatography to separate flavoprotein as a part of the sequential separation process of multiple egg white proteins.[44] However, all the methods are complicated and only useful for laboratory preparations.

Ovomacroglobulin (ovostatin) was purified using ammonium sulfate precipitation,[65,66] gel filtration (Sephadex G-200), Sepharose CL-4B, and then DEAE-cellulose chromatography,[67] or polyethylene glycol precipitation and chromatography on Ultragel AcA 34, DEAE-cellulose, and Sephacryl S-300 columns[68] after extracting it from egg white using 1% NaCl in Tris-HCl buffer, pH 7.5. However, these methods are complex, give low recovery, and are time-consuming and costly owing to the application of multiple chromatography steps. Geng *et al.* used a combination of PEG precipitation and gel filtration to separate ovomacroglobulin.[69] They diluted egg white with an equal volume of distilled water, and then ovomucin and most of the ovalbumin were removed from the egg white using two-step PEG precipitation. The precipitate was dissolved and further purified using gel filtration chromatography. The ovomacroglobulin obtained had a purity of 97.0% and a yield of 62.5%. To further improve the purification method for ovomacroglobulin, Geng *et al.* used Q Sepharose Fast Flow anion exchange chromatography and then Sephacryl S-200, instead of gel filtration chromatography.[70] They indicated that the new method took less time to separate and had a higher separation yield than their earlier method, but both of the methods were limited to laboratory-scale preparation.

Matsushima first isolated ovoinhibitor using its precipitation characteristics in half-saturated ammonium sulfate, trichloroacetic acid (2.6%), and acetone.[71] He distinguished it from ovomucoid and reported that the inhibitor was much more effective than ovomucoid in inhibiting trypsin. Rhodes *et al.* prepared the trypsin inhibitor-containing fraction (ovomucoid-rich) using salt fractionation, and trichloroacetic acid and acetone, and then separated ovoinhibitor by subjecting the crude ovomucoid preparation to gel filtration and ion exchange chromatography.[26] Davies *et al.* also separated ovoinhibitor using several steps of ammonium sulfate precipitation along with gel filtration and DEAE-cellulose ion exchange chromatography, but neither purity nor yield data were reported.[72] However, no recent research on the separation of ovoinhibitor from egg white is available.

Avidin is a minor egg white protein with a strong biotin-binding ability.[73] Although the biological function of avidin is not fully known, it is believed to serve as a defensive protein against biotin-requiring microorganisms.[74] Fraenkel-Conrat *et al.* first separated avidin with high activity by adsorbing avidin on bentonite, followed by selective elution with phosphate buffer, and then fractionation with $(NH_4)_2SO_4$.[75] Dhyse was the first to separate avidin in a large amount using a successive differential precipitation method.[76] However, the activity of the separated avidin was only about 20% of that of pure avidin, and the yield was also very low (23%). Later, several separation methods were developed using ion exchange chromatography or affinity chromatography. Melamed and Green used CM-cellulose resin to separate crude avidin from egg white first, and then ion exchange HPLC and other protein purification strategies after that.[77] The affinity chromatography of Cuatrecasas and Wilchek used a biotin–Sepharose column,[78] and that of the Heney and Orr used 2-iminobiotin-6-aminohexyl–Sepharose 4B.[79] Both methods used avidin–biotin complex formation, and the avidin separated showed over 95% yield and 99% purity. However, the affinity chromatography materials are very expensive and their lifetimes are somewhat limited. Lately, Fan *et al.* developed a new separation method for avidin using water-dispersible ferric oxide nanoparticles.[80] This method was much easier to apply on a larger scale than the affinity chromatography and the obtained avidin had >90% purity. Piskarev *et al.* (1990) used ion exchange HPLC after rough avidin isolation using successive differential $(NH_4)_2SO_4$ and organic solvent precipitations.[81] However, the amount of avidin recovered in a single run was low. Preparative electrophoresis was also developed to purify avidin through a sequential two-step protocol.[82] The avidin recovery was around 65%, and 0.1% lysozyme was detected in the final avidin fraction. Avidin fusion proteins have also been developed to expand the existing avidin–biotin technology.[83,84] Durance and Nakai used a single column cation exchange method, which allowed the simultaneous recovery of lysozyme and avidin from undiluted egg white.[85] They fed undiluted liquid egg white through the cation exchange column, involving the accumulation of avidin and lysozyme through several cycles of egg white application and lysozyme elution. After 16 cycles of egg white application and lysozyme elution, they recovered avidin with 75% yield and 40% purity. To increase the purity of avidin, they subsequently applied the crude avidin on a CM-cellulose cation exchange column and separated avidin with 85% purity. This is one of the best and most practical methods to separate lysozyme and avidin together; it is scalable and can be employed in an actual egg-breaking plant.

Cystatin was first separated using a three-step purification method.[86] This method used precipitation of ovomucin, followed by separation of cystatin using affinity chromatography on carboxymethylated papain–Sepharose, and then chromatofocusing. CM sepharose[87] and papain–Sepharose in combination with gel filtration[88] were also used to separate cystatin. However, owing to the low level of separation efficiency for most of the published methods, more simple and economical methods should be developed in the future. A summary of methods used for the separation of egg white proteins is shown in Figure 17.1.

17.3 Functional Characteristics and the Potential Uses of Egg White Proteins

Not only the separated egg proteins but also their hydrolysis products have many functional properties. Over the past few years, various functional peptides that have beneficial health effects have been developed from plant as well as animal proteins. Some researchers used whole egg white itself as a

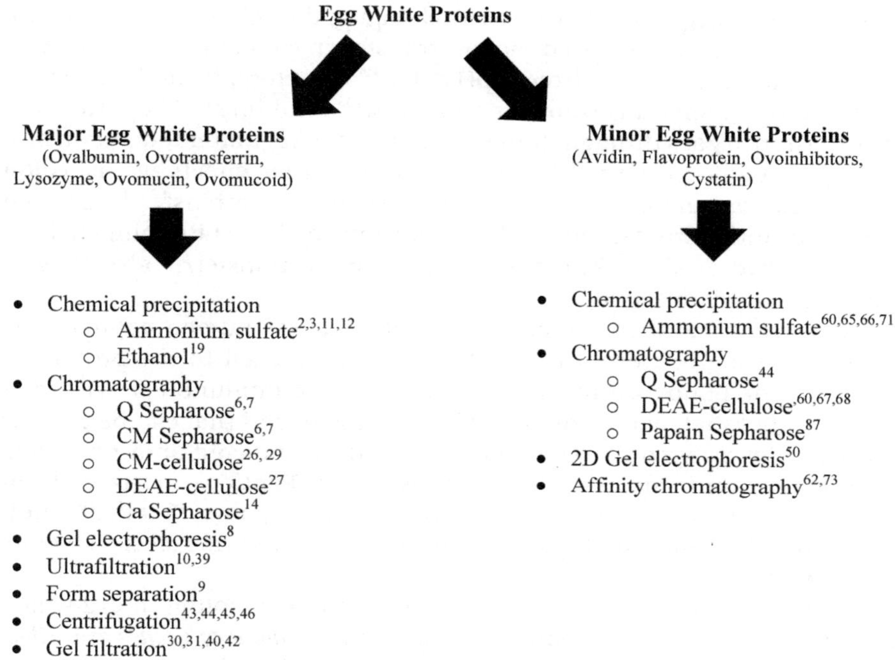

Figure 17.1 Summary of separation techniques used to separate egg white proteins.

substrate for enzymatic hydrolysis and produced bioactive peptides.[89–91] However, separated proteins can also be hydrolyzed easily to produce functional peptides using various enzymes, such as pepsin, papain, trypsin, and α-chymotrypsin, under different conditions.

Human blood albumin is reported as an excellent drug carrier, indicating that ovalbumin also has the potential to be used as a drug carrier.[92] Ovalbumin was reported to have tumor necrosis-releasing factors, which can be applied in tumor suppression.[93] The hydrolysates of ovalbumin were reported to have potent antioxidant, metal-chelating, and ACE-inhibitory activities.[91,94]

Ovotransferrin has strong antimicrobial activity in foods.[95,96] Babini and Livermore showed that ovotransferrin increased the activity of piperacillin/tazobactam against *Escherichia coli* through the iron-chelating activity of the protein.[97] In addition, ovotransferrin was reported to suppress *Pseudomonas* sp., *E. coli* and *Streptococcus mutans*.[98] Recently, ovotransferrin was used to control *E. coli* O157 : H7 and *Listeria monocytogenes*, the major foodborne pathogens.[96,99] Another study showed that peptides derived from ovotransferrin (OTAP-92) could suppress bacteria by damaging their cell membrane.[100] Zhang *et al.* also reported that peptides produced from ovotransferrin could control selected microorganisms.[101] So, both ovotransferrin and its peptides can be used as antimicrobial agents in foods. Wu and Acer-Lopez (2012) reported that ovotransferrin has an antioxidant effect on poultry meat by changing the cellular redox environment.[102] Ko and Ahn reported that ovotransferrin could bind with iron and easily released the bound iron at pH < 4.5.[19] Therefore, it can be an excellent iron supplementing source for humans.[103] Ibrahim *et al.* reported that ovotransferrin goes through thiol-linked auto-cleavage after reduction, producing partially hydrolyzed products with very strong effects against colon and breast cancer cells.[104] Peptides derived from ovotransferrin showed very good antimicrobial activity,[100] but ovotransferrin lost its ability to bind iron after hydrolysis.[102] Peptides derived from ovotransferrin also showed potent antioxidant activity.

Ovomucoid has strong allergenic effects in some human populations. However, it is not clear if the carbohydrates attached to the protein or the disulfide bonds within the protein cause the immunoreactivity.[105] It was reported that ovomucoid has a biospecific ligand that can be used as a drug delivery agent.[106] The hydrolysates of ovomucoid showed strong antioxidant and metal-chelating activities.[58] Peptides derived from ovomucoid showed immune-modulating activity against T-cells,[106] indicating that they have high potential to be used as pharmaceutical agents for humans.

Lysozyme is one of the major bacteriolytic proteins found in egg white. Lysozyme can control foodborne pathogens like *L. monocytogenes* and *Clostridium botulinum*,[107] which are two major pathogens in the food industry. It also effectively controls toxin formation from *C. botulinum* in fish, poultry, and some vegetables. It is reported that some modifications of lysozyme, using chemical and thermal treatments, increased its antimicrobial properties. Lysozyme not only inhibits microbial growth but also has antiviral, anti-inflammatory, and therapeutic effects.[106] Recently, lysozyme was used as a nitrate replacement in Italian-type sausages, which could reduce the use of nitrate in curing salts by 50%.[108] The World Health Organization (WHO) and many countries allow the use of lysozyme in food as a preservative, and it is currently used in kimchi pickles, sushi, Chinese noodles, cheese, and wine production.[109]

Ovomucin shows strong inhibitory activities against *E. coli*, *Bacillus* sp., *Pseudomonas* sp., and other food poisoning bacteria.[46] It has excellent emulsifying and foaming characteristics.[1] Foaming and emulsifying characteristics are important for the texture of bakery products. Therefore, adding ovomucin to bakery products can enhance not only the nutritional level but also the texture of the product. Recently, the peptides produced from ovomucin under high pH and heat treatment were shown to have strong antioxidant activities so can be used as potential natural antioxidants in the food industry.[110,111] Therefore, not only the proteins in egg white but also their peptides can be used in the food industry as agents to reduce oxidation of lipids in foods. Ovomucin is reported to have anti-tumor activity and antiviral effects.[46,112] Therefore, ovomucin can be used to control tumor growth. Ovomucin is also known to enhance the surface migration of primordial germ cells, which helped the expression of primordial germ cells (PGC) from E3 to E7 in male embryo cells.[113] Peptides derived from ovomucin showed macrophage-stimulating activities *in vitro*, indicating that they are good candidates for pharmaceutical use in humans.[106]

Ovomacroglobulin, also called ovostatin, is a 650 kDa egg white protein consisting of four 180 kDa subunits with proteinase inhibitory activity.[114,115] Ovomacroglobulin is part of the α2M family, but its proteinase specificity is different from that of the other α2M proteins and it is not recognized by the mammalian α2M receptor.[116] Ovomacroglobulin has been demonstrated to possess broad-spectrum inhibitory activity against various types of proteases as well as some other important biological activities. Unlike ovomucoid and ovoinhibitor, ovomacroglobulin inhibits proteinases of all four mechanistic classes. Besides, it has many kinds of biological activities, such as antibacterial, inhibiting sepsis, accelerating wound healing, and anti-inflammatory.[70,117–119] Therefore, egg white ovomacroglobulin has the potential to be used as a pharmaceutical agent. Geng *et al.* reported that ovomacroglobulin promoted fibroblast migration by altering the gene expression of β-integrin, E-cadherin, and cytoskeletal proteins, reducing intercellular aggregation and strengthening the cytoskeleton.[120] The findings are useful for understanding the role of ovomacroglobulin in wound healing and the pathological processes of cancer, but the detailed mechanisms of ovomacroglobulin in these processes are not clear yet.

Ovoinhibitor is a serine proteinase (Kaze-type) that inhibits the activity of trypsin, chymotrypsin, pronase, subtilisin, elastase, and *Aspergillus oryzae* alkaline proteinase, but does not inhibit papain and pepsin.[121,122] It has a molecular weight of 49 kDa and is comprised of seven domains, six of which are the a-type, and the seventh, which occupies the C-terminus, is a b-type. One molecule of ovoinhibitor can inhibit two molecules of trypsin and two of chymotrypsin, but the two trypsin-binding sites are not equivalent.[123] The advantage of having many domains that inhibit proteinases is that the protein provides greater protection against microorganisms because a wider range of proteinases can be inhibited.[124] Therefore, if ovoinhibitor can be separated in large quantities, it has high potential to be used as an antimicrobial agent. Begum *et al.* reported that conjugating ovoinhibitor with galactomannan improved its heat stability and emulsifying capacity while maintaining its enzyme inhibitory capability.[125] Thus, the ovoinhibitor–galactomannan conjugate could play an important role in protecting foods from microorganisms.

G2 and G3 globulins are among the least investigated egg white proteins from the biochemical standpoint. They are similar in their molecular weight but differ in their mobility in non-denaturing gels, their pI, and their sensitivities to chymotrypsin and V8 proteinase.[126] It is known that globulins play an important role in the foaming properties of egg white: Johnson and Zabik reported that solutions containing G2 and G3 globulins produced a large angel cake with excellent texture.[127] However, their exact biological functions are not known well.[1]

17.4 Summary and Future Research on Egg White Proteins

Poultry eggs contain numerous functional proteins, but the practical use of these proteins in the industry is highly limited. Separation of egg white proteins was done for many years, but still simple, economical, and sequential methods with better yield and purity are needed to the industry if the separated proteins are going to be used in food and pharmaceutical industries to increase their values. However, the separation protocol should not use toxic chemicals. Among egg white proteins, lysozyme is currently used as an antimicrobial agent in the food industry, and other proteins have strong potential, such as ovalbumin as a drug carrier, ovotransferrin as an antimicrobial agent or iron carrier, and ovomucin and ovomucoid as antimicrobial and immunomodulating agents. However, potential uses have not been identified for the rest of the proteins. On the other hand, peptides derived from these proteins have shown cytotoxic, anticancer, immunomodulating, ACE-inhibitory, antimicrobial, and antioxidant activities, and have high potential to be used in the pharmaceutical, nutraceutical, and food industries. The industrial applications of egg white proteins, as well as their enzyme hydrolysates, are in their infancy, even though some research on the use of egg proteins has been published in recent years. Thus, more research may need to be done to commercialize the use of these peptides. The future directions for research on egg white proteins include developing simple, economical and scalable methods that can separate multiple egg components, production of functional peptides from the separated components, physicochemical characterization of the peptides with specific functions, and testing the functional efficacy of egg white proteins as well as their peptides using animals and humans and in food systems. Addition of value and diversification of the use of egg products will increase the use of egg and significantly improve the sustainability of the poultry egg industry around the world.

References

1. W. J. Stadelman and O. J. Cotterill, *Egg Science and Technology*, 4th edn, 2001.
2. F. G. Hopkins, *J. Physiol.*, 1900, **25**, 306–330.
3. H. Chick and C. J. Martin, *Biochem. J.*, 1913, **7**, 380–398.
4. R. B. Rhodes, P. R. Azari and R. E. Feeney, *J. Biol. Chem.*, 1958, **230**, 399–408.
5. S. Mandeles, *J. Chromatogr.*, 1960, **3**, 256–264.
6. T. Croguennec, F. Nau, S. Pezennec, M. Piot and G. Brulé, *Eur. Food Res. Technol.*, 2001, **212**, 296–301.
7. Y. Sakakibara and H. Yanagisawa, *Bull. Aichi Univ. Educ.*, 2007, **56**, 45–49.

8. C. Desert, C. G. Dubiard, F. Nau, G. Jan, F. Val and J. Mallard, *J. Agric. Food Chem.*, 2001, **49**, 4553–4561.
9. T. M. Ward, R. A. Edwards and R. D. Tanner, *Appl. Biochem. Biotechnol.*, 2007, **136**, 927–934.
10. D. Datta, S. Bhattacharjee, A. Nath, R. Das, C. Bhattacharjee and S. Datta, *Sep. Purif. Technol.*, 2009, **66**, 353–361.
11. E. D. N. S. Abeyrathne, H. Y. Lee and D. U. Ahn, *Poultry Sci.*, 2014, **94**, 1001–1009.
12. H. Fraenkel-Conrat and R. Feeney, *Arch. Biotechnol.*, 1950, **29**, 101–113.
13. S. A. Al-Mashikhi and N. Nakai, *Agric. Biol. Chem.*, 1987, **51**, 2881–2887.
14. M. C. M. Chung, S. L. Chan and S. Shimizu, *Int. J. Biochem.*, 1991, **23**, 609–616.
15. A. C. Awade, S. Moreau, D. Mollé, G. Brulé and J. L. Maubois, *J. Chromatogr. A*, 1994, **677**, 279–288.
16. M. C. Vachier, M. Piot and A. C. Awade, *J. Chromatogr.*, 1995, **664**, 201–210.
17. A. C. Awade and T. Efstathiou, *J. Chromatogr. B*, 1999, **723**, 69–74.
18. A. Tankrathok, S. Daduang, R. Patramanon, T. Arakai and S. Thammasirirak, *Prep. Biochem. Biotechnol.*, 2009, **39**, 380–399.
19. K. Y. Ko and D. U. Ahn, *Poultry Sci.*, 2008, **87**, 1441–1450.
20. E. D. N. S. Abeyrathne, H. Y. Lee and D. U. Ahn, *Poultry Sci.*, 2014, **94**, 1010–1017.
21. H. Lineweaver and C. W. Murray, *J. Biol. Chem.*, 1947, **171**, 565–581.
22. E. Fredericq and H. F. Deutsch, *J. Biol. Chem.*, 1949, **181**, 499–510.
23. R. H. Forsythe and J. F. Foster, *J. Biol. Chem.*, 1950, **184**, 385–392.
24. S. Tanabe, S. Tesaki and M. Watanabe, *Biosci., Biotechnol., Biochem.*, 2000, **64**, 2005–2007.
25. A. N. Yousif and J. W. Kan, *Anal. Biochem.*, 2002, **311**, 93–97.
26. M. B. Rhodes, N. Bennett and R. E. Feeney, *J. Biol. Chem.*, 1960, **235**, 1686–1693.
27. J. G. Davies, C. J. Mapes and J. W. Donovan, *Biochemistry*, 1971, **10**, 39–42.
28. N. C. Price and J. Nairn, *Exploring Proteins: A student guide to experimental skills and methods*, Oxford Univ. Press, 2009.
29. R. H. Strang, *Biochem. Educ.*, 1984, **12**, 57–59.
30. I. Safarik, Z. Sabatkova, T. Oldrich and M. Safarikov, *Food Technol. Biotechnol.*, 2007, **45**, 355–359.
31. H. C. Chiu, C. W. Lin and S. Y. Suen, *J. Membr. Sci.*, 2007, **290**, 259–266.
32. G. L. Weaver, M. Kroger and F. Katz, *J. Food Sci.*, 1977, **42**, 1084–1087.
33. R. A. A. Muzzarelli, G. Barontini and R. Rochetti, *Biotechnol. Bioeng.*, 1978, **20**, 87–94.
34. H. Yamada, T. Fukumura, Y. Ito and T. Imoto, *Anal. Biochem.*, 1985, **146**, 71–74.

35. M. del Pilar Ferraris, U. A. Gonzalez, C. F. Aguilar and J. A. Rodriguez, *J. Chromatogr. B*, 2016, **2016**, 129–133.
36. R. Islam, J. Kite, A. S. Baker, J. A. Ching and M. R. Islam, *Afr. J. Biotechnol.*, 2006, **5**, 1902–1908.
37. R. Ghosh, S. S. Silva and J. Cui, *Biochem. Eng. J.*, 2000, **6**, 19–24.
38. Y. Wan, J. Lu and Z. Cui, *Purif. Technol.*, 2006, **48**, 133–142.
39. H. M. Chang, C. C. Yang and Y. C. Chang, *J. Agric. Food Chem.*, 2000, **48**, 161–164.
40. J. Hiidenhovi, J. Makinen, R. Hupaathti and E. L. Ryhanen, *J. Agric. Food Chem.*, 2002, **50**, 2840–2845.
41. D. A. Omana and J. Wu, *Poultry Sci.*, 2009, **88**, 2224–2234.
42. J. Hiidenhovi, H. S. Aro and V. Kankare, *J. Agric. Food Chem.*, 1999, **47**, 1004–1008.
43. D. S. Robinson and J. B. Monsey, *Biochem. J.*, 1975, **147**, 55–62.
44. C. Guérin-Dubiard, M. Pasco, A. Hietanen, A. Quiros del Bosque, F. Nau and T. Croguennec, *J. Chromatogr. A*, 2005, **1090**, 58–67.
45. D. A. Omana and J. Wu, *J. Agric. Food Chem.*, 2009, **57**, 3596–3603.
46. D. A. Omana, J. Wang and J. Wu, *J. Chromatogr. B*, 2010, **878**, 1771–1776.
47. J. Wang and J. Wu, *Process Biochem.*, 2012, **47**, 94–98.
48. R. W. Sleigh, G. J. H. Melrose and M. B. Smith, *Biochim. Biophys. Acta*, 1973, **310**, 453–460.
49. D. S. Robinson and J. B. Monsey, *Biochem. J.*, 1971, **121**, 537–547.
50. R. Huopalahti, R. L. Fandino, M. Anton and R. Schade, *Bioactive Egg Compounds*, Springer, NY, 2007, pp. 3–66.
51. C. Rabouille, M. A. Aon, G. Muller, J. Cartaud and D. Thomas, *Biochem. J.*, 1990, **266**, 697–706.
52. Y. Shibusawa, S. Kihira and Y. Ito, *J. Chromatogr. B: Biomed. Sci. Appl.*, 1998, **709**, 301–305.
53. Y. Shibusawa, S. Lino, H. Shindo and Y. Ito, *J. Liq. Chromatogr. Relat. Technol.*, 2001, **24**, 2007–2016.
54. F. Geng, Q. Huang, X. Wu, G. Ren, Y. Shan, G. Jin and M. Ma, *Sep. Purif. Technol.*, 2012, **96**, 75–80.
55. J. Brand, E. Dachmann, M. Pichler, S. Lotz and U. Kulozik, *Sep. Purif. Technol.*, 2016, **161**, 44–52.
56. E. D. N. S. Abeyrathne, H. Y. Lee and D. U. Ahn, *Korean J. Food Sci. Anim. Resour.*, 2013, **33**, 501–507.
57. E. D. N. S. Abeyrathne, H. Y. Lee, J. S. Ham and D. U. Ahn, *Poultry Sci.*, 2013, **92**, 1091–1097.
58. E. D. N. S. Abeyrathne, H. Y. Lee, C. Jo, J. W. Suh and D. U. Ahn, *Poultry Sci.*, 2015, **94**, 2280–2287.
59. J. Brand, M. Pichler and U. Kulozik, *J. Food Eng.*, 2014, **132**, 48–54.
60. R. E. Feeney, F. C. Stevens and D. T. Osuga, *J. Biol. Chem.*, 1963, **238**, 1415–1418.
61. Q. Qu, X. Juan, X. Wu, F. Shi and L. L. Wang, *Chin. Chem. Lett.*, 2012, **23**, 1389–1392.
62. E. Li-Chan and S. Nakai, *CRC Crit. Rev. Poult. Biol.*, 1989, **2**, 21–58.

63. J. A. Froehlich Jr, A. H. Merrill, C. O. Clagett and D. B. McCormick, *Biochem. Physiol.*, 1980, **66B**, 397–401.
64. P. F. Rao, S. T. Liu, Z. Wei, J. C. Li, R. M. Chen, G. R. Chen and Y. Q. Zheng, *J. Food Biochem.*, 1997, **20**, 473–479.
65. H. T. Miller and R. E. Feeney, *Biochemistry*, 1966, **5**, 952–957.
66. J. W. Donovan and T. M. White, *Biochemistry*, 1971, **10**, 32–38.
67. T. Kitamoto, M. Nakashima and A. Ikai, *J. Biochem.*, 1982, **92**, 1679–1682.
68. H. Nagase, E. D. Harris Jr, J. F. Woessner and K. Brew, *J. Biol. Chem.*, 1983, **258**, 7481–7489.
69. F. Geng, X. Huang, M. Ma, L. Jia and X. W. Zhang, *Asian J. Chem.*, 2013, **25**, 2683–2686.
70. F. Geng, X. Huang, N. Yan, L. Jia and M. Ma, *J. Sep. Sci.*, 2013, **36**, 3717–3722.
71. K. Matsushima, *Science*, 1958, **127**, 1178–1179.
72. J. G. Davies, J. Zahnely and J. W. Donovan, *Biochemistry*, 1969, **8**, 2044–2053.
73. F. Garret-Flaudy and R. Freitag, *Biotechnol. Bioeng.*, 2000, **71**, 223–234.
74. J. Korpela, M. Kulomaa, P. Tuohimaa and A. Vaheri, *EMBO J.*, 1983, **2**, 1715–1719.
75. H. Fraenkel-Conrat, N. S. Snell and E. D. Ducay, *Arch. Biochem. Biophys.*, 1952, **39**, 80–96.
76. F. G. Dhyse, *Proc. Soc. Exp. Biol. Med.*, 1954, **85**, 515–517.
77. M. D. Melamed and N. M. Green, *Biochem. J.*, 1963, **89**, 591–599.
78. P. Cuatrecasas and M. Wilchek, *Biochem. Biophys. Res. Commun.*, 1968, **33**, 235–239.
79. G. Heney and G. A. Orr, *Anal. Biochem.*, 1981, **114**, 92–96.
80. J. Fan, J. Lu, R. Xu, R. Jiang and Y. Gao, *J. Colloid Interface Sci.*, 2003, **266**, 215–218.
81. V. E. Piskarev, A. M. Shuster, A. G. Gabibov and A. G. Rabinkov, *Biochem. J.*, 1990, **265**, 301–304.
82. D. Rothemund, T. Thomas and D. B. Rylatt, *Protein Expression Purif.*, 2002, **26**, 149–152.
83. K. J. Airenne and M. S. Kulomaa, *Gene*, 1995, **167**, 63–68.
84. K. J. Airenne, V. S. Marjomäki and M. S. Kulomaa, *Biol. Eng.*, 1999, **16**, 87–92.
85. T. D. Durance and S. Nakai, *J. Food Sci.*, 1988, **53**, 1096–1101.
86. A. Anastasi, M. A. Brown, A. A. Kembhavi, M. J. Nicklin, C. A. Sayers, D. C. Sunter and A. J. Barrett, *Biochem. J.*, 1983, **211**, 129–138.
87. B. Gerhartz, R. A. Engh, R. Mentele, C. Eckerskorn, R. Torquato, J. Wittmann, H. J. Kolb, W. Machileidt, H. Fritz and E. A. Auersward, *FEBS Lett.*, 1997, **412**, 551–558.
88. T. Trziszka, Y. Saleh, W. Kopeae, M. Siewinski and E. Wesierska, *Int. J. Poult. Sci.*, 2004, **3**, 471–477.
89. W. Chiang, M. Lee, W. Guo and T. Tsai, *J. Food Drug Anal.*, 2006, **14**, 385–390.

90. M. Miguel and A. Aleixandre, *J. Nutr.*, 2006, **136**, 1457–1460.
91. M. Miguel, M. J. Alonso, M. Salaices, A. Aleixandre and R. Loez-Fandino, *Food Chem.*, 2007, **104**, 163–168.
92. F. Kratz, *J. Controlled Release*, 2008, **132**, 171–183.
93. J. K. N. Nolan, J. W. Zhang, S. Hayakawa and Y. Mine, *J. Agric. Food Chem.*, 2000, **48**, 6261–6266.
94. E. D. N. S. Abeyrathne, H. Y. Lee, C. Jo, K. C. Nam and D. U. Ahn, *Poultry Sci.*, 2014, **93**, 2678–2686.
95. F. Giansanti, L. Leboffe, G. Pitari, R. Ippoliti and G. Antonini, *Biochim. Biophys. Acta*, 2012, **1820**, 218–225.
96. F. Giansanti, L. Leboffe, F. Angelucci and G. Antonini, *Nutrients*, 2000, **7**, 9105–9115.
97. G. S. Babini and M. L. David, *J. Antimicrob. Chemother.*, 2000, **45**, 105–109.
98. P. Valenti, G. Antonini, M. R. R. Fanelli, N. Orsi and E. Antonini, *Antimicrob. Agents Chemother.*, 1982, 840–841.
99. K. Y. Ko, A. F. Mendonca and D. U. Ahn, *Poultry Sci.*, 2009, **87**, 1649–1658.
100. H. R. Ibrahim, Y. Sugmito and T. Akoi, *Biochim. Biophys.*, 2000, **1553**, 196–205.
101. T. Zhang, J. Zheng, H. Ye, Y. Yu, P. Zhao and J. Liu, *Chem. Res. Chin. Univ.*, 2011, **27**, 361–365.
102. J. Wu and A. Acer-Lopez, *Food Res. Int.*, 2012, **46**, 480–487.
103. F. B. Abdallah and J. M. Chaine, *Eur. J. Biochem.*, 1999, **263**, 912–920.
104. H. R. Ibrahim and T. Kiyono, *J. Agric. Food Chem.*, 2009, **57**, 11383–11390.
105. T. Gu, J. Matsuda, K. Tsuruta and R. Nakamura, *J. Food Sci.*, 1985, **50**, 592–594.
106. J. K. N. Nolan, M. Phillips and Y. Mine, *J. Agric. Food Chem.*, 2005, **53**, 8421–8431.
107. R. C. Radziejewska, G. Leśnierowski and J. Kijowski, *Pol. J. Food Nutr. Sci.*, 2008, **58**, 05–10.
108. I. A. H. M. E. Herath, J. M. P. Jayasinghe, D. U. Ahn and E. D. N. S. Abeyrathne, *Funct. Foods Health Dis.*, 2015, **5**, 320–330.
109. Y. Mine, F. Ma and S. Lauriau, *J. Agric. Food Chem.*, 2004, **52**, 1088–1094.
110. E. D. N. S. Abeyrathne, H. Y. Lee and D. U. Ahn, *Poultry Sci.*, 2013, **92**, 3292–3299.
111. E. D. N. S. Abeyrathne, H. Y. Lee, C. Jo, J. W. Suh and D. U. Ahn, *Food Chem.*, 2016, **192**, 107–113.
112. T. Oguro, K. Watanabe, H. Tani, H. Ohishi and T. Ebina, *Food Sci. Technol. Res.*, 2000, **5**, 179–185.
113. W. Halfter, B. Schurer, H. M. Hasselhorn, B. Christ, E. Gimpel and H. H. Epperlein, *Development*, 1996, **122**, 915–923.
114. J. W. Donovan and T. M. White, *Biochemistry*, 1971, **10**, 32–38.
115. A. Molla, T. Oda and H. Maeda, *J. Biochem.*, 1987, **101**, 199–205.

116. K. L. Nielsen, L. Scottup-Jensen, H. Nagasse, H. C. Thogersen and M. Etzerodt, *J. DNA Sequence*, 1994, **5**, 111–119.
117. A. Ikai, M. Nakashima and Y. Aoki, *Biochem. Biophys. Res. Commun.*, 1989, **158**, 831–836.
118. Y. Ofuji, T. Suzuki, H. Yoshi, K. Hara and M. Adachi, *Eur. PMC*, 1992, **14**, 13–22.
119. K. Maruo, T. Akaike, T. Ono and H. Maeda, *Infect. Immunol.*, 1988, **66**, 866–869.
120. F. Geng, X. Huang and M. Ma, *J. Sci. Food Agric.*, 2015, **96**, 3188–3194.
121. W. H. Liu, G. E. Means and R. E. Feeney, *Biochim. Biophys. Acta*, 1971, **229**, 176–185.
122. D. V. Vadehra, K. R. Nath and R. Forsythe, *Crit. Rev. Food Sci. Nutr.*, 1973, **4**, 193–309.
123. J. C. Zahnley, *J. Biol. Chem.*, 1974, **249**, 4282–4285.
124. L. Stevens, *Comp. Biochem. Biophysiol. Part B Comp. Biochem.*, 1991, **100**, 1–9.
125. S. Begum, A. Saito, X. Xu and A. Kato, *Biosci., Biotechnol., Biochem.*, 2003, **67**, 1897–1902.
126. L. Stevens and D. Duncan, *Br. Poult. Sci.*, 1988, **29**, 665–669.
127. T. M. Johnson and M. E. Zabik, *J. Food Sci.*, 1981, **46**, 1231–1236.
128. C. Davis and R. Reeves, RIRDC Publication, 2002, No. 02/094.
129. T. Croguennec, A. Renault, S. Beaufils, J. J. Dubois and S. Pezennec, *J. Colloid Interface Sci.*, 2007, **315**, 627–636.
130. J. Gautron, F. Nau, K. Mann, C. Guérin-Dubiard, S. Rehault, M. T. Hincke and Y. Nys, *Worlds Poult. Sci. J.*, 2007, **63**, 82–90.

CHAPTER 18

Advances in the Separation of Functional Egg Proteins – Egg Yolk Proteins

X. HUANG[a], E. D. N. S. ABEYRATHNE[b] AND D. U. AHN*[c]

[a]Huazhong Agricultural University, College of Food Science & Technology, Egg Processing Technology Local Joint National Engineering Research Center, National R&D Center for Egg Processing, No. 1 Shizishan Street, Wuhan, Hubei 430070, China; [b]Uva Wellassa University, Department of Animal Science, Badulla 90000, Sri Lanka; [c]Iowa State University, Department of Animal Science, Ames, IA 50010, USA
*E-mail: duahn@iastate.edu

18.1 Introduction

Egg yolk protein is mainly composed of lipovitellins (36%, α- and β-forms), livetins (38%, α-, β-, and γ-forms), low-density lipoproteins (LDL, 17%), and phosvitin (8.8%). Among these egg yolk proteins, γ-livetin (γ-globulin or immunoglobulin Y) and phosvitin are the most important value-added proteins, and also the most extensively studied. Immunoglobulin Y (IgY) is the major antibody in egg and antibodies to specific antigens can be produced by immunizing chickens with the antigens. Therefore, IgY can be used as an antimicrobial agent to cure various animal and human diseases.[1] Phosvitin is one of the most unique proteins in nature: one molecule of phosvitin, which

Food Chemistry, Function and Analysis No.14
Eggs as Functional Foods and Nutraceuticals for Human Health
Edited by Jianping Wu

Published by the Royal Society of Chemistry, www.rsc.org

Table 18.1 Protein and lipid composition of egg yolk.[a, 80–82]

Proteins (16.6%)	Lipids (31%)
Lipovitellins (α- and β-): 36%	Neutral lipids: 66%
- α-Lipovitellins: 13%	Phospholipids: 30%
- β-Lipovitelins: 23%	- PC: 78%
Livetins: 38%	- PE: 17%
- α-Livetin (serum albumin): 7.0%	- Sphingomyelin: 2.5%
- β-Livetin (glycoprotein): 20.2%	- Phosphatidylinositol: 0.5%
- γ-Livetin (γ-globulin): 10.8%	Cholesterol: 4%
Phosvitin: 8–11%	Carotenoids (carotenes)
Low-density lipoproteins: 17%	Xanthophylls (lutein, zeaxanthin)

[a]Percent of liquid yolk.

is composed of 217 amino acids, contains 123 serine residues, most of which are phosphorylated.[2] Therefore, phosvitin has very strong metal-chelating capacities, which makes it an excellent candidate for a natural antioxidant or antibacterial agent. Phosvitin is known to be involved in bone calcification, and thus can be used as a calcium/iron supplementing agent for animals and humans.[3,4] The rest of the major egg yolk proteins include lipovitellins and livetins (α- and β-form) and LDL, but not much is known of their separation methods, functions, and utilization (Table 18.1).

This chapter will cover the advances in separation methods for the selected proteins from egg yolk, and discuss their potential for food and non-food applications.

18.2 Separation of Functional Proteins from Egg Yolk

Immunoglobulin Y (IgY, also called γ-livetin) and phosvitin are the two most important value-added proteins in egg yolk. IgY is one of the major egg yolk proteins derived from chicken serum IgG.[5] There are many advantages of using laying hens (egg) to produce immunoglobulins: The amount of IgY in chicken egg yolk is approximately 5–7 mg mL^{-1}, of which 1–10% is expected to be antigen-specific. More than 20 eggs can be produced from one laying hen per month, which is equivalent to 300 mL of serum (1.5–2.1 g of IgY).[6] Therefore, the productivity of one chicken is equal to that of a large mammal (*e.g.*, sheep or goat), indicating that the production of immunoglobulin using chickens is much more economical than using mammals.[7–9] In addition, egg yolk antibodies (IgY) have better immune responsiveness to mammalian antigens than those from mammals because of the long phylogenic distance between chickens and mammals. Furthermore, chicken antibodies do not react with either rheumatoid factor (RF) or human anti-mouse IgG antibody (HAMA).[10–15] Thus, interference from these factors can be eliminated. Chicken antibodies do not activate or recognize the mammalian (human) complements,[12] and thus prevent false positive responses.

Furthermore, animal welfare can be improved because invasive blood collection from animals can be avoided. The separation of immunoglobulins from the egg is simpler and easier, and the isolated immunoglobulins are more stable and resistant to pH and temperature abuse than those from the blood. Therefore, chicken has higher potential than mammals for antibody production,[7,8] which opened the door for IgY application to immunotherapy and immunoprophylaxis for several bacterial and viral infections in humans and animals. However, the applications and efficiency of IgY are not yet fully appreciated.[1]

Several published IgY purification methods from egg yolk are available, but most of them are for laboratory scale and are complicated.[16–19] One of the main difficulties in separating IgY from egg yolk is its high lipid content.[20] To remove lipids and improve the extraction and separation efficiencies of IgY from egg yolk, various methods, such as adding xanthan[21] or carrageenan gum,[22] and dilution with acidic water,[23] have been used. Among the approaches, extracting IgY with 10 volumes of acidic water is the most popular because most of the water-insoluble components in egg yolk can be easily precipitated at low ionic strength conditions and with minimal use of chemicals. The extracted IgY is then precipitated using $(NH_4)_2SO_4$ or sodium sulfate.[18,23] Additionally, precipitation of IgY from egg yolk extracts using polyethylene glycol,[17] pectin,[25] dextran sulfate,[15] and ammonium sulfate[24] have also been used. However, many of these approaches have limitations for the commercial production of IgY owing to low yield and purity, and large volume increases from the dilution. Ultrafiltration has been used to reduce the volume of the IgY extract,[25,26] but the efficacy of ultrafiltration can be significantly affected by the amount of lipids in the extract. To improve the purity of IgY separated, affinity chromatography or ion exchange chromatography are often employed.[19,27]

Over the past 60 years, various methods for separating phosvitin from egg yolk have been developed, primarily using a three-step process: lipid removal from yolk using organic solvents, such as methanol, ether, chloroform, hexane, and ethanol, extraction of phosvitin from the lipid-free fraction using NaCl solution, and then precipitating the extracted phosvitin using $MgSO_4$ or $(NH_4)_2SO_4$.[28–31] For further purification of extracted phosvitin, anion exchange and affinity chromatography methods have been commonly used.[32–34] However, lipid removal before separating phosvitin uses many non-food-grade solvents, such as chloroform, methanol, or ether, and thus the phosvitin separated cannot be accepted for human use. Moreover, the solvents caused denaturation and modification of phosvitin's structure, which led to low phosvitin recovery and loss of functions.[30] To overcome the drawbacks, new approaches to separate phosvitin from egg yolk have been tested: Zhang *et al.* and Lei *et al.* used polyethylene glycol, heat treatment, and carbonate–bicarbonate buffer to separate phosvitin.[33,34] However, those methods used anion exchange chromatography or dialysis for further purification, which has limitations for application for industry-scale production. Recently, a simple, efficient, and scalable sequential separation method for IgY and phosvitin from egg yolk without using solvents has been developed.[35] This method opened the door for commercial-scale production of phosvitin and IgY from egg yolk because the method is simple and economical, uses no harmful chemicals, and the yield and purity of the phosvitin separated were high (>95% yield and >90% purity).[36]

There are many other proteins in egg yolk, including lipovitellins (α- and β-form), livetins (α- and β-form), LDL, and yolkin. Lipovitellins (HDLs) are present in two forms (α- and β-form) and are localized in yolk granules. Lipovitellins are complexed with phosvitin through phosphocalcic bridges to form the granular structure.[37] Lipovitellins are made up of 75–80% proteins and 20–25% of lipids, which are composed of 65% phospholipids, 30% triglycerides, and 5% cholesterol.[38] Lipovitellins are usually extracted using salt precipitation: Joubert and Cook first diluted egg yolk with 0.4 M $MgCl_2$ to break the lipovitellins–phosvitin complex, and then diluted the egg yolk further to precipitate phosvitin.[28] The precipitated phosvitin was removed by centrifugation, and the supernatant was further diluted with the same volume of 0.05 M $MgCl_2$ to precipitate the lipovitellin-rich fraction. The precipitant was collected, dissolved in 10% NaCl solution, and ultracentrifuged. After collecting the precipitant, lipovitellins was further purified on a hydroxyapatite column. An ion exchange chromatography method was also used to separate the lipovitellins after extracting them from the yolk.[39]

Low-density lipoproteins are the main constituents of yolk and are mainly located in the plasma fraction, even though a small fraction of LDL is also included in the granules of yolk.[37] LDLs constitute two-thirds of egg yolk lipids because it is composed of 11–17% protein and 83–89% lipids.[40] LDLs are known as the main contributor to the emulsifying properties of egg yolk. Initially, LDL was separated using ultracentrifugation, but the ammonium precipitation method (40% saturation) is preferred because the ultracentrifugation method is extremely time-consuming, requires very expensive equipment, and the yield is very low.[37,41]

Livetins, which include α, β, and γ-forms, represents about 9.3% of hen egg yolk proteins.[42] The livetins in egg yolk were separated by diluting egg yolk with acidified water (10× dilution and final pH 5.0).[43] The residual lipoproteins in the supernatant were further removed by adding gums, dextran, and cellulose.[16,21,44] The water-soluble supernatant that contains livetins was passed through an ultrafiltration cartridge (molecular weight cut-off size of 30 kDa) to concentrate them. Among the livetins, IgY (γ-livetin) is the major component and has been discussed above. α-Livetin is also known as chicken serum albumin with a molecular weight of 70 kDa and an isoelectric point between 4.3 and 5.7.[45] β-Livetin is a 45 kDa glycoprotein, but not much information is available for this protein. The specific separation methods for each of the α- and β-livetins are not well established.

Yolkin is not a protein but polypeptide complexes found in egg yolk with a molecular weight of 1–35 kDa. Polanowski *et al.* first developed a sequential separation method for IgY and yolkin. They diluted egg yolk with nine volumes of distilled water to extract the IgY- and yolkin-containing fraction and removed lipoproteins and lipids by centrifugation.[46] The residual lipoproteins in the supernatant were removed using

0.01% charcoal and pH adjustment (pH 4.0), and then the IgY and yolkin were precipitated using 40% saturated $(NH_4)_2SO_4$. The precipitant was collected and dialyzed in distilled water first, and then 0.1 M phosphate buffer at pH 7.2. After centrifugation, the supernatant was concentrated using ultrafiltration, and the IgY and yolkin were separated using a Sephacryl S-100 gel filtration column. The results indicated that the majority of the separated yolkins were in the molecular range of 16–23 kDa, but some samples had yolkins with MW of 15 and 35 kDa. Recently, Zambrowicz *et al.* developed an alternative simple and rapid separation method for yolkins.[47] In this method, they used the same protocol to extract IgY and yolkins from egg yolk, remove all the impurities from the extract using charcoal, and precipitate IgY and yolkins using ammonium sulfate as before, but used ethanol and acetone (50–70% final concentration), instead of size exclusion chromatography to precipitate IgY after dialysis. They found that 50% ethanol or acetone was the optimal concentration for the separation of yolkins, but 50% ethanol was better than 50% acetone. The yield of yolkins separated using 50% ethanol was higher than that of the previous size exclusion method, and the separated yolkins showed similar cytokine-inducing activity to those obtained using the size exclusion chromatography method. A summary of methods used for the separation of egg yolk proteins is shown in Figure 18.1.

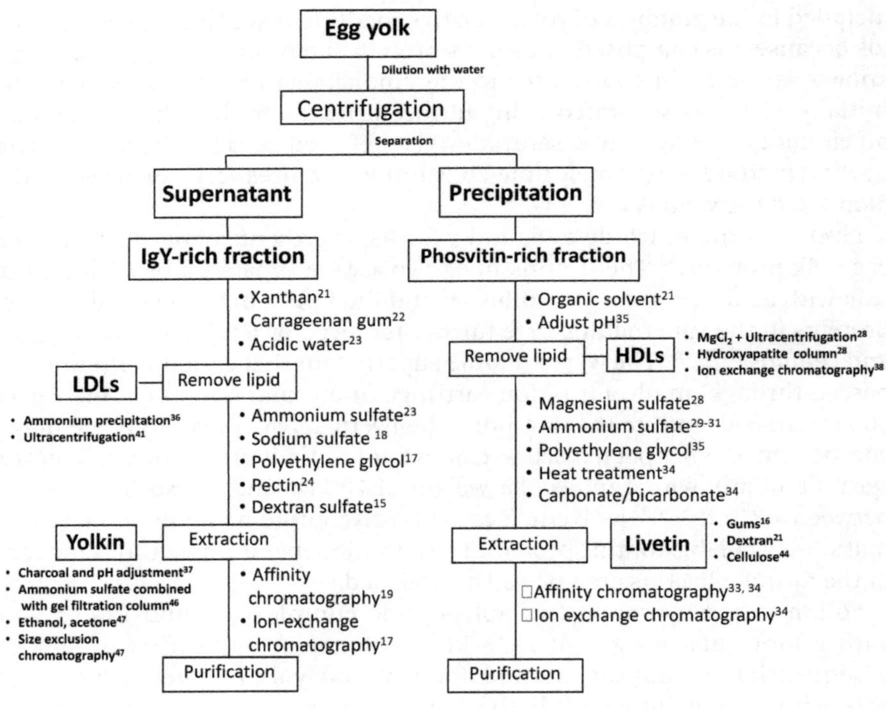

Figure 18.1 Summary of methods used to separate egg yolk proteins.

18.3 Functional Characteristics and Potential Uses of Egg Yolk Proteins

In recent years, as an alternative to antibiotics for growth improvement, IgY has attracted considerable attention.[48,49] Oral administration of IgY over mammalian IgG to treat oral and many other human diseases possesses many advantages, such as convenience, performance, and yield. However, the practical application of IgY is facing various challenges, such as the stability of IgY during processing, storage, and in the digestive tract.[50,51] Purified IgY solutions can be stored in frozen conditions for a few years without much loss of activity.[15,52] IgY is stable at pH 4–11, but loses its activity rapidly at temperature >70 °C, pH <3.5, or pH >12.0.[1,53] This loss of activity is owing to the conformational changes that influence the antigen-binding site in immunoglobulins. IgY is relatively resistant to trypsin and chymotrypsin, but very sensitive to pepsin digestion at low pH (pH < 4.5).[54,55] The IgY in yolk and egg suspensions showed higher antibody activity than that of the purified antibody solutions when incubated with digestive enzymes because of the buffering effect of the other proteins present in the egg yolk and egg suspension. However, the stability of IgY in the gut depends on various other factors, including enzyme levels, transit time, and diet, and encapsulation can improve the retention of biological activity in the gut.[56,57] Addition of stabilizers, such as non-reducing sugars, complex carbohydrates, or sorbitol, can also increase the heat, processing, and acid stability of IgY.[6,58]

Phosvitin is a major protein in egg yolk (9% of yolk protein) and 57% of the amino acid residues in phosvitin are serine (123 out of 217 amino acid residues).[59,60] Almost all the serine residues in phosvitin are phosphorylated, and thus phosvitin has an extremely strong and high metal-binding capacity.[61,62] Phosvitin is believed to carry and provide metal ions during embryo development,[63] but the bioavailability of metals bound to phosvitin molecules when consumed as food is very low.[64,65] Ji *et al.* reported that the water-soluble proteins in egg yolk (presumably phosvitin) stimulated bone formation in osteoblastic MC3T3-E1 cell line by activating the proliferation and differentiation of osteoblastic MC3T3-E1 cells, and by inhibiting bone resorption in osteoclast precursor cells.[66] Li *et al.* reported that phosvitin was involved in the bone formation of the chicken embryo through dephosphorylation.[67] Phosvitin is also reported to enhance mineralization both *in vivo* and *in vitro*, in which the degree of phosphorylation played a critical role.[68–71] Liu *et al.* suggested that phosvitin is involved in chicken bone formation using calcium ion adsorption and phosvitin–Ca-induced mineralization.[72] Lee *et al.* reported that phosvitin showed a potent immune-enhancing activity by stimulating the production of pro-inflammatory mediators.[35] Jung *et al.* reported that phosvitin inhibited the tyrosinase activity and melanin synthesis in melanoma cells.[73] These results indicate that phosvitin has the potential to be used as a melanogenesis inhibitor in the cosmetics industry, which is seeking natural bioactive compounds as hyper-pigmentation inhibitors for human skin. Moon *et al.* reported that phosvitin inhibited the growth of all the cancer cell lines tested in a dose-dependent manner but showed no effects to leucocytes.[74] Among the cancer cell lines tested, MCF-7 and SK-MES-1 were the least sensitive to phosvitin, while HeLa, AGS, and HepG2 were the most sensitive. The protective effects of phosvitin against damage to human leukocytes indicated that phosvitin has high potential as an anti-cancer agent for humans. Phosvitin is reported to increase the production of NO in RAW 264.7 macrophages. Phosvitin also increased the expression of mRNA for iNOS, TNF-α, and IL-1β in the RAW 264.7 macrophages by 46.25, 9.09, and 85.18 times the levels of the control, respectively. These results indicate that phosvitin has the potential to be used as an immune-enhancing agent.[35] Because phosvitin has a strong metal-binding capacity, it can inhibit metal-catalyzed lipid oxidation by inhibiting the hydroxyl radical formation from the Fenton reaction.[4,37,75] Phosvitin exhibits excellent emulsifying and emulsion-stabilizing properties and thus can be used as a preservative for food and an emulsifier/emulsion stabilizer.[76,77]

Fragmenting phosvitin into small peptides using enzymatic hydrolysis can dramatically increase the bioavailability of metals bound to the peptides. However, more details about the phosphopeptides are discussed elsewhere in this book. IgY from egg yolk is accompanied by a polypeptide complex that has immunomodulatory functions and has been called yolkin.[82] Yolkins are derived from vitellogenin and are known to play important roles in the developing embryo because they have cytokine-inducing activity. Yolkins are known to possess significant immunological activities and are potent inducers of TNF-α production and cytokine IL-1β, II-6, and IL-10 release.[46] They are also reported to stimulate nitric oxide release from macrophages, mitigate the behavioral symptoms of aging, and support cognitive learning and memory in rats.[78,79] However, all the research on yolkins is from a single research group, and more research is necessary to confirm the functions of these bioactive compounds in egg yolk.

18.4 Summary and Future Research on Egg Yolk Proteins

Poultry eggs contain numerous functional proteins, the functional properties of which are very well known. However, the practical use of these proteins in industry is highly limited. While the separation of some egg yolk proteins, such as IgY and phosvitin, has been studied for many years, the industrial applications of the separated egg yolk proteins need more research. If the separated proteins are mainly targeted for use in the food and pharmaceutical industries to increase their values, the separation protocol should not use toxic chemicals. In addition to egg yolk proteins, the peptides derived from phosvitin and IgY have cytotoxic, anticancer, immune-modulating, antimicrobial, anti-inflammatory, and antioxidant activities, and have high potential for use in the pharmaceutical, nutraceutical, and food industries. The future research of egg yolk proteins, as well as their enzyme hydrolysates, includes developing simple, economical, and scalable methods that can separate multiple egg components, as well as production of functional peptides from the separated components. The physicochemical characterization of peptides with specific functions and testing the functional efficacy of egg yolk proteins as well as their peptides in animals, humans, and food systems are also needed. The addition of value and the diversification of the use of egg yolk products will significantly improve the sustainability of the egg industry around the world.

References

1. H. Hatta, K. Tsuda, S. Akachi, M. Kim and T. Yamamoto, *Biosci., Biotechnol., Biochem.*, 1993, **57**, 450.
2. D. K. Mecham and H. S. Olcott, *J. Am. Chem. Soc.*, 1949, **71**, 3670.
3. S. M. A. Khan, S. Nakamura, M. Ogawa, E. Akita, H. Azakami and A. Kato, *J. Agric. Food Chem.*, 2000, **48**, 1503.
4. S. Ishikawa, Y. Yano, K. Arihara and M. Itoh, *Biosci., Biotechnol., Biochem.*, 2004, **68**, 1324.
5. J. Kovacs-Nolan and Y. Mine, *Avian Poult. Biol. Rev.*, 2004, **15**, 25.
6. M. Shimizu, H. Nagashima, K. Hashimoto and T. Suzuki, *J. Food Sci.*, 1994, **59**, 763.
7. R. Fayer and M. C. Jenkins, *Poult. Sci.*, 1992, **71**, 1637.
8. L. Svendsen, A. Crowley, L. H. Ostergaard, G. Stodulski and J. Hau, *Eur. PMC*, 1995, **45**, 89.
9. A. Michael, S. Meenatchisundaram, G. Parameswari, R. Subbraj, R. Selvakumaran and S. Ramalingam, *Indian J. Sci. Technol.*, 2010, **3**, 468.
10. R. Schade, E. G. Calzado, R. Sarmiento, P. A. Chacana, J. Porankiewicz-Asplund and H. R. Terzolo, *ATLA, Altern. Lab. Anim.*, 1991, **33**, 1.
11. A. Larsson, A. Karlsson-Parra and J. Sjoquist, *Clin. Chem.*, 1991, **37**, 411.
12. A. Larsson, P. E. Wejaker, P. O. Forsberg and T. Landahl, *J. Immunol. Methods*, 1992, **156**, 70.
13. D. Carlander, J. Stalberg and A. Larssen, *Upsala J. Med. Sci.*, 1999, **104**, 170.
14. M. Karlsson, H. Kollberg and A. Larssen, *World's Poult. Sci. J.*, 2004, **60**, 341.
15. R. Schade, E. G. Calzado, R. Sarmiento, P. A. Chacana, J. Porankiewicz-Asplund and H. R. Terzolo, *ATLA, Altern. Lab. Anim.*, 2005, **33**, 129.
16. J. C. Jensenius, I. Anderson, J. Hau, M. Cronc and C. Koch, *J. Immunol. Methods*, 1981, **46**, 63.
17. A. Polson, T. Coetzer, J. Krugar, E. Von Maltzahn and K. J. Van der Merwe, *Immunol. Invest.*, 1985, **14**, 323.
18. E. M. Akita and S. Nakai, *J. Food Sci.*, 1992, **57**, 629.

19. D. Dong, H. Liu, Q. Xiao and R. Li, *J. Chromatogr. B: Anal. Technol. Biomed. Life Sci.*, 2008, **870**, 51.
20. P. Hansen, J. A. Scoble, B. Hanson and N. J. Hoogenraad, *J. Immunol. Methods*, 1998, **215**, 1.
21. H. Hatta, J. S. Sim and S. Nakai, *J. Food Sci.*, 1988, **53**, 425.
22. H. Hatta, M. Kim and T. Yamamoto, *Agric. Biol. Chem.*, 1990, **54**, 2531.
23. E. M. Akita and S. Nakai, *J. Immunol. Methods*, 1993, **160**, 207.
24. H. M. Chang, C. C. Yang and Y. C. Chang, *J. Agric. Food Chem.*, 2000, **48**, 161.
25. F. J. Hernandez-Campos, E. Brito-De la Fuente and B. Torrestiana-Sanchez, *J. Agric. Food Chem.*, 2010, **58**, 187.
26. J. Liu, J. Yang, H. Xu, H. Zhu, J. Qu, J. Lu and Z. Cui, *Int. J. Food Eng.*, 2011, **7**, 1556.
27. K. Y. Ko and D. U. Ahn, *Poult. Sci.*, 2007, **86**, 400.
28. F. J. Joubert and W. H. Cook, Preparation and characterization of phosvitin from hen egg yolk, *Can. J. Biochem. Physiol.*, 1958, **36**, 399.
29. J. N. Losso and S. A. Nakai, in *Egg Uses and Processing Technologies – New Developments*, ed. J. S. Sim and S. Nakai, CAB International, Wallingford, UK, 1994, p. 150.
30. O. Castellani, V. Martinet, E. David-Briand, C. Guerin-Dubiard and M. Anton, *J. Chromatogr. B*, 2003, **791**, 273.
31. K. Y. Ko, K. C. Nam, C. Jo, E. J. Lee and D. U. Ahn, *Poult. Sci.*, 2011, **90**, 1096.
32. C. Connelly and G. Taborsky, *J. Biol. Chem.*, 1961, **236**, 1364.
33. B. Lei and J. Wu, *J. Chromatogr. A*, 2012, **1223**, 41.
34. J. Zhang, J. Sun, Y. Liu, J. Li, Y. Su, W. Xia and Y. Yang, *J. Chromatogr. B: Anal. Technol. Biomed. Life Sci.*, 2012, **893**, 121.
35. J. H. Lee, S. H. Moon, H. S. Kim, E. Park, D. U. Ahn and H. D. Paik, *Poult. Sci.*, 2017, **96**, 3872.
36. H. Y. Lee, E. D. N. S. Abeyrathne, I. Choi, J. W. Suh and D. U. Ahn, *Poult. Sci.*, 2014, **93**, 2668.
37. R. Shade and P. A. Chacana, in *Bioactive Egg Compounds*, ed. R. Huopalahti, R. Lopez-Fandino, M. Anton and R. Schade, Springer-Verlag Berlin Heidelberg, 2007, ch. 5, p. 25.
38. W. H. Cook and W. G. Martin, *Can. J. Biochem. Physiol.*, 1962, **40**, 1273.
39. M. W. Radomski and W. H. Cook, *Can. J. Biochem.*, 1964, **42**, 1203.
40. W. G. Martin, J. Augustyniak and W. H. Cook, *Biochim. Biophys. Acta*, 1964, **84**, 714.
41. M. Moussa, V. Martinet, A. Trimeche, D. Tainturier and M. Anton, *Theriogenology*, 2002, **57**, 1695.
42. M. Chalamaiah, Y. Esparza, F. Temelli and J. Wu, *Food Biosci.*, 2017, **18**, 38.
43. D. U. Ahn, S. H. Lee, H. Singam, E. J. Lee and J. C. Kim, *Food Sci. Biotechnol.*, 2006, **15**, 189.
44. H. Yokoyama, R. C. Peralta, T. Horikosh, J. Horaoka, M. Ikemori and Y. Kodama, *Poult. Sci.*, 1993, **72**, 275.

45. J. Williams, *Biochem. J.*, 1962, **83**, 346.
46. A. Polanowski, A. Zabłocka, A. Sosnowska, M. Janusz and T. Trziszka, *Biol. Chem.*, 2013, **394**, 879.
47. A. Zambrowicz, A. Zabłocka, L. Bobak, M. Macała, M. Janusz, A. Polanowski and T. Trziszka, *Food Chem.*, 2017, **230**, 705.
48. M. E. Cook and D. L. Trott, *World's Poult. Sci.*, 2010, **66**, 215.
49. M. E. Cook, *J. Appl. Poult. Res.*, 2004, **13**, 106.
50. J. Kovacs-Nolan and Y. Mine, *Annu. Rev. Food Sci. Technol.*, 2012, **3**, 163.
51. X. Li, L. Wang, Y. Zhen, S. Li and Y. Xu, *J. Anim. Sci. Biotechnol.*, 2015, **6**, 40.
52. A. Larsson, R. Balow, T. L. Lindahl and P. Forsberg, *Poult. Sci.*, 1993, **72**, 1807.
53. S. K. Lee, J. H. Han and E. A. Decker, *Food Chem. Toxicol.*, 2002, **67**, 37.
54. M. Shimizu, Y. Miwa, K. Hashimoto and A. Goto, *Biosci., Biotechnol., Biochem.*, 1993, **57**, 1445.
55. P. Schmidt, A. Hafner, G. H. Reubel, R. Wanke, V. Franke, U. Lösch and E. Dahme, *Zoonoses*, 1989, **36**, 661.
56. J. Kovacs-Nolan, M. Phillips and Y. Mine, *J. Agric. Food Chem.*, 2005, **53**, 8421.
57. X. Y. Li, L. J. Jin, T. A. McAllister, K. Stanford, J. Y. Xu, Y. N. Lu, Y. H. Zhen, Y. X. Sun and Y. P. Xu, *J. Agric. Food Chem.*, 2007, **55**, 2911.
58. Z. W. Jaradat and R. R. Marquardt, *Food Agric. Immunol.*, 2000, **12**, 263.
59. G. M. W. Cook, *Biol. Rev.*, 1968, **43**, 363.
60. G. Taborsky and C. Mok, *J. Biol. Chem.*, 1967, **242**, 1495.
61. B. M. Byrne, A. D. Van Het Schip, J. A. Van de Klundert, A. C. Arnberg, M. Gruber and G. Ab, *Biochemistry*, 1984, **23**, 4275.
62. M. A. Sattar-Khan, S. Nakamura, M. Ogawa, E. Akita, H. Azakami and A. Kato, *J. Agric. Food Chem.*, 2000, **48**, 1503.
63. G. Taborsky, *Biochemistry*, 1963, **2**, 260.
64. K. J. Albright, D. T. Gordon and O. J. Cotterill, *J. Food Sci.*, 1984, **49**, 78.
65. S. I. Ishikawa, S. Tamaki, K. Arihara and M. Itoh, *J. Food Sci.*, 2007, **72**, 412.
66. M. Y. Ji, K. H. Leem, M. J. Kim and H. K. Kim, *Biosci., Biotechnol., Biochem.*, 2007, **71**, 1327.
67. C. Li, F. Geng, X. Huang, M. Ma and X. Zhang, *Poult. Sci.*, 2014, **93**, 3065.
68. X. Zhang, F. Geng, X. Huang and M. Ma, *J. Cryst. Growth*, 2015, **409**, 44.
69. X. Zhang, F. Geng, X. Huang and M. Ma, *J. Inorg. Biochem.*, 2016, **159**, 76.
70. X. Zhang, X. Huang and M. Ma, *Int. J. Biol. Macromol.*, 2017, **101**, 712.
71. Q. Liu, C. Li, F. Geng, X. Huang and M. Ma, *J. Sci. Food Agric.*, 2017, **97**, 4532.
72. J. Liu, D. Czernick, S. C. Lin, A. Alasmari, D. Serge and E. Salih, *Dev. Biol.*, 2013, **381**, 256.
73. S. Jung, D. H. Kim, J. H. Son, K. Nam, D. U. Ahn and C. Jo, *Food Chem.*, 2012, **135**, 993.
74. S. H. Moon, J. H. Lee, M. H. Lee, E. J. Park, D. U. Ahn and H. D. Paik, *Poult. Sci.*, 2014, **93**, 2013.
75. C. L. Lu and R. C. Baker, *Poult. Sci.*, 1986, **65**, 2065.

76. S. L. Chung and K. L. Ferrier, *J. Food Sci.*, 2010, **57**, 40.
77. S. M. A. Khan, E. E. Babiker, H. Azakami and A. Kato, *J. Agric. Food Chem.*, 1998, **46**, 4977.
78. A. Polanowski, A. Zabłocka, A. Sosnowska, M. Janusz and T. Trziszka, *Poult. Sci.*, 2012, **91**, 3091.
79. M. Lemieszewska, M. Jakubik-Witkowska, B. Stańczykiewicz, A. Zambrowicz, A. Zabłocka, A. Polanowski and J. Rymaszewska, *Arch. Immunol. Ther. Exp.*, 2016, **64**, 425.
80. W. J. Stadelman and O. J. Cotterill, *Egg Science and Technology*, 4th edn, 2001.
81. M. Anton, in *Bioactive Egg Compounds*, Springer-Verlag Berlin Heidelberg, 2007, ch. 1.
82. H. H. Sunwoo and N. Gujral, in *Handbook of Food Chemistry*, Springer, Berlin, Heidelberg, 2018.

CHAPTER 19

Value-added Uses of Eggshell and Eggshell Membranes

TAMER A. E. AHMED[a,b], GARIMA KULSHRESHTHA[†b] AND MAXWELL T. HINCKE*[b,c]

[a]Medical Biotechnology Department, Genetic Engineering and Biotechnology Research Institute, City of Scientific Research and Technology Applications (SRTA-City), Alexandria, Egypt; [b]Department of Cellular and Molecular Medicine, Faculty of Medicine, University of Ottawa, Ottawa, Ontario, Canada, K1H 8M5; [c]Department of Innovation in Medical Education, Faculty of Medicine, University of Ottawa, Ottawa, Ontario, Canada, K1G 5Z3
*E-mail: mhincke@uottawa.ca

19.1 Introduction

Worldwide, chicken eggs are a vital part of the daily human diet and serve as a low-cost and high-quality nutrient resource. In 2011, global egg production was approximately 70.7 million metric tons, up from 37.4 million metric tons in 1990.[1,2] In industrialized countries, about 30% of shell eggs are diverted to breaker processing plants.[3] High quantities of eggshell residue from such plants are still disposed of as waste in landfills without any pretreatment.[4] The eggshell membrane (ESM) is associated with the eggshell (ES) and is also a byproduct of the food industry.[5] Eggshells are considered industrial

[†]Co-first author.

Food Chemistry, Function and Analysis No.14
Eggs as Functional Foods and Nutraceuticals for Human Health
Edited by Jianping Wu

Published by the Royal Society of Chemistry, www.rsc.org

waste when not properly managed as they can serve as a substrate for microbial growth.[4] In addition, the costs associated with disposal of egg waste will climb with inflation in landfill taxes. Major applications of ES waste from industrial processes are in agriculture to correct the pH of acid soil and in animal feed as a source of calcium.[6,7] Although such applications are of economic value, ES byproducts are still undervalued and many studies have been undertaken to functionally characterize eggshell for potential value-added applications.[8]

The avian ES is composed of the calcareous outer layer lined by the ESM; the shell and membrane together constitute about 10% of egg weight. Calcium carbonate ($CaCO_3$) comprises 95% of the ES weight, while proteins, glycoproteins, and proteoglycans are about 3.5%.[9] The ESM is around 1% of egg weight and is a bilayered proteinaceous fibrous meshwork.[10] Technically, ESM is composed of three layers: the outer ESM, the inner ESM, and the limiting membrane.[11] ESM is considered a functionally equivalent extracellular matrix (ECM), which is constituted mainly of proteins (90%), of which 10% are collagens and the remainder are other proteins and glycoproteins containing lysine-derived cross-links.[10,12]

This chapter presents an overview of the technological capacities of chicken ES and ESM, including their functional characteristics, followed by different processing methods for constructing compatible ES- and ESM-based platforms for potential value-added applications.

19.2 Composition of Eggshell and Eggshell Membranes

19.2.1 Composition of Eggshell

The mineralized shell is a natural porous bioceramic composed of calcium carbonate as a solid barrier against physical stress. ES is a highly ordered structure with four morphologically distinct regions that form sequentially upon the ESM in the final segments of the hen oviduct, beginning with the innermost mammillary zone, the palisades, and the vertical crystal layer, followed by the cuticle as the outermost layer.[13–15] The eggshell cuticle is deposited on the surface of the egg during the termination phase of shell calcification and consists of proteins, phosphate mineral, phosphoproteins, sulfated polysaccharides, and lipids.[16,17] Its coverage is uneven in chicken eggs with a variable thickness of 0–10 μm.[18] The completeness of the cuticle is a heritable trait in poultry and is associated with resistance to bacterial penetration.[19] Physicochemical analysis of industrial eggshell waste revealed that eggshell is an alkaline (pH 8.3 ± 0.1), calcium-rich material with 1% magnesium carbonate, 1% calcium phosphate, and a low percentage of organic matter.[20]

Eggshell mineralization is controlled precipitation of calcium carbonate initiated at nucleation sites on the outer membrane fibers within the uterine lumen, during three stages: initiation (~5 h), rapid mineralization (~12 h), and termination (~1.5 h). During the first stage of mineralization, organic aggregates are deposited at nucleation sites, where deposits of amorphous calcium carbonate become progressively transformed into the calcitic mammillary cones, which comprise the inner mammillary layer of the calcified shell (~100 μm in thickness).[14,21] In the second stage, the rapid growth of polycrystalline calcite takes place and the bases of the mammillary cones merge to form the palisade layer (~300 μm).[22] In the last stage, arrest of calcification occurs and the palisade layer ends with a high-density vertical crystal layer, followed by cuticle deposition.

19.2.2 Composition of Eggshell Membranes

The avian ESM fibers are assembled and secreted from the tubular gland cells in the white isthmus segment of the oviduct, and consist of an outer membrane (50–70 μm) and an inner membrane (15–26 μm).[23] ESM fibers are highly cross-linked and folded around the surface of the rotating egg white prior to shell mineralization.[24] The ESM is composed mainly of proteins (~90%), lipids (~3%), and carbohydrates (~2%).[10,25] ESM fibers contain various structural proteins, including collagens and cysteine-rich eggshell membrane proteins (CREMPs), in addition to a significant content of bioactive protein components.[5] ESM is greatly stabilized by extensive desmosine, isodesmosine, and disulfide cross-linkages, making the identification of its protein constituents by standard proteomic approaches technically challenging.[23,25,26] Scanning electron micrographs (SEM) of the ES and associated ESM are shown in Figure 19.1.

19.3 Functions of ES and ESM

19.3.1 Functions of ES

The calcified eggshell protects the embryo from mechanical damage, regulates the loss of moisture, is a source of calcium during embryonic development, and allows gaseous and heat exchange with the environment.[13,27,28] Proteomics studies of ES have identified a wide range of antimicrobial proteins, including lysozyme, ovotransferrin, and avian β-defensins (AvBDs), that prevent microbial contamination of the egg interior during and after its formation, as well as regulatory proteins that control mineralization and eggshell quality. Such proteins are useful markers for genetic selection to improve hen performance in terms of shell quality and egg resistance to pathogens.[29–32] These functional characteristics of eggshell are the basis for development of value-added commercial products from eggshell.

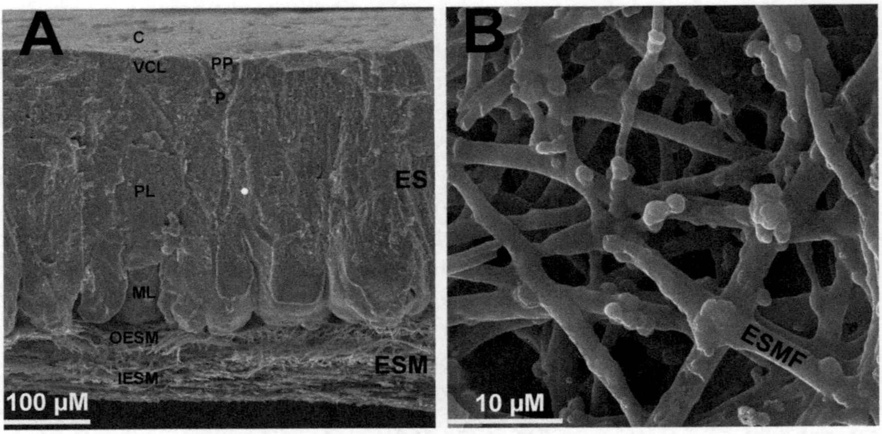

Figure 19.1 Morphology of the eggshell and eggshell membranes revealed by scanning electron microscopy (SEM). (**A**) Eggshell cross-fractured to show the calcified eggshell (ES), constituted of cuticle (C), vertical crystal layer (VCL), palisade layer (PL), and mammillary layer (ML); with the associated eggshell membranes (ESM), composed of outer eggshell membrane (OESM) and inner eggshell membrane (IESM). (**B**) Higher magnification of the ESM fibers (ESMF). P is an eggshell pore while PP is the pore plug. (Nano Imaging Facility, Carleton University, Ottawa, Canada.)

19.3.2 Functions of ESM

The primary functions of ESM are to surround the egg white and provide structural support upon which biomineralization occurs for shell formation. In addition, ESM along with the ES act as physicochemical barriers against pathogen invasion and thus are critical for avian reproduction and food safety. Functional annotation analysis of ESM protein constituents that are relatively specific for the eggshell membrane, compared to egg white, indicated the presence of various important functionalities, including structural molecule activity/ECM structural constituents (collagens), macromolecular complex assembly/chromosome organization (histones), cell adhesion (fibronectin 1, protocadherin 1, contactin, and collagens), motor activity (dyneins and kinesins), cell morphogenesis involved in differentiation, cytokinesis during cell cycle, and phosphopyruvate hydratase activity.[23]

19.4 Characterization of ES and ESM

19.4.1 Characterization of ES

19.4.1.1 Proteomics

Extensive proteomic analysis has identified the protein constituents of ES. Acetic acid is generally utilized to decalcify the ES to release the soluble protein matrix for further study.[33–35] Merging the proteomes established by these studies allowed the identification of more than 480 proteins in the ES matrix, with at least 390 that are relatively unique compared to ESM.[23]

19.4.1.2 Amino Acid Composition

The amino acid composition of ES is generally comparable to that of ESM; however, the ESM content of hydroxyproline, hydroxylysine, and cysteine suggests elevated levels of collagen and cysteine-rich proteins.[36]

19.4.2 Characterization of ESM

19.4.2.1 Proteomics

The protein constituents of ESM derived from both fertilized and unfertilized eggs have been identified using various extraction/solubilization conditions and proteomic analyses.[23,37–39] A comprehensive ESM proteome of almost 500 proteins was established by merging various ESM proteomes and then compared to the egg white and eggshell proteomes to identify proteins that are relatively or highly specific to ESM.[23,37,38,40] Analysis of the relative abundance of proteins identified in the ESM proteome, based on total spectral counts of the unique peptides, indicated that ESM is largely constituted of CREMPs (30%) and collagen X (10%), in addition to the bioactive constituents lysyl oxidase-like protein 2 (LOXL2) (30%) and lysozyme C (LYZ) (10%).[5] The presence of collagen X and lysozyme in ESM has been verified by immunochemistry.[41,42]

19.4.2.2 Amino Acid Composition

Amino acid analysis of ESM powder showed that proline/hydroxyproline and lysine/hydroxylysine constitute around 10% and 5% of ESM by weight, respectively, suggesting that collagens are significant constituents of ESM.[5] However, ESM contains around 10% glycine while the canonical G-X-Y repeats of collagen confirm the presence of 25% glycine in avian collagens. Moreover, the high cysteine content of ESM (~10%) is clearly inconsistent with the average of 1% cysteine observed in avian collagens. The overall amino acid composition of ESM is similar to the available CREMP amino acid sequences and indicates that CREMPs are a prominent constituent of ESM.[5,38]

19.5 ES- and ESM-based Formats

19.5.1 ES-based Applications

Eggshell can be processed to produce different derivatives, such as calcium carbonate, calcium oxide, and hydroxyapatite, for environmental and economical applications.

19.5.1.1 Calcium Carbonate

Eggshell is mainly calcium carbonate, which can be utilized as an alternative to geological $CaCO_3$ for various applications.[43] Powdered eggshell produced by drying and milling is a source of $CaCO_3$ for low-value applications. Removal of ESM from the eggshell is achieved by acid treatment or with flotation methods. A yield of 96% ESM and 99% ES can be achieved utilizing water in a countercurrent column with air pumped from the bottom for membrane separation.[44] Several other membrane separation techniques using vacuum suction, pulse energy system, or ethylenediaminetetraacetic acid (EDTA)/hexane chemical extraction have been documented to optimize the efficiency, reusability, and purity of the byproducts.[9,45,46] Pure calcite can be prepared from eggshell by heat treatment (300 °C) or with diluted bleach. Alternatively, ES calcite can be transformed into lime by heating to 750 °C. While bleach treatment is unsustainable and not environmentally friendly, heat treatment shows potential for scaling up with the estimated cost to produce ground $CaCO_3$ of \$75–350 ton^{-1}.[47]

ES-derived $CaCO_3$ is a raw material that can be used to produce more soluble forms of calcium, such as calcium citrate, which can be produced directly from digestion of ES using citric acid or from calcium hydroxide by acid–base reaction.[48] The sequential chemical process involves washing and cleaning of eggshells, grinding, centrifugation, organic acid (acetic or lactic acid) treatment, citric acid replacement reaction, filtration, washing with ethanol, and drying.[49] Alternatively, dilute HCl can be used to obtain pure (99%) calcium citrate. In recent years, research efforts have been directed towards production of nanocalcium citrate to improve calcium bioavailability.[50] Eggshell calcium nanopowder (ESNP) and nanocalcium citrate particles can be synthesized from eggshell *via* a top–down approach; pulsed air-flow pulverizing or ball milling have produced ESNP of 20 nm.[50,51]

19.5.1.2 Calcium Oxide

Eggshells are a sustainable source of calcium oxide (CaO) which is an effective catalyst in the chemical sector/industry. High calcium oxide-based catalytic activity (98%) is attained with eggshell calcination temperatures >800 °C.[52] ES-derived CaO exhibited superior catalytic activity compared to that from mollusk shell, due to the better porosity and higher surface area of ES.[53]

19.5.1.3 Hydroxyapatite

Naturally occurring hydroxyapatite (HA, $Ca_{10}(PO_4)_6(OH)_2$) is a calcium phosphate biomaterial used for bone tissue engineering. ES-derived HA (EHA) is synthesized by hydrothermal treatment with $Ca_3PO_4{\cdot}H_2O$ at elevated temperatures (1050 °C).[54] Rapid microwave irradiation, sol–gel precipitation, and high energy mechanochemical activation have also been reported for EHA production. Microwave irradiation requires a chelating agent, EDTA, to form a Ca–EDTA complex, which subsequently reacts with phosphate under microwave irradiation to generate flower-like hydroxyapatite nanostructures. The resulting product showed homogeneity and high crystallinity, with biocompatibility comparable to bone graft substitutes.[55] Single-phase ES-based nano-hydroxyapatite of high crystallinity can be obtained by mechanochemical activation with ES calcination followed by ball milling and mixing with dicalcium hydrogen phosphate dihydrous (DCPD) or phosphoric acid (H_3PO_4). Such ES-derived nano-hydroxyapatite showed stability at high temperatures with optimal osteoblast cell adhesion.[56]

19.5.2 ESM-based Applications

The large-scale separation of ESM from ES is a crucial step for ESM availability on an industrial scale.[11] Eggshell membranes are technically constituted of outer and inner layers; the inner layer can be manually separated, while the outer ESM fibers are strongly integrated into the tips of the mammillary cones of the inner ES.[11] To remove the bilayered ESM from ES, an acid treatment is required.[40] The separation of intact ESM can be carried out by dissolving the shell totally in acid or by filling the shell interior with acid to dissolve the bases of the mammillary cones.[11,40] Alternatively, ESM can be separated from ES using a dissolved air flotation (DAF) strategy. Using a DAF separation unit, it is possible to recover 96% of ESM from ES waste.[44]

ESM possesses a complex network of stable and water-insoluble fibers with a high surface area.[3] The insolubility and difficult manipulability of intact ESM have limited its utilization for various applications.[5] The surface area of ESM can be increased by grinding to a powder, leading to a decrease in ESM particle size and improved adsorption capacity.[57] The solubility of ESM is hindered by disulfide bonds and isodesmosine/desmosine cross-linkages. To overcome this limitation, soluble forms of ESM have been prepared by chemical treatment.[58] One strategy is the dissolution of ESM by performic acid oxidation followed by pepsin digestion.[59] Various bioactive soluble forms of ESM have been produced by reductive dissolution of the ESM fibers,[10] for example, using aqueous 3-mercaptopropionic acid (3-MPA) at elevated temperatures. Another approach involves treatment with a 3 : 1 mixture of NaOH–ethanol.[60] ESM can also be hydrolyzed *via* bacterial fermentation[61] or protease digestion.[62–64] The resultant ESM hydrolysates possess various bioactivities, including antibacterial, antioxidant, and angiotensin-converting enzyme (ACE) inhibitory activities.[61,63,64] Several forms of ESM, including intact, powdered, solubilized and digested, have been evaluated for various applications (Table 19.1).

Table 19.1 Summary of the various forms of processed ESM and their applications.

ESM form	Applications	Reference number
Intact	Adsorption	11,164–166,169,171,173–175, 178,180,181,184–186
	Biosensors	11,194–216
	Chemical processing support	9,11,217–223
	Electrochemical cells	224–226
	Food supplement	231
	GTR	11,162,234–239,241–244
	Medical technology	254,255
	Mucoadhesion assessment	256–258
Powdered	Adsorption	3,11,57,65,163,167,168,170, 172,176,177,182,183
	Anti-inflammatory agent	189,191
	GTR	5,11,112,233,240
Solubilized	Adsorption	11,179
	Antibacterial agent	187
	Anti-inflammatory agent	190,193
	Antioxidant	64,193
	Cosmetics	9,187
	GTR	10–12,25,26,58,59,245–253
Digested	Antibacterial agent	61
	Anti-inflammatory agent	188,192
	Antioxidant	63
	Food supplement	11,227–230
	GTR	11,232

19.6 Value-added Applications of ES and ESM

19.6.1 Applications of ES

19.6.1.1 Adsorption

Ground ES powder has been well documented as a low-cost sorbent for CO_2 capture, adsorption of heavy metals, and removal of organic pollutants and dyes from waste water.[9,65] Modified ES (using fabrication or chemical processing) and extracted components from powdered ES have also been considered as promising sorbents.

19.6.1.1.1 Adsorption of CO_2. Calcinated ES for CO_2 capture technologies possesses high sorption capacity at elevated temperatures and long-term durability.[66,67] In addition, zirconium (Zr)-doped CaO-based sorbents prepared from waste ES showed a CO_2 capture efficiency of 88%.[68] Furthermore, a low-cost CaO-based sorbent incorporated with 10% bauxite tailings showed enhanced ability to capture CO_2, with carbonation conversion of more than 55% after 40 cycles.[69] Biodegradable calcinated eggshell–sodium alginate beads have been applied to capture CO_2 in a fixed-bed reactor.[70]

19.6.1.1.2 Adsorption of Inorganic Pollutants. ES adsorbs heavy metals owing to the carbonate group with its cation-exchange and -binding properties; moreover, calcium aids in ion exchange with metal ions.[71,72] ES waste has thus been used as a low-cost activation agent to improve the heavy metal adsorption capacities of commercial carbon.[73] ES mixed with organic material has been used for capturing lead Pb(II) from aqueous solution. Addition of ES increases the solution pH, resulting in the precipitation of metals on the ES surface.[74] In addition, ES immobilized in a fixed bed simultaneously removes heavy metals and reduces the acidity of acid mine drainage.[75] ES-derived $Ca(OH)_2$ nanosheets decorated with Mn_3O_4 quantum dots showed high removal efficiency for trace lead levels from wastewater and outperformed many other Mn-based nanomaterials prepared from synthetic chemicals.[76] Finally, hydroxyapatite from ES was successfully used to remove lead contaminants from mineral water and energy drinks.[77]

19.6.1.1.3 Adsorption of Organic Pollutants. ES can remove organic pollutants such as toxic dyes from textile wastewater. A biocomposite adsorbent synthesized from ES waste showed high affinity for synthetic dyes, such as Remazol Red, in aqueous solution. Immobilization of ES on porous polymeric materials, such as poly(vinyl alcohol) (PVA) and alginate, improved its mechanical properties. The adsorption capacity is dependent on pH, particle size, adsorbent dosage, and temperature.[78] Amino acid-modified ES particles (AA-ESP) were useful for removal of styrylpyridinium dyes from aqueous waste.[79] Biosorption by ES involves surface phenomena such as physical adsorption, alkaline fading, and microprecipitation.[80] Many studies have shown the use of ES to synthesize low-cost nano-sorbents for removal purposes. For instance, multiwall carbon nanotubes were decorated on calcinated ES (CES) for treating organic waste in aqueous solution.[81] Green synthesis of metal nanocomposites (Cu and Fe_3O_4) on an ES surface proved effective in decontamination of dyes including 4-nitrophenol, methyl orange, Congo red, methylene blue, and rhodamine.[82] Sol–gel TiO_2 decorated on ES nanocrystal was validated as an engineered adsorbent for purifying of dyes from contaminated water.[83]

19.6.1.2 Antimicrobial

Proteomic and transcriptomic analysis of chicken ES has identified a diversity of antimicrobial molecules, which are targets for development of novel antimicrobials.[30,32,84] These proteins are inexpensive and readily available sources of bioactive molecules for utility in food production and for human and animal health.[31] C-type lectin-like proteins, chicken ES ovovcleidin-17 and its goose ortholog, ansocalcin, showed bactericidal activity against *Staphylococcus aureus* and *Pseudomonas aeruginosa*.[85] In addition, lipophilic ES cuticle extracts demonstrated potent bactericidal activity against both

Gram-positive and Gram-negative pathogenic bacteria.[15] Furthermore, ES porphyrin pigments have been utilized therapeutically as photosensitizers for photo-inactivation of bacteria; toxic reactive oxygen species (ROS) generated during photosensitization by porphyrins was the predominant mechanism of action.[86] Moreover, calcinated ES possesses rapidly acting antimicrobial activities against viral and bacterial poultry pathogens.[87] Finally, many studies have utilized ES as a biotemplate to fabricate antimicrobial nanostructures owing to its efficient biocompatibility and biodegradability. For example, ES composites with silver or TiO_2 nanoparticles have been fabricated for antimicrobial water filtration and pathogen removal.[88–90]

19.6.1.3 Catalysis

ES and ES-derived calcium oxide are useful in base-catalyzed reactions, such as biodiesel production and synthesis of bioactive compounds.

19.6.1.3.1 Biodiesel Production. Biodiesel is synthesized through *trans*-esterification of triglycerides with methanol using a homogenous solid acid and/or base catalyst. The increase in pH and complexity of separation of the product, toxicity, corrosion, and environmental pollution are major disadvantages to a homogenous catalyst. However, a highly active, reusable, heterogeneous catalyst based upon CaO from calcination of waste ES has found utility in biodiesel synthesis.[52,53,91]

Biodiesel from *Jatropha curcas* oil using ES-CaO catalyst was produced at 90% yield with six times reuse of the catalyst.[92] A significantly enhanced biodiesel yield using an ES-derived catalyst was achieved by microwave irradiation.[93] Alternatively, ES has been combined with sodium silicate (Na_2SiO_3) to produce a novel solid-based CaO–SiO_2 catalyst by biomimetic silicification. As the amount of Si in the catalyst increased, its activity gradually decreased; however, reusability was significantly improved.[94] In addition, a solid-based catalyst produced from ES (SBES) achieved a biodiesel yield of 99% from food-grade soybean oil. SBES exhibited stronger basicity than CaO and had reusability of >10 cycles. KOH generated in the modification process enhanced the basicity and catalytic ability of the catalyst.[95] Recently, a green and low-cost biodiesel production method with soybean oil and vegetable oil demonstrated high-activity *trans*-esterification at room temperature with calcined ES to obtain fatty acid methyl ester yields of >97% with good stability and reusability profiles.[96]

An improved process to produce biodiesel from microalgal biomass using a heterogeneous ES-derived CaO nanocatalyst demonstrated advantages including increased availability of active sites, high specific surface area, shorter reaction time, easy separation, better recovery, and resistance to saponification.[97] More recently, an ES-derived calcium catalyst was prepared by wet-impregnation in the presence of a molybdenum–zirconium (Mo–Zr) mixed salt. This modified catalyst produced biodiesel from waste cooking palm oil (WCPO) with >90% yield and with reduced Ca^{2+} leaching into the product.[98]

19.6.1.3.2 Synthesis of Bioactive Compounds. ES has been used as a natural heterogeneous catalyst for the synthesis of various biologically important scaffolds, including benzothiazoles, chromenones, lactulose, and pyrans.

Benzothiazoles. Benzothiazoles exhibit antitumor, antimicrobial, and leukotriene D4 (LTD_4) receptor antagonistic activities, as well as anticancer and anti-allergy properties. Calcinated ES is an appealing green catalyst for synthesis of 2-arylbenzothiazoles, compared to pure CaO, with respect to yield (92% *vs.* 30%) and reaction time (16 min *vs.* 5 h).[99]

Chromenones. Chromenones are used as pigments, cosmetics, and potential biodegradable agrochemicals. Powdered ES is a catalyst in the synthesis of 7,8-dihydro-4*H*-chromen-5(6*H*)-ones *via* the Knoevenagel–cyclocondensation reaction, with a higher yield (90–98%) compared to $CaCO_3$ (70%).[100] Particle size and porosity are critical for biocatalyst efficiency; nano ES powder showed increased catalytic activity for green synthesis of 2-aminochromenes (93–98%) compared to milled ES powder (85%) and commercial $CaCO_3$ (69–80%).[101]

Lactulose. Lactulose is synthesized by the isomerization of lactose and has various nutritional, pharmaceutical, and medical applications.[102] Powdered ES has been used as a food-grade catalyst to isomerize lactose from cheese whey permeate (WP) to lactulose, followed by β-galactosidase (*Bacillus circulans*)-catalyzed conversion of lactulose into lactulose-derived oligosaccharides with potential prebiotic properties.[103,104] Lactulose produced *via* ES-mediated catalysis has also been used to generate bioactive peptides with antioxidant activity by the Maillard reaction.[105]

Pyran Derivatives. Pyran derivatives display a wide range of biological and pharmacological activities, including antimicrobial, antiviral, and anticancer. Low-yielding conventional synthesis of pyran derivatives utilizes expensive reagents, prolonged reaction times, and acidic/harsh reaction conditions; therefore, development of natural heterogeneous catalysts for green chemistry methods is the focus of intensive research. Both ES powder and nano-bio calcite/nano-CaO are efficient catalysts for synthesis of pyrano [4,3-*b*]pyran scaffolds, with both nano-catalysts demonstrating a higher catalytic activity compared to powdered ES (yields of 90–98% *vs.* 65–86%, respectively).[106,107] Loading with transition metal ions such as copper to synthesize multifunctional biocatalysts can improve/manipulate the catalytic properties of powdered ES. ES-supported $Cu(OH)_2$ nano-ribbons provided a high catalytic activity (>93%) for the green synthesis of pyrano [4,3-*b*]pyrans.[108]

19.6.1.4 Guided Tissue Regeneration

Calcium is an essential component of bone metabolism and structure; ES-derived $CaCO_3$ is a promising and inexpensive bone substitute material.[8] For instance, ES-derived grafting material enhanced new bone formation in rats.[109] ES calcium carbonate is a biocompatible biofiller or packing material for maxillofacial and cranial fractures.[110–113] Heat-stable ES biofillers reduced surface roughness and improved adhesion strength of acrylic resins.[114,115] In addition, ES particles have been 3D-printed into a polymer scaffold[116] and have been used in conjunction with acids to form a cement.[117]

The calcified eggshell contains an organic matrix containing >500 proteins, proteoglycans, and glycoproteins, including ovocleidin-116, the chicken ortholog of matrix extracellular phosphoglycoprotein (MEPE), collagens, and osteopontin (OPN), which play important roles in bone calcification by increasing osteoblast binding and adhesion.[118,119] ES-derived hydroxyapatite (EHA) is suitable for many biografting applications.[120,121] EHA speeds up bone repair and has been used for bone augmentation, implant coating, and as a filler in bone/teeth.[122–124] Synthetic hydroxyapatite in nanostructural format improves biomaterial–cell interactions for clinical applications. For instance, enhanced osteogenesis is associated with the nanostructured surface design of macroporous hydroxyapatite bioceramic scaffolds, *via* activation of extracellular signal-regulated kinase (ERK) and p38 mitogen-activated protein kinase (MAPK) signaling pathways.[125] Ciprofloxacin-loaded hydroxyapatite–polycaprolactone nanocomposite film produced from ES is suitable for filling bone defects and showed potential as a drug delivery system in osteomyelitis patients.[126] Pure nanocrystalline HAp produced *via* ultrasound-mediated chemical synthesis showed superior mechanical properties and osteogenic capacity compared to commercially available hydroxyapatite.[127] A novel bone regenerative material with surface nano-texture was prepared from ES calcium carbonate (NT-ES) by phosphoric acid treatment. NT-ES particles were non-cytotoxic and supported a proliferative response from murine RAW264.7 macrophages and mesenchymal stem cells, with a significant increase in cell density.[128]

19.6.1.5 Food Supplement

19.6.1.5.1 Human Food Supplement. Chicken ES has a high calcium content (381 ± 89 mg Ca g^{-1} eggshell: ~40%) and is promoted as a natural source of calcium and other elements (strontium and fluoride) in health foods to improve bone mineral density, especially in the context of osteoporosis.[129–131] The concentrations of toxic elements in ES including Pb, Al, Cd, and Hg are either undetectable or are under the detection limit (<0.5 μg mL^{-1}).[132] However, ES calcium is less bioavailable in crude carbonate form. Other calcium salts, such as citrate and formate, showed superior ability to deliver calcium to the bloodstream after oral administration and offered significant advantages as dietary calcium supplements.[133,134] Synthesis of nanocalcium carbonate has gained attention to increase the bioavailability and absorption of calcium.[50] Calcium citrate nano-fortified milk powder gives enhanced absorption and bioavailability of calcium and is associated with improved bone stiffness and strength in osteoporotic rats.[135]

19.6.1.5.2 Livestock Food Supplement. ES powder was approved in 1982 by the Association of American Feed Control Officials as a feed additive for both pet and livestock animals. ES transformation from poultry industry residues into high-quality poultry feedstock involves drying at high temperature (80 °C) followed by crushing and milling, which is critical for microbial inactivation and moisture removal.[49] ES particles can serve as a calcium source for laying hens to maintain ES quality in their eggs and to improve bone mineralization.[9] Dietary inclusion of ES improves feed conversion and egg production in hens, particularly in the later laying period of production.[136] ES has calcium levels comparable to geologic $CaCO_3$ (limestone), but chicken ES calcium is a better calcium source in soya protein-based diets for growing piglets.[7]

19.6.1.6 Purified Calcium Carbonate from ES

Eggshell-derived calcium carbonate is an ideal replacement for $CaCO_3$ mined from non-renewable sources. It has various industrial applications based on the purity grade.

19.6.1.6.1 Construction Sector. Purified ES $CaCO_3$ is a low-cost alternative raw material for the cement industry, and it improved the packing and densification properties of soil–cement bricks.[137,138] In addition, ES mortar produced from eggshell waste demonstrated accelerated hydration compared to conventional limestone, which increased the early strength of the cement.[139] ES powder improves the compressive strength of concrete material.[140,141]

19.6.1.6.2 Glass Fabrication. ES supplementation improves the thermal properties, crystallization behavior, and mechanical properties of glass.[142] Addition of eggshell powder induced an increase in the elastic modulus, hardness, and fracture toughness of soda–lime–silica (SLS) glasses.[143] In addition, a $CaO–MgO–SiO_2$ semi-crystalline bioactive glass was successfully formed from rice husk and ES.[144] In another study, discarded glass bottles were successfully converted into glass foams using ES as a foaming agent.[145]

19.6.1.7 Soil Amendments

Powdered ES can stabilize and immobilize heavy metals in soil, improve soil quality, and reduce waste disposal costs in landfill sites. In addition, this approach has additional environmental benefits of simultaneously tackling soil remediation, since ES possesses low levels of toxic components in comparison to other natural sources of calcium and nitrogen. Heavy metals can be immobilized in soil by adsorption, precipitation/co-precipitation, and complexation using organic or inorganic amendments.[146,147] Lime-based materials such as ES limit the mobility (bioavailability) of heavy metals by transforming their readily available forms to less accessible and more stable fractions in the soil.[6,9,148,149] For instance, ES can immobilize Pb and Cd in both alkaline and acidic soils.[43] ES waste in combination with fertilizers can immobilize Pb and Cd in neutral soil, owing to the formation of Pb hydroxide or lanarkite or co-precipitation with iron (Fe) and aluminum (Al) oxyhydroxides.[150]

ES can be recycled into a value-added compost to overcome calcium deficiencies in soil. In addition, its carbonate content can improve the pH of acidic soil (by liming) to improve the bioaccessibility of essential nutrients required for the normal growth of plants.[151] For example, co-composting with ES raised the soil pH and immobilized Pb and Zn by more than 95%, in addition to suppressing eco-toxicity, in contaminated acidic soil.[20] In a composting process, the major energy input to raise the temperature of the composting matrix for pathogen inactivation is derived from organic decomposition of the initial mixture; this exothermic process does not occur with ES owing to its inorganic nature. However, the incorporation of 30% (w/w) ES into organic material did not reduce the capacity of the composting mixture to reach sanitizing temperatures, and the ES-enriched compost attained physical, chemical, and phytotoxic properties suitable for soil incorporation.[152]

Co-composting is an attractive ES treatment option to remove biotic contaminants such as antibiotic-resistant bacteria (ARB) and antibiotic resistance genes (ARGs) from contaminated soils. Endogenous soil ARBs can colonize plants through epidermal wounds and surface tissue pores, and thereby pose a direct threat to human health through food-chain accumulation. Calcined eggshell amendment can mitigate mixed soil pollutants of antibiotics, heavy metals, ARB, and ARGs in cultivated soil and landfill leachates.[153] The greatest removal of *Escherichia coli* and gentamycin-resistant gene (*gmrA*) was achieved by ES combined with sulfate and calcination.[47,154]

19.6.1.8 Other Applications

Other industrial applications of purified calcium carbonate include manufacturing of paints, dyes, papers, plastics, and rubber.[155–157] ES as a coating material gives brightness and smoothness to paper. ES-derived calcium carbonate enhanced the optical density of inkjet color pigments while decreasing the black ink density and the gloss of the coated paper.[44] Furthermore, ES had been used as a filler for synthetic polymers to enhance their physical and mechanical properties. Thermal insulation composite foams have been prepared with natural rubber as a matrix phase and an ES powder dispersed phase.[158] Eco-friendly polypropylene carbonate (PPC) composite films synthesized using ES showed improved tensile strength, mechanical properties, and thermal stability.[159] ES-based intumescent flame protective coatings possessed effective fire resistance performance, including thermal stability, char formation, fire propagation, water resistance, and adhesion strength.[160] Addition of eggshell powder resulted in superior water resistance and

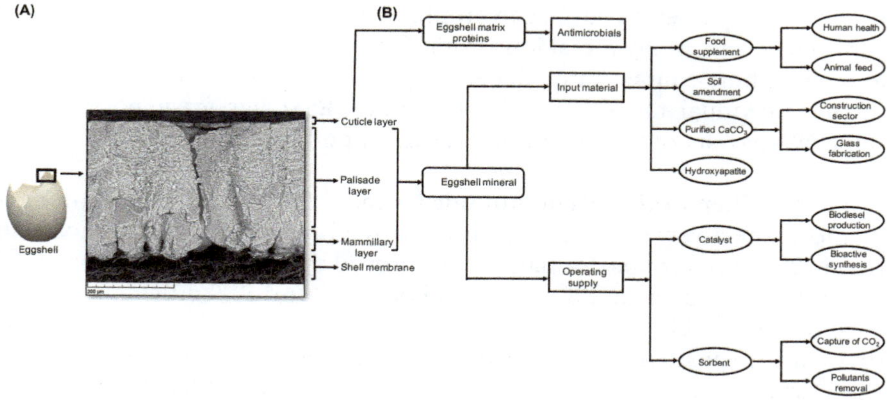

Figure 19.2 Scheme for eggshell exploitation. (**A**) Image and SEM micrograph of eggshell. (**B**) Classification of diverse applications for eggshell mineral and eggshell matrix proteins.

thermal stability of thermoplastic starch (TPS), compared to calcium carbonate, owing to improved interaction between organic ES components and the TPS matrix.[161] SEM of structurally different layers of ES along with the diverse applications of eggshell mineral and matrix proteins are illustrated in Figure 19.2.

19.6.2 Applications of Eggshell Membranes

Various physical properties of ESM, including its porous fibrous nature, large surface area, gaseous exchange capacity, great water-permeability, and stability, have facilitated its utilization in various biochemical and biophysical applications, including adsorption, chemical processing support, biosensors, and electrochemical cell production, along with medical technology.[9,10,162] In addition, ESM combines important characteristics, including adhesion capability, antibacterial activity, biocompatibility, antioxidant and anti-inflammatory activities, and nontoxicity, which make it a potential biomaterial for various biomedical applications,[5,162] including cosmetics, wound healing, GTR, and drug mucoadhesion assessment.[5,162]

19.6.2.1 Adsorption

Sufficient clean water and sanitation are significant problems affecting 30–60% of people worldwide owing to striking increases in population, industrialization, agricultural activity, and inappropriate use of natural resources.[163,164] Different low-cost byproducts derived from agriculture and industry along with natural materials have been evaluated as adsorbents for heavy metals and dyes, including ES and the associated ESM from egg-breaking plants.[65] ESM has a great capacity to bind phenols and various dyes.[163] ESM possesses surface hydrophilic amino and carboxyl groups, and can concentrate heavy metal ions from dilute aqueous solution in high yield and with short contact time, depending on the pH and the characteristics of the individual metal ion.[164,165] Therefore, ESM has great potential for removal/recovery of metal ions and for water pollution control.[165]

19.6.2.1.1 Removal of Metal Anionic Forms. ESM removed oxyanions of Se more effectively (~90%) than those of As; however, chemical modification of carboxyl groups dramatically improved the As^{5+} sorption capacity.[166] Similarly, thiol-bearing ESMs adsorb both Se^{4+} and Se^{6+} efficiently; Se^{6+} is retained reversibly, possibly *via* ionic interactions, while Se^{4+} is reduced to Se and deposited.[167] In addition, ESM has been assessed as an adsorbent for Au^{3+} and Pt^{2+}, approaching 55% and 25% of ESM weight at pH 4, respectively.[165] In a related study, ESM has been evaluated for its ability to adsorb gold ions Au^{+} (dicyanoaurate) and Au^{3+} (tetrachloroaurate) from solution and electroplating wastewater, with maximum adsorption capacities of 147 and 618 mg g^{-1} ESM dry weight, respectively. Selective recovery of gold from electroplating waste water in the presence of various cations was observed.[168] ESM, with and without glutaraldehyde cross-linking, is effective for removal of gold–cyanide ion ($Au(CN)_2^{-}$).[169] ESM can also adsorb cyanide ions (CN^{-}) from synthetic and industrial waste waters, with up to ~90% cyanide removal.[170]

Chromium (Cr^{6+}) is carcinogenic and mutagenic to living organisms, and hence more hazardous than other heavy metals. Native ESM and layered double hydroxide/eggshell membrane (LDH/ESM)-based constructs (MgAl–CO_3^{2-}–LDH/ESM and MgAl–Cl^{-}–LDH/ESM) have been evaluated as adsorbents for Cr^{6+} removal. The MgAl–Cl^{-}–LDH/ESM composite membrane had a higher adsorption capacity than ESM and MgAl–CO_3^{2-}–LDH/ESM, even when the Cr^{6+} solution pH was not further adjusted by addition of acid, reflecting practical significance in wastewater.[171] In a related study, ESM showed selective retention of Cr^{6+} through a reductive sorption process, while Cr^{3+} retention was very limited.[172] Similarly, arsenic (As^{5+}) could be easily extracted using ESM as a solid-phase extraction (SPE) adsorbent.[173] In addition, boron was adsorbed efficiently to both ESM and methyl esterified eggshell membrane (MESM).[163]

19.6.2.1.2 Removal of Metal Cationic Forms. ESM has been evaluated as an adsorbent for Pd^{2+} and U^{6+} (as UO_2^{2+})[65] but demonstrates superior capacity for removal of actinides, especially U^{6+} and thorium (Th^{4+}).[174,175] ESM selectivity can be achieved by controlling the pH of the solution.[174] Differential adsorption capacity of ESM has been demonstrated ($Ag^{+} > Cd^{2+} > Zn^{2+}$), and ESM is suitable for pre-concentration of silver in polymetallic ore samples.[176,177]

Functionalization of ESM modifies its capacity for binding Al^{3+} (magnetite-doped ESM), Cu^{2+} (polyethyleneimine-ESM), and Hg^{2+} (soluble eggshell membrane proteins (SEP) doped with reduced graphene oxide, SEP-rGO).[178–180]

19.6.2.1.3 Removal of Nanoparticles. Production of nanomaterials is currently the focus of intensive research; however, nanoparticles may pose risk to the environment and human health, and the toxicity of silver and gold nanoparticles to mammalian cells is well known. ESM biotemplated with NiO metal oxide can extract gold and silver nanoparticles (Au and Ag NPs) efficiently from spiked water samples.[164]

19.6.2.1.4 Removal of Organic Compounds and Gases. ESM shows great potential as a solid-phase extraction (SPE) adsorbent owing to the presence of surface functional groups and it is a biocompatible material that degrades easily, producing minor secondary environmental pollutants.[181] ESM efficiently absorbs textile dyes (Direct Red 80 (RD80), Acid Blue 25 (AB25)), C.I. Reactive Yellow 205 (a sulfonated reactive azo dye) and the reactive dyes *p*-chlorophenol (*p*-CP), 2,4-dichlorophenol (2,4-DCP), and 3,5-dichlorophenol (3,5-DCP).[57,182,183] In contrast, ESM particles exhibited poor capacity for adsorption of the basic dye methylene blue.[3] To enhance the solid-phase extraction capability of ESM towards Sudan I–IV, it was modified by co-adsorption of sodium dodecylbenzenesulfonate (SDBS; an anionic surfactant) with Triton X-100 (TX100; a nonionic surfactant). Co-adsorption of TX100 and SDBS at a ratio of 2 : 8 improved the extraction capacity of ESM towards Sudan I–IV due to the formation of mixed hemimicelles.[184] Methyl-esterification of ESM (MESM) significantly increased its surface area and shifted its negative surface charge to positive at all pH values, which increased the Sulfur Blue anionic dye sorption capacity.

The efficacy of ESM as an SPE bio-adsorbent for linear alkylbenzene sulfonates (LAS) as a model of organic pollutants was investigated. Near the isoelectric point of ESM, ESM was able to capture C10–C13 LAS homologues through hydrophobic interactions.[181] A novel SPE adsorbent was created using ESM as a template for a mixed hemimicelle/admicelle LAS adsorbent and demonstrated removal of carcinogenic polycyclic aromatic hydrocarbons (PAHs) from aqueous environmental samples. The mixed hemimicelle/admicelle adsorbent exhibited high extraction efficiency for PAHs and good selectivity with respect to natural organic matter.[185]

ESM can adsorb atmospheric CO_2, with reuse following acetic acid regeneration (6 g CO_2 g^{-1} ESM).[186]

19.6.2.2 Antibacterial Agent

In the egg, ESM is a physical and chemical barrier against pathogen invasion; antimicrobial proteins identified in the ESM proteome include lysozyme, avian β-defensins, and histones.[23] ESM hydrolysates produced *via* NaOH–ethanol hydrolysis are active against bacterial strains including *Staphylococcus aureus*, *Bacillus subtilis*, *Klebsiella pneumoniae*, *E. coli*, and *Serratia marcescens*.[187] In addition, ESM hydrolysate produced by *Lactobacillus plantarum*-mediated fermentation showed antibacterial activity against *Streptococcus agalactiae*, *E. coli*, *Salmonella typhimurium*, and *S. aureus*.[61]

19.6.2.3 Anti-inflammatory Agent

Consumption of ESM is reported to reduce pro-inflammatory cytokines, liver fibrosis, and joint pain in osteoarthritic patients.[188] The immunomodulatory effects of processed ESM powder (PEP) and the ESM-derived carbohydrate fraction were evaluated *in vitro* using monocytic cell lines; they reduced the activity of nuclear factor-κB (NF-κB) along with down-regulation of toll-like receptor 4 (TLR-4), intercellular adhesion molecule 1 (ICAM-1), and cell surface glycoprotein (CD44) expression in a lipopolysaccharides (LPS)-induced inflammation model. PEP and its carbohydrate fraction differentially regulate cytokine secretion as PEP decreased inflammation by increasing secretion of the anti-inflammatory cytokine interleukin-10 (IL-10), while the carbohydrate fraction reduced secretions of the pro-inflammatory cytokines IL-1β and IL-6.[189] In contrast, various hydrolysates of ESM (fermentation, enzymatic, or chemical) increase NF-κB levels in THP-1 cells in the absence of LPS.[188] Different formulations of the commercially available ESM powder NEM® reduce the production of tumor necrosis factor α (TNF-α) by peripheral blood mononuclear cells (PBMC) in response to stimulation by pokeweed mitogen (PWM). These findings suggested that immunomodulation by NEM® could potentially avoid the side effects exhibited by currently available anti-inflammatory drugs.[190] In addition, ESM powder has been evaluated *in vitro* as a possible intervention against inflammatory bowel disease (IBD); it up-regulated growth factors to attenuate LPS-induced inflammatory cytokine production and improve Caco-2 cell proliferation. Furthermore, in a mouse model of dextran sodium sulfate (DSS)-induced colitis, ESM significantly enhanced gene expression of inflammatory mediators, intestinal epithelial cell proliferation, and antimicrobial peptides[191] ESM hydrolysate inhibits secretion *in vitro* of the pro-inflammatory cytokine IL-8. *In vivo* treatment with ESM hydrolysate reduced DSS-induced weight loss, signs of colitis, and secretion of IL-6, along with the attenuation of IL-10-mediated severe intestinal inflammation.[192] Finally, ESM powder has been shown to prevent liver fibrosis and cirrhosis in a rat model of carbon tetrachloride (CCl_4)-induced liver injury.[193]

19.6.2.4 Antioxidant

ESM hydrolysate has been evaluated as a functional food ingredient to control cardiovascular disease; it possesses antioxidant activity and inhibits ACE *in vitro*.[64] In a related study, SEP exhibited scavenging activities for superoxide and hydroxyl radicals, and prevented hydroxyl radical-induced DNA damage, suggesting the potential application of ESM as a cost-effective antioxidant.[63] Dietary supplementation with ESM alleviates oxidative stress, liver enzymes, and collagen accumulation in the CCI_4-induced liver injury model in Wistar rats. ESM showed an anti-fibrotic effect through suppression of oxidative stress and promotion of collagen degradation by inhibiting hepatic stellate cells (HSCs) transformation.[193]

19.6.2.5 Biosensors

ESM has been utilized for the fabrication of biosensors for various target compounds, including inorganic and organic compounds as well as biomacromolecules and dyes.[194–216]

19.6.2.5.1 Biosensor for Inorganic Compounds. An amperometric biosensor was fabricated from carbonized ESM (CESM), gold nanoparticles (AuNPs), and horseradish peroxidase (HRP), which showed superior electrochemical redox behavior and exhibited good biocompatibility and accuracy along with high sensitivity for hydrogen peroxide (H_2O_2) detection.[212] In a related study, a DNAzyme-based chemiluminescence (CL) biosensor for efficient detection of H_2O_2 was developed *via* immobilization of DNAzyme (DNA oligonucleotide with peroxidase activity) on ESM, which showed high catalytic activity in strong alkaline medium as compared to typical HRP-based H_2O_2 biosensors.[195] A graphene oxide-doped ESM (GO-ESM) platform was used to coat carbon ceramic electrodes (CCE) and then modified with Prussian blue *via* a simple dip-coating strategy to prepare a H_2O_2 electrochemical sensor that was capable of detecting H_2O_2 in spiked milk samples.[199]

19.6.2.5.2 Dyes. A solid-surface fluorescence biosensor fabricated by immobilizing acriflavine (AY) on ESM was evaluated for the rapid detection of Sudan I–IV. Under optimal conditions, the fluorescence of AY-ESM could be efficiently quenched by Sudan I–IV and showed lower detection limits, higher sensitivity, and selectivity, along with superior stability, as compared to in solution-based detection systems.[197]

19.6.2.5.3 Macromolecules. ESM was evaluated as a matrix to develop a label-free immunoassay system for the determination of immunoglobulin G (IgG) in human serum. Rabbit anti-human IgG (Ab) was immobilized on ESM; the target human IgG antigen (Ag) and poly(diallyldimethylammonium chloride) (PDDA) were captured through immunoreaction and electrostatic interaction, respectively. The light-scattering signal produced by PDDA is directly related to the concentration of target Ag and gave results comparable to those obtained by the general immunonephelometric method.[202] In a related study, a sandwich immunoassay biosensor was fabricated by immobilization of rabbit anti-human IgG (primary antibody) onto ESM membrane and evaluated for the detection of human IgG (HIgG) in serum. The detection scheme depends on the capture of HIgG by ESM-immobilized rabbit anti-human IgG for detection by goat anti-human IgG labeled with fluorescein isothiocynate (FITC, secondary antibody). The fabricated biosensor showed a prolonged lifetime with a detection range of 20–100 ng mL^{-1}. The biosensor exhibited a linear response and generated results comparable to immunonephelometry.[204] Another sandwich immunosensor using ESM as a matrix was evaluated for the detection of human immunoglobulin M (HIgM) in serum. Goat anti-human IgM antibody (primary antibody) was immobilized on ESM to capture HIgM for detection by a second FTIC-labeled goat anti-human IgM (secondary antibody). This sandwich biosensor exhibited superior storage stability and a linear detection range of 5–60 ng mL^{-1} with a detection limit of 4.3 ng mL^{-1}, which is comparable to other immunonephelometric methods.[203] In addition, haptoglobin (Hp)- and 3-aminophenylboronic acid (APBA)-modified ESM has been assessed as a three-dimensional (3D) label-free electrochemical detection system for multiple diabetes markers. This system achieved high precision for the simultaneous detection of total and glycated hemoglobin (HbA1c) with acceptable reproducibility. However, the overall shelf life of the system was under a month.[194] ESM functionalized with *n*-butyl acetate or acetic acid is suitable as a matrix for immobilization of oligonucleotides for subsequent detection of target DNA. Modification of ESM with *n*-butyl acetate shifted the lower limit of detection of the biosensor to 10 nM of target DNA.[200]

19.6.2.5.4 Organic Molecules. A glucose biosensor was developed by covalent immobilization of glucose oxidase (GOx) on ESM in combination with an oxygen electrode. The detection mechanism depends on the depletion of dissolved oxygen content owing to the reaction of glucose oxidase with glucose. This glucose biosensor exhibited a fast and linear response, good specificity, high sensitivity, and good storage stability (4 months shelf life), and has been used to determine glucose in commercial glucose preparations and wines.[209] Similarly, GOx immobilized onto ESM showed a linear detection response of 1–1000 mM for glucose with a shelf life of 6 weeks.[201] In a related study, a combination of gold nanoparticles (AuNPs) with ESM has been utilized to immobilize glucose oxidase(GOx) for glucose biosensing with a linear response range of 20 μM to 0.8 mM glucose.[213,215] A CL flow-through glucose biosensor was fabricated by immobilizing GOx and horseradish peroxidase (HRP) on ESM, based on the enzymatic oxidation of glucose to D-gluconic acid and H_2O_2, which in turn oxidizes luminol to produce CL emission in the presence of HRP, with successful application for the determination of glucose in human serum.[196] Finally, a non-enzymatic glucose biosensor was developed for detection of glucose in clinical samples including urine and serum by modifying ESM (as a template) with hierarchical porous Au networks (HPANs) serving as an electrocatalyst for glucose oxidization.[216]

An alcohol biosensor was fabricated by immobilizing ethanol oxidase–chitosan on ESM, based on the ethanol-dependent consumption of dissolved oxygen, for detection of ethanol in wine.[208] Similarly, an aspartame optical biosensor was prepared by immobilization of α-chymotrypsin and alcohol oxidase onto ESM in combination with oxygen-sensitive optode membrane as the transducer; the sensor exhibited a detection range of 0.056 to 3.07 mM.[210] A uric acid biosensor was fabricated by the immobilization of uricase on ESM in combination with an oxygen electrode, to detect the depletion of dissolved oxygen owing to the action of uricase on uric acid.[214] Furthermore, a biosensor for detection of organophosphorus pesticides (OPs) in fruit samples was developed by immobilizing CdTe quantum dots (QDs) and a bi-enzyme complex (acetylcholinesterase (AChE)–choline oxidase (ChOx)). The detection mechanism depends on the inhibition of enzymatic activity by OPs with a subsequent reduction in H_2O_2. The decreased H_2O_2 resulted in diminished quenching of fluorescent CdTe QDs.[211]

Tyrosinase immobilized on ESM was utilized as a biosensor for dopamine with a linear response and a detection limit of 25 μM.[206] Similarly, an optical biosensor using ESM-immobilized tyrosinase was evaluated for the detection of L-tyrosine (L-Tyr), based on the enzymatic oxidation of L-Tyr to dopaquinone, and its interaction with 3-methyl-2-benzothiazolinonehydrazone.[198] In addition, a salbutamol biosensor was fabricated by the immobilization of *R*-phycoerythrin (*R*-PE), with a detection strategy based on the decrease in the fluorescence intensity in the presence of salbutamol.[205] Finally, ESM ashes generated by microwave-assisted processing are a green, rapid, fluorescent, and water-soluble source of carbon nanodots (C-Dots) for detection of glutathione.[207]

19.6.2.6 Chemical Processing Support

ESM is a natural solid-phase support for chemical processing in a variety of applications, including catalysis, medical imaging, and optics.[9] ESM in combination with *n*-dodecanethiol has been utilized to produce $BaCrO_4$ biomimetic nano-superstructures with branch-like and feather-like morphologies that exhibited different optical properties from bulk materials.[217] ESM has been coated with ZrO_2 *via* a sol–gel coating procedure and subsequent calcination to produce hierarchically ordered thin films with a macroporous network structure comprising crystalline ZrO2 tubes.[218] In addition, ESM has been evaluated for the development of functional nanomaterials. ESM fibers containing active functional groups including amine, hydroxyl, and imine were utilized to prepare PbS nanoclusters. In this model, ESM served as the reactive substrate and ESM biomacromolecules served as the surfactant, while PbS nanocrystallites were *in situ* assembled into well-distributed nanoparticle aggregations. This hybrid PbS–ESM nanocomposite could be utilized in nanostructured devices, optoelectronic fields, and semiconductor industries.[219] Furthermore, ESM has been utilized to fabricate hierarchical biomorphic mesoporous TiO_2 with interwoven meshwork conformation and a hierarchical porous structure of intersecting fibers assembled by nanocrystallites.[220] Moreover, ESM has been utilized to separate racemic amino acids and their derivatives by electrodialysis.[221] ESM decorated with Ag NPs has been evaluated as a surface-enhanced Raman scattering platform after synthesis *in situ* by reduction of silver nitrate with ascorbic acid.[222] Finally, oxidized ESM has been utilized to immobilize *Burkholderia cepacia* lipase (BCL) for ester hydrolysis and *trans*-esterification. BCL stably bonded to oxidized ESM with enhanced catalytic activity.[223]

19.6.2.7 Cosmetics

ESM contains bioactive components, including collagens, proteoglycans, and glycosaminoglycans, that show great potential in cosmeceuticals.[9] The effect of ESM hydrolysates (ESMH) on wrinkle, UV, and moisture protection has been evaluated *in vitro* and *in vivo*. Human fibroblasts exposed to ultraviolet-B radiation (UV–B) and with ESMH showed increased collagen and decreased expression of matrix metalloproteinases (MMPs). Treatment of human keratinocytes with ESMH led to enhanced release of hyaluronic acid. Mice exposed to UV-B to induce wrinkles before treatment with ESMH showed reduced skin damage compared to non-treated mice, suggesting potential applications in functional cosmetic materials.[187] Various patents have been issued for ESM hydrolysate alone or in combination with other ingredients for cosmetic applications.[9]

19.6.2.8 Electrochemical Cells

Owing to the microporous architecture of ESM, carbonized ESM is a natural polysulfide reservoir for highly reversible Li–S batteries. Sucrose modification of carbonized ESM improves electrical conductivity without altering the microporosity. A novel ESM-based reservoir localized the dissolved polysulfides and stabilized the electrochemical reaction within the cathode region, along with promotion of high discharge capacity, long-term cycle stability, and high sulfur loading.[224] A 3D fibrous ESM-based lightweight supercapacitor showed outstanding electrochemical performance, including low resistance, fast charge–discharge capability, and good cycling stability.[225,226]

19.6.2.9 Food Supplement

A commercial method has been developed to effectively separate ESM from eggshells to create a shell-free ESM dietary supplement (NEM®) powder.[227] The safety of NEM® was evaluated using *in vitro* and *in vivo* toxicological studies with human cells, various *S. typhimurium* strains, and oral administration in a rat model.[228] The positive effect of NEM® on collagen-induced arthritis was demonstrated in a rat model of inflammation and rheumatoid arthritis.[229] Furthermore, the efficacy and safety of NEM® as a therapeutic supplementation for pain and stiffness associated with joint disorders were evaluated in human clinical studies.[227,230] Finally, outer ESM (OESM) has been evaluated as a delivery system for polysaccharide–protein microcapsules incorporated with vitamin E. The combined OESM–microcapsule delivery system demonstrated significantly superior controlled release properties as compared to microcapsules alone.[231]

19.6.2.10 Guided Tissue Regeneration

19.6.2.10.1 Bone Tissue Regeneration. ESM has been evaluated for bone regeneration as it contains collagens known to play a regulatory role in osteoblastic growth and differentiation.[232] In addition, ESM has been shown to mineralize *in vitro*.[41] Although ESM exhibits limited regenerative capacity and early collapse of the membranes in animal models,[112,232,233] it has been used as an interpositional material in rabbit osteotomized ulnar experiments as an active barrier against bone bridging.[234]

19.6.2.10.2 Nerve Tissue Regeneration. Owing to its proteinaceous nature and structural properties, ESM is a potential biomaterial for nerve tissue engineering applications. A double network fibrous construct composed of ESM combined with polycaprolactone fumarate (PCLF) showed superior mechanical features as compared to native ESM. In addition, the construct (ESM–PCLF) promoted attachment, proliferation, and spreading of neurogenic PC12 cells.[235] An ESM tube conduit improved nerve regeneration and promoted functional recovery of the injured sciatic nerve in a rat model.[236]

19.6.2.10.3 Wound Healing. ESM is widely used in traditional Chinese medicine for the management of wounds and burn injuries.[10,12] The first significant study to assess the efficacy of ESM as a biological dressing was carried out in the early 1980s in a rabbit model, where the formation of well-organized collagenous tissue was demonstrated in treated wounds.[237] An ESM biological dressing applied to the rat full-thickness excisional wound model demonstrated significantly accelerated healing at early stages.[238] In addition, a copper-containing bioactive glass–eggshell membrane (Cu-BG–ESM) nanocomposite showed antibacterial and angiogenic activity *in vitro*, as well as improved angiogenesis and re-epithelialization in full-thickness skin defects in a mouse model.[162] Similarly, a nano-silver-decorated microfibrous eggshell membrane (EM–AgNPs) possesses antimicrobial activity against *E. coli* and *S. aureus in vitro*. In a murine full-thickness skin wound model, EM–AgNPs promoted re-epithelialization, granulation tissue formation, and wound healing *via* enhancing cell proliferation and controlling inflammatory response.[239] Recently, PEP has been evaluated for the promotion of wound healing using a mouse excisional wound splinting model and wound histopathologic scoring. PEP significantly accelerated wound closure at days 3, 7 and 10. Histologic analysis showed improved granulation tissue formation and higher levels of collagen deposition at day 10 in wounds treated with PEP, with limited inflammatory reaction.[5] Moreover, PEP has been shown to promote fibroblast and keratinocyte proliferation, to enhance the differentiation of fibroblast into myofibroblasts, and to regulate the activity of various matrix metalloproteinases.[240]

ESM has been used as a biological dressing for wound healing in various clinical settings.[237,241–244] The application of ESM to a human skin graft donor site and skin burn promoted satisfactory re-epithelialization.[237] In addition, ESM has been used for the satisfactory healing of a full-thickness traumatic lip laceration.[244] Similarly, ESM has been assessed clinically as a biological dressing to promote infection-free healing and pain relief in human split-thickness skin graft donor sites, demonstrating cost-effective promotion of healing, wound protection, and pain relief.[243,244] Furthermore, an ESM-based patch to treat tympanic membrane perforation in human subjects demonstrated significantly improved healing compared to spontaneous healing controls.[241,242]

SEP showed superior ability to support GTR as compared to the native ESM.[58] NIH3T3 cell morphology, adhesion, and proliferation after seeding onto SEP films were comparable to cells seeded onto type I collagen films.[245,246] However, the manipulation of SEP to form various shapes and formats is technically difficult. Furthermore, SEP-based constructs possess poor mechanical features. To overcome these limitations, SEP can be blended with various natural and synthetic materials to produce films and fibers with satisfactory mechanical properties.[58] SEP in combination with pepsin-solubilized collagen (PSC) promoted the reconstruction of highly ordered collagen matrices that are capable of resisting various solubilization conditions.[59] Superfine particles of SEP blended with polyurethane (PU) resulted in the formation of nanofibers with enhanced mechanical properties.[10] Furthermore, blending of SEP with chitosan,[247] poly(lactic acid) (PLA),[248–250] PVA,[25] and poly(propylene carbonate) (PPC)[249] led to the formation of films with enhanced mechanical properties and satisfactory biocompatibility with NIH3T3 cells (*i.e. in vitro* cell model). SEP combined with poly(ξ-caprolactone) (PCL)[251,252] or PSC[26] promotes the adhesion and proliferation of human dermal fibroblasts (HDF) *in vitro*. An SEP–poly(lactic-*co*-glycolic acid) (PLGA) electrospun membrane, which had a uniform and interconnected porous network structure, showed improved mechanical properties and promoted the attachment, spreading, and proliferation of murine fibroblast cells.[253] Finally, a water-soluble alkaline-digested form of eggshell membrane (ASESM) immobilized on phosphorylcholine showed a fibrous surface that promoted the adhesion of HDF.[12]

19.6.2.11 Medical Technology

The chicken egg has been used as a cost-effective surgical tool to train residents in acquisition of surgical skills required for temporal bone drilling. Residents were trained through drilling and dissection of the eggshell without compromising the eggshell membrane.[254] In addition, ESM has been evaluated as an eye protectant during 5-aminolevulinic acid photodynamic therapy (ALA-PDT) for eyelid actinic keratosis in human subjects. ESM provided good protection for eyes during ALA-PDT therapy, with reduced discomfort, redness, and itching, without interfering with ALA penetration or the PDT effect.[255]

19.6.2.12 Mucoadhesion Assessment

ESM has been used for *in vitro* evaluation of the mucoadhesion capacity of various drugs,[256] yielding reliable data in terms of detachment force and work of adhesion.[257] Tablets prepared from ethylcellulose showed a two-fold increase of adhesiveness to ESM as compared to hard fat tablets.[258] Finally,

ESM was utilized to evaluate the mucoadhesion properties of acyclovir (an antiviral drug)-loaded mucoadhesive microspheres (ACV-ad-ms). Adherence of microspheres to ESM yielded similar results as for adherence to mouse stomach mucosa.[256]

19.7 Commercialization

Various applications of ES and ESM are illustrated in Figure 19.3. A number of processes for harvesting and exploitation of ES and ESM have been patented.[9] However, despite intense research to identify novel biological and biomedical applications of ES/ESM, there remains a gap between identification of ES/ESM-based biomaterials at the laboratory scale and its implementation at a commercial scale. Table 19.2 shows value-added applications of ES

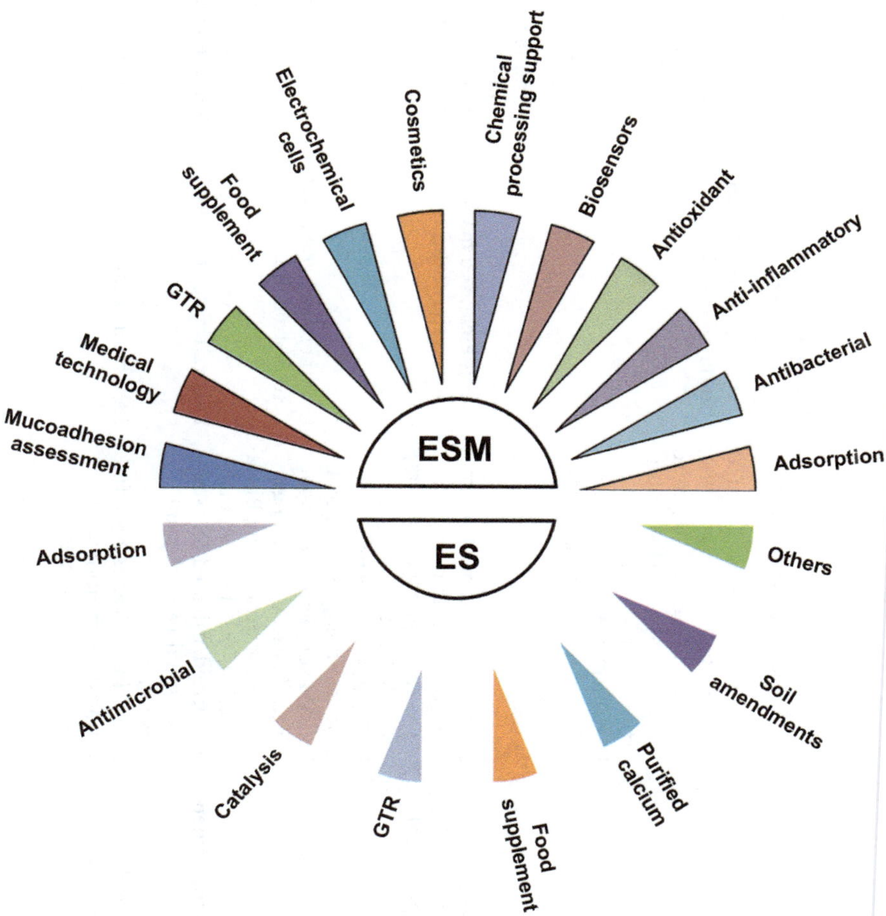

Figure 19.3 Scheme summarizing range of applications for ES and ESM.

Table 19.2 Comparative assessment. Value-added products from processed eggshell (ES)/eggshell membrane (ESM).

Value-added application	Product source/description	Stage of development/ operation level	Product function/advantage	Estimated market: Investment/ Benefit[a]
Human joint health	Utilize ESM to develop natural products for pharmaceuticals, *e.g.*: Ovomet®, Eggnovo, Navarra, Spain; NEM®, Stratum nutrition ESM Technologies, MO, USA; Biovaflex®, Biova, LLC, IA, USA	Commercialized market, industrial scale	Ovomet® claims: Reduced inflammation, regenerate cartilage NEM® claims: Improve joint mobility and production of cartilage and connective tissues Biovalex® claims: Reduces lower back pain in 5 days, promotes natural anti-inflammatory response from free radical-induced damage to the joints	High/High
Human nutritional supplement	ES-derived calcium carbonate as food supplement, *e.g.*: Ovocet®, Eggnovo, Navarra, Spain; NEM ESC®, Stratum Nutrition ESM Technologies, MO, USA	Commercialized market, industrial scale	Ovocet® claims: Strengthen bones ESC® claims: Facilitate calcium absorption and maintain healthy bone mineral density	High/High
Animal feed	ES/ESM supplements for pet health, *e.g.*: Ovopet®, Eggnovo, Navarra, Spain; BiovaPlex®, Biova, LLC, IA, USA	Commercialized market, industrial scale	Ovopet®– pet joint claims: reduce inflammation, regenerate cartilage BiovaPlex® claims: Support essential joint and skin health needs	High/High
Soil amendment	Pulverized, calcined ES as a natural lime-based soil conditioner	Laboratory scale	Remineralizes soil and controls pH	Low/Medium
Biodiesel Production	ES/calcined ES as catalyst for transesterification of triglycerides with methanol	Laboratory scale	Enhances the yield (96.7–99.1%), reusable solid catalyst	—

Skin care	Water-soluble ESM as a nutri-cosmetic ingredient for skin health, *e.g.*: BiovaBio™, Biovaderm®, Biova, LLC, IA, USA; Ovoderm®, Eggnovo, Navarra, Spain	Commercialized market, industrial scale	Ovoderm® claims: Promote hydration, firmness, and cutaneous regeneration BiovaBio™ claims: Increases skin elasticity and reduces roughness, reduce free radical and oxidative damage associated with aging Biovaderm® claims: Reduces appearance of fine lines and wrinkles, improves moisture retention and hydrates skin	High/High
Purified $CaCO_3$	ES-derived $CaCO_3$ free of organic solvents for construction sector cement, glass, paint, dye, and mortar ingredients	Pilot scale	Improves the packing and densification properties of soil–cement material, accelerates hydration, improves the thermal properties, crystallization behavior, and mechanical properties of glass	High/High
Biomaterial composite	Hydroxyapatite from ES for orthopedic and dental implants	Laboratory scale	High compatibility with human soft tissue, enhances bone repair	High/High
Wound healing	ESM-derived biological dressing for skin burns, skin graft donor sites, and chronic wounds, *e.g.*: DermaRep™, Biovotec, Oslo, Norway (product launch 2019)	Commercialized market, industrial scale	A novel, low-cost biological wound dressing that promotes re-epithelialization and granulation tissue formation	High/High
Bioplastics	Powdered ES as an economical plastic filler, *e.g.*: Eggshell powder by just Egg processing plant Leicester, UK is used by Silvergate Plastics, Wrexham, UK	Commercialized market, industrial scale	Less dense and lighter, economical, and environmental friendly product	High/High

[a]Estimated market (Investment): Low – investing up to $500K USD in the installation of the application; Medium – investing more than $500K USD in the installation of the application; High – investing more than $1M USD in the installation of the application. Estimated market (Benefit): Low – economic benefit ≤ established cost for the treatment of residues; Medium – economic benefit ≤ 5 × established cost for the treatment of residues; High – economic benefit > 5 × established cost for the treatment of residues.

and ESM with their advantages, economic benefits, and investment required. A variety of ESM supplements are available, such as Kordel's BiovaFlex® eggshell membrane; Swanson ultra-natural eggshell membrane,[49] and Jamieson natural eggshell membrane (NEM®).[188,190,227–230] Development of novel technologies, including micro- and nano-fabrication, to produce ES/ESM-based functional platforms is necessary to transform ESM-based research to the commercial scale.

19.8 Conclusion and Prospects

Chicken egg processing plants produce considerable amounts of ES and ESM waste, which is a useful resource as raw materials for various applications and secondary processing. This chapter summarizes the applications of ES and ESM as valuable bio-resources in different fields from low to high value. The reuse of ES and ESM waste can reduce the risk of microbial contamination and the cost of landfill disposal. The recycling of ES will preserve a non-renewable biological source of calcium, while the reuse of ESM generates various beneficial protein-based interventions. ES and ESM exhibit unique physicochemical and biological properties, which cannot be chemically synthesized. This overview of ES and ESM applications could form the basis for pilot studies to confirm technological and economic feasibility before industrial-scale implementation. Many *in vitro* biological applications of ES waste have been described, while *in vivo* studies are essential in order to justify claims of human health benefits. However, ESM has been assessed extensively *in vitro* and evaluated *in vivo* for GTR as well as for human food supplements. The development of ES as a physical platform is important for promoting its utilization in diverse fields, including biological, biomedical, agricultural, and environmental. The processing of ESM into various forms will diversify its utilization for different applications. There is a need to prepare micro- or nano-scale units of ES and ESM to increase the bioavailability of the biologically active components, in order to preserve and enhance their unique structures and bioactivities.

Acknowledgements

Preparation of this chapter was supported by funding from the Natural Sciences and Engineering Research Council to MTH (NSERC-discovery RGPIN/2016-04410 and NSERC CRD CRDPJ/514335-2017).

References

1. FAO, *FAO Statistical Pocketbook*, 2015, vol. 2015.
2. K. Thomson, *Land use policy*, 2003, **20**, 375.
3. W. T. Tsai, J. M. Yang, C. W. Lai, Y. H. Cheng, C. C. Lin and C. W. Yeh, *Bioresour. Technol.*, 2006, **97**, 488.

4. W. Russ, and M. Schnappinger, in *Utilization of By-Products and Treatment of Waste in the Food Industry*, 2007, p. 1.
5. T. A. E. Ahmed, H.-P. Suso, A. Maqbool and M. T. Hincke, *Mater. Sci. Eng., C*, 2019, **95**, 192.
6. H. J. Park, S. W. Jeong, J. K. Yang, B. G. Kim and S. M. Lee, *J. Environ. Sci.*, 2007, **19**, 1436.
7. A. Schaafsma and G. M. Beelen, *J. Sci. Food Agric.*, 1999, **79**, 1596.
8. J. Neunzehn, T. Szuwart and H. P. Wiesmann, *Head Face Med.*, 2015, **11**, 12.
9. C. M. Cordeiro and M. T. Hincke, *Recent Pat. Food, Nutr. Agric.*, 2011, **3**, 1.
10. L. Chen, J. Kang and S. Sukigara, *Biomed. Mater. Eng.*, 2014, **24**, 1979.
11. M. Balaz, *Acta Biomater.*, 2014, **10**, 3827.
12. E. Ohto-Fujita, T. Konno, M. Shimizu, K. Ishihara, T. Sugitate, J. Miyake, K. Yoshimura, K. Taniwaki, T. Sakurai, Y. Hasebe and Y. Atomi, *Cell Tissue Res.*, 2011, **345**, 177.
13. M. T. Hincke, Y. Nys, J. Gautron, K. Mann, A. B. Rodriguez-Navarro and M. D. McKee, *Front. Biosci.*, 2012, **17**, 1266.
14. Y. Nys, M. T. Hincke, J. L. Arias, J. M. Garcia-Ruiz and S. E. Solomon, *Avian Poult. Biol. Rev.*, 1999, **10**, 143.
15. O. Wellman-Labadie, S. Lemaire, K. Mann, J. Picman and M. T. Hincke, *J. Agric. Food Chem.*, 2010, **58**, 10156.
16. R. G. Board and N. A. Halls, *Br. Poult. Sci.*, 1973, **14**, 69.
17. A. B. Rodriguez-Navarro, N. Dominguez-Gasca, A. Munoz and M. Ortega-Huertas, *Poult. Sci.*, 2013, **92**, 3026.
18. A. L. Romanoff and A. J. Romanoff, *The Avian Egg*, Wiley, New York, 1942, vol. 918.
19. M. M. Bain, K. McDade, R. Burchmore, A. Law, P. W. Wilson, M. Schmutz, R. Preisinger and I. C. Dunn, *Anim. Genet.*, 2013, **44**, 661.
20. M. A. Soares, M. J. Quina and R. M. Quinta-Ferreira, *J. Environ. Manage.*, 2015, **164**, 137.
21. A. B. Rodriguez-Navarro, P. Marie, Y. Nys, M. T. Hincke and J. Gautron, *J. Struct. Biol.*, 2015, **190**, 291.
22. J. L. Arias, D. J. Fink, S. Q. Xiao, A. H. Heuer and A. I. Caplan, *Int. Rev. Cytol.*, 1993, **145**, 217.
23. T. A. Ahmed, H. P. Suso and M. T. Hincke, *J. Proteomics*, 2017, **155**, 49.
24. M. L. Rose and M. T. Hincke, *Cell. Mol. Life Sci.*, 2009, **66**, 2707.
25. F. Yi, J. W. Lu, Z. X. Guo and J. Yu, *J. Biomater. Sci., Polym. Ed.*, 2006, **17**, 1015.
26. T. Ino, M. Hattori, T. Yoshida, S. Hattori, K. Yoshimura and K. Takahashi, *Biosci., Biotechnol., Biochem.*, 2006, **70**, 865.
27. C. A. Lunam and J. Ruiz, *Br. Poult. Sci.*, 2000, **41**, 584.
28. N. H. C. Sparks, *Microbiology of the Avian Egg*, Springer, US, Boston, 1994, pp. 25–42.
29. F. Baron, S. Jan, F. Gonnet, M. Pasco, J. Jardin, B. Giudici, M. Gautier, C. Guerin-Dubiard and F. Nau, *J. Food Prot.*, 2014, **77**, 955.

30. M. Rose-Martel, J. Du and M. T. Hincke, *J. Proteomics*, 2012, **75**, 2697.
31. M. Rose-Martel and M. T. Hincke, in *Egg Innovations and Strategies for Improvements*, Elsevier, 2017, pp. 157–163.
32. O. Wellman-Labadie, J. Picman and M. T. Hincke, *Br. Poult. Sci.*, 2008, **49**, 125.
33. K. Mann, B. Macek and J. V. Olsen, *Proteomics*, 2006, **6**, 3801.
34. P. Marie, V. Labas, A. Brionne, G. Harichaux, C. Hennequet-Antier, Y. Nys and J. Gautron, *J. Proteomics*, 2015, **126**, 140.
35. C. Sun, G. Xu and N. Yang, *Proteomics*, 2013, **13**, 3523.
36. T. Nakano, N. I. Ikawa and L. Ozimek, *Poult. Sci.*, 2003, **82**, 510.
37. C. M. Cordeiro and M. T. Hincke, *J. Proteomics*, 2016, **130**, 11.
38. V. K. Kodali, S. A. Gannon, S. Paramasivam, S. Raje, T. Polenova and C. Thorpe, *PLoS One*, 2011, **6**, e18187.
39. S. Makkar, R. Liyanage, L. Kannan, B. Packialakshmi, J. O. Lay Jr and N. C. Rath, *J. Agric. Food Chem.*, 2015, **63**, 9888.
40. M. Rose-Martel, S. Smiley and M. T. Hincke, *J. Proteomics*, 2015, **116**, 81.
41. J. L. Arias, O. Nakamura, M. S. Fernandez, J. J. Wu, P. Knigge, D. R. Eyre and A. I. Caplan, *Connect. Tissue Res.*, 1997, **36**, 21.
42. M. T. Hincke, J. Gautron, M. Panheleux, J. Garcia-Ruiz, M. D. McKee and Y. Nys, *Matrix Biol.*, 2000, **19**, 443.
43. Y. S. Ok, S. S. Lee, W. T. Jeon, S. E. Oh, A. R. Usman and D. H. Moon, *Environ. Geochem. Health*, 2011, **33**(Suppl 1), 31.
44. S. Yoo, J. S. Hsieh, P. Zou and J. Kokoszka, *Bioresour. Technol.*, 2009, **100**, 6416.
45. J. H. MacNeil, Penn State Research Foundation. Method and apparatus for separating a protein membrane and shell material in waste egg shells, *US Pat.* 7007806B2, 2006.
46. J. H. MacNeil, Penn State Research Foundation. Hatchery eggshell waste processing method and device, *US Pat.* 6899294B2, 2005.
47. D. Cree and A. Rutter, *ACS Sustainable Chem. Eng.*, 2015, **3**, 941.
48. Z. Xi and M. Meihu, *China Agric. Sci.*, 2010, **43**, 1031.
49. D. A. Oliveira, P. Benelli and E. R. Amante, *J. Cleaner Prod.*, 2013, **46**, 42.
50. M. Al Mijan, D. H. Kim and H. S. Kwak, *Int. J. Food Sci. Technol.*, 2014, **49**, 1751.
51. S. Huang, J. C. Chen, C. W. Hsu and W. H. Chang, *Nanotechnology*, 2009, **20**, 375102.
52. Z. Wei, C. Xu and B. Li, *Bioresour. Technol.*, 2009, **100**, 2883.
53. N. Viriya-Empikul, P. Krasae, B. Puttasawat, B. Yoosuk, N. Chollacoop and K. Faungnawakij, *Bioresour. Technol.*, 2010, **101**, 3765.
54. E. M. Rivera, M. Araiza, W. Brostow, V. M. Castano, J. Dıaz-Estrada, R. Hernández and J. R. Rodrıguez, *Mater. Lett.*, 1999, **41**, 128.
55. G. S. Kumar, A. Thamizhavel and E. K. Girija, *Mater. Lett.*, 2012, **76**, 198.
56. A. A. Hamidi, M. N. Salimi and A. H. M. Yusoff, *AIP Conf. Proc.*, 2017, **1835**, 020045.

57. M. Arami, N. Yousefi Limaee and N. M. Mahmoodi, *Chemosphere*, 2006, **65**, 1999.
58. M. K. Sah and S. N. Rath, *Mater. Sci. Eng., C*, 2016, **67**, 807.
59. K. Takahashi, K. Shirai, M. Kitamura and M. Hattori, *Biosci., Biotechnol., Biochem.*, 1996, **60**, 1299.
60. Y. L. Li, Extraction of egg membrane extract useful in cosmetics, *CN Pat.* CN111514A, 1995.
61. S. Jain and A. K. Anal, *J. Food Sci. Technol.*, 2017, **54**, 1062.
62. M. Cheng, S. Takenaka, S. Aoki, S. Murakami and K. Aoki, *J. Biosci. Bioeng.*, 2009, **107**, 373.
63. X. Huang, Y. Zhou, M. Ma, Z. Cai and T. Li, *J. Agric. Food Chem.*, 2010, **58**, 12137.
64. A. Santana, A. Melo, T. Tavares and I. M. Ferreira, *Food Funct.*, 2016, **7**, 4597.
65. J. Carvalho, J. Araujo and F. Castro, *Waste Biomass Valorization*, 2011, **2**, 157.
66. M. Ives, R. C. Mundy, P. S. Fennell, J. F. Davidson, J. S. Dennis and A. N. Hayhurst, *Energy Fuels*, 2008, **22**, 3852.
67. T. Witoon, *Ceram. Int.*, 2011, **37**, 3291.
68. M. Mohammadi, P. Lahijani and A. Mohamed, *Chem. Eng. J.*, 2014, **243**, 455.
69. S. Shan, A. Ma, Y. Hu, Q. Jia, Y. Wang and J. Peng, *Environ. Pollut.*, 2016, **208**, 546.
70. S. Hosseini, F. E. Babadi, S. M. Soltani, M. K. Aroua, S. Babamohammadia and A. M. Moghadam, *Process Saf. Environ. Prot.*, 2017, **109**, 387.
71. M. Ahmad, A. R. A. Usman, S. S. Lee, S. C. Kim, J. H. Joo, J. E. Yang and Y. S. Ok, *J. Ind. Eng. Chem.*, 2012, **18**, 198.
72. W. Zheng, X. M. Li, Q. Yang, G. M. Zeng, X. X. Shen, Y. Zhang and J. J. Liu, *J. Hazard. Mater.*, 2007, **147**, 534.
73. A. Guijarro-Aldaco, V. Hernández-Montoya, A. Bonilla-Petriciolet, M. A. Montes-Morán and D. I. Mendoza-Castillo, *Ind. Eng. Chem. Res.*, 2011, **50**, 9354.
74. M. A. R. Soares, S. Marto, M. J. Quina, L. Gando-Ferreira and R. Quinta-Ferreira, *Water, Air, Soil Pollut.*, 2016, **227**, 150.
75. T. Zhang, Z. Tu, G. Lu, X. Duan, X. Yi, C. Guo and Z. Dang, *J. Environ. Manage.*, 2017, **188**, 1.
76. Y. Wu, J. Wei, S. Guo, K. Yu, Z. Zhuang and Y. Yu, *J. Mater. Chem. A*, 2017, **5**, 20448.
77. O. Kaplan Ince, M. Ince, V. Yonten and A. Goksu, *Food Chem.*, 2017, **214**, 637.
78. M. F. Elkady, A. M. Ibrahim and M. M. Abd El-Latif, *Desalination*, 2011, **278**, 412.
79. P. S. Guru and S. Dash, *J. Dispersion Sci. Technol.*, 2013, **34**, 1099.
80. D. Podstawczyk, A. Witek-Krowiak, K. Chojnacka and Z. Sadowski, *Bioresour. Technol.*, 2014, **160**, 161.

81. E. N. Seyahmazegi, R. Mohammad-Rezaei and H. Razmi, *Chem. Eng. Res. Des.*, 2016, **109**, 824.
82. M. Nasrollahzadeh, S. M. Sajadi and A. Hatamifard, *Appl. Catal., B*, 2016, **191**, 209.
83. M. A. El-Kemary, I. M. El-Mehasseb, K. R. Shoueir, S. E. El-Shafey, O. I. El-Shafey, H. A. Aljohani and R. R. Fouad, *J. Dispersion Sci. Technol.*, 2018, **39**, 911.
84. J. Gautron, M. T. Hincke, K. Mann, M. Panheleux, M. Bain, M. D. McKee, S. E. Solomon and Y. Nys, *J. Biol. Chem.*, 2001, **276**, 39243.
85. O. Wellman-Labadie, R. Lakshminarayanan and M. T. Hincke, *FEBS Lett.*, 2008, **582**, 699.
86. S. Ishikawa, K. Suzuki, E. Fukuda, K. Arihara, Y. Yamamoto, T. Mukai and M. Itoh, *FEBS Lett.*, 2010, **584**, 770.
87. M. Ota, C. Toyofuku, C. Thammakarn, N. Sangsriratanakul, M. Yamada, K. Nakajima, M. Kitazawa, H. Hakimullah Hakim, S. Alam, D. Shoham and K. Takehara, *J. Vet. Med. Sci.*, 2016, **78**, 831.
88. V. Apalangya, V. Rangari, B. Tiimob, S. Jeelani and T. Samuel, *Appl. Surf. Sci.*, 2014, **295**, 108.
89. B. J. Tiimob, G. Mwinyelle, W. Abdela, T. Samuel, S. Jeelani and V. K. Rangari, *J. Agric. Food Chem.*, 2017, **65**, 1967.
90. T. Yadav, A. A. Mungray and A. K. Mungray, *Environ. Nanotechnol. Monit. Manage.*, 2018, **9**, 50.
91. N. Viriya-Empikul, P. Krasae, W. Nualpaeng, B. Yoosuk and K. Faungnawakij, *Fuel*, 2012, **92**, 239.
92. S. B. Chavan, R. R. Kumbhar, D. Madhu, B. Singhd and Y. C. Sharma, *RSC Adv.*, 2015, **5**, 63596.
93. P. Khemthong, C. Luadthong, W. Nualpaeng, P. Changsuwan, P. Tongprem, N. Viriya-empikul and K. Faungnawakij, *Catal. Today*, 2012, **190**, 112.
94. G. Chen, R. Shan, S. Li and J. Shi, *Fuel*, 2015, **153**, 48.
95. D. Zeng, Q. Zhang, S. Chen, S. Liu, Y. Chen, Y. Tian and G. Wang, *J. Environ. Chem. Eng.*, 2015, **3**, 560.
96. A. Piker, B. Tabah, N. Perkas and A. Gedanken, *Fuel*, 2016, **182**, 34.
97. P. R. Pandit and M. H. Fulekar, *J. Environ. Manage.*, 2017, **198**, 319.
98. N. Mansir, S. H. Teo, U. Rashid and Y. H. Taufiq-Yap, *Fuel*, 2018, **211**, 67.
99. A. V. Borhade, B. K. Uphade and A. G. Gadhave, *Res. Chem. Intermed.*, 2016, **42**, 6301.
100. E. Mosaddegh and A. Hassankhani, *Catal. Commun.*, 2013, **33**, 70.
101. E. Mosaddegh, *Ultrason. Sonochem.*, 2013, **20**, 1436.
102. A. Aït-Aissa and M. Aïder, *Int. J. Food Sci. Technol.*, 2014, **49**, 1245.
103. M. Corzo-Martinez, P. Copovi, A. Olano, F. J. Moreno and A. Montilla, *J. Sci. Food Agric.*, 2013, **93**, 1591.
104. A. Montilla, M. D. del Castillo, M. L. Sanz and A. Olano, *Food Chem.*, 2005, **90**, 883.

105. M. Nooshkam and A. Madadlou, *Food Chem.*, 2016, **192**, 831.
106. E. Mosaddegh and A. Hassankhani, *Chin. J. Catal.*, 2014, **35**, 351.
107. E. Mosaddegh, A. Hassankhani, S. Pourahmadi and D. Ghazanfari, *Int. J. Green Nanotechnol.*, 2013, **5**, 1.
108. E. Mosaddegh, A. Hassankhani and H. Karimi-Maleh, *Mater. Sci. Eng., C*, 2015, **46**, 264.
109. A. Uraz, S. E. Gultekin, B. Senguven, B. Karaduman, I. P. Sofuoglu, S. Pehlivan, Y. Capan and K. Eren, *J. Clin. Exp. Dent.*, 2013, **5**, e23.
110. M. Baliga, P. Davies and L. Dupoirieux, *Rev. Stomatol. Chir. Maxillofac.*, 1998, **99**(Suppl 1), 86.
111. L. Dupoirieux, M. Neves and D. Pourquier, *J. Oral Maxillofac. Surg.*, 2000, **58**, 40.
112. E. Durmus, I. Celik, A. Ozturk, Y. Ozkan and M. F. Aydin, *J. Int. Med. Res.*, 2003, **31**, 223.
113. V. S. Kattimani, P. S. Chakravarthi, N. R. Kanumuru, V. V. Subbarao, A. Sidharthan, T. S. S. Kumar and L. K. Prasad, *J. Int. Oral Health*, 2014, **6**, 15.
114. S. C. Onwubu, A. Vahed, S. Singh and K. M. Kanny, *J. Prosthet. Dent.*, 2017, **117**, 310.
115. M. C. Yew, N. H. Ramli Sulong, M. K. Yew, M. A. Amalina and M. R. Johan, *Prog. Org. Coat.*, 2013, **76**, 1549.
116. P. Dadhich, B. Das, P. Pal, P. K. Srivas, J. Dutta, S. Ray and S. Dhara, *ACS Appl. Mater. Interfaces*, 2016, **8**, 11910.
117. R. Jayasree, T. S. Sampath Kumar, K. Pavani Siva Kavya, P. Rakesh Nankar and D. Mukesh, *Bioceram. Dev. Appl.*, 2015, **5**, 1000084.
118. Y. C. Chien, M. T. Hincke and M. D. McKee, *Cells Tissues Organs*, 2009, **189**, 38.
119. M. T. Hincke, Y. C. Chien, L. C. Gerstenfeld and M. D. McKee, *J. Histochem. Cytochem.*, 2008, **56**, 467.
120. G. Gergely, F. Wéber, I. Lukács, A. L. Tóth, Z. E. Horváth, J. Mihály and C. Balázsi, *Ceram. Int.*, 2010, **36**, 803.
121. V. Kattimani, K. P. Lingamaneni, P. S. Chakravarthi, T. S. Kumar and A. Siddharthan, *J. Craniofac. Surg.*, 2016, **27**, 112.
122. N. Elizondo-Villarreal, A. Martínez-De-La-Cruz, R. O. Guerra, J. L. Gómez-Ortega, L. M. Torres-Martínez and V. M. Castaño, *Water, Air, Soil Pollut.*, 2012, **223**, 3643.
123. D. L. Goloshchapov, V. M. Kashkarov, N. A. Rumyantseva, P. V. Seredin, A. S. Lenshin, B. L. Agapov and E. P. Domashevskaya, *Ceram. Int.*, 2013, **39**, 4539.
124. S. C. Wu, H. C. Hsu, S. K. Hsu, Y. C. Chang and W. F. Ho, *Ceram. Int.*, 2015, **41**, 10718.
125. L. Xia, K. Lin, X. Jiang, Y. Xu, M. Zhang, J. Chang and Z. Zhang, *J. Mater. Chem. B*, 2013, **1**, 5403.
126. R. Nithya and N. Meenakshi Sundaram, *Int. J. Nanomed.*, 2015, **10**(Suppl 1), 119.

127. V. H. Ingole, K. Hany Hussein, A. A. Kashale, K. Ghule, T. Vuherer, V. Kokol, J. Y. Chang, Y. C. Ling, A. Vinchurkar, H. N. Dhakal and A. V. Ghule, *J. Biomed. Mater. Res., Part A*, 2017, **105**, 2935.
128. N. Calvert, S. Proulx, T. Ahmed, M. Hincke and I. Catelas, 33rd Annual Meeting of the Canadian Biomaterials Society, Winnipeg, Manitoba, Canada, 2017, (Poster114179).
129. L. R. Brun, M. Lupo, D. A. Delorenzi, V. E. Di Loreto and A. Rigalli, *Int. J. Food Sci. Nutr.*, 2013, **64**, 740.
130. J. Rovensky, M. Stancikova, P. Masaryk, K. Svik and R. Istok, *Int. J. Clin. Pharmacol. Res.*, 2003, **23**, 83.
131. A. Schaafsma and I. Pakan, *Bratisl. Lek. Listy*, 1999, **100**, 651.
132. A. Schaafsma, I. Pakan, G. J. Hofstede, F. A. Muskiet, E. Van Der Veer and P. J. De Vries, *Poult. Sci.*, 2000, **79**, 1833.
133. R. P. Hanzlik, S. C. Fowler and D. H. Fisher, *J. Pharmacol. Exp. Ther.*, 2005, **313**, 1217.
134. K. Sakhaee, T. Bhuket, B. Adams-Huet and D. S. Rao, *Am. J. Ther.*, 1999, **6**, 313.
135. A. Erfanian, H. Mirhosseini, B. Rasti, M. Hair-Bejo, S. Bin Mustafa and M. Y. Abd Manap, *J. Agric. Food Chem.*, 2015, **63**, 5795.
136. N. Gongruttananun, *Poult. Sci.*, 2011, **90**, 524.
137. D. L. Greene, R. Isaac, M. Neuwirth and F. D. Bitan, *J. Spinal Disord. Tech.*, 2007, **20**, 229.
138. A. J. Olarewaju, M. O. Balogun and S. O. Akinlolu, *EJGE*, 2011, **16**, 899.
139. P. Pliya and D. Cree, *Constr. Build. Mater.*, 2015, **95**, 1.
140. F. Ujin, K. S. Ali and Z. Y. Hanur Harith, *Key Eng. Mater.*, 2017, **728**, 402.
141. T. Y. Yu, D. S. Ing, C. S. Choo and M. A. Azed, *Int. J. Adv. Sci., Eng. Inf. Technol.*, 2017, **7**, 1798.
142. T. S. Kang and S. J. Lee, *J. Korean Ceram. Soc.*, 2017, **54**, 395.
143. B. Aktas, M. Albaskara, K. Dogru and S. Yalcin, *Acta Phys. Pol., A*, 2017, **132**, 436.
144. E. R. Essien, V. N. Atasie and E. U. Udobang, *Bull. Mater. Sci.*, 2016, **39**, 989.
145. M. T. Souza, B. G. O. Maia, L. B. Teixeira, K. G. de Oliveira, A. H. B. Teixeira and A. P. Novaes de Oliveira, *Process Saf. Environ. Prot.*, 2017, **111**, 60.
146. M. Farrell, W. T. Perkins, P. J. Hobbs, G. W. Griffith and D. L. Jones, *Environ. Pollut.*, 2010, **158**, 55.
147. J. H. Park, D. Lamb, P. Paneerselvam, G. Choppala, N. Bolan and J. W. Chung, *J. Hazard. Mater.*, 2011, **185**, 549.
148. M. Ashrafi, S. Mohamad, I. Yusoff and F. Shahul Hamid, *Environ. Sci. Pollut. Res. Int.*, 2015, **22**, 223.
149. S. S. Lee, S. A. M. Abd El-Azeem, J. E. Lim, A. U. Rajapaksha, K. R. Kim, Y. H. Lee, Y. B. Lee, Y. Y. Chang and Y. S. Ok, *Chem. Ecol.*, 2013, **29**, 501.

150. M. Ahmad, Y. Hashimoto, D. H. Moon, S. S. Lee and Y. S. Ok, *J. Hazard. Mater.*, 2012, **209–210**, 392.
151. M. J. Quina, M. A. R. Soares, A. A. Ribeiro, A. P. Marques, I. H. Costa and M. C. Magalhães, *Waste Biomass Valorization*, 2014, **5**, 87.
152. M. A. Soares, M. J. Quina and R. Quinta-Ferreira, *Environ. Technol.*, 2016, **37**, 2773.
153. M. Ye, M. Sun, Y. Feng, X. Li, A. P. Schwab, J. Wan, M. Liu, D. Tian, K. Liu, J. Wu and X. Jiang, *J. Agric. Food Chem.*, 2016, **64**, 5446.
154. M. Ye, M. Sun, X. Chen, Y. Feng, J. Wan, K. Liu, D. Tian, M. Liu, J. Wu, A. P. Schwab and X. Jiang, *Waste Manage.*, 2017, **63**, 275.
155. S. Kirboga and M. Öner, *Powder Technol.*, 2013, **249**, 95.
156. N. Tangboriboon, W. Pannangpetch, K. Aranyik, K. Petcharoen and A. Sirivat, *Prog. Rubber, Plast. Recycl. Technol.*, 2015, **31**, 189.
157. B. J. Tiimob, S. Jeelani and V. K. Rangari, *J. Appl. Polym. Sci.*, 2016, **133**, 43124.
158. A. S. M. Bashir, Y. Manusamy, T. L. Chew, H. Ismail and S. Ramasamy, *J. Vinyl Addit. Technol.*, 2017, **23**, 3.
159. Y. Feng, B. Ashok, K. Madhukar, J. Zhang, J. Zhang, K. O. Reddy and A. V. Rajulu, *Int. J. Polym. Anal. Charact.*, 2014, **19**, 637.
160. M. C. Yew, N. H. Ramli Sulong, M. K. Yew, M. A. Amalina and M. R. Johan, *Sci. World J.*, 2014, **2014**, 1–9.
161. M. Bootklad and K. Kaewtatip, *Carbohydr. Polym.*, 2013, **97**, 315.
162. J. Li, D. Zhai, F. Lv, Q. Yu, H. Ma, J. Yin, Z. Yi, M. Liu, J. Chang and C. Wu, *Acta Biomater.*, 2016, **36**, 254.
163. M. A. Al-Ghouti and M. Khan, *J. Environ. Manage.*, 2018, **207**, 405.
164. R. Mallampati and S. Valiyaveettil, *Nanoscale*, 2013, **5**, 3395.
165. K. Suyama, Y. Fukazawa and Y. Umetsu, *Appl. Biochem. Biotechnol.*, 1994, **45–46**, 871.
166. S. Ishikawa, S. Sekine, N. Miura, K. Suyama, K. Arihara and M. Itoh, *Biol. Trace Elem. Res.*, 2004, **102**, 113.
167. T. Yang, M. L. Chen, X. W. Hu, Z. W. Wang, J. H. Wang and P. K. Dasgupta, *Analyst*, 2011, **136**, 83.
168. S. Ishikawa, K. Suyama, K. Arihara and M. Itoh, *Bioresour. Technol.*, 2002, **81**, 201.
169. S. Ishikawa and K. Suyama, *Appl. Biochem. Biotechnol.*, 1998, **70–72**, 719.
170. G. Asgari and A. Dayari, *Data Brief*, 2018, **16**, 442.
171. X. Guo, F. Zhang, Q. Peng, S. Xu, X. Lei, D. G. Evans and X. Duan, *Chem. Eng. J.*, 2011, **166**, 81.
172. A.-M. Zou, X.-W. Chen, M.-L. Chen and J.-H. Wang, *J. Anal. At. Spectrom.*, 2008, **23**, 412.
173. Y. Zhang, W. Wang, L. Li, Y. Huang and J. Cao, *Talanta*, 2010, **80**, 1907.
174. S. Ishikawa, K. Suyama, K. Arihara and M. Itoh, *Biol. Trace Elem. Res.*, 2002, **86**, 227.
175. S. Ishikawa, K. Suyama and I. Satoh, *Appl. Biochem. Biotechnol.*, 1999, **77–79**, 521.

176. M. Balaz, J. Ficeriova and J. Briancin, *Chemosphere*, 2016, **146**, 458.
177. X. Cheng, K. Shao, S. Shen, S. Hu and H. Qiu, *Geostand. Geoanal. Res.*, 2011, **35**, 461.
178. H. Abdolmohammad-Zadeh and Z. Talleb, *Microchim. Acta*, 2014, **181**, 1797.
179. H. Razmi, S. J. Musevi and R. Mohammad-Rezaei, *Microchim. Acta*, 2016, **183**, 555.
180. X. Zou and Y. Huang, *Anal. Methods*, 2013, **5**, 6486.
181. W. Wang, B. Chen, Y. Huang and J. Cao, *J. Chromatogr. A*, 2010, **1217**, 5659.
182. B. Koumanova, P. Peeva, S. J. Allen, K. Gallagher and M. Healy, *J. Chem. Technol. Biotechnol.*, 2002, **77**, 539.
183. N. Pramanpol and N. Nitayapat, *Nat. Sci.*, 2006, **40**, 192.
184. Y. Li, A. Wang, Y. Bai and S. Wang, *J. Sep. Sci.*, 2017, **40**, 2591.
185. W. Wang, B. Chen and Y. Huang, *J. Agric. Food Chem.*, 2014, **62**, 8051.
186. A. Banerjee, S. Panda, M. Sidhantha, S. Chakrabarti, B. Chaudhuri and S. Bhattacharjee, *Int. J. Global Warming*, 2010, **2**, 252.
187. J. Yoo, K. Park, Y. Yoo, J. Kim, H. Yang and Y. Shin, *Korean J. Food Sci. Anim. Resour.*, 2014, **34**, 26.
188. K. J. Ruff, P. L. Durham, A. O'Reilly and F. D. Long, *J. Inflammation Res.*, 2015, **8**, 49.
189. T. T. Vuong, S. B. Ronning, H. P. Suso, R. Schmidt, K. Prydz, M. Lundstrom, A. Moen and M. E. Pedersen, *J. Inflammation Res.*, 2017, **10**, 83.
190. K. F. Benson, K. J. Ruff and G. S. Jensen, *J. Med. Food*, 2012, **15**, 360.
191. H. Jia, M. Hanate, W. Aw, H. Itoh, K. Saito, S. Kobayashi, S. Hachimura, S. Fukuda, M. Tomita, Y. Hasebe and H. Kato, *Sci. Rep.*, 2017, **7**, 43993.
192. Y. Shi, P. Rupa, B. Jiang and Y. Mine, *Int. J. Mol. Sci.*, 2014, **15**, 22728.
193. H. Jia, W. Aw, K. Saito, M. Hanate, Y. Hasebe and H. Kato, *Sci. Rep.*, 2014, **4**, 7473.
194. Y. Boonyasit, O. Chailapakul and W. Laiwattanapaisal, *Anal. Chim. Acta*, 2016, **936**, 1.
195. W. Chen, B. Li, C. Xu and L. Wang, *Biosens. Bioelectron.*, 2009, **24**, 2534.
196. B. Li, D. Lan and Z. Zhang, *Anal. Biochem.*, 2008, **374**, 64.
197. Y. Li, A. Wang, Y. Bai and S. Wang, *Food Chem.*, 2017, **237**, 966.
198. Y. J. Li, *J. AOAC Int.*, 2010, **93**, 1912.
199. R. Mohammad-Rezaei, H. Razmi and S. Dehgan-Reyhan, *Colloids Surf., B*, 2014, **118**, 188.
200. P. G. Ray and S. Roy, *Mater. Sci. Eng., C*, 2016, **59**, 404.
201. A. K. Singh, A. Roychoudhury and S. K. Jha, *Anal. Sci.*, 2016, **32**, 1077.
202. J. Tang, L. Han, Y. Yu, J. Kang and Y. Zhang, *Luminescence*, 2011, **26**, 634.

203. J. Tang, L. Han, Y. Yu, J. Kang and Y. Zhang, *J. Fluoresc.*, 2011, **21**, 339.
204. J. Tang, J. Li, J. Kang, L. Zhong and Y. Zhang, *Sens. Actuators, B*, 2009, **B 140**, 200.
205. J. Tang, Z. Liu, J. Kang and Y. Zhang, *Anal. Bioanal. Chem.*, 2010, **397**, 3015.
206. S. Tembe, B. S. Kubal, M. Karve and S. F. D'Souza, *Anal. Chim. Acta*, 2008, **612**, 212.
207. Q. Wang, X. Liu, L. Zhang and Y. Lv, *Analyst*, 2012, **137**, 5392.
208. G. Wen, Y. Zhang, S. Shuang, C. Dong and M. M. Choi, *Biosens. Bioelectron.*, 2007, **23**, 121.
209. B. Wu, G. Zhang, S. Shuang and M. M. Choi, *Talanta*, 2004, **64**, 546.
210. D. Xiao and M. M. Choi, *Anal. Chem.*, 2002, **74**, 863.
211. G. Xue, Z. Yue, Z. Bing, T. Yiwei, L. Xiuying and L. Jianrong, *Analyst*, 2016, **141**, 1105.
212. D. Zhang, H. Zhao, Z. Fan, M. Li, P. Du, C. Liu, Y. Li, H. Li and H. Cao, *PLoS One*, 2015, **10**, e0130156.
213. Y. Zhang, W. Jia, M. Cui, C. Dong, S. Shuang, Y. Kwan and M. M. Choi, *Biotechnol. J.*, 2011, **6**, 492.
214. Y. Zhang, G. Wen, Y. Zhou, S. Shuang, C. Dong and M. M. Choi, *Biosens. Bioelectron.*, 2007, **22**, 1791.
215. B. Zheng, L. Qian, H. Yuan, D. Xiao, X. Yang, M. C. Paau and M. M. Choi, *Talanta*, 2010, **82**, 177.
216. S. L. Zhong, J. Zhuang, D. P. Yang and D. Tang, *Biosens. Bioelectron.*, 2017, **96**, 26.
217. J. Liu, Q. Wu, Y. Ding and Y. Yi, *Bull. Korean Chem. Soc.*, 2004, **25**, 1775.
218. D. Yang, L. Qi and J. Ma, *J. Mater. Chem.*, 2003, **13**, 1119.
219. H. Su, J. Han, N. Wang, Q. Dong, D. Zhang and C. Zhang, *Smart Mater. Struct.*, 2008, **17**, 015045.
220. Q. Donga, H. Sua, W. Caoa, D. Zhanga, Q. Guob and Y. Laic, *J. Solid State Chem.*, 2007, **180**, 949.
221. Y. Kondo and M. Yoshikawa, *Membrane*, 2001, **26**, 228.
222. P. Y. Lin, C. W. Hsieh, P. C. Tsai and S. Hsieh, *ChemPhysChem*, 2014, **15**, 1577.
223. C. Jiang, C. Cheng, M. Hao, H. Wang, Z. Wang, C. Shen and L. Z. Cheong, *Int. J. Biol. Macromol.*, 2017, **105**, 1328.
224. S. H. Chung and A. Manthiram, *Adv. Mater.*, 2014, **26**, 1360.
225. J. Geng, H. Wu, A. M. Al-Enizi, A. A. Elzatahry and G. Zheng, *Nanoscale*, 2015, **7**, 14378.
226. H. Yu, Q. Tang, J. Wu, Y. Lin, L. Fan, M. Huang, J. Lin, Y. Li and F. Yu, *J. Power Sources*, 2012, **206**, 463.
227. K. J. Ruff, D. P. DeVore, M. D. Leu and M. A. Robinson, *Clin. Interventions Aging*, 2009, **4**, 235.
228. K. J. Ruff, J. R. Endres, A. E. Clewell, J. R. Szabo and A. G. Schauss, *Food Chem. Toxicol.*, 2012, **50**, 604.

229. K. J. Wedekind, K. J. Ruff, C. A. Atwell, J. L. Evans and A. M. Bendele, *Mod. Rheumatol.*, 2017, **27**, 838.
230. K. J. Ruff, A. Winkler, R. W. Jackson, D. P. DeVore and B. W. Ritz, *Clin. Rheumatol.*, 2009, **28**, 907.
231. Z. Chai, Y. Li, F. Liu, B. Du, T. Jiao, C. Zhang and X. Leng, *J. Agric. Food Chem.*, 2013, **61**, 589.
232. L. Dupoirieux, D. Pourquier, M. C. Picot and M. Neves, *Int. J. Oral Maxillofac. Surg.*, 2001, **30**, 58.
233. L. Dupoirieux, D. Pourquier, M. C. Pico and M. Neves, *J. Craniomaxillofac. Surg.*, 1999, **27**, 314.
234. J. I. Arias, A. Gonzalez, M. S. Fernandez, C. Gonzalez, D. Saez and J. L. Arias, *J. Tissue Eng. Regener. Med.*, 2008, **2**, 228.
235. N. Golafshan, H. Gharibi, M. Kharaziha and M. Fathi, *Biofabrication*, 2017, **9**, 025008.
236. G. H. Farjah, B. Heshmatian, M. Karimipour and A. Saberi, *Iran. J. Basic Med. Sci.*, 2013, **16**, 901.
237. K. Maeda and Y. Sasaki, *Burns. Incl. Therm. Inj.*, 1982, **8**, 313.
238. F. Guarderas, Y. Leavell, T. Sengupta, M. Zhukova and T. L. Megraw, *Adv. Skin Wound Care*, 2016, **29**, 131.
239. M. Liu, G. Luo, Y. Wang, R. Xu, Y. Wang, W. He, J. Tan, M. Xing and J. Wu, *Sci. Rep.*, 2017, **7**, 436.
240. T. T. Vuong, S. B. Rønning, T. A. E. Ahmed, K. Brathagen, V. Høst, M. T. Hincke, H.-P. Suso and M. E. Pedersen, *PLoS One*, 2018, **13**, e0201975.
241. H. J. Jun, K. H. Oh, J. Yoo, W. G. Han, J. Chang, H. H. Jung and J. Choi, *Acta Otolaryngol.*, 2014, **134**, 250.
242. J. Y. Jung, H. C. Yun, T. M. Kim, J. W. Joo, I. S. Song, Y. C. Rah, J. Chang, G. J. Im and J. Choi, *J. Audiol. Otol.*, 2017, **21**, 39.
243. J. Y. Yang, S. S. Chuang, W. G. Yang and P. K. Tsay, *Chang Gung Med. J.*, 2003, **26**, 153.
244. Y. Zadik, *Wilderness Environ. Med.*, 2007, **18**, 230.
245. F. Yi, Z. X. Guo, L. X. Zhang, J. Yu and Q. Li, *Biomaterials*, 2004, **25**, 4591.
246. F. Yi, J. Yu, Z.-X. Guo, L.-X. Zhang and Q. Li, *Macromol. Biosci.*, 2003, **3**, 234.
247. Q. L. Qi, Q. Li, J. W. Lu, Z. X. Guo and J. Yu, *Chin. J. Polym. Sci.*, 2009, **27**, 387.
248. J. W. Lu, Q. Li, Q. L. Qi, Z. X. Guo and J. Yu, *J. Biomed. Mater. Res., Part A*, 2009, **91**, 701.
249. X. Xiong, Q. Li, J. W. Lu, Z. X. Guo, Z. H. Sun and J. Yu, *J. Biomater. Sci., Polym. Ed.*, 2012, **23**, 1217.
250. X. Xiong, Q. Li, J. W. Lu, Z. X. Guo and J. Yu, *J. Appl. Polym. Sci.*, 2010, **117**, 1955.
251. J. Jia, Y. Y. Duan, J. Yu and J. W. Lu, *J. Biomed. Mater. Res., Part A*, 2008, **86**, 364.
252. G. H. Kim, T. Min, S. A. Park and W. D. Kim, *Bioinspiration Biomimetics*, 2008, **3**, 016006.

253. J. Jia, G. Liu, Z. X. Guo, J. Yu and Y. Duan, *J. Nanomater.*, 2012, **2012**, 282736.
254. J. M. Meléndez García, A. S. Araujo Da Costa, T. Rivera Schmitz, C. M. Chiesa Estomba and M. I. Hamdan Zavarce, *Otol. Neurotol.*, 2014, **35**, 941.
255. Y. Zhang, G. Zhang, D. Yang, Y. Lai, L. Zhang, P. Wang, X. Zhouzhong and X. Wang, *Photodiagn. Photodyn. Ther.*, 2016, **15**, 156.
256. Y. Tao, Y. Lu, Y. Sun, B. Gu, W. Lu and J. Pan, *Int. J. Pharm.*, 2009, **378**, 30.
257. B. Parodi, E. Russo, P. Gatti, S. Cafaggi and G. Bignardi, *Drug Dev. Ind. Pharm.*, 1999, **25**, 289.
258. Y. Ikeuchi-Takahashi, N. Watanabe, M. Sasatsu and H. Onishi, *Drug Dev. Ind. Pharm.*, 2013, **39**, 1254.

Subject Index